Sleep Medicine in Clinical Practice

Sleep Medicine in Clinical Practice

Editor: Cersei Nash

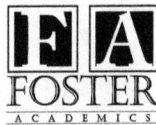

FA FOSTER ACADEMICS

www.fosteracademics.com

www.fosteracademics.com

FA FOSTER
ACADEMICS

Cataloging-in-Publication Data

Sleep medicine in clinical practice / edited by Cersei Nash.
    p. cm.
Includes bibliographical references and index.
ISBN 978-1-63242-719-9
    1. Sleep disorders. 2. Sleep--Physiological aspects. 3. Sleep disorders--Treatment.
4. Sleep therapy. I. Nash, Cersei.
RC547 .S54 2019
616.849--dc23

Foster Academics,
118-35 Queens Blvd., Suite 400,
Forest Hills, NY 11375, USA

ISBN 978-1-63242-719-9 (Hardback)

Contents

Permissions

List of Contributors

Index

Preface

Every book is initially just a concept; it takes months of research and hard work to give it the final shape in which the readers receive it. In its early stages, this book also went through rigorous reviewing. The notable contributions made by experts from across the globe were first molded into patterned chapters and then arranged in a sensibly sequential manner to bring out the best results.

Sleep medicine is a field of medicine that deals with sleep disorders, their diagnosis and management. Sleep medicine requires a specialist to treat a diverse plethora of disorders, such as Kleine-Levin syndrome, sleep apnea, narcolepsy, circadian rhythm disturbances, etc. Sleep disorders are divided into three main groups, primary sleep disorders, those associated with substance abuse or a medical condition and those that are secondary to mental disorders. A thorough medical history check, previous medication review, evaluation of the patient's Epworth Sleepiness Scale (ESS), polysomnography, a multiple sleep latency test, etc. are used for diagnosing sleep disorders. Practitioners of sleep medicine seek to address both the underlying cause of the disorder and the sleep problem itself. Various methodologies such as cognitive behavioral therapy, patient education about sleep hygiene, etc. are used for the management of sleep disorders. This book is a compilation of chapters that discuss the most vital concepts and emerging trends in the field of sleep medicine. It aims to shed light on some of the unexplored aspects of sleep medicine and the recent researches in this field. For all those who are interested in this field, this book can prove to be an essential guide.

It has been my immense pleasure to be a part of this project and to contribute my years of learning in such a meaningful form. I would like to take this opportunity to thank all the people who have been associated with the completion of this book at any step.

Editor

High incidence of posterior nasal cavity obstruction in obstructive sleep apnea patients

Carlos Torre[1,2,3*], Robson Capasso[1], Soroush Zaghi[1], Ryan Williams[1] and Stanley Yung-Chuan Liu[1]

Abstract

Background: Nasal obstruction is a common problem in patients with obstructive sleep apnea (OSA). Systematic evaluation of nasal obstruction remains challenging due to the high number of variables and factors that contribute to nasal obstruction. Nasal examination by means of anterior rhinoscopy is limited to the evaluation of anterior septal deviation, internal nasal valve angle, and inferior turbinate size, but obstruction due to posterior septal deviation and nasal polyposis may go undiagnosed. The primary objective of this study was to determine the incidence of posterior nasal obstruction in OSA patients. Specifically, we were interested in other causes of posterior nasal obstruction that were difficult to assess by anterior rhinoscopy examination alone, and that required nasal endoscopy for identification.

Methods: This is a retrospective case series study. Flexible fiberoptic examination of the nasal cavity was performed on 274 consecutive OSA patients evaluated at the Stanford Sleep Surgery Clinic. Examination video files were recorded and later reviewed and scored by a single investigator blinded to the patients' subjective nasal complaints. Anatomic features that contribute to posterior nasal obstruction were noted.

Results: Posterior septal deviation was the most common incidental finding in OSA patients with posterior nasal obstruction. Other causes included nasal polyposis, nasal mucosal inflammation, and purulent mucosal discharge. In total, there were 73/274 (26.6%) patients for whom nasal endoscopy provided findings that directed management.

Conclusion: Nasal endoscopy provides additional diagnostic information in a significant number of OSA patients who complain of nasal obstruction. Our findings suggest the use of nasal endoscopy for OSA patients who complain of nasal obstruction or CPAP intolerance, despite unremarkable anterior rhinoscopy examination.

Keywords: Obstructive Sleep Apnea (OSA), Nasal obstruction, Nasal endoscopy, Posterior septal deviation, Nasal polyposis, Chronic rhinosinusitis, Continuous positive airway pressure (CPAP)

Background

Obstructive sleep apnea (OSA) is a disorder caused by the repetitive collapse of the upper airway during sleep resulting in either partial or complete airflow obstruction (Strollo and Rogers 1996). Nasal obstruction is related to OSA in several ways: 1) reduces airflow through the collapsible airway, therefore increasing upper airway resistance, 2) forces patients to become oral breathers during sleep, which leads to narrowing of the airway, and 3) interferes with the nasal reflexes that stimulate ventilation (de Sousa Michels et al. 2014; Georgalas 2011). The nose also serves as a major conduit for the treatment of OSA with continuous positive airway pressure (CPAP) therapy (Georgalas 2011; Stepnowsky and Moore 2003; Ebben et al. 2012). Nasal obstruction can therefore interfere with the medical treatment of OSA.

For OSA patients, nasal obstruction may be treated with the goal of reducing snoring and airway collapse, or to improve CPAP tolerance. Data on OSA patients treated for nasal obstruction alone has shown consistent

* Correspondence: cat139@miami.edu
[1]Division of Sleep Surgery, Department of Otolaryngology-Head & Neck Surgery, Stanford Hospital and Clinics, Stanford, CA, USA
[2]Division of Sleep Medicine, Department of Psychiatry and Behavioral Sciences, Stanford Hospital and Clinics, Stanford, CA, USA
Full list of author information is available at the end of the article

improvement in subjective symptoms such as daytime somnolence and snoring despite minimal change in their sleep study results (Bican et al. 2010). Nasal surgery alone has also been shown to significantly impact CPAP tolerance and adherence (Poirier et al. 2014; Powell et al. 2001).

Systematic evaluation of nasal obstruction remains challenging due to the high number of factors that contribute to nasal obstruction. Nasal examination by anterior rhinoscopy allows evaluation of anterior septal deviation, internal nasal valve angle, and inferior turbinate size. Frequently, this limited examination of the anterior nasal cavity does not correlate with patient symptoms. Patients may complain of nasal obstruction despite no signs of objective anatomical abnormalities in the nasal cavity when examined with anterior rhinoscopy alone. Other etiologies for nasal obstruction such as posterior septal deviation or chronic sinusitis with or without polyposis may go undiagnosed. Structural and inflammatory problems often coexist and need to be addressed concurrently in order to reestablish normal nasal function (Rotenberg and Pang 2015; El Rassi et al. 2015).

We therefore aimed to evaluate different causes of posterior nasal cavity obstruction that are difficult, if not impossible, to asses by anterior rhinoscopy. The high incidence of posterior nasal cavity obstruction in this study suggests the use of nasal endoscopy in all OSA patients who also complain of nasal obstruction or CPAP intolerance.

Methods

This was a retrospective case series of 274 consecutive OSA patients examined using flexible fiberoptic examination at the Stanford Sleep Surgery Clinic. The protocol for this study was approved by the Institutional Review Board and Hospital Research Ethics Committee of Stanford University. Examination video files were recorded, reviewed, and then scored by a single investigator blinded to the patients' subjective nasal complaints. Presence of posterior septal deviation, nasal crusting, erythema, swelling, scar band, purulent drainage, thick mucus, and nasal polyposis was noted.

Results

Demographic data of the subjects are summarized in Table 1. The mean age was 42.1 +/- 14.8 years and the mean BMI 27.5 +/- 5.7 kg/m². All patients had a positive diagnosis for OSA with a mean Apnea-Hypopnea Index (AHI) of 31.6 +/- 25.3 events/hr, Apnea Index of 7.5 +/- 15.4 events/hr, Oxygen Desaturation Index of 15.4 +/- 22.0 events/hr, and Lowest Oxygenation Saturation of 86.7 +/- 6.6%. Majority of the patients complained of excessive daytime somnolence with a mean Epworth Sleepiness Scale Score of 10.1 +/- 5.2 (mean +/- SD).

Table 1 Patient characteristics

Patient characteristics	Mean ± SD
Age, yr	42.1 ± 14.8
Body mass index, kg/m²	27.5 ± 5.7
Epworth Sleepiness Sclae	10.1 ± 5.2
Apnea hypopnea index, per hr	31.6 ± 25.3
Apnea index, per hr	7.5 ± 15.4
Oxygen desaturation index, per hr	15.4 ± 22.0
Lowest oxygen saturation, %	86.7 ± 6.6

SD standard deviation

Table 2 shows the different causes of incidental posterior nasal obstruction that were identified in this patient population. Posterior nasoseptal deviation was the most common cause of posterior nasal obstruction (55/274, 20.0%). The majority presented with unilateral obstruction, although there was one case with bilateral nasoseptal deviation (Fig. 1). There were also 5 cases of combined anterior and posterior septal deviation (5/274, 1.8%).

A significant number of patients also had inflammatory problems leading to nasal obstruction (Fig. 2). The most common inflammatory problem identified was nasal polyposis (11/274, 4.0%), followed by edematous nasal mucosa inflammation (2/274, 0.7%), and purulent mucosal discharge (1/274, 0.36%). In total, there were 73/274 (26.6%) patients for whom nasal endoscopy provided findings that directed management.

Discussion

Nasal obstruction can be caused by structural abnormalities (e.g. deviated nasal septum, enlarged turbinates and nasal valve collapse) or by inflammatory mucosal disease (rhinitis, chronic rhinosinusitis with or without nasal polyps) (Lee et al. 2013; Prasad et al. 2013). Correction of nasal obstruction is unquestionably a priority in the management of OSA patients, regardless of whether it leads to an improvement in OSA severity based on objective polysomnography respiratory parameters. There

Table 2 Posterior Nasal Obstruction Findings

Location	Total	Percentage(%)
Total	73/274	26.6
Isolated Posterior Septal Deviation	55/274	20
Right	19	—
Left	35	—
Bilateral	1	—
Combined Anterior and Posterior Septal Deviations	5/274	1.8
Nasal Polyposis	11/274	4
Purulent Discharge	1/274	0.36
Mucosal Inflammation	2/274	0.7

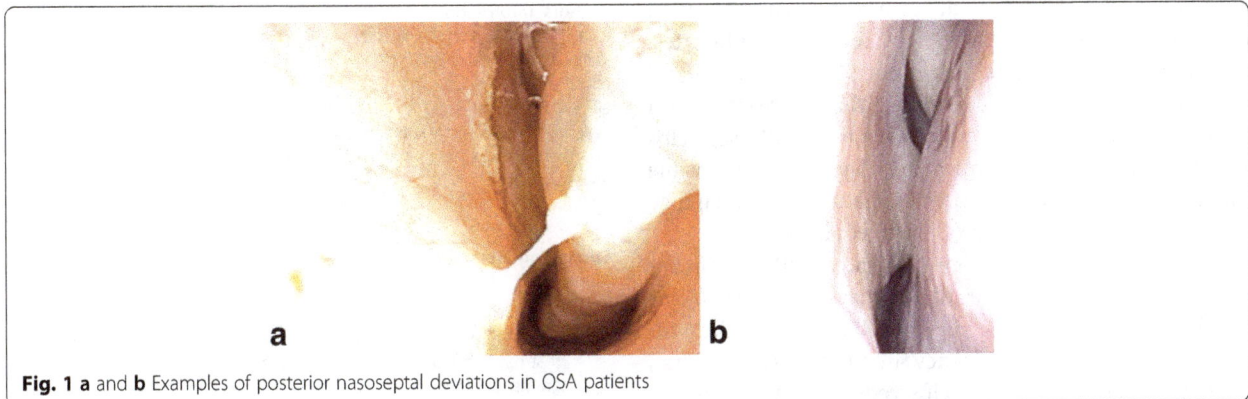

Fig. 1 a and **b** Examples of posterior nasoseptal deviations in OSA patients

is extensive evidence showing that nasal obstruction not only decreases quality of life, but that it also contributes to snoring, plays an important role in the pathophysiologic mechanisms leading to OSA, and represents an obstacle for effective treatment with CPAP therapy in OSA patients (de Sousa Michels et al. 2014; Bican et al. 2010). Currently, nasal examination of OSA patient in most medical practices is limited to anterior rhinoscopy, which fails to identify other sites and sources contributing to nasal obstruction.

There are several mechanisms by which nasal obstruction contributes to the pathogenesis of OSA. Following the Sterling resistor model, elevated nasal resistance increases negative pressure in the oropharyngeal airway downstream, thus contributing to airway collapse (Smith et al. 1988; Park 1993). Increased nasal resistance also results in compensatory oral breathing, which leads to an unstable airway with increased total resistance (Phillips 2006; Akbay et al. 2013). Finally, decreased nasal airflow blunts the activation of the nasal-ventilatory reflex important in the maintenance of adequate muscle tone, breathing frequency, and minute lung ventilation (Mcnicholas; Douglas et al. 1983). One of the priorities in the management of OSA patients should be the reestablishment of efficient nasal breathing.

Mouth breathing is a problem oftentimes ignored in the management of OSA. Oral breathing resulting from nasal obstruction may lead to a closed cycle where nasal respiration ends up becoming worse due to profound anatomic derangement. Continuous oral breathing often leads to a transverse maxillary deficiency that deepens the palatal arch. The high arched palate may compress the septum in a cranio-caudal orientation, thus resulting in a displaced septum (Akbay et al. 2013). Most of the posterior septal deviation that cannot be visualized using anterior rhinoscopy alone are not from traumatic insult, but from pressure exerted by a high arched palate during active craniofacial skeletal development. Since many OSA patients present with a high arched palate, we infer that many of these patients would present with posterior septal deviations.

It is common to see OSA patients with impaired nasal breathing to also present with inflammatory mucosal disease. It is estimated that 58% of OSA patients are affected by rhinitis (Gelardi et al. 2012). Over 70% of patients with chronic rhinosinusitis (CRS) report poor sleep quality, and the degree of sleep disturbance correlates with decreased overall quality of life (QOL) (Rotenberg and Pang 2015). Sleep impairment in CRS exerts a greater relative influence on the decision to pursue endoscopic sinus surgery (ESS) when compared to rhinologic specific symptom domains (El Rassi et al. 2015).

A possible explanation for this is that a night-time under-ventilated nose (due to apnea) may be at increased risk of infections and inflammation. The findings from Gelardi et al. support this theory. They found that

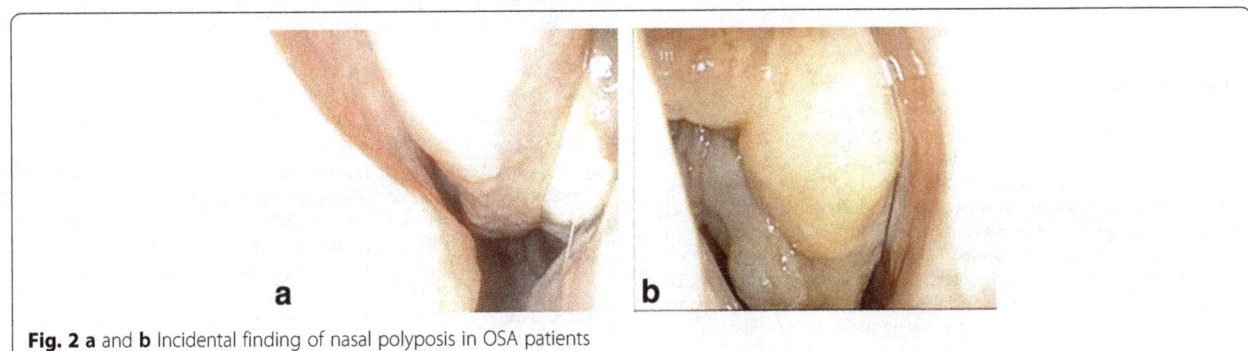

Fig. 2 a and **b** Incidental finding of nasal polyposis in OSA patients

regular CPAP treatment induces a significant reduction of cell infiltration (neutrophils, eosinophils, lymphocytes, and muciparous cells), which is not seen in non-treated patients. This supports the theory that increased nasal ventilation, in some cases secondary to CPAP use, helps reduce some of the enzymes (ex. elastasis) responsible for the production of free radicals that cause cell damage and mucosal inflammation (Gelardi et al. 2012).

Nasal surgery has not been correlated with significant improvement in post-operative Apnea-Hypopnea Index (AHI). However, ample evidence supports the re-establishment of nasal patency in OSA patients. First, decreased nasal resistance helps reduce CPAP pressures and improves its tolerance (Poirier et al. 2014). Other studies have also shown an improvement in overall sleep architecture with increases in non-REM stage 3 and 4, and REM sleep (Sériès and St Pierre 1992). Finally, nasal surgery is known to have a positive effect in the snoring complaints of OSA patients (Fairbanks 1984).

Conclusions
The observations made in this study support the fact that a significant number of OSA patients with normal anterior rhinoscopy examination may still have other etiology of nasal obstruction that can be visualized by nasal endoscopy. These findings, and the implications of nasal obstruction in the pathogenesis and treatment of OSA, warrant the use of routine nasal endoscopy in this population. We propose that OSA patients complaining of nasal obstruction or CPAP intolerance need to be offered nasal endoscopic evaluation to further define clinical strategies for treatment.

Abbreviations
AHI: Apnea-Hypopnea Index; CPAP: Continuous positive airway pressure; CRS: Chronic rhinosinusitis; ESS: Endoscopic sinus surgery; OSA: Obstructive sleep apnea; QOL: Quality of life

Acknowledgements
None.

Funding
None.

Authors' contributions
All authors met the four criteria for authorship established by the International Committee of Medical Journal Editors: CT was responsible for the conception, design, analysis, and drafting the work, revising the work and reviewing the manuscript. SL, RW, and RC had substantial contributions to the acquisition of data for the work as well as drafting the work, revising the work and reviewing the manuscript. SZ had substantial contributions to data analysis, interpretation of data for the work, and revising the work critically for important intellectual content. Additionally, all authors provided final approval of the version to be published and agreed to be accountable for all aspects of the work in ensuring including the accuracy and/or integrity of the work.

Authors' information
All authors in this manuscript, except for Dr. Ryan Williams, are fellowship trained sleep surgeons graduated from Stanford University. We believe that one of the priorities in the management of OSA patients should be the re-establishment of efficient nasal breathing. The goal of this study was to show that among OSA patients, there is a significant number presenting with other causes of nasal obstruction that are hard, if not impossible, to identify by means of anterior rhinoscopy.

Competing interests
None.

i. No financial and no material support for this research and work.
ii. Authors have no financial interests in any companies or other entities that have an interest in the information in the Contribution (e.g., grants, advisory boards, employment, consultancies, contracts, honoraria, royalties, expert testimony, partnerships, or stock ownership in medically-related fields).

Author details
[1]Division of Sleep Surgery, Department of Otolaryngology-Head & Neck Surgery, Stanford Hospital and Clinics, Stanford, CA, USA. [2]Division of Sleep Medicine, Department of Psychiatry and Behavioral Sciences, Stanford Hospital and Clinics, Stanford, CA, USA. [3]Department of Otolaryngology-Head and Neck Surgery, University of Miami, Miller School of Medicine, Miami, Florida, USA.

References
Akbay E, Cokkeser Y, Yilmaz O, Cevik C. The relationship between posterior septum deviation and depth of maxillopalatal arch. Auris Nasus Larynx. 2013;40(3):286–90.

Bican A, Kahraman A, Bora I, Kahveci R, Hakyemez B. What is the efficacy of nasal surgery in patients with obstructive sleep apnea syndrome? J Craniofac Surg. 2010;21(6):1801–6.

de Sousa Michels D, da Mota Silveira Rodrigues A, Nakanishi M, Sampaio ALL, Venosa AR. Nasal involvement in obstructive sleep apnea syndrome. Int J Otolaryngol. 2014;2014(2014):717419.

Douglas NJ, White DP, Weil JV, Zwillich CW. Effect of breathing route on ventilation and ventilatory drive. Respir Physiol. 1983;51:209–18.

Ebben MR, Oyegbile T, Pollak CP. The efficacy of three different mask styles on a PAP titration night. Sleep Med. 2012;13(6):645–9.

El Rassi E, Mace JC, Steele TO, Alt JA, Smith TL. Improvements in sleep-related symptoms after endoscopic sinus surgery in patients with chronic rhinosinusitis. Int Forum Allergy Rhinol. 2015;00:1–9.

Fairbanks DN. Snoring: surgical vs. nonsurgical management. Laryngoscope. 1984; 94(9):1188–92.

Gelardi M, Carbonara G, Maffezzoni E, Marvisi M, Quaranta N, Ferri R. Regular CPAP utilization reduces nasal inflammation assessed by nasal cytology in obstructive sleep apnea syndrome. Sleep Med. 2012;13(7):859–63.

Georgalas C. The role of the nose in snoring and obstructive sleep apnoea: an update. Eur Arch Oto-Rhino-Laryngology. 2011;268(9):1365–73.

Lee DC, Shin JH, Kim SW, et al. Anatomical analysis of nasal obstruction: nasal cavity of patients complaining of stuffy nose. Laryngoscope. 2013;123(6):1381–4.

Mcnicholas WT, Coffey M, Boyle T. Effects of nasal airflow on breathing during sleep in normal humans. Am Rev Respir Dis. 1993;147(3):620–3.

Park SS. Flow-regulatory function of upper airway in health and disease: A unified pathogenetic view of sleep-disordered breathing. Lung. 1993;171(6):311–33.

Phillips BA. Mouth breathing compromises adherence to nasal continuous positive airway pressure therapy. Yearb Pulm Dis. 2006;2006:239–40.

Poirier J, George C, Rotenberg B. The effect of nasal surgery on nasal continuous positive airway pressure compliance. Laryngoscope. 2014;124(1):317–9.

Powell NB, Zonato AI, Weaver EM, et al. Radiofrequency treatment of turbinate hypertrophy in subjects using continuous positive airway pressure: a randomized, double-blind, placebo-controlled clinical pilot trial. Laryngoscope. 2001;111(10):1783–90.

Prasad S, Varshney S, Bist SS, Mishra S, Kabdwal N. Correlation study between nasal septal deviation and rhinosinusitis. Indian J Otolaryngol Head Neck Surg. 2013;65(4):363–6.

Rotenberg BW, Pang KP. The impact of sinus surgery on sleep outcomes. Int Forum Allergy Rhinol. 2015;5(4):329–32.

Sériès F, St Pierre SCG. Effects of surgical correction of nasal obstruction in the treatment of obstructive sleep apnea. Am Rev Respir Dis. 1992;146(5 Pt 1):1261–5.

Smith PL, Wise RA, Gold AR, Schwartz AR. Upper airway pressure-flow relationships in obstructive sleep apnea. Permut J Appl Physiol Publ. 1988;1(2):789–95.

Stepnowsky CJ, Moore PJ. Nasal CPAP treatment for obstructive sleep apnea: developing a new perspective on dosing strategies and compliance. J Psychosom Res. 2003;54(6):599–605.

Strollo Jr PJ, Rogers RM. Obstructive sleep apnea. N Engl J Med. 1996;334:99–104.

2

Is purpose in life associated with less sleep disturbance in older adults?

Arlener D. Turner[*], Christine E. Smith and Jason C. Ong

Abstract

Background: Previous work has shown that purpose in life can be protective against numerous negative health outcomes including sleep disturbances. Given that sleep disturbances are common among older adults and African Americans, the aim of the present study was to examine the relationship between purpose in life, overall sleep quality, and the presence of sleep disorders in a community-based bi-racial sample of older adults.

Methods: Participants were 825 non-demented older African Americans ($n = 428$) and Whites ($n = 397$) from two cohort studies, the Minority Aging Research Study (MARS) and the Rush Memory and Aging Project (MAP). Participants completed a 32-item questionnaire assessing sleep quality and symptoms of Sleep Apnea, Restless Leg Syndrome (RLS) and REM Behavior Disorder (RBD). Purpose in life was assessed with a 10-item measure modified from Ryff & Keyes's scales of Psychological Well Being.

Results: In a series of hierarchical multiple linear regressions controlling for the demographic covariates of age, sex, race, and education, higher levels of purpose in life were associated with better sleep quality at baseline. Using longitudinal follow-up data, higher levels of purpose in life was associated with lower risk of sleep apnea at baseline, 1-year follow-up, and 2-year follow-up, as well as reduced symptoms of RLS at 1-year and 2-year follow-up.

Conclusions: These findings provide support for the hypothesis that a higher level of meaning and purpose in life among older adults is related to better sleep quality and appears to be protective against symptoms of sleep apnea and RLS.

Keywords: Purpose in life, Sleep quality, Sleep apnea, Restless leg syndrome, REM behavior disorder, Older adults, African Americans

Background

Disturbances in sleep are common in older adults, with an estimated 32–45% of older adults reporting some sleep complaint such as difficulty falling or staying asleep, or disrupted sleep (Ancoli-Israel 2009; Beaudreau et al. 2012; Kim et al. 2015). Also, almost 40% of older adults suffer from a sleep disorder (Kim et al. 2015; Jaussent et al. 2011), with the most common primary sleep disorders in the elderly being sleep-disordered breathing, REM behavior disorder (RBD) and restless legs syndrome (RLS) (Ancoli-Israel 2009; Foley et al. 2004; Kim et al. 2013). In addition to older adults being more prone to sleep disturbances and disorders, risk appears to vary among racial groups. Specifically, African

Americans have been found to have higher prevalence rates of sleep disturbance than Whites (Patel et al. 2010; Pigeon et al. 2011; Ruiter et al. 2011), including increased susceptibility to the development of sleep-disordered breathing and higher severity rates when diagnosed (Cohen-Zion et al. 2004; Redline et al. 1997). Having disturbed sleep or a sleep disorder is concerning in and of itself since the accompanying fatigue has been linked with dangerous public safety issues such as drowsy driving (Chen et al. 2014; Hossain and Shapiro 2002). Furthermore, sleep disturbances have been associated with higher rates of mental and physical health problems, cognitive impairment and even mortality (Ancoli-Israel 2009; Kim et al. 2015; Foley et al. 2004). Specific physical health and mental health problems that have been associated with sleep disturbances/disorders, especially in older adults, include depression, heart

---

* Correspondence: arlener.turner@northwestern.edu
Department of Neurology, Northwestern University Feinberg School of Medicine, 710 North Lake Shore Drive, Abbott Hall, Room 1005, Chicago 60611, IL, USA

disease, and impaired physical functioning (Ancoli-Israel 2009; Kim et al. 2015; Foley et al. 2004).

Studies on positive psychology have revealed the possible interplay between positive psychological well-being and physiological functioning (Phelan et al. 2010; Ryff et al. 2004). Purpose in life is one of the major factors in positive psychological well-being (Ryff 1989; Ryff and Keyes 1995). Purpose in life is generally conceptualized as one's sense of meaning and directedness in his/her life, essentially having aspirations and goals for the future and feeling that experiences in life are meaningful (Ryff 1989; Ryff and Keyes 1995; Ryff 2014). Previous works have shown that purpose in life is independently linked to numerous positive health outcomes and healthy behaviors, as well as longevity (Kim et al. 2013; Boyle et al. 2009; Boyle et al. 2010a; Boyle et al. 2010b; Boyle et al. 2012; Krause 2009; Roepke et al. 2014). For example, having higher levels of purpose in life has been associated with a reduced risk of stroke (Kim et al. 2013), Alzheimer's disease (Boyle et al. 2010a; Boyle et al. 2012), disability (Boyle et al. 2010b), and all-cause mortality (Boyle et al. 2009; Krause 2009). Purpose in life, though trait-like, is dynamic and research suggests change in this construct is induced by psychological and social influences. It has been suggested via clinical intervention that purpose in life is a construct that can be consciously cultivated and enhanced (Ryff 2014; Burrow and Hill 2011).

A limited number of studies have examined the association between purpose in life and sleep. A cross-sectional examination of older women indicated that those with higher purpose in life showed less body movement during sleep—a proxy for better sleep quality (Ryff et al. 2004). In a second cross-sectional examination, it was reported that in middle aged adults, lower purpose in life was associated with problematic sleep duration (either excessive or inadequate hours of sleep) (Hamilton et al. 2006). In a final cross-sectional study it was demonstrated that after adjusting for demographic covariates and negative psychological states such as psychological distress, higher purpose in life scores were associated with fewer sleep problems in a sample of British civil servants (Steptoe et al. 2008). In the first longitudinal examination, the focus was on identifying subgroups of people and identifying their sleep trajectories over time. The researchers found that while there was an overall decline in sleep quality over time, individuals with higher baseline levels of purpose in life were least likely to be in the group with disrupted sleep (Phelan et al. 2010). Finally, a recent study by Kim, Hershner, & Strecher (Kim et al. 2015) found that higher purpose in life was associated with a reduction in incidence of sleep disturbances after adjusting for age, sex, education, race/ethnicity, health behaviors, physical functioning, and

baseline level of sleep disturbance in a nationally representative sample of older adults (Kim et al. 2015). One shortcoming of these studies is the use of a general measure of sleep disturbance or sleep quality. It is unclear if purpose in life is associated with specific sleep disorders beyond poor sleep quality. Such a finding would indicate that the construct of purpose in life could have clinical utility. In addition, previous studies have not examined possible differences in race, which could be important given the elevated levels of sleep disturbances in older adults and African Americans.

The present study expands on previous work by including a cohort study of African Americans and extending deeper into specific types of sleep disturbances, including insomnia, sleep-disordered breathing, REM behavior disorder (RBD), and restless legs syndrome (RLS). The first aim of the study is to replicate previous findings by examining the relationship between purpose in life and sleep quality. The second aim of this study is to examine the relationship between purpose in life and symptoms of three common sleep disorders in older adults (sleep apnea, RLS, and RBD) in a community based bi-racial sample of older adults. It was hypothesized that higher levels of purpose in life would be associated with better sleep quality and lower risk of sleep disorders at baseline, as well as change in sleep quality and risk of sleep disorders at follow-up.

Methods
Participants
The sample for this study was pooled from two ongoing longitudinal epidemiological cohort studies of aging and cognition, the Minority Aging Research Study (MARS) and the Rush Memory and Aging Project (MAP). Both cohort studies were approved by the Rush University Medical Center Institutional Review Board and had similar recruitment techniques and operational methods.

MARS is a longitudinal community-based cohort study of risk factors for cognitive decline that enrolls older community dwelling African Americans without known dementia. Participants are recruited from community based organizations, churches, senior-subsidized housing facilities in the greater Chicago area, and the Clinical core of the Rush Alzheimer's Disease Center. All MARS participants signed an informed consent agreeing to annual clinical evaluations, as previously described (Barnes et al. 2012).

MAP (88% White) is a longitudinal clinical-pathologic cohort study of older adults that enrolls older community dwelling adults without known dementia who agree to brain autopsy at death. Participants were recruited from Chicago area retirement and senior-subsidized housing facilities. All MAP participants signed an informed consent agreeing to annual clinical evaluations and organ donation, as previously described (Bennett et al. 2012).

At the time of analysis, 1195 (534 MARS; 661 MAP) individuals were enrolled in one of the cohort studies with complete baseline information. We excluded 274 (68 MARS; 206 MAP) individuals who did not have at least two clinical evaluations to measure change over time from their baseline assessment to a subsequent yearly follow-up. We also excluded 96 (38 MARS; 58 MAP) individuals who had more than 1 year between their baseline evaluation and first follow-up. The remaining 825 (428 MARS; 397 MAP) individuals were included in the analyses.

Purpose in life

Purpose in life was assessed at baseline using a modified 10-item measure derived from Ryff's and Keyes's scales of Psychological Well-Being (Ryff and Keyes 1995; Boyle et al. 2009). Individuals rated their agreement with each of the 10 items on a 5-point scale ranging from 1—strongly disagree to 5—strongly agree. Sample items included: "I feel good when I think of what I've done in the past and what I hope to do in the future" and "some people wander aimlessly through life, but I am not one of them." Scores are averaged to yield a mean score ranging from 1 to 5 with higher scores indicating higher levels of purpose in life.

Sleep quality and symptoms of sleep disorders

Sleep quality and the possible presence of sleep disorders were assessed using a 32-item questionnaire derived from three validated sleep measures, the Pittsburgh Sleep Quality Index (PSQI; (Buysse et al. 1989)), the Berlin Questionnaire (Redline and Strohl 1998) and the Mayo Sleep Questionnaire (MSQ; (Boeve et al. 2002)). Participants were given the sleep questionnaire with an addressed and stamped envelope at the end of their annual visit and were instructed to complete the questionnaire and return it via the stamped envelope.

Sleep Quality was measured using a modified version of the PSQI that assessed 6 components of sleep rather than the original 7 (all but the "Sleep Quality" component was assessed). Additionally, adjustments were made with regard to specific questions in order to avoid redundancy and over taxing of the older adult cohort (see (Turner et al. 2016) for full description of scale). The sum of the 6 components ranges from 0 to 16 with higher scores indicating poorer sleep quality (Turner et al. 2016). Sleep apnea risk was assessed using the Berlin Questionnaire, which was scored as previously published and validated (Netzer et al. 1999), indicating either a high or low risk for sleep apnea (Turner et al. 2016). Consistent with previous work (Rongve et al. 2010), the possible presence of Restless Leg Syndrome

(RLS) was measured using questions 2 and 3 from the MSQ (Turner et al. 2016). In addition, the MSQ was also used to assess for REM Behavior Disorder (RBD) via questions 1a–e, scored as previously published and validated (Turner et al. 2016; Boeve et al. 2011).

Demographic covariates

Other variables used in the analyses included demographic variables of age, sex, years of education, and race.

Data analysis

Analyses were conducted utilizing the Statistical Package for the Social Sciences software version 23 (IBM and Statistical Package for the Social Sciences (SPSS) (SPSS) 2015). Statistical significance was set at alpha = 0.05. Frequency and descriptive analyses were conducted to identify missing data, outliers, means, and standard deviations across all demographic and study variables.

Individuals undergo annual clinical assessments, therefore, to identify change over time in the continuous variable of sleep quality, change scores were derived by subtracting the baseline score from each yearly follow-up (i.e. next annual clinical evaluation) score. Thus change score 1 is the change in sleep quality from baseline to 1-year follow-up, and so forth, for a total of three change scores across all sleep-related outcomes.

To determine if purpose in life independently predicted baseline sleep quality or change in sleep quality over time we conducted a series of hierarchical linear multiple regressions. The first step of each model included the demographic covariates age, sex, race, and years of education, and the second step included the covariates and purpose in life. In order to determine if purpose in life was associated with symptoms of sleep apnea, RLS and/or RBD at baseline and at follow-up time points 1–3 we conducted a series of hierarchical logistic regression analyses controlling for age, sex, race, and years of education.

Results

The majority of the 825 respondents were female (77.3%), a little more than half (53.7%) were African American, age ranged from 60.84 to 99.81 with a mean of 79.02 (SD = 7.46), and participants had an average of 15.14 (SD = 3.07) years of education. At baseline the respondents' sleep quality was slightly disturbed (modified PSQI mean score = 5.93 ± 2.81; Table 1). Approximately 42% of participants were at high risk for sleep apnea and approximately a quarter of the sample (23.6%) endorsed symptoms of RLS. A lower proportion of participants (7.0%) endorsed symptoms of RBD (see Table 1).

Hierarchical multiple linear regression was conducted to determine if purpose in life independently predicted

Is purpose in life associated with less sleep disturbance in older...

9

Table 1 Frequencies, means, and standard deviations among sleep variables

	Baseline $n = 825$		1-year Follow-Up $n = 825$		2-year Follow-Up $n = 554$		3-year Follow-Up $n = 247$	
	Mean (SD)/N(%)	Range	Mean (SD)/N(%)	Range	Mean (SD)/N(%)	Range	Mean (SD)/N(%)	Range
Sleep Quality Total Score	5.93 (2.81)	0–15	5.92 (2.89)	0–14	5.86 (2.91)	0–14	5.94 (2.91)	0–15
High Sleep Apnea Risk	346 (41.9%)		341 (41.3%)		225 (27.3%)		100 (12.1%)	
High Restless Leg Syndrome Risk	195 (23.6%)		189 (22.9%)		137 (16.6%)		48 (5.8%)	
High REM Behavior Disorder Risk	58 (7.0%)		60 (7.3%)		41 (5.0%)		28 (3.4%)	

baseline sleep quality. Analyses indicated that at step 1, the covariate race contributed significantly to the regression model, [$F_{(4809)} = 2.408$, $p = .048$], and accounted for 1.2% of the variance in sleep quality. Introducing purpose in life in step 2 explained an additional 4.3% of the variance in sleep quality. This change in R^2 was significant, [$F_{(5808)} = 9.383$, $p < .001$] (see Table 2).

Hierarchical linear multiple regression was also used to determine whether purpose in life predicted change in sleep quality from baseline to 1-year follow-up. Analyses indicated that at step 1 no covariates contributed significantly to the regression. While introducing purpose in life in step 2 did not result in the model being statistically significant, the individual predictor purpose in life predicted change in sleep quality from baseline to the first follow-up assessment ($t = 2.344$, $p = .019$), such that for every unit increase in purpose in life there was an increase in change in sleep quality from baseline to 1-year follow-up by 0.449 units ($\beta = .449$, $p = 0.019$) (see Table 2). No significant relationships were found between purpose in life and change in sleep quality from baseline to 2-year or 3-year follow-up.

A series of hierarchical logistic regressions adjusting for the demographic covariates of age, sex, race, and years of education were conducted to determine if purpose in life was associated with risk of sleep apnea. Regression analyses for baseline revealed that in step 1 only the covariate age significantly contributed to the model, which accounted for 2.9% of the variance (Nagelkerke $R^2 = .029$, $X^2_{(4)} = 17.71$, $p = .001$) of sleep apnea risk, with increasing age being associated with a decreased likelihood of risk of sleep apnea (OR .965, 96% CI .945–.985). In step 2 introducing purpose in life explained an additional 1.3% of the variance (Nagelkerke $R^2 = .042$, $X^2_{(5)} = 25.41$, $p < .001$) of risk of sleep apnea, with increasing levels of purpose in life being associated with decreased risk of sleep apnea (OR .630, CI 95% .454–.875) (see Table 3). Similarly, at 1-year follow-up, regression analyses showed age was the only significant covariate in step 1; the model accounted for 2.9% of the variance (Nagelkerke $R^2 = .029$, $X^2_{(4)} = 17.56$, $p = .002$) of sleep apnea risk, with increasing age being associated with a decreased likelihood of risk of sleep apnea (OR .963, 96% CI .943–.983). Adding purpose in life in step 2 explained an additional 0.6% of the variance (Nagelkerke $R^2 = .035$, $X^2_{(5)} = 21.61$, $p = .001$) of risk of

sleep apnea, with increasing levels of purpose in life being associated with decreased risk of sleep apnea (OR .719, CI 95% .520–.993) (see Table 3). Regression analyses for 2-year follow-up also revealed similar results, in step 1 age was the only significant covariate, the model accounted for 2.5% of the variance (Nagelkerke $R^2 = .025$, $X^2_{(4)} = 10.36$, $p = .035$) of sleep apnea risk, with increasing age being associated with a decreased likelihood of risk of sleep apnea (OR .973, 96% CI .948–1.000). Introducing purpose in life in step 2 explained an additional 1.3% of the variance (Nagelkerke $R^2 = .038$, $X^2_{(5)} = 15.82$, $p = .007$) of risk of sleep apnea, with increasing levels of purpose in life being associated with decreased risk of sleep apnea (OR .604, CI 95% .395–.925) (see Table 3). The logistic regression analysis for sleep apnea risk at 3-year follow-up was not significant.

A series of hierarchical logistic regressions controlling for the demographic covariates of age, sex, race, and years of education were also conducted to determine if purpose in life was associated with RLS symptoms. Purpose in life did not significantly predict possible RLS at baseline (see Table 4). However, at 1-year follow-up regression analyses revealed that at step 1 no covariates contributed significantly to the regression, but, introducing purpose in life in step 2 explained 2.7% of the variance (Nagelkerke $R^2 = .027$, $X^2_{(5)} = 14.69$, $p = .012$) of RLS symptoms, with increasing levels of purpose in life being associated with a decreased likelihood of having possible RLS (OR .524, 95% CI .361–.762) (see Table 4). For 2-year follow-up regression analyses revealed that at step 1, no covariates contributed significantly to the regression. However, introducing purpose in life in step 2 explained 4.5% of the variance (Nagelkerke $R^2 = .045$, $X^2_{(5)} = 17.11$, $p = .004$), with increasing purpose in life being associated with a decreased likelihood of having possible RLS (OR .396, 95% CI .245–.639) (see Table 4). The logistic regression analyses for RLS symptoms at 3-year follow-up was not significant (see Table 4).

The series of hierarchical logistic regression analyses for possible presence of RBD at baseline, 1-year follow-up, 2-year follow-up and 3-year follow-up all yielded non-significant results.

Discussion

In a bi-racial sample of over 800 older adults the present findings provide support for the hypothesis that purpose

Table 2 Hierarchical Multiple Linear Regression Analyses of Purpose in Life and Sleep Quality

		B	SE	β	p	F	R^2
Sleep Quality at Baseline (n = 814)	Step 1					**2.41$_{(4)}$***	**.012**
	Sex	−.324	.234	−.049	.167		
	Years of Education	−.016	.032	−.018	.618		
	Age	.004	.014	.012	.755		
	Race	**.534**	**.210**	**.095**	**.011**		
	Step 2					**9.383$_{(5)}$****	**.055**
	Sex	−.298	.229	−.045	.193		
	Years of Education	.023	.032	.026	.471		
	Age	−.016	.014	−.042	.261		
	Race	**.548**	**.206**	**.097**	**.008**		
	Purpose in Life	**−1.326**	**.218**	**−.220**	**.000**		
Sleep Quality Change Baseline to 1-Year Follow-up (n = 814)	Step 1					.556$_{(4)}$	.003
	Sex	−.119	.202	−.021	.555		
	Education	−.029	.028	−.037	.293		
	Age	−.011	.012	−.034	.367		
	Race	−.074	.181	−.407	.684		
	Step 2					1.546$_{(5)}$	.009
	Sex	−.128	2.01	−.022	.526		
	Years of Education	−.043	.028	−.055	.132		
	Age	−.004	.012	−.012	.746		
	Race	−.078	.180	−.016	.665		
	Purpose in Life	**.449**	**.192**	**.087**	**.019**		
Sleep Quality Change Baseline to 2-Year Follow-up (n = 550)	Step 1					.857$_{(4)}$	.006
	Sex	.098	.245	.017	.689		
	Education	−.032	.034	−.040	.352		
	Age	.018	.016	.050	.269		
	Race	.265	.226	.053	.240		
	Step 2					.855$_{(5)}$	.008
	Sex	.087	.245	.015	.724		
	Years of Education	−.039	.035	−.049	.270		
	Age	.021	.016	.058	.205		
	Race	.261	.226	.052	.249		
	Purpose in Life	.235	.255	.041	.357		
Sleep Quality Change Baseline to 3-Year Follow-up (n = 245)	Step 1					.593$_{(4)}$	.012
	Sex	−.398	.357	−.072	.266		
	Education	.014	.054	.016	.801		
	Age	.007	.025	.018	.787		
	Race	.412	.345	.081	.234		
	Step 2					.693$_{(5)}$	.013
	Sex	−.388	.358	−.071	.279		
	Years of Education	.022	.057	.026	.702		
	Age	.003	.026	.008	.914		
	Race	.396	.347	.078	.255		
	Purpose in Life	−.183	.363	−.036	.615		

Four separate regression analyses. * = $p \leq .05$, ** = $p \leq .01$, bolding is used to emphasize significant predictors within the models

Is purpose in life associated with less sleep disturbance in older...

11

Table 3 Hierarchical Multiple Logistic Regression Analyses of purpose in life and risk of sleep apnea

		β	SE	p	Odds ratio	95% CI	X^2	Nagelkerke R^2
Risk of Sleep Apnea at Baseline (n = 808)	Step 1						**17.707**$_{(4)}$**	**.029**
	Sex	.282	.172	.101	1.325	.947–1.856		
	Years of Education	−.053	.024	.028	.348	.904–.994		
	Age	**−.036**	**.010**	**.001**	**.365**	**.945–.985**		
	Race	−.252	.155	.104	.778	.574–1.053		
	Step 2						**25.408**$_{(5)}$**	**.042**
	Sex	.294	.173	.089	1.341	.956–1.881		
	Years of Education	−.040	.025	.102	.961	.915–1.008		
	Age	**−.043**	**.011**	**.000**	**.957**	**.937–.978**		
	Race	−.248	.156	.111	.780	.575–1.059		
	Purpose in Life	**−.462**	**.168**	**.006**	**.630**	**.454–.875**		
Risk of Sleep Apnea at 1-Year Follow-Up (n = 810)	Step 1						**17.563**$_{(4)}$**	**.029**
	Sex	.187	.171	.274	1.206	.862–1.688		
	Years of Education	−.036	.024	.132	.965	.920–1.011		
	Age	**−.038**	**.011**	**.000**	**.963**	**.943–.983**		
	Race	−.002	.154	.990	.998	.737–1.351		
	Step 2						**21.608**$_{(5)}$*	**.035**
	Sex	.195	.172	.257	1.215	.867–1.702		
	Years of Education	−.026	.024	.282	.974	.929–1022		
	Age	**−.043**	**.011**	**.000**	**.958**	**.937–.978**		
	Race	.001	.155	.996	1.001	.739–1.356		
	Purpose in Life	**−.331**	**.165**	**.045**	**.719**	**.520–.993**		
Risk of Sleep Apnea at 2-Year Follow-Up (n = 548)	Step 1						**10.360**$_{(4)}$*	**.025**
	Sex	.296	.203	.146	1.344	.903–2.002		
	Years of Education	−.045	.029	.124	.956	.903–1.012		
	Age	**−.027**	**.014**	**.047**	**.973**	**.948–1.000**		
	Race	.175	.189	.354	1.191	.823–1.724		
	Step 2						**15.816**$_{(5)}$**	**.038**
	Sex	.322	.205	.116	1.380	.924–2.060		
	Years of Education	−.030	.030	.312	.971	.916–1.028		
	Age	**−.034**	**.014**	**.016**	**.967**	**.941–.994**		
	Race	.184	.190	.332	1.202	.829–1.743		
	Purpose in Life	**−.503**	**.217**	**.020**	**.604**	**.395–.925**		
Risk of Sleep Apnea at 3-Year Follow-Up (n = 242)	Step 1						3.983$_{(4)}$	.022
	Sex	−.056	.307	.856	.946	.518–1.728		
	Years of Education	−.033	.047	.479	.967	.882–1.060		
	Age	−.032	.022	.142	.969	.928–1.011		
	Race	.154	.299	.607	1.167	.649–2.097		
	Step 2						4.094$_{(5)}$	.023
	Sex	−.051	.308	.869	.951	.520–1.738		
	Years of Education	−.029	.049	.556	.972	.883–1.069		
	Age	−.034	.022	.132	.967	.925–1.010		
	Race	.147	.300	.625	1.158	.643–2.085		
	Purpose in Life	−.104	.312	.739	.901	.489–1.661		

Four separate regression analyses. * = p ≤ .05, ** = p ≤ .01, bolding is used to emphasize significant predictors within the models

Table 4 Hierarchical Multiple Logistic Regression Analyses of Purpose in Life and Possible Presence of RLS

		β	SE	p	Odds ratio	95% CI	X^2	Nagelkerke R^2
Possible presence of RLS at Baseline (n = 814)	Step 1						$8.189_{(4)}$	.015
	Sex	−.315	.208	.131	.730	.485–1.098		
	Years of Education	−.043	.028	.129	.958	.906–1.013		
	Age	.019	.012	.109	1.019	.996–1.043		
	Race	.043	.179	.808	1.044	.735–1.483		
	Step 2						$11.758_{(5)}*$	.022
	Sex	−.307	.209	.141	.736	.489–1.108		
	Education	−.032	.029	.263	.968	.915–1.025		
	Age	.014	.012	.263	1.014	.990–1.038		
	Race	.050	.180	.782	1.051	.739–1.494		
	Purpose in Life	−.355	.188	.059	.701	.485–1.013		
Possible presence of RLS at 1-Year Follow-Up (n = 814)	Step 1						$3.105_{(4)}$	.006
	Sex	−.087	.203	.667	.916	.616–1.364		
	Years of Education	−.045	.028	.111	.956	.904–1.010		
	Age	−.002	.012	.884	.998	.975–1.021		
	Race	−.117	.179	.514	.890	.626–1.264		
	Step 2						$14.688_{(5)}**$	.027
	Sex	−.073	.204	.722	.930	.623–1.388		
	Years of Education	−.026	.029	.367	.974	.920–1.031		
	Age	−.012	.012	.326	.988	.964–1.012		
	Race	−.109	.181	.547	.897	.629–1.279		
	Purpose in Life	**−.646**	**.191**	**.001**	**.524**	**.361–.762**		
Possible presence of RLS at 2-Year Follow-Up (n = 550)	Step 1						$2.218_{(4)}$	.006
	Sex	−.196	.237	.407	.822	.517–1.307		
	Years of Education	−.026	.033	.422	.974	.913–1.039		
	Age	−.004	.015	.808	.996	.967–1.026		
	Race	−.204	.211	.334	.816	.539–1.234		
	Step 2						$17.106_{(5)}**$	.045
	Sex	−.148	.240	.538	.862	.539–1.380		
	Years of Education	.001	.034	.979	1.001	.937–1.069		
	Age	−.015	.016	.319	.985	.955–1.015		
	Race	−.184	.214	.390	.832	.546–1.266		
	Purpose in Life	**−.927**	**.244**	**.000**	**.396**	**.245–.639**		
Possible presence of RLS at 3-Year Follow-Up (n = 245)	Step 1						$4.132_{(4)}$	.027
	Sex	−.696	.425	.102	.499	.217–1.148		
	Years of Education	.005	.058	.938	1.005	.897–1.125		
	Age	.012	.026	.641	1.012	.963–1.064		
	Race	−.348	.355	.327	.706	.352–1.417		
	Step 2						$4.138_{(5)}$	.027

Table 4 Hierarchical Multiple Logistic Regression Analyses of Purpose in Life and Possible Presence of RLS *(Continued)*

Sex	−.694	.426	.103	.500	.217–1.151
Years of Education	.006	.061	.922	1.006	.893–1.133
Age	.011	.027	.675	1.011	.959–1.066
Race	−.350	.357	.326	.705	.350 −1.417
Purpose in Life	−.030	.381	.936	.970	.460–2046

Four separate regression analyses. * = p ≤ .05, ** = p ≤ .01, bolding is used to emphasize significant predictors within the models, *RLS* Restless Leg Syndrome

in life is related to sleep quality with indications that it could be a potentially useful clinical tool for assessing older adults. We found that higher levels of purpose in life at baseline predicted better sleep quality at baseline as well as increased change in sleep quality over a 1-year period, a finding that is consistent with previous studies (Kim et al. 2015; Phelan et al. 2010; Ryff et al. 2004; Hamilton et al. 2006; Steptoe et al. 2008). Furthermore, these findings are consistent with anecdotal observations that people who have meaning and purpose in their waking activities appear to sleep well at night. It appears that for both African American and White American older adults, the more meaning and purpose one has in daytime activities, the better one tends to sleep at night. Collectively, the emerging data indicates the benefits of positive psychology on sleep health.

To our knowledge, this study is the first to demonstrate a relationship between purpose in life and the risk for symptoms of common sleep disorders in older adults. We found that higher levels of purpose in life were generally protective against the occurrence of sleep apnea and RLS as well as the onset of sleep apnea and RLS over the following 1 to 2 years. One interpretation of our findings is that individuals with a high purpose in life tend to have better overall mental and physical health. The premise of positive psychological well-being includes the notion that improved well-being will be accompanied by the optimal functioning of the persons' physiological systems (Phelan et al. 2010; Ryff et al. 2004). Also research has indicated that individuals who are high in components of psychological well-being other than purpose in life such as positive affect have fewer physical symptoms and better overall health (Fredman et al. 2014). Research by Ancoli-Isreal suggests a strong association between sleep difficulties and cardiac disease (Ancoli-Israel 2009), this research also posits that comorbidities associated with aging, such as medical and psychiatric illness, like cardiac disease and depression, foster the decreased ability to sleep in older adults rather than increasing age alone. Therefore, the protective factor we are seeing with purpose in life at baseline for sleep quality and sleep apnea (as well as a trending result for RLS) may be a consequence of fewer

medical comorbidities (Ryff et al. 2004). Another possibility is that individuals with higher levels of purpose in life tend to engage in more healthy behaviors. For example, studies have shown that people with more purpose in life are more likely to exercise, participate in preventative behaviors, such as doctor visits, and seek out adequate relaxation (Holahan et al. 2008; Kim et al. 2014; Holahan et al. 2011). It is possible that engagement in these types of healthy behaviors by the individuals who are high in purpose in life could lead to reduced risk of developing sleep apnea and RLS symptoms.

Our findings should be interpreted with some limitations. First, our findings are based on self-report, which are open to recall bias and subjective interpretation of sleep symptoms. Also, though this is a community-based sample, the educational attainment status of the sample is relatively high and it is possible that these higher levels of educational attainment may reflect a healthier population with higher levels of purpose in life and less severe sleep problems, as well as, greater access to health care. It is also possible that given the higher levels of educational attainment, this sample was more inclined engage in behaviors related to a healthier lifestyle, as research has suggested that in older adults in the United States, higher socioeconomic status, especially as measured via educational attainment, has been associated with choosing healthier lifestyle behaviors, specifically healthy diet choices and increased physical exercise (Kim et al. 2004). In addition, the proportion of those with RBD was relatively low (7% of the sample), which might have limited power to detect changes over time. Finally, while our analyses revealed statistical significance at the $p < .001$ level on several analyses, the amount of variance explained is relatively low. Therefore, future research should examine the magnitude of the effects relative to other known risk factors for sleep disturbances in older adults.

Conclusion

Despite these limitations, this study has several important advances. First, we examined the relationship between purpose in life and risk of specific sleep disorders. In addition, we had a large sample size of over 800 older adults that included a large proportion of African Americans (53.7%), greatly increasing the generalizability of our findings. Finally, these findings indicate that the construct of purpose in life may have utility in a clinical setting. When evaluating older adults for sleep issues, assessing for purpose in life could provide insights into sleep quality, the presence of sleep apnea, and to a lesser degree RLS. Further investigation into possible mechanisms on purpose in life and other benefits of positive psychology and sleep health are needed. For instance research should examine the link between purpose in life and specific symptoms of insomnia, such as nocturnal symptoms versus daytime symptoms. This could help identify potential mechanisms for the impact of positive psychology on insomnia. Moreover, future research could examine the use of interventions using positive psychology to target purpose in life in older adults. For example, mindfulness-based therapies (Ong 2016) and Acceptance and Commitment Therapies (Dalrymple et al. 2010) include values and cultivation of compassion that could enhance purpose in life (Ong et al. 2012).

Abbreviations
MAP: Memory and Aging Project; MARS: Minority Aging Research Study; MSQ: Mayo Sleep Questionnaire; PSQI: Pittsburgh Sleep Quality Index; RBD: REM Behavior Disorder; RLS: Restless Leg Syndrome

Acknowledgements
The authors thank the participants of the Minority Aging Research Study, the participants of the Memory and Aging Project and the Rush Clinical Core for their invaluable contributions. We would also like to thank Drs. Patricia Boyle and Lisa Barnes for assisting in the development of this idea and the collaboration with the Rush Alzheimer's Disease Center's Research Resource Sharing Hub.

Funding
This research was supported by National Institute on Aging Grant Numbers R01AG22018, P30G10161, R01AG17917, P20MD6886 and the Illinois Department of Public Health.

Authors' contributions
ADT was a major contributor in the idea conception for the manuscript, analyzing and interpreting the data as well as writing the manuscript. CES was a major contributor in analyzing and interpreting data. JCO was a major contributor in the conception of the manuscript and review and revision of the manuscript for intellectual content. All authors read and approved the final manuscript.

Competing interests
The authors declare that they have no competing interests.

References
Ancoli-Israel S. Sleep and its disorders in aging populations. Sleep Med. 2009; 10(Suppl 1):S7–S11.

Barnes LL, et al. The Minority Aging Research Study: ongoing efforts to obtain brain donation in African Americans without dementia. Curr Alzheimer Res. 2012;9(6):734–45.

Beaudreau SA, et al. Validation of the Pittsburgh sleep quality index and the Epworth sleepiness scale in older black and white women. Sleep Med. 2012; 13(1):36–42.

Bennett DA, et al. Overview and findings from the rush Memory and Aging Project. Curr Alzheimer Res. 2012;9(6):646–63.

Boeve B, et al. Validation of a questionnaire for the diagnosis of REM sleep behavior disorder. Neurology. 2002;58(SUPPL. 3):A509.

Boeve BF, et al. Validation of the Mayo Sleep Questionnaire to screen for REM sleep behavior disorder in an aging and dementia cohort. Sleep Med. 2011; 12(5):445–53.

Boyle PA, et al. Purpose in life is associated with mortality among community-dwelling older persons. Psychosom Med. 2009;71(5):574–9.

Boyle PA, et al. Effect of a purpose in life on risk of incident Alzheimer disease and mild cognitive impairment in community-dwelling older persons. Arch Gen Psychiatry. 2010a;67(3):304–10.

Boyle PA, Buchman AS, Bennett DA. Purpose in life is associated with a reduced risk of incident disability among community-dwelling older persons. Am J Geriatr Psychiatry. 2010b;18(12):1093–102.

Boyle PA, et al. Effect of purpose in life on the relation between Alzheimer disease pathologic changes on cognitive function in advanced age. Arch Gen Psychiatry. 2012;69(5):499–505.

Burrow AL, Hill PL. Purpose as a form of identity capital for positive youth adjustment. Dev Psychol. 2011;47(4):1196–206.

Buysse DJ, et al. The Pittsburgh Sleep Quality Index: a new instrument for psychiatric practice and research. Psychiatry Res. 1989;28(2):193–213.

Chen X, Gelaye B, Williams MA. Sleep characteristics and health-related quality of life among a national sample of American young adults: assessment of possible health disparities. Qual Life Res. 2014;23(2):613–25.

Cohen-Zion M, et al. Cognitive changes and sleep disordered breathing in elderly: differences in race. J Psychosom Res. 2004;56(5):549–53.

Dalrymple KL, et al. Incorporating principles from acceptance and commitment therapy into cognitive-behavioral therapy for insomnia: A case example. J Contemp Psychother, 2010. 40(4): p. 209–217.

Foley D, et al. Sleep disturbances and chronic disease in older adults: results of the 2003 National Sleep Foundation Sleep in America Survey. J Psychosom Res. 2004;56(5):497–502.

Fredman L, et al. Positive affect is associated with fewer sleep problems in older caregivers but not noncaregivers. Gerontologist. 2014;54(4):559–69.

Hamilton NA, et al. Sleep and psychological well-being. Soc Indic Res. 2006;82(1): 147–63.

Holahan CK, Holahan CJ, Suzuki R. Purposiveness, physical activity, and perceived health in cardiac patients. Disabil Rehabil. 2008;30(23):1772–8.

Holahan CK, et al. Purposiveness and leisure-time physical activity in women in early midlife. Women Health. 2011;51(7):661–75.

Hossain JLS, Shapiro CM. The Prevalence, Cost Implications, & Management of Sleep Disorders. Sleep Breath. 2002;6(2):85–102.

IBM, Statistical Package for the Social Sciences (SPSS). 2015.

Jaussent I, et al. Insomnia symptoms in older adults: associated factors and gender differences. Am J Geriatr Psychiatry. 2011;19(1):88–97.

Kim S, Symons M, Popkin BM. Contrasting socioeconomic profiles related to healthier lifestyles in China and the United States. Am J Epidemiol. 2004; 159(2):184–91.

Kim ES, et al. Purpose in life and reduced incidence of stroke in older adults: 'The Health and Retirement Study'. J Psychosom Res. 2013;74(5):427–32.

Kim ES, et al. Life satisfaction and frequency of doctor visits. Psychosom Med. 2014;76(1):86–93.

Kim ES, Hershner SD, Strecher VJ. Purpose in life and incidence of sleep disturbances. J Behav Med. 2015;38(3):590–7.

Krause N. Meaning in life and mortality. J Gerontol B Psychol Sci Soc Sci. 2009; 64(4):517–27.

Netzer NC, et al. Using the Berlin Questionnaire to identify patients at risk for the sleep apnea syndrome. Ann Intern Med. 1999;131(7):485–91.

Ong JC. Mindfulness-Based Therapy for Insomnia. Washington, DC: American Psychological Association; 2016.

Ong JC, Ulmer CS, Manber R. Improving sleep with mindfulness and acceptance: a metacognitive model of insomnia. Behav Res Ther. 2012;50(11):651–60.

Patel NP, et al. "Sleep disparity" in the population: poor sleep quality is strongly associated with poverty and ethnicity. BMC Public Health. 2010;10:475.

Phelan CH, et al. Psychosocial predictors of changing sleep patterns in aging women: a multiple pathway approach. Psychol Aging. 2010;25(4):858–66.

Pigeon WR, et al. Elevated sleep disturbance among blacks in an urban family medicine practice. J Am Board Fam Med. 2011;24(2):161–8.

Redline S, Strohl KP. Recognition and consequences of obstructive sleep apnea hypopnea syndrome. Clin Chest Med. 1998;19(1):1–19.

Redline S, et al. Racial Differences in Sleep-disordered Breathing in African-Americans and Caucasians. Am J Respir Crit Care Med. 1997;155:186–92.

Roepke AM, Jayawickreme E, Riffle OM. Meaning and health: a systematic review. Appl Res Qual Life. 2014;9(4):1055–79.

Rongve A, Boeve BF, Aarsland D. Frequency and correlates of caregiver-reported sleep disturbances in a sample of persons with early dementia. J Am Geriatr Soc. 2010;58(3):480–6.

Ruiter ME, et al. Normal sleep in African-Americans and Caucasian-Americans: A meta-analysis. Sleep Med. 2011;12(3):209–14.

Ryff CD. Happiness Is Everything, or Is It? Explorations on the Meaning of Psychological Well-Being. J Pers Soc Psychol. 1989;57(6):1069–81.

Ryff CD. Psychological well-being revisited: advances in the science and practice of eudaimonia. Psychother Psychosom. 2014;83(1):10–28.

Ryff CDK, Keyes CL. The Structure of Psychological Well-Being Revisited. J Pers Soc Psychol. 1995;69(4):719–27.

Ryff CD, Singer BH, Dienberg Love G. Positive health: connecting well-being with biology. Philos Trans R Soc Lond B Biol Sci. 2004;359(1449):1383–94.

Steptoe A, et al. Positive affect, psychological well-being, and good sleep. J Psychosom Res. 2008;64(4):409–15.

Turner AD, Lim AS, Leurgans SE, Bennett DA, Buchman AS, Barnes LL. Self-Reported Sleep in Older African Americans and White Americans. Ethn Dis. 2016;26(4):521–8.

3

An assessment of online information related to surgical obstructive sleep apnea treatment

Christopher J. Gouveia[1*], Hannan A. Qureshi[1], Robert C. Kern[1], Stanley Yung-Chuan Liu[2] and Robson Capasso[2]

Abstract

Background: Patients are accessing online health information frequently and using it to guide treatment decisions. Few studies have been done assessing obstructive sleep apnea (OSA) information, and no studies have examined surgical resources for these patients.

Methods: This was a cross-sectional analysis. "Sleep surgery" and "sleep apnea surgery" were entered into Google, MSN Bing, and Yahoo! search engines. The first 25 results of each individual search were evaluated. Each unique site was assessed for content quality, accessibility, usability, reliability, and readability using validated instruments. The date of last update for each site was also documented.

Results: "Sleep surgery" was searched for an average of 1,703,991 (SD = 166,585) times per month from June 2015 to June 2016. 33 unique websites were identified. Sites were most often academically/government affiliated (10/33, 30.3%), health information sites (8/33, 24.2%), or non-profit/hospital related (8/33, 24.2%). The mean overall DISCERN score for quality was "good," at 56.6 (range, 22–79). The mean overall LIDA score for accessibility, usability, and reliability was "moderate," at 123.9 (range, 97–152). The mean Flesch Reading Ease score for readability was 49.77 (range 22.7–74.3); 7/33 (21.2%) scored above 60, the recommended range for average visitors. 60.6% (20/33) of the sites had been updated since January 1, 2014. There was no significant correlation between a websites' position on a browser's search and its DISCERN, LIDA, FRE, or total score.

Conclusions: With patients' increasing reliance on Internet information, efforts to understand and improve websites' quality and usefulness present unique opportunities in OSA surgery and beyond.

Keywords: Obstructive sleep apnea, OSA, Sleep surgery, Internet, Online resources

Background

The Internet is an increasingly important resource for patients seeking health information. An estimated 8 of 10 Internet users pursue online medical education, with 85% utilizing search engines to find it (Fox S. Health topics. Pew Internet and American Life Project. http://pewinternet.org/Reports/2011/Health Topics.aspx. Viewed Feb 27 2016; Ybarra and Suman 2006). However, studies have shown poor quality and inaccurate information on websites regarding numerous different medical and surgical conditions (Biermann et al. 2000; Impicciatore et al. 1997; Soot et al. 1999). This is concerning in an environment where nearly three-fourths of patients using the Internet say their findings influence their treatment decisions (Rainie and Fox S. The Online Health Care Revolution: The Internet's powerful influence on "health seekers". http://www.pewinternet.org/2000/11/26/the-online-health-care-revolution. Viewed March 3 2016).

Obstructive sleep apnea (OSA) is a major public health burden (Yaggi et al. 2005; Peker et al. 2002) with substantial socioeconomic impact (Kapur 2010; Mulgrew et al. 2007; Omachi et al. 2009). Patients with OSA are treated by a variety of specialists including internists, neurologists,

* Correspondence: Christopher.gouveia@northwestern.edu
[1]Department of Otolaryngology, Head and Neck Surgery, Northwestern University Feinberg School of Medicine, 676 N. St. Claire, Suite 1325, Chicago, IL 60611, USA
Full list of author information is available at the end of the article

psychiatrists, and otolaryngologists. The most commonly prescribed initial treatment is continuous positive airway pressure (CPAP), but more than 50% of patients fail, which suggests surgery as a promising alternative (Gay et al. 2006). Indeed, sleep surgery is being performed at increasing rates nationwide (Ishman et al. 2014). Due to the risk and variability in outcomes of different management options for OSA, the potential harms from misinformation can be catastrophic. To date, no studies have examined the quality of web-based information related to OSA surgery.

The main objective of this study is to assess the online sites visited by patients performing online searches for OSA surgery information using several validated instruments. Our hypothesis is that the topic would have a dearth of high quality information and overall be lacking in useful resources. Identifying this and focusing on areas of need would be valuable in setting future priorities for patient education efforts. Additionally, conducting this analysis would provide guidance for providers and patients on suggested websites for OSA treatment information.

Methods

This study received approval by the Northwestern University Institutional Review Board.

Search engine query

"Sleep surgery" was chosen as the initial search term and entered into Google, MSN Bing, and Yahoo! search engines. Utilizing Google AdWords (Google AdWords Keyword Planner. https://adwords.google.com/Keyword Planner. Viewed January 1 2015), the most commonly associated search term "sleep apnea surgery" was identified and also entered into the three search engines to allow for a broad review of sites patients would encounter. Inclusion in the study required that a website be free, written in English, non-duplicate, and a source of online health information. Search engine query and collection of websites was performed on June 1, 2016.

The first 25 results of each browser search meeting inclusion criteria were evaluated. Each unique site was assessed for content quality, accessibility, usability, reliability, and readability using validated instruments. The last update for each site was also documented.

Validated assessment instruments

For quality, the DISCERN instrument was used (Charnock et al. 1999; Shepperd et al. 2002). This 16-item questionnaire is a validated tool that measures quality of online health information (Kaicker et al. 2010; Batchelor and Ohya 2009). Questions included are "is it clear what sources of information were used to compile the publication?" and "does it describe the benefits/risks of

treatments?" Each question is rated on a 5-point scale. The maximum score for the DISCERN instrument was 80. Each website was categorized as "excellent" (68–80), "good" (55–67), "fair" (42–54), "poor" (29–41), or "very poor" (16–28).

For accessibility, usability, and reliability, the LIDA instrument was used. This 41-item questionnaire is a validated tool to examine these three domains of quality for Internet resources (Minervation. The Minervation validation instrument for healthcare web- sites. Available at: http://www.minervation.com/lida-tool/. Accessed March 20 2015). Questions 1-6 pertain to accessibility and assess a site's code and setup for compliance with World Wide Web Consortium standards, as well as need for registration. Usability is assessed in questions 7–24, which examine website clarity, consistency of layout, and browsing/interactive abilities. Lastly, questions 25–41 assess reliability with questions focusing on frequency of updates, conflicts of interest, and accuracy of content. The maximum score for each domain is 60, 54, and 51 respectively. Each question assessed by raters is rated on a 0 ("Never") to 3 ("Always") scale. The raw scores for each category were converted into percentages, and were classified as "high" (>90%), "moderate" (50–90%), or "low" (< 50%).

For readability, the Flesch Reading Ease (FRE) score was used. Each site's text was copied and pasted into a Microsoft Word 2010 (Microsoft Inc., Redmond, Washington) document (Microsoft Corporation 2010). All efforts were made to remove author names, hyperlinks, nonstandard text formatting, dates, and abbreviations to prevent low-skewing of scores (Goslin and Elhassan 2013). The grammar check function of Word software calculates FRE score on a 0–100 scale with higher scores indicating increased ease of reading.

Data collection and analysis

After the search engine query was performed, two authors (C.G. and H.Q.) evaluated each website independently. The scores for each question were then averaged to give an overall score that was utilized for results and statistical analysis. SPSS version 21 (SPSS Inc., Chicago, IL) was used for summary data and statistical analysis. Inter-observer reliability was measured separately for the DISCERN and LIDA instruments using the Cohen's weighted-kappa coefficient, with significance set at > 0.6. Differences in mean scores between types of websites were analyzed using the Wilcoxon rank sum test, with threshold for significance set at $p < 0.05$. The correlation between DISCERN, LIDA, FRE, and total score with the position a website appeared on each browser search was analyzed using the Spearman correlation coefficient.

Results

"Sleep surgery" was searched for an average of 1,703,991 (SD = 166,585) times per month from June 2015 to June 2016. The most commonly associated search term "sleep apnea surgery" was searched an average of 1,818,541 (SD = 159,541) times per month from June 2015 to June 2016.

Of the 150 websites identified using the Google, MSN Bing, and Yahoo search engines, 33 (22.0%) unique websites met inclusion criteria. Reasons for exclusion of the other 117 websites included duplicate searches (n = 88, 75.2%), news story (n = 15, 8.5%), advertisements/commercials (n = 5, 4.3%), online videos (n = 3, 2.6%), nonfunctioning or hacked site (n = 3, 2.6%), research journal website (n = 2, 1.7%), and online discussion forums (n = 1, 0.9%). Most websites were academically/government affiliated (10/33, 30.3%), health information sites (8/33, 24.2%), or non-profit/hospital related (8/33, 24.2%), as shown in Fig. 1.

Inter-observer reliability for the DISCERN instrument was significant (k = 0.688). The mean overall DISCERN score for quality was "good," at 56.6 (range, 22–79; SD = 14.0). The DISCERN instrument rated 7/33 (21.2%) websites as "excellent," 13/33 (39.4%) as "good," 9/33 (27.3%) as "fair," 2/33 (6.1%) as "poor," and 2/33 (6.1%) as "very poor." Figure 2 displays the number of websites in each DISCERN category.

Inter-observer reliability for the LIDA instrument was significant (k = 0.814). The mean overall LIDA score for accessibility, usability, and reliability was "moderate," at 123.9 (75.1%; range, 97–152; SD = 14.2). The distribution of LIDA scores for accessibility, usability, and reliability for all 33 websites is shown in Fig. 3.

The mean score for accessibility was "moderate" at 48.2 (80.3%) (SD = 4.4). Only 2/33 (6.1%) had "high" LIDA accessibility scores and the remaining 31/33 (93.9%) had "moderate" scores. The mean score for usability was "moderate" at 42.3 (78.3%) (SD = 7.3) for all 33 websites. There were 5/33 (15.1%) websites with "high" LIDA usability scores, 27/33 (81.8%) with "moderate"

scores, and 1/33 (3.0%) with "low" usability scores. The mean score for reliability for all 33 websites was "moderate" at 33.4 (65.5%) (SD = 10.7). 5/33 (15.1%) websites had "high" LIDA reliability scores, 21/33 (63.6%) with "moderate" scores, and 7/33 (21.2%) with "low" reliability scores. The number of websites rated "high," "moderate," or "low" in each LIDA instrument category is displayed in Fig. 4.

The mean FRE score for readability was 49.8 (range 22.7–74.3, SD 13.3). 7/33 (21.2%) websites scored above 60, the recommended range for average visitors (Van der Marel et al. 2009; D'Alessandro et al. 2001). 20/33 (60.6%) of sites had been updated since January 1, 2014.

The websites with the top 5 aggregate total of the DISCERN, LIDA, and FRE scores are listed in Table 1. Two of these five websites are academic/government-sponsored sites, whereas the remaining three are health information sites. There were no significant differences between mean scores for all academic versus non-academic websites in DISCERN score (p = 0.98), LIDA score (p = 0.50), FRE score (p = 0.57), and aggregate total score (p = 0.92). There was no significant linear correlation between a websites' rank in each browser search and its DISCERN score, LIDA score, FRE score, and aggregate total.

Discussion

An estimated one-third of all adults and children with sleep disorders first present to an otolaryngologist, of whom many are diagnosed with OSA (Yaremchuk and Wardrop 2010). These patients utilize Internet resources in important ways: more than half seek contact with a medical professional because of information they have found online (Ybarra and Suman 2006; Pusz and Brietzke 2012) and more than 70% report it significantly influences their treatment decisions (Rainie and Fox S. The Online Health Care Revolution: The Internet's powerful influence on "health seekers". http://www.pewinternet.org/2000/11/26/the-online-health-care-revolution. Viewed March 3 2016). Search engines are the mode of choice for patients seeking information on the web (Ybarra and Suman 2006), but at present there are no studies examining the quality and usefulness of these resources for sleep surgery. This is important as surgical procedures for OSA carry unique benefits and risks, and are being performed in record levels nationwide (Ishman et al. 2014).

In our study examining online resources for OSA surgery, there is, unsurprisingly, significant heterogeneity in the quality and utility of websites. Overall though, the results of this study are encouraging. Quality was 'excellent' or 'good' for the majority of websites studied (29/33, 87.9%). The average DISCERN score of 56.6 is higher than any other topic examined within the otolaryngology literature, including OSA (Goslin and Elhassan 2013; Pusz and

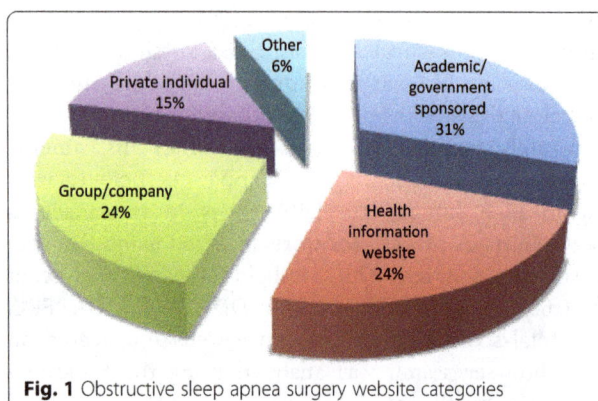

Fig. 1 Obstructive sleep apnea surgery website categories

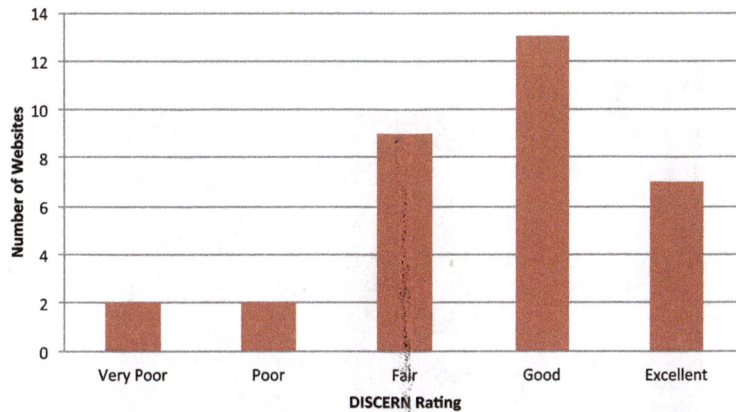

Fig. 2 Number of websites in each DISCERN instrument category for quality

Brietzke 2012; Langille et al. 2012; Alamoudi and Hong 2015; McKearney 2013).

These encouraging results carried over to non-quality measures as well. The majority of sites studied had at least "moderate" accessibility, usability, and reliability. This compares favorably to a previous study examining LIDA in other otolaryngologic disorders (Goslin and Elhassan 2013). This study also found that the vast majority of sites have moderate ratings for all three non-quality measures, with reliability having the widest range of scores- this reflects the homogenous nature of sites when it comes to user interface and interactivity, but heterogeneity when examining frequency of updates and sources of information. No studies examining LIDA or similar measures in OSA specifically have ever been performed.

There remain several shortcomings of online resources for OSA surgery. Numerous sites in our study scored "low" for their reliability. Average readability score was 49.8 and less than one-fourth of sites had a readability score above 60, which is often cited as the minimum

recommended for patients (Van der Marel et al. 2009; D'Alessandro et al. 2001). Further, nearly 40% (13/33) of sites had not been updated since January 1, 2014. These are concerning findings: even the most comprehensive, quality online materials will be unhelpful and potentially dangerous if they are unable to be understood by patients or outdated. This is especially true in sleep surgery, as it is an evolving field with new paradigms occurring frequently (Lin et al. 2008; Kezirian 2011).

Why are top browser searches not scoring well on quality and adjunctive measures of usefulness? The Wikipedia site for "sleep surgery" was one of the top 2 searches in all browser queries, however was not one of the top scoring websites. When examining this site's score breakdown, its LIDA is close to top websites, but its quality score (56) is much lower. Comparing individual domain scores, the site suffered from not having a more thorough discussion of treatment options, especially of surgical risks, medical management, and overall impact on quality of life. It is worth noting that on a

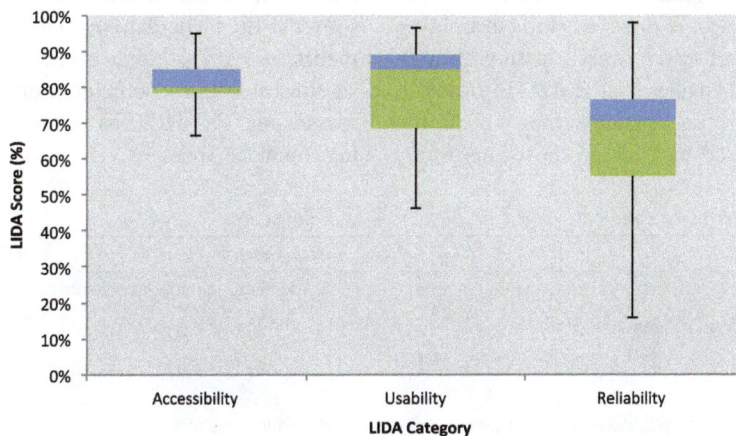

Fig. 3 Box-and-whisker plot of the distribution of LIDA scores (%) for each LIDA category in all websites

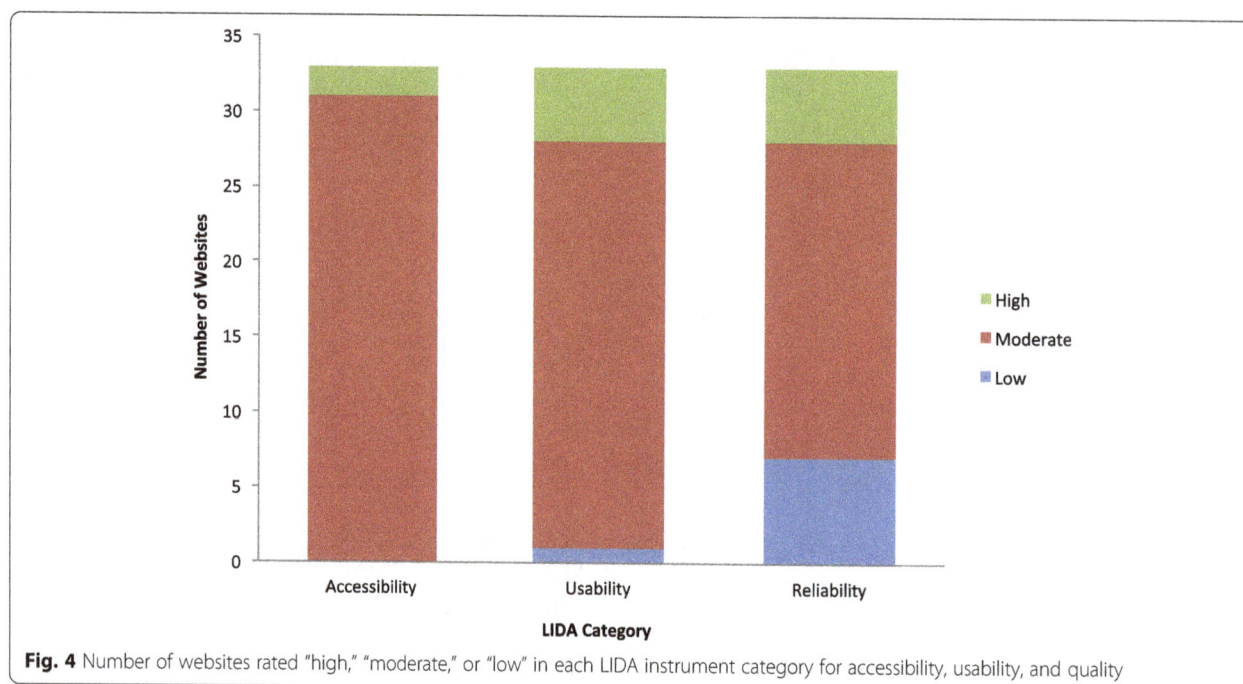

Fig. 4 Number of websites rated "high," "moderate," or "low" in each LIDA instrument category for accessibility, usability, and quality

more contemporary review of the website, some of these issues seem to have improved. Examining sites that we, anecdotally, often recommend to patients (entnet.org, sleepeducation.org), found that they suffered mostly from lower LIDA scores for usability and reliability versus our top scoring websites. We continue to feel there is utility to all of these resources individually, but it highlights the challenges to clinicians and patients when utilizing online information.

This study has several limitations. First, we chose the term 'sleep surgery' by consensus of the authors. It was felt that this would represent a simple, common-language phrase that would be frequently used by patients seeking further information about surgery for OSA. Consideration was given to selecting 'sleep apnea treatment' or simply 'sleep apnea,' but the authors felt this would examine resources focusing on non-surgical issues related to OSA, or those favoring CPAP therapy. A previous study examining quality in OSA sites found lower overall quality, though more frequent updates (Langille et al. 2012). In order to best include other sites these patients may encounter, Google AdWords was used to find the most commonly

associated search term, which was 'sleep apnea surgery.' Given the significant amount of website overlap amongst these terms, our findings likely represent the majority of information sources patients would find on their searches. We executed our search with only 3 search engines, although they represent nearly all United States activity (Top 15 Most Popular Search Engines: EBiz. www.ebizmba.com/articles/search-engines. Viewed Feburary 24 2016). Searches were limited to the first 25 sites from each search because nearly all users click within the first 2–3 results pages (Goslin and Elhassan 2013).

Our study utilized the DISCERN, LIDA, and FRE instruments to measure quality, accessibility, usability, reliability, and readability, which all have shortcomings in their respective domains. However, they are the few tested and validated tools for analyzing online health resources. In particular, the DISCERN and LIDA instruments rely on subjective scoring- however, our study's significant kappa-coefficients on these respective tests is reassuring. The FRE has inherent limitations in examining medical websites, as many complex jargon terms

Table 1 Top 5 websites in terms of aggregate total DISCERN, LIDA, and FRE scores

Website URL	Website type	DISCERN	LIDA	FRE	Total
http://umm.edu/health/medical/reports/articles/obstructive-sleep-apnea	Academic/government sponsored	79	145	53.6	277.6
http://www.medicinenet.com/sleep_apnea/page9.htm	Health information website	74	148	54.7	276.7
http://www.mayoclinic.org/diseases-conditions/sleep-apnea/basics/definition/con-20020286	Health information website	73	146	54.6	273.6
http://www.webmd.com/sleep-disorders/tc/sleep-apnea-surgery	Health information website	61.5	141	69.4	271.9
https://www.nhlbi.nih.gov/health/health-topics/topics/sleepapnea	Academic/government sponsored	61	134	74.3	269.3

cannot simply be replaced which skews to lower scores. This applies to all websites evaluated, however, so comparisons remain helpful. Other scoring systems, like the Flesch-Kincaid Grade Level or Gunning Frequency of Gobbledygook, can be used- but there is a high correlation with FRE and they have similar limitations. These instruments were chosen to provide a broad overview of website quality and adjunctive measures on the topic of OSA surgery, and we feel that they are effective in this.

The present study provides a useful overview of online health resources for patients pursuing sleep surgery. Overall, the quality and utility of these websites is strong, and greater than prior investigations in other fields of otolaryngology. Future research is needed to determine the etiology of this finding, and to assess its impact on patient experience and outcomes. This information can help direct physicians when discussing OSA surgery with patients, as well as healthcare providers developing online medical education.

Conclusions

Patients utilize online resources for information on their health conditions and treatments options. On the topic of OSA surgery, the quality and usefulness of current online materials are good overall, and rated higher than other otolaryngologic topics analyzed with the same metrics. Physicians must stay abreast of Internet content to assist in patient education and guidance.

Acknowledgements
We would like to thank Amy Yang M.S. of the Northwestern University Biostatistics Collaboration Center for her assistance with statistical analysis.

Funding
The authors have no external funding sources responsible for this research.

Authors' contributions
CG came up with study idea, was involved in data collection, data analysis, manuscript preparation, and final approval. HQ was involved in data collection, data analysis, and final manuscript approval. RK was involved in study creation, data analysis, and final manuscript approval. SL and RC were involved in study creation, data analysis, manuscript preparation, and final manuscript approval.

Competing interests
The authors declare that they have no competing interests.

Author details
[1]Department of Otolaryngology, Head and Neck Surgery, Northwestern University Feinberg School of Medicine, 676 N. St. Claire, Suite 1325, Chicago, IL 60611, USA. [2]Department of Otolaryngology, Head and Neck Surgery, Stanford University Medical Center, Stanford, CA, USA.

References

Alamoudi U, Hong P. Readability and Quality assessment of websites related to microtia and aural atresia. IJPO. 2015;79(2):151–6.

Batchelor JM, Ohya Y. Use of the DISCERN instrument by patients and health professionals to assess information resources on treatments for asthma and atopic dermatitis. Allergol Int. 2009;58:141–5.

Biermann JS, Golladay GJ, Greenfield MLVH, Baker LH. Evaluation of cancer information on the Internet. Cancer. 2000;86:381–90.

Charnock D, Shepperd S, Needham G, Gann R. DISCERN: an instrument for judging the quality of written consumer health information on treatment choices. J Epidemiol Community Health. 1999;53:105–11.

D'Alessandro DM, Kingsley P, Johnson-West J. The readability of pediatric patient education materials on the World Wide Web. Arch Pediatr Adolesc Med. 2001;155:807–12.

Fox S. Health topics. Pew Internet and American Life Project. http://pewinternet.org/Reports/2011/Health Topics.aspx. Viewed Feb 27, 2016

Gay P, Weaver T, Loube D, et al. Evaluation of positive airway pressure treatment for sleep related breathing disorders in adults. Sleep. 2006;29(3):381–401.

Google AdWords Keyword Planner. https://adwords.google.com/KeywordPlanner. Viewed January 1, 2015.

Goslin RA, Elhassan HA. Evaluating Internet Health Resources in Ear, Nose, and Throat Surgery. Laryngoscope. 2013;123:1626–31.

Impicciatore P, Pandolfini C, Casella N, Bonati M. Reliability of health information for the public on the World Wide Web: systematic survey of advice on managing fever in children at home. BMJ. 1997;314:1875–9.

Ishman SL, Ishii LE, Gourin CG. Temporal trends in sleep apnea surgery: 1993-2010. Laryngoscope. 2014;124(5):1251–8.

Kaicker J, Debono VB, Dang W, et al. Assessment of the quality and variability of health information on chronic pain websites using the DISCERN instrument. BMC Med. 2010;8:59.

Kapur VK. Obstructive sleep apnea: diagnosis, epidemiology, and economics. Respir Care. 2010;55:1155–67.

Kezirian EJ. Nonresponders to pharyngeal surgery for obstructive sleep apnea: insights from drug-induced sleep endoscopy. Laryngoscope. 2011;121(6):1320–6.

Langille M, Veldhuyzen S, Shanavaz SA, Massoud E. Systematic evaluation of obstructive sleep apnea websites on the internet. J Otolaryngol Head Neck Surg. 2012;41(4):265–72.

Lin HC, Friedman M, Chang HW, Gurpinar B. The efficacy of multilevel surgery of the upper airway in adults with obstructive sleep apnea/hypopnea syndrome. Laryngoscope. 2008;118(5):902–8.

McKearney TC. McKearney RM The quality and accuracy of internet information on the subject of ear tubes. IJPO. 2013;77:894–7.

Microsoft Corporation. Microsoft Office 2010 Standard Edition: Word [computer program]. Redmond, WA: Microsoft Corp; 2010.

Minervation. The Minervation validation instrument for healthcare web- sites. Available at: http://www.minervation.com/lida-tool/. Accessed March 20, 2015.

Mulgrew AT, Ryan CF, Fleetham JA, et al. The impact of obstructive sleep apnea and daytime sleepiness on work limitation. Sleep Med. 2007;9:42–53.

Omachi TA, Claman DM, Blanc PD, Eisner MD. Obstructive sleep apnea: a risk factor for work disability. Sleep. 2009;32(6):791–8.

Peker Y, Hedner J, Norum J, Kraiczi H, Carlson J. Increased incidence of cardiovascular disease in middle-aged men with obstructive sleep apnea: a 7-year follow-up. Am J Respir Crit Care Med. 2002;166:159–65.

Pusz MD, Brietzke SE. How good is Google? The quality of otolaryngology information on the internet. Otolaryngol Head Neck Surg. 2012;147(3):462–5.

Rainie L, Fox S. The Online Health Care Revolution: The Internet's powerful influence on "health seekers". http://www.pewinternet.org/2000/11/26/the-online-health-care-revolution. Viewed March 3, 2016.

Shepperd S, Charnock D, Cook A. A 5-star system for rating the quality of information based on DISCERN. Health Info Libr J. 2002;19:201–5.

Soot LC, Goneta GL, Edwards JM. Vascular surgery and the internet: a poor source of patient-oriented information. J Vasc Surg. 1999;30:84–91.

Top 15 Most Popular Search Engines: EBiz. www.ebizmba.com/articles/search-engines. Viewed Feburary 24, 2016.

Van der Marel S, Duijvestein M, Hardwick JC, et al. Quality of web-based information on inflammatory bowel diseases. Inflamm Bowel Dis. 2009;15:1891–6.

Yaggi HK, Concato J, Kernan WN, Lichtman JH, Brass LM, Mohsenin V. Obstructive sleep apnea as a risk factor for stroke and death. N Engl J Med. 2005;353:2034–41.

4

Relationships and CPAP adherence among women with obstructive sleep apnea

Kelly Glazer Baron[1*], Heather E. Gunn[2], Lisa F. Wolfe[3] and Phyllis C. Zee[3]

Abstract

Background: Obstructive sleep apnea contributes to daytime sleepiness, poor quality of life and increased risk for heart disease and hypertension among women. Continuous positive airway pressure improves sleepiness and quality of life and may reduce health risks but few studies have evaluated predictors of adherence among women. The goal of this study was to evaluate the role of relationship factors in women's continuous positive airway pressure (CPAP) adherence and change in relationship quality among married/partnered women.

Methods: Women recently diagnosed with obstructive sleep apnea completed relationship quality, social support questionnaires and spousal involvement interviews. CPAP adherence was collected at 12 weeks.

Results: Data were available for 16 women. Average CPAP adherence was 3.6 SD = 2.7 h per night. Women with higher reports of social support had higher adherence. None of the unmarried/partnered participants were adherent to the recommendation of CPAP use ≥ 4 h per night at 12 week follow-up. Marital status was not associated with demographic, disease severity or social support measures. Relationship conflict among married/partnered participants was associated with lower adherence. In qualitative surveys, encouragement and support were the two most commonly reported types of partner involvement. Relationship quality did not change between baseline and 3 months.

Conclusion: Results suggest relationship factors are robust predictors of CPAP adherence among women with obstructive sleep apnea.

Keywords: Obstructive apnea, Continuous positive airway pressure, Adherence

Background

Obstructive sleep apnea (OSA) prevalence rapidly increases among middle aged women, and prevalence of moderate to severe OSA is 6% of postmenopausal women (Redline et al. 2014). Consequences of OSA include daytime sleepiness, depressive symptoms, decreased quality of life as well as increased risk for cardiovascular disease, diabetes and stroke (Doherty et al. 2005; Engleman et al. 1994; Marin et al. 2005, 2012). The main treatment for OSA is continuous positive airway pressure (CPAP), in which the patient wears a mask connected to a small machine that pushes humidified air into the airway, thus preventing airway collapse during sleep. Despite the benefits of continuous positive airway pressure (CPAP) for health and quality of life, 46–83% of OSA patients are non-adherent (Weaver

and Grunstein 2008). Understanding women's CPAP use is important because women with untreated OSA have increased risk of hypertension, stroke and cardiovascular death. Two studies have highlighted elevated cardiovascular mortality and stroke in samples of women with OSA (Campos-Rodriguez et al. 2012, 2014). Few studies have focused on women with OSA and only a handful of those examine CPAP adherence (Ye et al. 2009). Three studies have demonstrated that women have poorer adherence compared to men (Joo and Herdegen 2007; Pelletier-Fleury et al. 2001; Woehrle et al. 2011). In an urban public hospital, for example, women were 1.72 times more likely to be non-adherent to CPAP even when adjusting for age and race (Joo and Herdegen 2007). However, one study reported higher adherence in women (Sin et al. 2002) and two studies have reported no relationship between gender and adherence (Gagnadoux et al. 2011; McArdle et al. 1999).

* Correspondence: kgbaron@rush.edu
[1]Department of Behavioral Sciences, Rush University Medical Center, 1653 W. Congress Parkway, Chicago, IL 60612-3833, USA
Full list of author information is available at the end of the article

Given that so few studies have explored effects of gender in adherence rates, even fewer studies have explored the role of gender in CPAP adherence. Relationship quality is a factor known to affect adherence to many different medical treatments, such as medication and dialysis adherence (DiMatteo 2004; Gove et al. 1990; Lewis and Butterfield 2007). However few studies have evaluated the role of social support and relationship quality in CPAP and none have been conducted among female patients. Despite compelling evidence linking relationships and social support to health (Uchino 2006; House et al. 1988; Walen and Lachman 2000), there is limited understanding of the role of relationships in CPAP treatment, especially among women. One study conducted in men and women found that having a bed partner was associated with greater CPAP adherence (Lewis et al. 2004). A recent study found that being married was associated with higher adherence in a sample of both women and men (Gagnadoux et al. 2011). However, these studies did not take into account relationship quality or they ways in which spouses were involved. We previously reported in a study of male patients with OSA, higher relationship conflict was associated with poorer adherence and collaborative spousal involvement by the spouse was associated with greater CPAP adherence (Baron et al. 2011; Baron KG 2008). Given that women are more physically and emotionally reactive to relationship conflict (Kiecolt-Glaser and Newton 2001) and both marital status and relationship quality have been associated with women's sleep quality (Gallo et al. 2003).

Therefore, the purpose of this study was to evaluate the role of relationship status and relationship quality in CPAP adherence among women with newly diagnosed OSA. We predicted that being married or partnered, as well as having higher relationship quality and higher general levels of social support would be associated with higher adherence. Our battery included known predictors of CPAP adherence (self-efficacy for CPAP), pre-sleep arousal, which has been related to relationship quality, and a measure of insomnia symptoms, which are more common among women. We also assessed partner support through open-ended questions with married or partnered participants to explore the helpful and unhelpful ways their partners were involved in CPAP treatment. Finally, we evaluated change in relationship quality among married/partnered participants over the first 3 months of starting CPAP.

Methods

Participants

This study was approved by the Northwestern University Institutional Review Board and all participants completed written informed consent. Women who were undergoing polysomnography due to suspected OSA were recruited for the study from the Northwestern Medical Center Sleep Disorders Laboratory. Patients were recruited at the diagnostic, split night or titration study and completed questionnaires before CPAP was set up at home. Inclusion criteria included: female gender and CPAP naïve. Exclusionary criteria included: diagnosis of chronic obstructive pulmonary disease, neurological disorders, use of supplemental oxygen, plan to undergo surgery in the next 3 months, use of other treatments for OSA (including bariatric surgery, upper airway surgery, or oral appliance), dementia, inability to read or write in English and unstable psychiatric disorders.

Procedure

Female participants undergoing diagnostic, split night, or CPAP titration studies aged 18–70 were recruited using flyers and phone calls. Participants who were interested in the study were invited to complete questionnaires in a one hour visit to the sleep research laboratory. Pre-treatment questionnaires were scheduled after an OSA diagnosis was confirmed via polysomnography but before CPAP was set up in their home. All PSG were conducted in the laboratory (no home PSG studies) and were scored using standard AASM criteria. Patients participated in the standard clinic protocol for titration and CPAP initiation. All participants had mask fittings and CPAP education with a sleep technician at the titration or split night study. Patients were assigned to durable medical equipment (DME) companies for CPAP set-up per the clinic's usual practices. The DME company representative again reviewed the use and care of the equipment as well as the importance of compliance. CPAP machine settings were determined by the ordering physician who was blinded to study enrollment status of each patient. Adherence was determined objectively, based on reports generated by querying the internal recording system that accompanies the CPAP devices. The data was obtained by electronic download at 10–12 weeks after treatment initiation.

Measures

Demographics: Age, gender, race, education, and income were assessed by self-report.

Depressive Symptoms: Depressive symptoms were assessed using the Center for Epidemiologic Studies Depression Scale, (CES-D; Radloff 1977). This 20-item measure is a commonly used and well-validated measure of depressive symptoms in which scores ≥ 16 are associated with clinically elevated depressive symptoms in middle-aged and older adults.

Subjective Sleepiness: The Epworth Sleepiness Scale (ESS) was used to assess self-reported subjective sleepiness at baseline (Johns 1991). In this questionnaire, participants rate the likelihood they would fall asleep in 8 different situations, such as being a passenger in a car. Scores range from 0–24 and scores >10 have been associated with excessive sleepiness (Johns 1991).

Relationship Quality: Relationship quality was measured by the Quality of Relationship Inventory (QRI) support and conflict subscales at baseline and follow-up (Pierce et al. 1991). The support subscale contained items related to emotional support in the marriage, such as "To what extent could you count on your spouse for help with a problem?" and "To what extent could you count on this person to listen to you when you are very angry at someone else?" The conflict subscale contained items related to the frequency and extent of marital conflict, such as, "How angry does your spouse make you feel?" and "How often do you have to work hard to avoid conflict with your spouse?" Subscales were scored as the average of the 7 support items and average of the 12 conflict items. Reported test-retest reliability correlations ranged from 0.48 to 0.79 (Pierce et al. 1997; Verhofstadt et al. 2006). This questionnaire in our sample demonstrated adequate internal consistency (Cronbach's alpha = 0.80 for the support subscale and 0.74 for the conflict subscale).

Social Support: Social support was measured using the Enhancing Recovery in Coronary Heart Disease Patients social support index (ESSI) (Mitchell et al. 2003). This 8 item questionnaire measures structural, instrumental, and emotional social support. Scores range from 8 to 34, with higher scores indicating greater social support. This measure had good internal consistency in our sample (Cronbach's alpha = 0.86). Although it was developed in cardiac patients, this measure has been used in other medical populations including cancer and HIV (Penedo et al. 2012; Mergenova et al. 2016).

Sleep Apnea Self-Efficacy: Self efficacy related to sleep apnea was measured by the Self Efficacy Measure for Sleep Apnea. This 26-item measure contains 3 subscales: risk perception of OSA (e.g., "chances of falling asleep driving"), outcome expectancies of CPAP (e.g., "job performance will improve"), and treatment self-efficacy (e.g., "I would use CPAP if it made my nose stuffy"). Patients completed this measure at baseline. In validation studies of OSA patients, this scale demonstrated good psychometric properties. Cronbach's alpha was reported as 0.90 for the total scale, 0.85–0.89 for the 3 subscales and reported test-retest reliabilities ranged from 0.68–0.77 (Weaver et al. 2003). In our sample, Cronbach's alpha was between 0.70 and 0.89.

Perceived important of OSA treatment: We assessed perceived importance for OSA treatment in one item: "How important is it to you that you are treated for OSA". Item responses range from 0 (not at all) to 5 (very motivated).

Pre-sleep Arousal was measured by the Pre-sleep arousal scale (Nicassio et al. 1985). This 16 item scale has two subscales "cognitive" and "somatic". Items for the cognitive arousal subscale include the feeling of having an active mind before sleep, anxious or depressed thoughts. The somatic pre-sleep arousal subscale includes physical feelings of anxiety and restlessness before sleep, such as a racing heart. Items are scored from 1 (not at all) to 4 (extremely). Scores range from 8–40. This scale has demonstrated adequate reliability and internal validity (Nicassio et al. 1985; Jansson-Frojmark and Norell-Clarke 2012).

Insomnia Symptoms were measured by the Insomnia Severity Index (ISI). This 5 item scale assesses symptoms of insomnia as well as satisfaction with quality of sleep and concern about the impact of sleep on quality of life (Morin 1993). Chronbach's alpha demonstrated adequate internal consistency (0.74) and this measure has been demonstrated to have adequate concurrent validity and sensitivity to improvements in sleep (Bastien et al. 2001).

Apnea severity was determined by the apnea severity index (apnea or hypopnea events per hour) on the diagnostic polysomnography or the diagnostic portion of the split night polysomnogram.

Data analysis

Data were analyzed using SPSS Version 20. Participant characteristics were described using means, standard deviations, and percentages. Associations between relationship status, quality, and CPAP adherence were evaluated using Pearson correlations and linear regression. All tests were 2-tailed and statistical significance was defined as $p < 0.05$.

Results

Sample characteristics

Sample characteristics are listed in Table 1. During the recruitment period, 384 women underwent polysomnography and study staff identified 129 women who met eligibility criteria for the study. Reasons for non-participation were not provided by most of the potential participants but those who did provide reasons reported: they were not starting CPAP ($n = 6$), they did not have time to participate ($n = 3$) and they already started CPAP at home ($n = 4$). Of the eligible women who were provided flyers and phone calls, 33 women volunteered for the study. Nine women dropped out without providing a reason before completing informed consent. A total of 24 women provided informed consent and completed baseline questionnaires for the study. There were no differences in age, BMI, insurance type, AHI between participants and non-participants. After enrollment, three participants declined CPAP treatment and data from one participant was removed from the analyses due to

Table 1 Participant Characteristics

N = 20	M (SD) or N (%)
Age	50 (10) years
Race/Ethnicity	
Black	6 (30%)
White	9 (45%)
Latina	4 (20%)
Other/more than one race	1 (5%)
Marital Status	
Married	7 (35%)
Living with a romantic partner	6 (30%)
Never married, living alone	5 (25%)
Other (separated, widowed)	2 (10%)
Apnea Hypopnea Index	20.5 (16.3) events/h
Epworth Sleepiness Scale	11.7 (5.0)
Body Mass Index	37.8 (10.8) kg/m^2
CPAP Adherence[a]	
Average use per night	3.7 (2.8) hours
Percentage with adherence ≥4 h, 70% of nights	6 of 16 (38%)

[a]CPAP adherence data were missing for 4 participants (unable to contact 3 participants, equipment failure in 1 participant)

prior CPAP use. Therefore, the resulting sample was 20 participants (with adherence data available for 16 of the 20 participants). Missing adherence data were due to inability to contact participant for download ($n = 3$) and one participant did not have a chip to record adherence. The sample was 45% ($n = 6$) non-Hispanic white. Over half of participants were married or living with a romantic partner ($n = 13$, 65%). There was a range of apnea severity but the average AHI was in the moderate range. Average subjective sleepiness was >10 and BMI was in the obese range. Average adherence was 3.7 h (SD = 2.8) and the range was 0.1 h to 7.8 h. Of the 16 participants with adherence data, 6 (38%) were considered adherent (CPAP ≥4 h on ≥ 70% of nights).

Associations with CPAP Adherence

Comparisons of characteristics of married/partnered vs. unmarried partnered participants are listed in Table 2. There was a trend for higher average nightly CPAP use among married/partnered participants compared to unmarried/unpartnered participants (4.6 h versus 2.1 h, $p < 0.08$). Using the Medicare adherence criteria of ≥4 h of use on 70% of nights, 40% of married or partnered participant and 100% of the unpartnered patients were nonadherent ($p < .05$). Unmarried/unpartnered participants reported greater CPAP self-efficacy ($p < .05$) but there were no other differences demographic, disease related, or psychosocial characteristics between married/partnered and unpartnered participants.

Table 2 Comparison of key variables for married/partnered versus unmarried/unpartnered participants

	Married or partnered women (N = 13) M (SD) or N (%)	Unmarried and unpartnered women (N = 7) M (SD) or N (%)
Age	50.8 (9.1)	48.7 (12.0)
Race		
White	7 (53)	2 (29)
Black	3 (23)	3 (43)
Hispanic/Latina	5 (15)	2 (29)
Other/More than 1 race	1 (8)	0 (0)
Apnea Hypopnea Index	16.2 (12.4)	28.4 (20.5)
Epworth Sleepiness Scale	11.7 (4.7)	11.7 (5.9)
Body Mass Index	35.0 (8.4)	42.7 (13.4)
Split night study	4 (57)	3 (23)
CPAP Adherence*		
Average use per night	4.6 (2.8)	2.1 (1.7)[†]
Adherence ≥4 h, 70% of nights	6 (60)	0 (0)*
Center for Epidemiologic Depression Scale (CES-D)	12.9 (6.6)	13.9 (4.3)
CPAP Self-Efficacy	27.4 (6.7)	34.6 (4.6)*
Perceived importance of treating OSA (1, not important-5, very important)	4.7 (0.9)	4.9 (0.4)
Insomnia Severity Index	15.5 (7.9)	20.4 (6.6)
Presleep Arousal Scale		
Cognitive	20.9 (10.2)	23.9 (9.4)
Somatic	16.5 (9.5)	19.5 (9.4)

*$p < .05$, [†]$p < .08$

Correlations between adherence, relationship quality, social support, self-efficacy, and pre-sleep arousal are listed in Table 3. Among married or partnered patients, relationship conflict was negatively associated with adherence ($r = -0.60$, $p < 0.05$, Fig. 1). Ratings of support in the relationship were unassociated with adherence. Greater perceived social support was positively associated with adherence among all participants ($r = 0.65$, $p < 0.05$, Fig. 2). In addition, both cognitive and somatic pre-sleep arousal were associated with poorer CPAP adherence ($r = -0.53$, $p < 0.05$, $r = -0.59$, $p < 0.05$,) and higher relationship conflict ($r = 0.66$, $p < 0.05$, $r = 0.53$, $p < 0.05$). Depressive symptoms were correlated with relationship conflict ($r = 0.58$, $p < 0.05$), social support ($r = -0.48$, $p < 0.05$), cognitive ($r = 0.60$, $p < 0.05$) and somatic pre-sleep arousal ($r = 0.63$, $p < 0.05$). Relationship support, depressive symptoms, insomnia symptoms, CPAP self- efficacy were not associated with CPAP adherence.

Table 3 Correlations between CPAP use, relationship quality and social support

	1.	2.	3.	4.	5.	6.	7.	8.	9.
1. CPAP Use	–	−.60*	.37	.65*	.30	.01	.01	−.53*	−.59*
2. Relationship conflict		–	−.25	−.47	−.33	−.01	.31	.66**	.53*
3. Relationship support			–	.09	−.02	−.13	−.34	−.41	−.46
4. Social support				–	−.14	.09	−.06	−.36	−.39
5. OSA risk					–	.28	−.23	−.13	−.06
6. CPAP expectations						–	.04	.23	.48
7. OSA self-efficacy							–	.21	.11
8. Cognitive pre-sleep arousal								–	.74
9. Physiological pre-sleep arousal									–

*$p < .05$, **$p < .01$

Qualitative responses about "helpful" and "unhelpful" spousal behaviors

One week after CPAP initiation, 7 participants provided responses to open ended questions about helpful and unhelpful ways their spouse or partner was involved in CPAP. The majority (6 of 7) of participants reported support and encouragement from their spouse/partner to use CPAP. Helpful types of involvement reported by participants included: asking about CPAP, problem solving, support, providing encouragement, using humor, helping the participant "realize the benefits" of CPAP, encouraging use to "better my health", helping the participant to feel less self-conscious about it, and checking to see if she is snoring at night. One participant reported her spouse was not involved in CPAP use and two participants report unhelpful types of involvement. Unhelpful types of involvement listed included: repeatedly asking if "it's working" and making fun of the participant (referring to it as a "Darth Vader" mask).

Change in relationship quality

Participants did not demonstrate changes in overall relationship quality, relationship support or conflict (Table 4).

Discussion

Results of this study demonstrate that both relationship status and relationship quality strongly predict women's CPAP adherence. We found a very strong link between relationship status (being married or living with a partner) and adherence, in that 40% of married/partnered participants were adherent according to the criteria set by Medicare whereas none of the unpartnered participants were adherent (≥4 h of CPAP use on 70% of nights). Furthermore, there was a strong correlation between ratings of conflict in the relationship (for married/partnered patients) as well as general levels of social support and CPAP adherence. Therefore, even in the case of unpartnered participants, higher levels of support from other sources was associated with better adherence.

In an attempt to explain the effects of relationship status on CPAP, we explored differences in demographic, physical, and psychological variables. CPAP self-efficacy was actually *higher* among unmarried/unpartnered participants. However, we did find associations between relationship quality and social support variables with depression and pre-sleep arousal. Although our sample size is too small to formally explore a mediation pathway, this may be one way relationship conflict interferes with CPAP adherence among women. Both cognitive

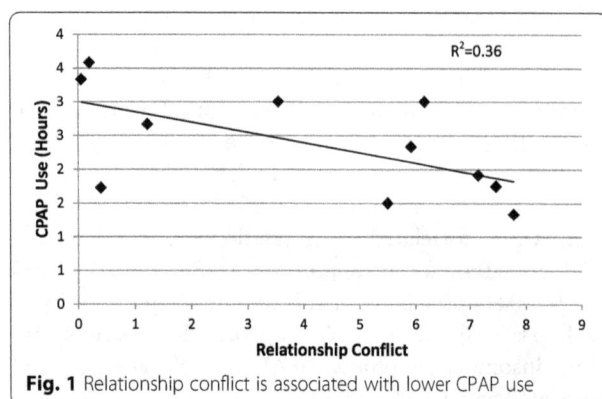
Fig. 1 Relationship conflict is associated with lower CPAP use

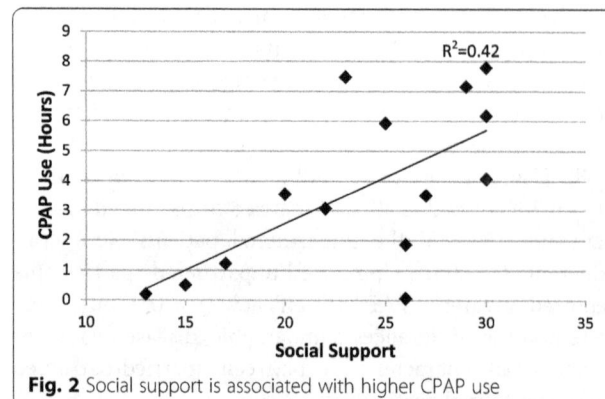
Fig. 2 Social support is associated with higher CPAP use

Table 4 Relationship quality measures at baseline and 3 month follow-up for married/partnered participants (N = 13)

	Baseline	3 Month follow-up
Relationship quality total score	60.3 (11.3)	59.7 (10.4)
Relationship support	3.5 (0.5)	3.4 (0.8)
Relationship conflict	2.0 (0.7)	2.1 (0.7)

P values are all non-significant

(e.g., active thoughts and worry) as well as somatic pre-sleep arousal (e.g., physical tension) were associated with poorer CPAP use. Poor marital quality may increase pre-sleep arousal, which may in turn negatively impact CPAP adherence. Because patients wear CPAP at bedtime, marital stress and lack of support may hinder women's motivation to use CPAP because they may be more preoccupied with other factors, such as managing relationship stress. It is also possible the feeling "wound up" cognitively or physiologically may interfere with the ability to tolerate CPAP in women. Previous studies have found that marital happiness is associated with better sleep quality in women, above and beyond depression (Troxel et al. 2007).

We also queried married/partnered participants about what they found to be helpful and unhelpful behaviors from their spouse or partner one week after starting CPAP. The majority reported that support and encouragement from their partner was an important factor in their CPAP adherence. In addition, patients reported their partners were involved in many different ways, including helping them feel less self-conscious and helping solve problems and check that they are wearing the CPAP properly (e.g., monitoring for snoring). All but one of the patients who responded to the open ended questions could generate examples of helpful spousal involvement. We received fewer answers on the item about unhelpful spousal involvement. It is possible that the women who did not provide responses to this question either did not experience unhelpful spousal involvement or were reluctant to report it. Our previous study of spousal involvement in men utilized a written survey and found that 57% of male patients reported their spouse attempted to scare them into using CPAP, which is typically viewed as a negative tactic (Baron et al. 2011).

Results of our study add to a broader context of the role of relationships in OSA and CPAP use as well as the role of gender in OSA treatment. The symptoms of OSA, including snoring, daytime sleepiness, and depressed mood, affect both patient and partner quality of life (Doherty et al. 2003; Reishtein et al. 2006; Cartwright 2008; Cartwright and Knight 1987; Baron et al. 2009). In male participants, relationship conflict was associated with poorer adherence and collaborative involvement from the spouse was associated with higher adherence (Baron et al. 2009, 2011). Results of this study cannot address gender differences per se; but, we can compare magnitude of correlations between studies. In our previously published study in men, the correlation between relationship conflict and adherence was -0.31 whereas in this current study in women, it is twice as strong (−0.61). Although relationship conflict may be deleterious for CPAP adherence in both men and women, it may have a greater negative impact on women's CPAP use. In addition, we reported a decrease in perceived relationship conflict among men who started CPAP, whereas in this study we did not observe a change in relationship measures among women.

Our results are limited by a small sample size and recruitment from a single center. It is possible we were unable to observe associations with adherence among some of the typical predictors (e.g., self-efficacy) due to low statistical power from samples size and/or lack of variability in the measures. This study was also unable to identify the frequency of symptoms such as claustrophobia, which may have affected adherence. Strengths of this study are in-depth assessment of spousal involvement and diversity of the sample in terms of age, race/ethnicity, and social structure. Future studies conducted in larger samples may elucidate the pathways between these interrelated variables, and inform the design of interventions that take into account relationship factors. Our results suggest that increasing helpful spousal involvement may be helpful for both men and women. We previously reported that collaborative involvement and support were associated with higher adherence (Baron et al. 2011, 2012). To date only one intervention has specifically involved spouses (Hoy et al. 1999) and found that increasing helpful involvement was one part of a successful intervention.

Conclusions

These data suggest that the context of a supportive relationship is highly important to women's CPAP use. Understanding of gender and social processes among women with OSA expands our knowledge and ability to modify risk factors for poor CPAP adherence in this population.

Acknowledgements

We gratefully acknowledge the contributions of Erin McGorry, Brittany Fondel and Nirmit Desai for their assistance with data collection and data entry.

Funding

This work was supported by the National Institutes of Health grants 1K23HL109110-01 and 5 K12 HD055884. The funding agencies were not involved in the design, data collection, analysis or interpretation of the manuscript.

Authors' contributions

KGB contributed to study design, data collection, data analysis and was the main author involved in writing the manuscript. HEG contributed to data collection and writing the manuscript. LFW and PCZ contributed to study design, interpretation of results and writing the manuscript. All authors read and approved the final manuscript.

Competing interests

The authors declare that they have no competing interests.

Author details

[1]Department of Behavioral Sciences, Rush University Medical Center, 1653 W. Congress Parkway, Chicago, IL 60612-3833, USA. [2]Department of Psychiatry, University of Pittsburgh, Pittsburgh, USA. [3]Center for Circadian and Sleep Medicine, Feinberg School of Medicine, Northwestern University, Chicago, USA.

References

Baron KG. Effects of relationship quality and social control on adherence to CPAP in patients with obstructive sleep apnea. Dissertation Abstracts International: Section B: The Sciences and Engineering. 2008. p. 68.

Baron KG, Smith TW, Czajkowski LA, Gunn HE, Jones CR. Relationship quality and CPAP adherence in patients with obstructive sleep apnea. Behav Sleep Med. 2009;7:22–36.

Baron KG, Smith TW, Berg CA, Czajkowski LA, Gunn H, Jones CR. Spousal involvement in CPAP adherence among patients with obstructive sleep apnea. Sleep Breath. 2011;15:525–34.

Baron KG, Gunn HE, Czajkowski LA, Smith TW, Jones CR. Spousal involvement in CPAP: does pressure help? Clin Sleep Med. 2012;8:147–53.

Bastien CH, Vallieres A, Morin CM. Validation of the insomnia severity index as an outcome measure for insomnia research. Sleep Med. 2001;2:297–307.

Campos-Rodriguez F, Martinez-Garcia MA, de la Cruz-Moron I, Almeida-Gonzalez C, Catalan-Serra P, Montserrat JM. Cardiovascular mortality in women with obstructive sleep apnea with or without continuous positive airway pressure treatment: a cohort study. Ann Intern Med. 2012;156:115–22.

Campos-Rodriguez F, Martinez-Garcia MA, Reyes-Nunez N, Caballero-Martinez I, Catalan-Serra P, Almeida-Gonzalez CV. Role of sleep apnea and continuous positive airway pressure therapy in the incidence of stroke or coronary heart disease in women. Am J Respir Crit Care Med. 2014;189:1544–50.

Cartwright RD. Sleeping together: a pilot study of the effects of shared sleeping on adherence to CPAP treatment in obstructive sleep apnea. J Clin Sleep Med. 2008;4:123–7.

Cartwright RD, Knight S. Silent partners: the wives of sleep apneic patients. Sleep. 1987;10:244–8.

DiMatteo MR. Social support and patient adherence to medical treatment: a meta-analysis. Health Psychol. 2004;23:207–18.

Doherty LS, Kiely JL, Lawless G, McNicholas WT. Impact of nasal continuous positive airway pressure therapy on the quality of life of bed partners of patients with obstructive sleep apnea syndrome. Chest. 2003;124:2209–14.

Doherty LS, Kiely JL, Swan V, McNicholas WT. Long-term effects of nasal continuous positive airway pressure therapy on cardiovascular outcomes in sleep apnea syndrome. Chest. 2005;127:2076–84.

Engleman HM, Martin SE, Deary IJ, Douglas NJ. Effect of continuous positive airway pressure treatment on daytime function in sleep apnoea/hypopnoea syndrome. Lancet. 1994;343:572–5.

Gagnadoux F, Le Vaillant M, Goupil F, Pigeanne T, Chollet S, Masson P, Humeau MP, Bizieux-Thaminy A, Meslier N. Influence of marital status and employment status on long-term adherence with continuous positive airway pressure in sleep apnea patients. PLoS ONE. 2011;6:e22503.

Gallo LC, Troxel WM, Matthews KA, Kuller LH. Marital status and quality in middle-aged women: Associations with levels and trajectories of cardiovascular risk factors. Health Psychol. 2003;22:453–63.

Gove WR, Style CB, Hughes M. The effect of marriage on the well-being of adults: a theoretical analysis. J Fam Issues. 1990;11:4–35.

House JS, Landis KR, Umberson D. Social relationships and health. Science. 1988; 241:540–5.

Hoy CJ, Vennelle M, Kingshott RN, Engleman HM, Douglas NJ. Can intensive support improve continuous positive airway pressure use in patients with the sleep apnea/hypopnea syndrome? Am J Respir Crit Care Med. 1999;159: 1096–100.

Jansson-Frojmark M, Norell-Clarke A. Psychometric properties of the pre-sleep arousal scale in a large community sample. J Psychosom Res. 2012;72:103–10.

Johns MW. A new method for measuring daytime sleepiness: the Epworth sleepiness scale. Sleep. 1991;14:540–5.

Joo MJ, Herdegen JJ. Sleep apnea in an urban public hospital: assessment of severity and treatment adherence. J Clin Sleep Med. 2007;3:285–8.

Kiecolt-Glaser JK, Newton TL. Marriage and health: his and hers. Psychol Bull. 2001;127:472–503.

Lewis MA, Butterfield RM. Social control in marital relationships: effect of one's partner on health behaviors. J Appl Soc Psychol. 2007;37:298–319.

Lewis KE, Seale L, Bartle IE, Watkins AJ, Ebden P. Early predictors of CPAP use for the treatment of obstructive sleep apnea. Sleep. 2004;27:134–8.

Marin JM, Carrizo SJ, Vicente E, Agusti AG. Long-term cardiovascular outcomes in men with obstructive sleep apnoea-hypopnoea with or without treatment with continuous positive airway pressure: an observational study. Lancet. 2005;365:1046–53.

Marin JM, Agusti A, Villar I, Forner M, Nieto D, Carrizo SJ, Barbe F, Vicente E, Wei Y, Nieto FJ, Jelic S. Association between treated and untreated obstructive sleep apnea and risk of hypertension. JAMA. 2012;307:2169–76.

McArdle N, Devereux G, Heidarnejad H, Engleman HM, Mackay TW, Douglas NJ. Long-term use of CPAP therapy for sleep apnea/hypopnea syndrome. Am J Respir Crit Care Med. 1999;159:1108–14.

Mergenova G, Shaw SA, Terlikbayeva A, Gilbert L, Gensburg L, Primbetova S, El-Bassel N. social support and HIV risks among migrant and non-migrant market workers in Almaty, Kazakhstan. J Immigr Minor Health. 2016.

Mitchell PH, Powell L, Blumenthal J, Norten J, Ironson G, Pitula CR, Froelicher ES, Czajkowski S, Youngblood M, Huber M, Berkman LF. A short social support measure for patients recovering from myocardial infarction: the ENRICHD social support inventory. J Cardiopulm Rehabil. 2003;23:398–403.

Morin CM. Insomnia: psychological assessment and management. New York: Guilford Press; 1993.

Nicassio PM, Mendlowitz DR, Fussell JJ, Petras L. The phenomenology of the pre-sleep state: the development of the pre-sleep arousal scale. Behav Res Ther. 1985;23:263–71.

Pelletier-Fleury N, Rakotonanahary D, Fleury B. The age and other factors in the evaluation of compliance with nasal continuous positive airway pressure for obstructive sleep apnea syndrome. A Cox's proportional hazard analysis. Sleep Med. 2001;2:225–32.

Penedo FJ, Traeger L, Benedict C, Thomas G, Dahn JR, Krause MH, Goodwin WJ. Perceived social support as a predictor of disease-specific quality of life in head-and-neck cancer patients. J Support Oncol. 2012;10:119–23.

Pierce GR, Sarason IG, Sarason BR. General and relationship-based perceptions of social support: are two constructs better than one? J Pers Soc Psychol. 1991; 61:1028–39.

Pierce GR, Sarason IG, Sarason BR, Solky-Butzel JA, Nagel LC. Assessing the quality of personal relationships. J Soc Pers Relat. 1997;14:339–56.

Radloff LS. The CES-D scale: a self-report depression scale for research in the general population. Appl Psychol Meas. 1977;1:385–401.

Redline S, Sotres-Alvarez D, Loredo J, Hall M, Patel SR, Ramos A, Shah N, Ries A, Arens R, Barnhart J, et al. Sleep-disordered breathing in hispanic/latino individuals of diverse backgrounds. The hispanic community health study/study of Latinos. Am J Respir Crit Care Med. 2014;189:335–44.

Reishtein JL, Pack AI, Maislin G, Dinges DF, Bloxham TJ, George CF, Greenberg H, Kader GA, Mahowald MW, Younger JB, Weaver TE. Sleepiness and relationships in obstructive sleep apnea. Issues Ment Health Nurs. 2006;27:319–30.

Sin DD, Mayers I, Man GC, Pawluk L. Long-term compliance rates to continuous positive airway pressure in obstructive sleep apnea: a population-based study. Chest. 2002;121:430–5.

Troxel WM, Robles TF, Hall M, Buysse DJ. Marital quality and the marital bed: examining the covariation between relationship quality and sleep. Sleep Med Rev. 2007;11:389–404.

Uchino BN. Social support and health: a review of physiological processes potentially underlying links to disease outcomes. J Behav Med. 2006;29:377–87.

Verhofstadt LL, Buysse A, Rosseel Y, Peene OJ. Confirming the three-factor structure of the quality of relationships inventory within couples. Psychol Assess. 2006;18:15–21.

Walen HR, Lachman ME. Social support and strain from partner, family, and friends: costs and benefits for men and women in adulthood. J Soc Pers Relat. 2000;17(1):5–30.

Weaver TE, Grunstein RR. Adherence to continuous positive airway pressure therapy: the challenge to effective treatment. Proc Am Thorac Soc. 2008;5: 173–8.

Weaver TE, Maislin G, Dinges DF, Younger J, Cantor C, McCloskey S, Pack AI. Self-efficacy in sleep apnea: instrument development and patient perceptions of obstructive sleep apnea risk, treatment benefit, and volition to use continuous positive airway pressure. Sleep. 2003;26:727–32.

Woehrle H, Graml A, Weinreich G. Age- and gender-dependent adherence with continuous positive airway pressure therapy. Sleep Med. 2011;12:1034–6.

Ye LC, Pien GW, Weaver TE. Gender differences in the clinical manifestation of obstructive sleep apnea. Sleep Med. 2009;10:1075–84.

5

Practical considerations for effective oral appliance use in the treatment of obstructive sleep apnea

Hiroko Tsuda[1,2*], Naohisa Wada[2] and Shin-ichi Ando[1]

Abstract

Oral appliance (OA) therapy is a promising alternative to continuous positive airway pressure (CPAP) for patients with obstructive sleep apnea (OSA). By holding the mandible in a forward position, an OA keeps the airway open and prevents collapse. The recently revised practice parameters of the American Academy of Sleep Medicine extend the indications for OA therapy, recommending that "sleep physicians consider prescription of an OA for adult patients with OSA who are intolerant of CPAP therapy or prefer alternative therapy." This manuscript reviews the practical considerations for effective OA therapy with a discussion of three factors: patient eligibility for OA therapy, device features, and requirements for OA providers. Identification of patients who are eligible for OA therapy is a key factor because the overall success rate of OA therapy is lower than that of CPAP. Conventional predictive variables have low sensitivity and specificity; however, new tools such as drug-induced sleep endoscopy and single-night polysomnographic OA titration have been developed. Other factors to consider when determining the indications for OA include the patient's oral health, evidence of inadequate treatment for older populations, and the risk of long-term dentofacial side effects. For the second factor, customization of OA features is a key component of treatment success, and no single OA design most effectively improves every situation. Although adjustment of the mandibular position is much more important than device selection, the adjustment procedure has not been standardized. Additionally, a pitfall that tends to be forgotten is the relationship between application of the mandibular position and device selection. Promising new technology has become commercially available in the clinical setting to provide objective adherence monitoring. Finally, the third factor is the availability of enough qualified dentists because sleep medicine is a relatively new and highly multidisciplinary field. Because OSA treatments such as CPAP and OA therapy are generally considered for continuous use, treatments should be carefully planned with attention to multiple aspects. Additionally, because OA therapy requires the cooperation of professionals with different areas of expertise, such as dentists and physicians with various specialties, everyone involved in OA therapy must understand it well.

Keywords: Obstructive sleep apnea, Oral appliance, Mandibular advancement

Background

Obstructive sleep apnea (OSA) is a major sleep disorder. Because of repeated complete or partial collapse of the upper airway during sleep, patients develop sleep fragmentation and oxygen desaturation. OSA is estimated to occur in approximately 24% of middle-aged men and 9% of women (Young et al. 1993).

Typical nocturnal signs and symptoms of OSA are snoring, observed apnea, waking with a sensation of choking or gasping, unexplained tachycardia, restless sleep, sweating during sleep, nocturia, bruxism, nocturnal gastroesophageal reflux, insomnia, disrupted sleep, sleep walking, and sleep terrors. Daytime symptoms of OSA include excessive daytime sleepiness, afternoon drowsiness, forgetfulness, impaired concentration and attention, personality changes, and morning headache (Cao et al. 2011). As a result, OSA increases the risk of motor vehicle accidents, cardiovascular morbidity, and

* Correspondence: htsuda@dent.kyushu-u.ac.jp
[1]Sleep Apnea Center, Kyushu University Hospital, Kyushu University, 3-1-1 Maidashi Higashiku, Fukuoka 812-8582, Japan
[2]Department of General Dentistry, Kyushu University Hospital, Kyushu University, 3-1-1 Maidashi Higashiku, Fukuoka 812-8582, Japan

all-cause mortality (Marshall et al. 2008; Young et al. 2002). Therefore, OSA requires effective, appropriate treatment to preserve overall health.

Continuous positive airway pressure (CPAP), which opens and splints the upper airway with controlled compressed air, is considered the gold standard treatment for OSA. Although CPAP is highly effective in decreasing respiratory events, low acceptance and adherence are weaknesses of this therapy (Sutherland et al. 2014a and b).

Many treatment options have been developed for patients who are not eligible for CPAP therapy, including oral appliance (OA) therapy, surgery, weight loss, exercise, nasal expiratory positive airway pressure therapy, oral pressure therapy, hypoglossal nerve stimulation, and pharmacologic treatment (Sutherland et al. 2015).

OA therapy, which holds the mandible in a forward position, works by keeping the airway open and preventing collapse. Previous imaging studies have revealed that mandibular advancement with the use of an OA enlarges the upper airway space, particularly in the lateral dimension of the velopharyngeal area (Chan et al. 2010a). Most types of OAs hold the mandible forward; therefore, they are called mandibular advancement splints, mandibular advancement devices (MADs), or prosthetic mandibular advancement. Except for the discussion about tongue-retaining devices (TRDs), the OAs in this review refer to MADs.

Recent comparisons between CPAP and OA in overnight sleep studies have shown that both treatments improve sleep-disordered breathing (SDB) (Sutherland et al. 2014a). CPAP is generally more effective than OA therapy, with a higher percentage of patients experiencing complete control of OSA. However, this greater efficacy does not necessarily translate into better health outcomes in clinical practice. The inferiority of OA therapy in reducing apneic events may be counteracted by greater treatment adherence because of more frequent nightly use of OA therapy compared with CPAP (Sutherland et al. 2014a).

The previous practice parameters of the American Academy of Sleep Medicine suggested OA therapy as a first-line treatment in patients with mild to moderate OSA and for patients with more severe OSA who fail treatment attempts with CPAP therapy (Kushida et al. 2006). In other words, first-line use of OA therapy was limited to mild to moderate OSA. The recently revised practice parameters have extended the indications for OA use, recommending that "sleep physicians consider prescription of an OA, rather than no treatment, for adult patients with OSA who are intolerant of CPAP therapy or prefer alternative therapy" (Ramar et al. 2015).

OA therapy differs from other treatment options. Patients cannot be given optimal care without crucial division of roles and collaboration between dentists and physicians with expertise in sleep medicine. In addition, OAs are generally custom-made and require delicate adjustment based on many factors, such as patients' symptoms of OSA and oral condition. Both proper device selection and skill regarding how to adjust these devices are needed for effective treatment. This review summarizes three important components of practical, effective OA therapy: (1) eligibility of patients for OA therapy, (2) device features, and (3) requirements for OA providers.

Patient eligibility for OA therapy
Predictors of treatment success
Determining which patients are eligible for OA therapy is one key factor of successful treatment because the total success rate of OA therapy is lower than that of CPAP, and the treatment process generally requires more time and higher cost. However, although many studies have explored the subject, no standardized parameters and procedures have been established to predict the treatment response before OA fabrication. Although female sex, young age, low body mass index, small neck circumference, low baseline apnea–hypopnea index (AHI), supine-dependent OSA, and obstruction area mainly in the oropharyngeal region during sleep are reportedly associated with treatment success, none of these parameters can predict the outcome of OA treatment, either singly or combination (Chan and Cistulli 2009).

Optimal CPAP pressure (Sutherland et al. 2014b; Tsuiki et al. 2010), videoendoscopy (Sasao et al. 2014), drug-induced sleep endoscopy (DISE) (Vroegop et al. 2013), and remotely controlled mandibular protrusion (RCMP) assessment, which involves titration of the mandibular position during a sleep study similar to CPAP titration (Remmers et al. 2013), have recently been introduced as new indicators or tools with which to predict treatment responders and are more effective than some conventional variables. These are favorable tools in the clinical setting under the appropriate circumstances, although some require extra cost and examination.

A few studies have explained why anatomical measurement can partially predict the treatment response, although OAs are considered to enlarge the upper airway space, particularly in the lateral dimension of the velopharyngeal area (Chan et al. 2010a). Vroegop et al. (Vroegop et al. 2014) reported variations in the obstruction area in 1249 patients who underwent DISE study. That study revealed that 68.2% of patients had multiple obstructive areas. Thus, the obstruction area is not the only narrow area in the airway; the airway dynamics dramatically change during sleep.

Another current area of research interest is the attempt to define pathophysiological phenotypes of OSA. In one study (Eckert et al. 2013), four key anatomical and non-anatomical mechanisms were measured in more than 50 individuals with OSA. The passive critical closing pressure, an indicator of collapsibility of the upper airway, was measured as an anatomic factor. Non-anatomic factors included the arousal threshold, loop gain, and upper airway dilator muscle responsiveness. The study results revealed that 81% of patients had a highly collapsible airway. With respect to non-anatomic factors, 36% of patients exhibited minimal genioglossus muscle responsiveness, 37% had a low arousal threshold, and 36% had high loop gain. One or more non-anatomic pathophysiologic traits were present in 69% of patients with OSA. In addition, non-anatomic features played an important role in 56% of patients with OSA. The findings of that study indicate that non-anatomic factors are important and may be even more important than anatomic features in some patients, although a prime predisposing factor in most patients with OSA is a highly collapsible airway. A study based on this concept recently showed that OA improved upper airway collapsibility without affecting muscle function, loop gain, or the arousal threshold (Edwards et al. 2016). This suggests that patients with better passive upper airway anatomy/collapsibility and low loop gain will obtain the greatest benefit from OA therapy (Edwards et al. 2016). Gray et al. (2016) reported that non-obese patients with OSA were more likely to have a low respiratory arousal threshold and that these patients were difficult to treat with CPAP. In another study, Nerfeldt and Friberg (2016) compared adherence to and treatment effects of OA therapy between patients with two types of OSA: those with mainly respiratory arousals ("arousers") and those with oxygen desaturations ("desaturaters"). The authors found that the 1-year adherence rate was significantly higher among arousers (85%) than desaturaters (55%), although the reduction in the AHI was similar in both groups. These results seem reasonable and can help to explain why we cannot predict the treatment response based on anatomic factors alone. Therefore, OSA phenotyping promises to be an important part of future treatment strategies.

Oral health of patients with OSA

A frequent barrier to OA therapy initiation is the patient's dental or oral health status. Petit et al. (2002) determined the contraindication rate in 100 consecutive patients referred for suspected OSA. In that survey, 34% of patients had a contraindication to OA therapy, and another 16% required close supervision and follow-up to avoid impairment of preexisting temporomandibular joint or dental problems. This is one of the inconvenient considerations involved in treatment decisions: many patients cannot use an OA or require time to complete dental treatment before the device can be prescribed. This is especially true in older patients, who have more dental concerns than do younger patients.

Several recent studies have suggested an association between tooth loss and OSA. One questionnaire-based survey found that 40.3% of edentulous participants had a high probability of having OSA Tsuda et al. (Epub). Another cross-sectional study of community-dwelling older adults revealed a significant association between denture use and an AHI of >15 (odds ratio, 6.29; confidence interval, 1.71–23.22; $P = 0.006$) (Endeshaw et al. 2004). A recent national health and nutrition examination study also revealed a relationship between the risk of OSA and certain oral health variables such as tooth loss, occlusal contacts, and denture use (Sanders et al. 2016). That study revealed that chance of developing a high risk for OSA increased by 2% for each additional lost tooth among adults aged 25 to 65 years.

Another dental problem in patients undergoing OA therapy is chronic periodontitis, which is the major cause of tooth loss (Phipps and Stevens 1995). Gunaratnam et al. (2009) reported a four-times-higher prevalence of periodontitis among patients with OSA than historical controls from a national survey. A recent large, community-based, cross-sectional study revealed that the adjusted odds of severe periodontitis was 40% higher in patients with subclinical SDB, 60% higher in those with mild SDB, and 50% higher in those with moderate/severe SDB compared with the non-apneic reference (Sanders et al. 2015). The novel association between mild SDB and periodontitis was most pronounced in young adults.

Dry mouth is a common symptom among patients with sleep apnea; it is also an important indicator of oral health (Oksenberg et al. 2006; Ruhle et al. 2011; Kreivi et al. 2010). Several reports have suggested that patients with dry mouth or salivary hypofunction have significantly more caries, fewer teeth, and more pain related to denture use than patients without these symptoms (Hopcraft and Tan 2010). Salivary output reaches its lowest levels during sleep, and the mouth breathing seen in patients with OSA can worsen dryness.

Sleep bruxism is a more concerning topic than OSA among dentists because it is one of the factors that causes prosthetic damage. An occlusal splint that covers only the maxillary dental arch is frequently prescribed for sleep bruxism without the need for a sleep study. Gagnon et al. (2004) estimated the effect of occlusal splints in patients with OSA. The authors reported that the AHI increased by >50% in 5 of 10 patients and that the sleeping time with snoring increased by 40% with use of the occlusal splint. This risk of aggravation associated with occlusal splints should be generally known because sleep bruxism is frequently seen in patients with OSA (Cao et al. 2011). Some authors have reported the treatment effects of OA therapy or CPAP for sleep bruxism (Landry-Schönbeck et al. 2009; Oksenberg and Arons 2002). However, some patients with OSA who exhibit sleep bruxism have reportedly broken their OA by the grinding events in the clinical setting. Because the relationship between OSA and sleep bruxism remains unclear, it may be a confounding factor in treatment decisions.

Healthy dentition is required for OA therapy, and patients with OSA are at high risk for developing the above-mentioned oral conditions. An alternative option for patients with inappropriate dentition is a TRD. A TRD features an extraoral flexible bulb and holds the tongue forward by suction. One type of TRD, the tongue-stabilizing device (TSD), is prefabricated. Because this device does not require the presence of teeth for retention, the patient's dental condition does not need to be considered. A TSD is suggested for patients who poorly tolerate an MAD; inadequate device retention is a potential issue that reduces the effectiveness of such devices in patients with normal dentition, although objective testing of MADs and TSDs have shown similar efficacy in terms of AHI reduction (Deane et al. 2009). A TSD is never the first-line device for OA therapy; however, these prefabricated devices have advantages for patients whose dentition is not appropriate for a MAD or for patients undergoing dental treatment.

Aging

The prevalence of OSA among older patients is higher than that among middle-aged patients (Young et al. 2002). Most treatment efficacy trials have examined individuals aged <65 years. There is insufficient evidence to support the efficacy of OA therapy in older people. This population has an increased prevalence of dental disease, including missing teeth and periodontitis. The current practice parameters suggest that a clear recommendation for MAS, MAD, or TSD as first-line treatment in patients with mild to moderate SDB cannot be made because of poor evidence. The practice parameters suggest that in the case of CPAP failure, second-line treatment with a MAS, MAD, or TSD is recommended in older patients with SDB after full assessment of the dental status (Netzer et al. 2016).

Nocturia is a frequently overlooked cause of poor sleep in older patients (Bliwise et al. 2009). Nocturia is relatively common in patients with OSA, and 28% of patients reportedly take four to seven nightly trips to the bathroom (Hajduk et al. 2003). OSA has been suggested

as an independent cause of frequent nocturia in older men (Guilleminault et al. 2004). In the clinical setting, some patients have reported that they discontinue CPAP use after removing the mask to go to the bathroom. Although nocturia may not be completely relieved with OSA therapy, OA therapy makes trips to the bathroom easier than does CPAP.

Side effects of OA therapy

Side effects of OA therapy are divided into two types: transient and permanent. During initiation of OA therapy, common adverse side effects include excessive salivation, mouth dryness, tooth pain, gum irritation, headaches, and temporomandibular joint discomfort. Although the reported frequencies of side effects vary greatly (Ferguson et al. 2006), symptoms are usually transient, lasting around 2 months.

When considering OA therapy as a treatment option, permanent side effects, mainly tooth movement, may be an important factor for some patients. Possible dental changes associated with OA therapy include decreased overbite (the vertical overlap of the lower teeth by the upper) and overjet (the horizontal overlap of the lower teeth by the upper), forward inclination of the lower incisors and backward inclination of the upper incisors, changes in anteroposterior occlusion, and a reduction in the number of occlusal contacts. A study of the long-term dental side effects during a decade of OA treatment revealed clinically significant and progressive changes in occlusion (Pliska et al. 2014). These side effects generally do not affect masticatory function, and many patients are unaware of any changes in their bite. Most patients concur that positive effects of OA treatment far outweigh any adverse effects related to dental changes (Marklund and Franklin 2007). However, tooth movement was found in 85.7% of patients in a 5-year analysis (Almeida et al. 2006). The possibility of occlusal change should be explained to patients, especially young patients, those with esthetic requirements, and those with narrow acceptance of occlusal change.

Tooth movement is a well-known side effect of OA therapy; however, dentofacial side effects of CPAP therapy are not yet well recognized. Cephalometric analysis of CPAP users during a 2-year period revealed significant craniofacial changes characterized by reduced maxillary and mandibular prominence and/or alteration of the relationship between the dental arches (Tsuda et al. 2010). Another research group reported a significant decrease in the number of occlusal contact points in the premolar region in patients using a CPAP device during a 2-year period (Doff et al. 2013). Patients treated with CPAP as well as those using an OA need thorough follow-up with a dental specialist experienced in the field of dental sleep medicine to ensure their oral health.

Eligibility for adjunctive therapy

OA therapy may be used as part of combination therapy or as monotherapy. Considering long-term treatment, it is important to consider each patient's OSA characteristics and lifestyle.

Positional therapy in patients with residual supine-dependent OSA undergoing OA therapy leads to greater therapeutic efficacy than either treatment modality alone (Dieltjens et al. 2015).

El-Solh et al. 2011 suggested combined therapy comprising CPAP and an OA based on their data suggesting that the optimal CPAP pressure was reduced with combination therapy, allowing all subjects in their study to tolerate CPAP.

A recent meta-analysis comparing the efficacy of CPAP, OA therapy, exercise training, and dietary weight loss revealed that exercise training, which significantly improves daytime sleepiness, could be used as an adjunct to CPAP or OA therapy (Iftikhar et al. 2017).

CPAP is difficult to use in patients with seasonal nasal congestion, during travel, and sometimes after evacuation in case of a disaster. An OA can be used as a temporary alternative to CPAP, although its efficacy may not be adequate for routine use. The treatment plan must be determined with consideration of multiple factors.

Appliance features

Appliance design

A variety of OAs have become available on the market. Devices are characterized according to their method of retention (mandible or tongue), fabrication (preformed or custom-made), adjustability (in both the vertical and anteroposterior dimensions), allowance of jaw movement (monoblock or twin-block), and flexibility of materials (soft elastic or hard acrylic). Few studies to date have compared the efficacy of different designs. A systematic review of the efficacy of OAs according to their design suggested that no single OA design most effectively improves polysomnographic indices, and careful consideration is needed because efficacy depends on the severity of OSA as well as the OA materials, method of fabrication, and type (monoblock/twin-block) (Ahrens et al. 2011).

Fabrication of a custom-made OA typically begins with the creation of dental casts of the patient's dentition and bite registration. These chair-side steps, including initiation or adjustment of the device after laboratory work, are generally conducted by an experienced dentist. This process therefore requires time and cost. In contrast, a device molded of thermoplastic polymer materials, a so-called "boil and bite" OA, is sometimes introduced as a low-cost and easily made alternative to a custom-made appliance. The patient bites into the softened material with a roughly advanced jaw position until this configuration sets with cooling. However, thermoplastic OAs are associated with insufficient mandibular protrusion and poor retention in the patient's mouth. A crossover study comparing the efficacy of thermoplastic and custom-made OAs showed that the post-treatment AHI was reduced only with the custom-made OA (Vanderveken et al. 2008). In addition, the thermoplastic device had a much lower rate of treatment success (60% vs 31%, respectively), and 82% of subjects preferred the customized OA at the end of the study. That study suggests that customization is a key component of treatment success. The most recent practice guideline also suggests that "a qualified dentist use a custom, titratable appliance over non-custom oral devices" (Ramar et al. 2015).

Differences in durability or the frequency of follow-up visits might influence device selection; however, data on which to base firm recommendations are lacking. One study of the side effects and technical complications of OAs during a 5-year follow-up period reported that patients made a mean of 2.5 unscheduled dental visits per year and a mean of 0.8 appliance repairs/relines per year with a dental technician (Martinez-Gomis et al. 2010). The most frequent problems among the study participants were acrylic breakage on the lateral telescopic attachment, poor retention, and the need for additional adjustments to improve comfort. Because these results may depend on the design of the device, more detailed evaluations are needed.

Titration procedure

Setting the mandibular position is critical to optimize OA therapy. It is generally thought that greater advancement is associated with a better treatment effect (Kato et al. 2000). However, a meta-regression analysis of different amounts of mandibular advancement in 13 randomized controlled trials showed that advancement amounts of >50% do not significantly influence the success rate (Bartolucci et al. 2016). Remmers et al. (2013) evaluated the ability to predict therapeutic success based on sleep studies using a remotely controlled mandibular protrusion device. The effective target protrusion position values were relatively small, with the smallest being 6% and the median being 68% of the patient's protrusive range. Based on these reports, it seems that some patients do not need a large amount of advancement and that their devices may be over-protruding the mandible. The applied mandibular position must be balanced because too much advancement increases the risk of side effects. Although it is clearly important to achieve an optimized mandibular position for treatment success, the titration procedure is not currently standardized (Chan et al. 2010b).

One review classified the titration procedures for OAs as follows: 1) subjective titration (titration solely based on the physical limits of the patient as indicated by self-reported evolution of symptoms and physical limits), 2) objective titration (initial overnight titration of mandibular advancement during polysomnography), and 3) multiparametric titration (combination of subjective and objective findings by a single-channel device, type III portable monitoring device, and polysomnography) (Dieltjens et al. 2012).

The most popular titration procedure in the clinical setting is based on the patient's subjective response to OA use. If a patient reports that snoring, sleepiness, or morning headache persist without side effects such as tooth pain or jaw muscle pain, the dentist advances the OA. Conversely, if the patient reports side effects, the jaw position of the OA is set back. These adjustments continue until a maximum subjective effect is achieved.

The problem associated with this titration procedure is the time-consuming steps needed and the risk of under-titration because of the absence of an objective parameter. Almeida et al. (2009) showed that subjective titration by self-reporting is often insufficient and that some patients miss the chance for successful treatment. Several subjects in their study had residual respiratory events after titration based on subjective responses; 17.4 to 30.4% of patients, depending on the definition of treatment success, could be treated with additional titration under a polysomnographic study. In the clinical setting, a follow-up sleep study is crucial to objectively verify satisfactory treatment and thus improve clinical outcomes.

Initial overnight titration may have additional benefits other than determining the titration protocol. The advantage of this type of titration is that in addition to estimating the optimal jaw position, it also predicts which patients will respond to treatment before beginning the customized OA fabrication. Because a low success rate is the biggest concern when making treatment decisions, accurate prediction of treatment responders is one of the most important issues in OA therapy. Thus, initial overnight titration is considered the most likely titration protocol to be standardized.

Several studies have estimated the accuracy and usefulness of overnight titration procedures (Table 1). One report used the appliance itself as a titration appliance (Raphaelson et al. 1998); others used a temporary appliance for the titration study and evaluated the treatment efficacy and accuracy of treatment prediction using a customized appliance with a titrated mandibular position (Remmers et al. 2013; Kuna et al. 2006; Dort et al. 2006; Tsai et al. 2004; Petelle et al. 2002; Zhou and Liu 2012).

Raphaelson et al. (1998) conducted initial overnight titration in six subjects by awakening the subjects each time the appliance was advanced. Although the authors did not report the amount of jaw advancement, they suggested that progressive jaw advancement could determine the optimal jaw position for eliminating sleep apnea and snoring.

Kuna et al. (2006) used a commercialized low-cost temporary titration appliance in their study. Although 42.9% of subjects achieved the criteria of successful treatment, such as an AHI of <10 and 50% reduction from the baseline AHI, none exhibited the same success rate with a prescribed appliance using the same jaw position estimated during the titration night. Following additional advancement, 47% of subjects achieved effective AHI reduction (AHI of <15 and 50% reduction from baseline AHI). The authors concluded that titration data cannot predict the efficacy of long-term appliance treatment.

Petelle et al. (2002) first reported a system for titration sleep studies using a hydraulic, remotely adjustable temporary appliance. Although the number of participants was small, three of seven reduced their AHI to <20 from a baseline AHI of 66.9 ± 32.4. These three patients exhibited similar results with a prescribed appliance, and two of the four patients who continued to have more than 20 obstructive events during the titration study also reduced their AHI to <20 with their prescribed appliance.

Tsai et al. (2004), Dort et al. (2006), and Remmers et al. (2013) used RCMPs in their studies. This titration system advances the mandible until obstructive respiratory events and snoring are eliminated. After the titration studies, the patients underwent another sleep study with a custom-made appliance. In the studies by Dort et al. (2006) and Remmers et al. (2013), the jaw position was estimated based on the RCMP study. In contrast, a conventional titration procedure was used by Tsai et al. (2004). Ten of 19 subjects (52.6%) in the study by Tsai et al. (2004), 16 of 33 (48.5%) in the study by Dort et al. (2006), and 58.2% in the study by Remmers et al. (2013) were treatment responders according to the definition of treatment success for each study. The positive and negative predictive values for treatment success were 90 and 89%, respectively, in the study by Tsai et al. (2004); 80 and 78%, respectively, in the study by Dort et al. (2006); and 94 and 83%, respectively, in the study by Remmers et al. (2013). Despite the high predictive rates found by Tsai et al. (2004), meaningful correlations were not found between the individual protrusion values determined by the RCMP and those at the end of the study. Remmers et al. (2013) also reported that 87.1% of their subjects were successfully treated with an estimated position; however, four subjects who were predicted to be treatment responders needed additional mandibular advancement on their fabricated final appliances.

Ferguson et al. (2006) reported that patients with mild to severe OSA have a 52% chance of controlling their sleep apnea with an OA. An overnight titration protocol seemed to result in higher treatment success rates than conventional procedures.

Zhou and Liu (2012) evaluated differences in treatment results between prescribed appliances. Titration was performed with a remote control device until a maximum reduction in the AHI was achieved. Patients received both monoblock and twin-block type appliances and underwent a sleep study to evaluate treatment efficacy. Although both appliances maintained the same jaw position based on the titration study data, the monoblock appliance reduced the AHI more than the twin-block appliance (baseline AHI, 26.4 ± 4.1; AHI with monoblock appliance, 6.6 ± 2.3; AHI with twin-block appliance, 9.9 ± 2.9). Forty-four percent of patients preferred the monoblock appliance, whereas 13% preferred the twin-block appliance.

When a single-night titration procedure is used to estimate the treatment response, RCMP studies might show acceptable results in clinical use. The limitation of this procedure is the lack of information about side effects, such as tooth or jaw pain, with long-term use. Some patients may not tolerate an OA because of excessive jaw advancement despite the fact that this achieves optimal positioning to eliminate respiratory events.

Considering the titration procedure, the difference between temporary appliances for titration and the prescribed final appliance should be mentioned. Zhou and Liu (2012) demonstrated different results with a monoblock versus twin-block appliance using the same jaw position during a single-night titration study. Similar interesting results have been reported in comparison studies of two different MADs (Geoghegan et al. 2015; Isacsson et al. 2016). Geoghegan et al. (2015) evaluated the effects of two different MADs (monoblock and twin-block) with the same bite registration as used in the study by Zhou and Liu (2012) and found that monoblock appliances reduced the AHI more than twin-block appliances. Conversely, in another study comparing monoblock and twin-block appliances, Isacsson et al. (2016) reported that both types significantly reduced the AHI and sleepiness to the same degree. Importantly, the mandible protruded an average of 3 mm more in the twin-block than monoblock appliance group. The reported average maximum protrusion in young adults is 8.0 mm (range, 2.5–13.5 mm) (Woelfel et al. 2014). To determine the optimal jaw position that controls OSA

Table 1 Prediction of treatment response with oral appliance

Authors, year of publication	Number of patients	Type of titration tray	Titration criteria	AHI or RDI (/h) baseline	AHI(/h) titration PSG	AHI(/h) OA	Type of OA	OA jaw position
Raphaelson et al. 1998	6	N/A					Silencer	
Dort et al. 2006	33	RCMP	Until obstructive events and snoring were eliminated	26.9 ± 18.3	N/A	N/A	Klearway	Evaluated position by titration
Kuna et al. 2006	21	EMA-T	• Snoring, apnea, hypopnea, were eliminated • Maximum tolerated advancement	33.5 ± 18.3	16.4 ± 13.0	24.6 ± 17.1 (titration position) 24.9 ± 18.8 (final position)	Klearway	• Evaluated position by titration • Additional advancement (final)
Tsai et al. 2004	19	RCMP	Elimination of majority of obstructive sleep apnea, hypopnea and oxygen desaturation	34.0 ± 4.88	N/A	17 ± 4.7	Klearway	Used conventional procedure
Petelle et al. 2002	7	temporary appliance	• Significant reduction of the incidence of sleep disordered breathing • Reaching position of maximum advancement of system • Position causing discomfort or pain	66.9 ± 32.4	26.1 ± 20.7	19.6 ± 20.2	Herbst	Evaluated position by titration
Zhou and Liu 2012	16	temporary appliance	Until the maximum AHI reduction was achieved	26.38 ± 4.13	N/A	6.58 ± 2.28 (monoblock) 9.87 ± 2.88 (SILENT NITE)	monoblock SILENTNITE	Evaluated position by titration
Remmers et al. 2013	67	RCMP	Elimination of majority of respiratory events in REM and NREM sleep in both the supine and lateral position	25.2 ± 14.8	N/A	N/A	SomnoDent	• Predicted effective target jaw position • 70% of A-P range of motion for predicted failure

AHI apnea–hypopnea index, *RDI* respiratory disturbance index, *RCMP* remotely controlled mandibular protrusion

Table 1 Prediction of treatment response with oral appliance *(Continued)*

Authors, year of publication	Prediction of treatment responder (%)				Treatment success with OA	Criterion of success	Remark
	Sensitivity	Specificity	Positive predictive value	Negative predictive value			
Raphaelson et al. 1998	N/A	N/A	N/A	N/A			Case report
Dort et al. 2006	75	82.4	80	77.8	49%	RDI < 15/h and RDI reduction of <30%	
Kuna et al. 2006	0 (AHI < 10) 75 (50%reduction)	55 (AHI < 10) 46 (50%reduction)	0 (AHI < 10) 46.1 (50%reduction)	92 (AHI < 10) 75 (50%reduction)	47	AHI < 15/h and >50% reduction inAHI	
Tsai et al. 2004	90	89	90	89	53	AHI < 15/h and AHI reduction of >30% and a subjective improvement in symptoms	
Petelle et al. 2002	0 (AHI < 10) 60 (AHI < 20)	100 (AHI < 10) 100 (AHI < 20)	N/A (AHI < 10) 100 (AHI < 20)	57 (AHI < 10) 50 (AHI < 20)	42.9 (AHI < 10) 68.9 (AHI < 20)	AHI < 10/h AHI < 20/h	
Zhou and Liu 2012	N/A	N/A	N/A	N/A	68.9 (monoblock) 56.3 (SILENT NITE)	AHI < 10 and >50% reduction in AHI	
Remmers et al. 2013	86	92	94	83	58	AHI < 10 and >50% reduction in AHI	

symptoms, titrations of the appliance are usually repeated by the dentist with minuscule advancements, such 0.25 to 1.00 mm. In terms of structure or mechanism, the jaw position that is applied with a monoblock appliance is identical to the bite registration if it is properly fabricated. Conversely, an adjustable or twin-block appliance allows mandibular movement including vertical opening with retroclination of the mandible. Although patients generally appreciate this flexibility, the protrusion achieved with a twin-block appliance is clearly less than the bite registration or that achieved with a monoblock appliance.

Because titration is a very sensitive procedure, bite registration and consideration of appliance characteristics are essential.

Objective adherence monitoring
Compared with CPAP, in which adherence can be objectively monitored, most adherence data for OA therapy has been limited to patients' self-reports. This lack of objective monitoring may be a concern of sleep physicians when referring patients for OA therapy, especially patients with serious morbidities requiring strict OSA management. Commercially available objective adherence monitors have recently been developed for OA therapy, representing a great advancement in both research and clinical practice (Vanderveken et al. 2013; Inoko et al. 2009; Bonato and Bradley 2013). Vanderveken et al. (2013) estimated the safety and feasibility of a microsensor (TheraMon) with on-chip integrated readout electronics. Their study was based on the assumption that the OA therapy was being used at a measured temperature of >35 °C. No microsensor-related adverse

events occurred during study period, and no statistically significant difference was found between the objective and self-reported compliance data (Vanderveken et al. 2013). Another commercially available sensor (Denti-Trac) with an internal battery, internal sensors, internal memory storage, and a method to retrieve information from the data logger was also recently introduced (Bonato and Bradley 2013). Both of these adherence monitors are small enough to embed in the OA without interrupting the patient's comfort and can be to attached to any type of OA. In the clinical setting, adherence monitors may motivate appliance use, and objective data can serve as a communication tool between the physician and dentist. Furthermore, objective data can be used for commercial drivers to prove treatment compliance for their reinstatement (Sutherland et al. 2014a).

Knowledge and skill related to dental sleep medicine among dentists
One of the roles of dentists in sleep medicine is providing OA therapy for patients with sleep apnea. The American Board of Dental Sleep Medicine (ABDSM), established in 2004, is an independent, nonprofit board of examiners that certifies dentists who treat snoring and OSA with OA therapy. Although more than 270 ABDSM diplomates are providing quality treatment for patients across the US (http://www.abdsm.org/About. aspx), more qualified dentists are needed in this field.

Difficulties have been encountered in developing educational programs in sleep medicine at academic institutions because the field is relatively new and highly multidisciplinary. In 2004, a questionnaire-based survey of 192 general dental practitioners revealed that 58% of dentists could not identify common signs and symptoms of OSA and that 55% did not know the therapeutic mechanism of OAs, despite the fact that 93% agreed that OSA constitutes a life-threatening illness (Bian 2004).

Simmons and Pullinger (2012) reported that the teaching time dedicated to sleep medicine in predoctoral dental programs in the US had increased to 3.92 h, but the authors still considered this to be insufficient. One of the authors of the present review conducted a similar survey of Japanese dental schools. Of the responding schools, 80.8% reported some educational time devoted to sleep medicine; the average was 3.8 instruction hours, which is similar to the findings in the survey by Simmons and Pullinger (2012). Most sleep medicine instruction was didactic (58.5%); only 11.5% of institutions reported a hands-on clinical laboratory experience (Tsuda et al. 2014).

For appropriate OA therapy, dentists need both technical skills to adjust the appliance and fundamental knowledge in areas such as pathophysiology, typical symptoms of OSA, sleep study interpretation, and alternate treatment options to communicate effectively with patients and sleep physicians. Sleep physicians' specialties vary and include respirology, otolaryngology, cardiology, neurology, and psychiatry, and their treatment strategies also vary. Each of these specialists should understand this multidisciplinary situation, and dentistry should also be recognized as a specialty in sleep medicine. Current practice guidelines recommend close cooperation between sleep physicians and qualified dentists to optimize patient care (Ramar et al. 2015).

Because healthcare systems differ among countries, original treatment strategies and educational curricula should be developed to maximize the quality and cost-effectiveness of treatment according to each country's situation. Importantly, the planning and execution of sleep medicine education in dental schools should be based not only on the dentist's limited role, but also on the dentist's role in general disease management within the healthcare system.

Conclusion

This manuscript reviewed practical considerations for effective OA therapy with assessment of three factors: patient eligibility for OA therapy, device features, and requirements for OA providers. Because neither CPAP nor OA therapy cures OSA, continuous use of these devices is required. Although OA therapy does not completely relieve respiratory events in all patients, the advantages and disadvantages of OA therapy differ from those of CPAP. Treatment decisions should be carefully planned with assessment of multiple factors. The three above-mentioned factors may seem to lack an interrelationship or to be of low importance, but treatment optimization is impossible without considering all of them, especially in the clinical setting (Fig. 1). Because OA therapy requires cooperation among professionals with different areas of expertise, such as dentists and physicians of many specialties, everyone involved in therapy must understand both the benefits and drawbacks or challenges of therapy.

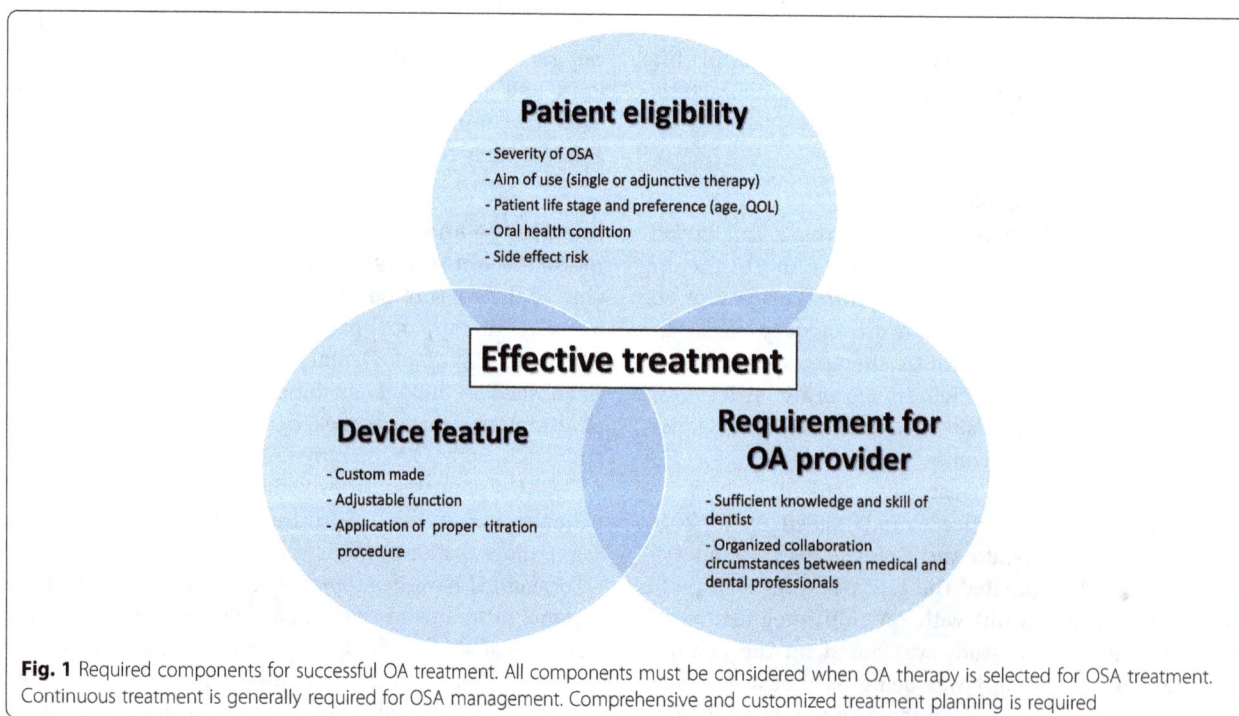

Patient eligibility
- Severity of OSA
- Aim of use (single or adjunctive therapy)
- Patient life stage and preference (age, QOL)
- Oral health condition
- Side effect risk

Effective treatment

Device feature
- Custom made
- Adjustable function
- Application of proper titration procedure

Requirement for OA provider
- Sufficient knowledge and skill of dentist
- Organized collaboration circumstances between medical and dental professionals

Fig. 1 Required components for successful OA treatment. All components must be considered when OA therapy is selected for OSA treatment. Continuous treatment is generally required for OSA management. Comprehensive and customized treatment planning is required

Abbreviations

AHI: Apnea–hypopnea index; CPAP: Continuous positive airway pressure; MAD: Mandibular advancement device; OA: Oral appliance; OSA: Obstructive sleep apnea; RCMP: Remotely controlled mandibular protrusion; SDB: Sleep-disordered breathing; TRD: Tongue-retaining device; TSD: Tongue-stabilizing device

Acknowledgements

None.

Funding

Not applicable.

Authors' contributions

HT interpreted the articles and was a major contributor in writing the manuscript. HT, NW, and SA read and approved the final manuscript.

Competing interests

HT and NW declare that they have no competing interest. SA has unrestricted research funding from Teijin Home Health Company and Philips Respironics Inc.

References

Ahrens A, McGrath C, Hagg U. A systematic review of the efficacy of oral appliance design in the management of obstructive sleep apnoea. Eur J Orthod. 2011;33(3):318–24.

Almeida FR, Lowe AA, Otsuka R, et al. Long-term sequellae of oral appliance therapy in obstructive sleep apnea patients: Part 2. Study-model analysis. Am J Orthod Dentofacial Orthop. 2006;129(2):205–13. Epub 2006/02/14. (Article in eng).

Almeida FR, Parker JA, Hodges JS, et al. Effect of a titration polysomnogram on treatment success with a mandibular repositioning appliance. J Clin Sleep Med. 2009;5(3):198–204.

Bartolucci ML, Bortolotti F, Raffaelli E, et al. The effectiveness of different mandibular advancement amounts in OSA patients: a systematic review and meta-regression analysis. Sleep Breath. 2016;20(3):911–9.

Bian H. Knowledge, opinions, and clinical experience of general practice dentists toward obstructive sleep apnea and oral appliances. Sleep Breath. 2004;8(2):85–90.

Bliwise DL, Foley DJ, Vitiello MV, et al. Nocturia and disturbed sleep in the elderly. Sleep Med. 2009;10(5):540–8. Pubmed Central PMCID: 2735085.

Bonato RA, Bradley DC. Introducing a novel micro-recorder for the detection of oral appliance compliance: DentiTrac. Sleep Diagn Ther. 2013;8:12–5.

Cao M, Guilleminault C, Kushida C. Clinical features and evaluation of obstructive sleep apnea and upper airway resistance syndrome. In: Principles and practice of sleep medicine. Philadelphia: Elsevier Saunders; 2011. p. 1206–18.

Chan AS, Cistulli PA. Oral appliance treatment of obstructive sleep apnea: an update. Curr Opin Pulm Med. 2009;15(6):591–6.

Chan AS, Sutherland K, Schwab RJ, et al. The effect of mandibular advancement on upper airway structure in obstructive sleep apnoea. Thorax. 2010a;65(8):726–32.

Chan AS, Phillips CL, Cistulli PA. Obstructive sleep apnoea–an update. Intern Med J. 2010b;40(2):102–6.

Deane SA, Cistulli PA, Ng AT, et al. Comparison of mandibular advancement splint and tongue stabilizing device in obstructive sleep apnea: a randomized controlled trial. Sleep. 2009;32(5):648–53. Pubmed Central PMCID: 2675900. Epub 2009/06/02. (Article in eng).

Dieltjens M, Vanderveken OM, Heyning PH, et al. Current opinions and clinical practice in the titration of oral appliances in the treatment of sleep-disordered breathing. Sleep Med Rev. 2012;16(2):177–85.

Dieltjens M, Vroegop AV, Verbruggen AE, et al. A promising concept of combination therapy for positional obstructive sleep apnea. Sleep Breath. 2015;19(2):637–44. Pubmed Central PMCID: 4873543.

Doff MH, Finnema KJ, Hoekema A, et al. Long-term oral appliance therapy in obstructive sleep apnea syndrome: a controlled study on dental side effects. Clin Oral Investig. 2013;17(2):475–82. Pubmed Central PMCID: 3579417.

Dort LC, Hadjuk E, Remmers JE. Mandibular advancement and obstructive sleep apnoea: a method for determining effective mandibular protrusion. Eur Respir J. 2006;27(5):1003–9. Epub 2006/05/19. (Article in eng).

Eckert DJ, White DP, Jordan AS, et al. Defining phenotypic causes of obstructive sleep apnea. Identification of novel therapeutic targets. Am J Respir Crit Care Med. 2013;188(8):996–1004. Pubmed Central PMCID: 3826282.

Edwards BA, Andara C, Landry S, Sands SA, Joosten SA, Owens RL, et al. Upper-airway Collapsibility and Loop Gain Predict the Response to Oral Appliance Therapy in Patients with Obstructive Sleep Apnea. Am J Respir Crit Care Med. 2016;194(11): 1413–22.

El-Solh AA, Moitheennazima B, Akinnusi ME, Churder PM, Lafornara AM. Combined oral appliance and positive airway pressure therapy for obstructive sleep apnea: a pilot study. Sleep Breath. 2011;15(2):203–8.

Endeshaw YW, Katz S, Ouslander JG, et al. Association of denture use with sleep-disordered breathing among older adults. J Public Health Dent. 2004;64(3): 181–3. Epub 2004/09/03. (Article in eng).

Ferguson KA, Cartwright R, Rogers R, et al. Oral appliances for snoring and obstructive sleep apnea: a review. Sleep. 2006;29(2):244–62. Epub 2006/02/24. (Article in eng).

Gagnon Y, Mayer P, Morisson F, et al. Aggravation of respiratory disturbances by the use of an occlusal splint in apneic patients: a pilot study. Int J Prosthodont. 2004;17(4):447–53. Epub 2004/09/24. (Article in eng).

Geoghegan F, Ahrens A, McGrath C, et al. An evaluation of two different mandibular advancement devices on craniofacial characteristics and upper airway dimensions of Chinese adult obstructive sleep apnea patients. Angle Orthod. 2015;85(6):962–8.

Gray E, McKenzie D, Eckert D. Obstructive Sleep Apnea Without Obesity is Common and Difficult to Treat: Evidence for a Distinct Pathophysiological Phenotype. J Clin Sleep Med. 2016;13(1):81–88.

Guilleminault C, Lin CM, Goncalves MA, et al. A prospective study of nocturia and the quality of life of elderly patients with obstructive sleep apnea or sleep onset insomnia. J Psychosom Res. 2004;56(5):511–5.

Gunaratnam K, Taylor B, Curtis B, et al. Obstructive sleep apnoea and periodontitis: a novel association? Sleep Breath. 2009;13(3):233–9. Epub 2009/ 02/10. (Article in eng).

Hajduk IA, Strollo Jr PJ, Jasani RR, et al. Prevalence and predictors of nocturia in obstructive sleep apnea-hypopnea syndrome–a retrospective study. Sleep. 2003;26(1):61–4.

Hopcraft MS, Tan C. Xerostomia: an update for clinicians. Aust Dent J. 2010;55(3): 238–44. quiz 353.

Iftikhar IH, Bittencourt L, Youngstedt SD, Ayas N, Cistulli P, Schwab R, et al. Comparative efficacy of CPAP, MADs, exercise-training, and dietary weight loss for sleep apnea: a network meta-analysis. Sleep Med. 2017;30:7–14

Inoko Y, Yoshimura K, Kato C, et al. Efficacy and safety of temperature data loggers in measuring compliance with the use of oral appliances. Sleep Biol Rhythms. 2009;7(3):188–92.

Isacsson G, Fodor C, Sturebrand M. Obstructive sleep apnea treated with custom-made bibloc and monobloc oral appliances: a retrospective comparative study. Sleep Breath. 2017;1:93–100

Kato J, Isono S, Tanaka A, et al. Dose-dependent effects of mandibular advancement on pharyngeal mechanics and nocturnal oxygenation in patients with sleep-disordered breathing. Chest. 2000;117(4):1065–72.

Kreivi HR, Virkkula P, Lehto J, et al. Frequency of upper airway symptoms before and during continuous positive airway pressure treatment in patients with obstructive sleep apnea syndrome. Respiration. 2010;80(6):488–94.

Kuna ST, Giarraputo PC, Stanton DC, et al. Evaluation of an oral mandibular advancement titration appliance. Oral Surg Oral Med Oral Pathol Oral Radiol Endod. 2006;101(5):593–603. Epub 2006/04/25. (Article in eng).

Kushida CA, Morgenthaler TI, Littner MR, et al. Practice parameters for the treatment of snoring and Obstructive Sleep Apnea with oral appliances: an update for 2005. Sleep. 2006;29(2):240–3. Epub 2006/02/24. (Article in eng).

Landry-Schönbeck A, de Grandmont P, Rompré PH, Lavigne GJ. Effect of an adjustable mandibular advancement appliance on sleep bruxism: a crossover sleep laboratory study. Int J Prosthodont. 2009;22(3):251–59.

Marklund M, Franklin KA. Long-term effects of mandibular repositioning appliances on symptoms of sleep apnoea. J Sleep Res. 2007;16(4):414–20. Epub 2007/11/27. (Article in eng).

Marshall NS, Wong KK, Liu PY, et al. Sleep apnea as an independent risk factor for all-cause mortality: the Busselton Health Study. Sleep. 2008;31(8):1079–85. Pubmed Central PMCID: 2542953.

Martinez-Gomis J, Willaert E, Nogues L, et al. Five years of sleep apnea treatment with a mandibular advancement device. Side effects and technical complications. Angle Orthod. 2010;80(1):30–6.

Nerfeldt P, Friberg D. Effectiveness of oral appliances in obstructive sleep apnea with respiratory arousals. J Clin Sleep Med. 2016;12(8):1159–65. Pubmed Central PMCID: 4957194.

Netzer NC, Ancoli-Israel S, Bliwise DL, Fulda S, Roffe C, Almeida F, et al. Principles of practice parameters for the treatment of sleep disordered breathing in the elderly and frail elderly: the consensus of the International Geriatric Sleep Medicine Task Force. Eur Respir J. 2016:ERJ-01975-2015.

Oksenberg A, Arons E. Sleep bruxism related to obstructive sleep apnea: the effect of continuous positive airway pressure. Sleep Med. 2002;3(6):513–5.

Oksenberg A, Froom P, Melamed S. Dry mouth upon awakening in obstructive sleep apnea. J Sleep Res. 2006;15(3):317–20.

Petelle B, Vincent G, Gagnadoux F, et al. One-night mandibular advancement titration for obstructive sleep apnea syndrome: a pilot study. Am J Respir Crit Care Med. 2002;165(8):1150–3. Epub 2002/04/17. (Article in eng).

Petit FX, Pepin JL, Bettega G, et al. Mandibular advancement devices: rate of contraindications in 100 consecutive obstructive sleep apnea patients. Am J Respir Crit Care Med. 2002;166(3):274–8. Epub 2002/08/03. (Article in eng).

Phipps KR, Stevens VJ. Relative contribution of caries and periodontal disease in adult tooth loss for an HMO dental population. J Public Health Dent. 1995; 55(4):250–2.

Pliska BT, Nam H, Chen H, Lowe AA, Almeida FR. Obstructive sleep apnea and mandibular advancement splints: occlusal effects and progression of changes associated with a decade of treatment. J Clin Sleep Med 2014; 10(12):1285-1291 publication of the American Academy of Sleep Medicine. 2014;10(12):1285.

Ramar K, Dort LC, Katz SG, Lettieri CJ, Harrod CG, Thomas SM, et al. Clinical Practice Guideline for the Treatment of Obstructive Sleep Apnea and Snoring with Oral Appliance Therapy: An Update for 2015. J Clin Sleep Med. 2015; 11(7):773–827.

Raphaelson MA, Alpher EJ, Bakker KW, et al. Oral appliance therapy for obstructive sleep apnea syndrome: progressive mandibular advancement during polysomnography. Cranio. 1998;16(1):44–50. Epub 1998/03/03. (Article in eng).

Remmers J, Charkhandeh S, Grosse J, et al. Remotely controlled mandibular protrusion during sleep predicts therapeutic success with oral appliances in patients with obstructive sleep apnea. Sleep. 2013;36(10):1517–25. Pubmed Central PMCID: 3773201, 25A.

Ruhle KH, Franke KJ, Domanski U, et al. Quality of life, compliance, sleep and nasopharyngeal side effects during CPAP therapy with and without controlled heated humidification. Sleep Breath. 2011;15(3):479–85.

Sanders AE, Essick GK, Beck JD, et al. Periodontitis and sleep disordered breathing in the Hispanic community health study/study of Latinos. Sleep. 2015;38(8): 1195–203. Pubmed Central PMCID: 4507724.

Sanders AE, Akinkugbe AA, Slade GD, et al. Tooth loss and obstructive sleep apnea signs and symptoms in the US population. Sleep Breath. 2016;20(3): 1095–102. Pubmed Central PMCID: 4947024.

Sasao Y, Nohara K, Okuno K, et al. Videoendoscopic diagnosis for predicting the response to oral appliance therapy in severe obstructive sleep apnea. Sleep Breath. 2014;18(4):809–15.

Simmons MS, Pullinger A. Education in sleep disorders in US dental schools DDS programs. Sleep Breath. 2012;16(2):383–92. Pubmed Central PMCID: 3306848.

Sutherland K, Vanderveken OM, Tsuda H, et al. Oral appliance treatment for obstructive sleep apnea: an update. J Clin Sleep Med. 2014a;10(2):215–27. Pubmed Central PMCID: 3899326.

Sutherland K, Phillips CL, Davies A, et al. CPAP pressure for prediction of oral appliance treatment response in obstructive sleep apnea. J Clin Sleep Med. 2014b;10(9):943–9. Pubmed Central PMCID: 4153122.

Sutherland K, Cistulli PA. Recent advances in obstructive sleep apnea pathophysiology and treatment. Sleep Biol Rhythms. 2015;13(1):26–40.

Tsai WH, Vazquez JC, Oshima T, et al. Remotely controlled mandibular positioner predicts efficacy of oral appliances in sleep apnea. Am J Respir Crit Care Med. 2004;170(4):366–70. Epub 2004/04/24. (Article in eng).

Tsuda H, Almeida FR, Tsuda T, et al. Craniofacial changes after 2 years of nasal continuous positive airway pressure use in patients with obstructive sleep apnea. Chest. 2010c;138(4):870–4.

Tsuda H, Ohmaru T, Higuchi Y. Requirement for sleep medicine education in Japanese pre-doctoral dental curriculum. Sleep Biol Rhythms. 2014;12(4): 232–4.

Tsuda H, Almeida FR, Walton JN, Lowe AA. Questionnaire-based study on sleep-disordered breathing among edentulous subjects in a university oral health center. Int J Prosthodont. 2010;23(6):503–6.

Tsuiki S, Kobayashi M, Namba K, et al. Optimal positive airway pressure predicts oral appliance response to sleep apnoea. Eur Respir J. 2010;35(5):1098–105.

Vanderveken OM, Devolder A, Marklund M, et al. Comparison of a custom-made and a thermoplastic oral appliance for the treatment of mild sleep apnea. Am J Respir Crit Care Med. 2008;178(2):197–202. Epub 2007/08/04. (Article in eng).

Vanderveken OM, Dieltjens M, Wouters K, et al. Objective measurement of compliance during oral appliance therapy for sleep-disordered breathing. Thorax. 2013;68(1):91–6. Pubmed Central PMCID: 3534260.

Vroegop AV, Vanderveken OM, Dieltjens M, et al. Sleep endoscopy with simulation bite for prediction of oral appliance treatment outcome. J Sleep Res. 2013;22(3):348–55.

Vroegop AV, Vanderveken OM, Boudewyns AN, et al. Drug-induced sleep endoscopy in sleep-disordered breathing: report on 1,249 cases. Laryngoscope. 2014;124(3):797–802.

Woelfel JB, Igarashi T, Dong JK. Faculty-supervised measurements of the face and of mandibular movements on young adults. J Adv Prosthodont. 2014;6(6): 483–90. Pubmed Central PMCID: 4279047.

Young T, Palta M, Dempsey J, et al. The occurrence of sleep-disordered breathing among middle-aged adults. N Engl J Med. 1993;328(17):1230–5. Epub 1993/ 04/29. (Article in eng).

Young T, Peppard PE, Gottlieb DJ. Epidemiology of obstructive sleep apnea: a population health perspective. Am J Respir Crit Care Med. 2002;165(9): 1217–39.

Zhou J, Liu YH. A randomised titrated crossover study comparing two oral appliances in the treatment for mild to moderate obstructive sleep apnoea/ hypopnoea syndrome. J Oral Rehabil. 2012;39(12):914–22.

Effect of postoperative positive airway pressure on risk of postoperative atrial fibrillation after cardiac surgery in patients with obstructive sleep apnea: a retrospective cohort study

Feihong Ding[1], Jimmy Kar-Hing Wong[2], Alice S. Whittemore[3] and Clete A. Kushida[1*]

Abstract

Background: Obstructive sleep apnea (OSA) is a known risk factor for postoperative atrial fibrillation (POAF) after cardiac surgery. However, whether better management of OSA reduces the risk of POAF remains unknown. The aim of this study was to determine if postoperative positive airway pressure (PAP) treatment for OSA reduces POAF risk after cardiac surgery. PAP included both continuous and bilevel positive airway pressure.

Methods: This retrospective cohort study was conducted at Stanford University teaching hospital. We included a total of 152 OSA patients with preoperative electrocardiography showing sinus rhythm who underwent coronary artery bypass grafting (CABG), aortic valve replacement, mitral valve repair/replacement, or combined valve and CABG surgery from October 2007 to September 2014. Postoperative PAP use status was determined by reviewing electronic health records. The primary outcome was time to incident POAF. We reviewed records from the time of surgery to hospital discharge. Multivariate Cox regression model was used to calculate the adjusted hazard ratio of postoperative PAP in association with risk of POAF.

Results: Of the 152 OSA patients included for analysis, 86 (57%) developed POAF, and 76 (50%) received postoperative PAP treatment. POAF occurred in 37 (49%) of the patients receiving postoperative PAP, compared with 49 (65%) of those not receiving postoperative PAP (unadjusted p value = 0.33). Multivariable Cox regression analysis of time to incident POAF did not show an association between postoperative PAP treatment and risk of POAF (adjusted hazard ratio: 0.93 [95%CI: 0.58 – 1.48]). There were no significant differences in other postoperative complications between the two groups.

Conclusions: The study did not find an association between postoperative PAP treatment and risk of POAF after cardiac surgery in patients with OSA. Future prospective randomized trials are needed to investigate this issue further.

Keywords: Obstructive sleep apnea, Positive airway pressure, Postoperative atrial fibrillation, Cardiac surgery

* Correspondence: clete@stanford.edu
[1]Division of Sleep Medicine, Department of Psychiatry and Behavioral Sciences, Stanford Sleep Medicine Center, 450 Broadway Street, MC 5704, Pavilion C, 2nd Floor, Redwood City, CA 94063-5704, USA
Full list of author information is available at the end of the article

Background

Postoperative atrial fibrillation (POAF) is a common complication following cardiac surgery, affecting 30% to 50% of patients (Yadava et al. 2014). Although generally well-tolerated and self-resolving, POAF is associated with multiple adverse outcomes: increased risk of stroke, increased short- and long-term mortality, prolonged hospitalizations, increased cost of care, and late recurrence of atrial fibrillation (Horwich et al. 2013; Phan et al. 2015; LaPar et al. 2014; Ahlsson et al. 2010). Multiple risk factors—including advanced age, previous atrial fibrillation, valve surgery, chronic obstructive pulmonary disease, and perioperative withdrawal of beta-blockers—are associated with POAF after cardiac surgery (Mathew et al. 2004), but few are modifiable. Several studies have shown that obstructive sleep apnea (OSA), with an estimated prevalence of up to 80% in the cardiac surgical population (Zhao et al. 2015), is an independent risk factor for POAF (Zhao et al. 2015; Wong et al. 2015; Uchôa et al. 2015; van Oosten et al. 2014; Qaddoura et al. 2014). However, whether OSA is a modifiable risk factor for POAF after cardiac surgery is unknown.

The most effective OSA treatments are continuous positive airway pressure (CPAP) or bilevel positive airway pressure (BPAP) (the term "positive airway pressure" or PAP denotes either CPAP or BPAP in this study). In nonsurgical OSA patients, PAP therapy has been shown to reduce the recurrence rate of atrial fibrillation (Qureshi et al. 2015). However, no studies have investigated the effect of postoperative PAP on POAF after cardiac surgery. Given the poor adherence to PAP treatment of OSA patients at home (Stepnowsky & Moore 2003), the postoperative period after cardiac surgery may provide an ideal opportunity for physicians to use PAP to reduce the risk of POAF in OSA patients. Therefore, this retrospective cohort study aimed to determine if postoperative PAP reduces POAF risk after cardiac surgery in OSA patients.

Methods

Study population

We included OSA patients who underwent coronary artery bypass grafting (CABG), aortic valve replacement, mitral valve replacement/repair, or combined valve and CABG surgery requiring cardiopulmonary bypass performed at Stanford University from October 2007 to September 2014. We reviewed electronic medical charts of consecutive patients. Cardiac parameters including atrial fibrillation history and POAF, and sleep-related data including OSA history and post-operative PAP use were reviewed by two different investigators. We considered patients to have OSA if: 1) two independent sources documented a prior diagnosis of OSA, 2) one source documented a prior diagnosis of OSA with explicit documentation of whether the patient was using nocturnal PAP, or 3) a sleep study in the medical record documented OSA (Wong et al. 2015). We considered patients to have received postoperative PAP

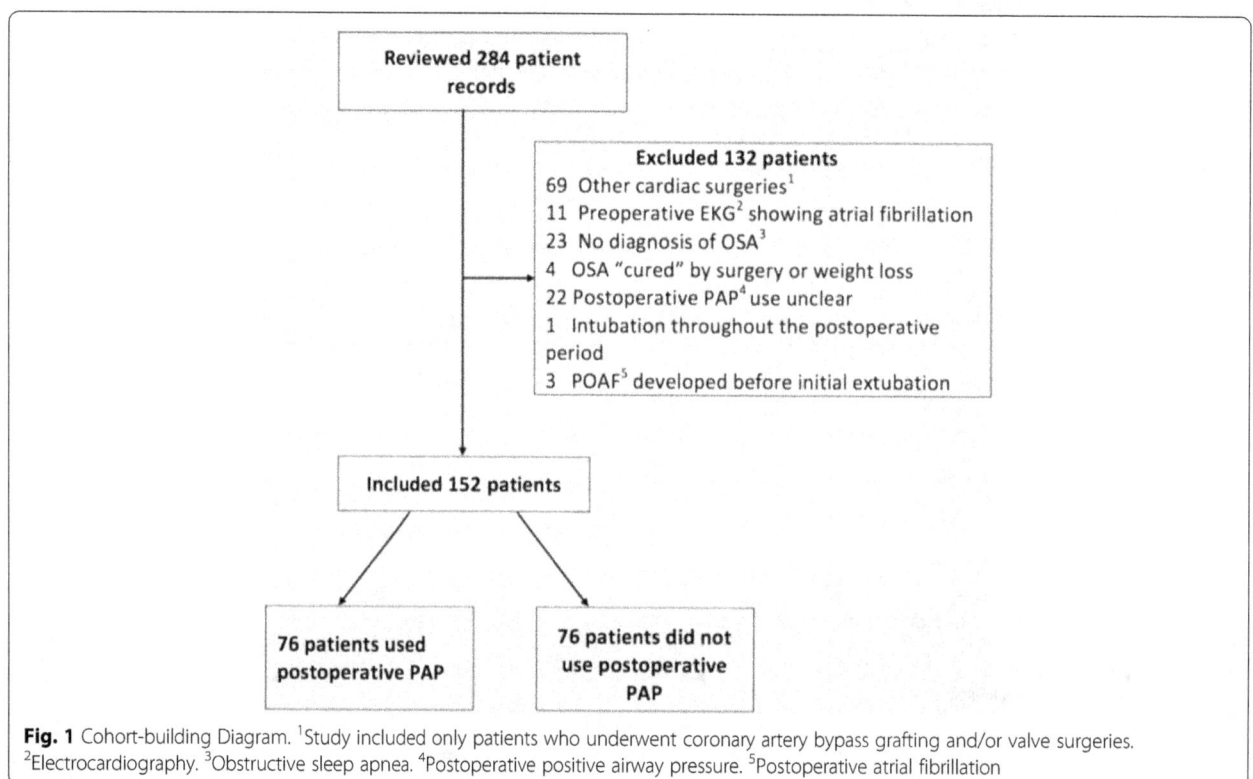

Fig. 1 Cohort-building Diagram. [1]Study included only patients who underwent coronary artery bypass grafting and/or valve surgeries. [2]Electrocardiography. [3]Obstructive sleep apnea. [4]Postoperative positive airway pressure. [5]Postoperative atrial fibrillation

Table 1 Descriptive Characteristics of the Study Groups, mean ± S.D. or N (%)

Characteristics	No Postoperative PAP[a]	Postoperative PAP	p value[b]
N	76 (50)	76 (50)	
Age (yrs.)	67.3 ± 10.4	63.7 ± 12.1	0.05
Male	53 (69.7)	64 (84.2)	0.03
White	53 (69.7)	56 (73.7)	0.59
Body Mass Index (kg/m^2)	32.1 ± 7.6	32.1 ± 7.1	0.99
Comorbidities			
Previous Atrial Fibrillation	16 (21.1)	16 (21.1)	1.00
Previous Cerebrovascular Event[c]	13 (17.1)	5 (6.6)	0.05
Previous Myocardial Infarction	16 (21.1)	6 (7.9)	0.02
COPD[d]	11 (14.5)	5 (6.6)	0.11
Hypertension	63 (82.9)	59 (77.6)	0.42
Hyperlipidemia	50 (65.8)	51 (67.1)	0.86
Perioperative Characteristics			
Elective Surgery	69 (90.8)	67 (88.2)	0.60
Valve Surgery	44 (57.9)	47 (61.8)	0.62
Preoperative IABP[e]	2 (2.6)	0 (0)	0.50
CPB time[f] (mins)	153.9 ± 59.3	174.4 ± 79.7	0.07
Aortic Cross-Clamp time (mins)	103.9 ± 44.7	121.2 ± 62.3	0.05
Post operative day of extubation	0.5 ± 0.8	0.6 ± 1.0	0.68
Home PAP use	17 (22.4)	62 (81.6)	<0.0001

[a]Positive airway pressure
[b]Student t tests, Chi-square tests or Fisher's exact tests were used to calculate the p value
[c]Cerebrovascular Event includes cerebral vascular accident and transient ischemic attack
[d]Chronic obstructive pulmonary disease
[e]Intra-aortic balloon counterpulsation pump
[f]Cardiopulmonary bypass time

if: 1) progress notes or sleep prescriptions explicitly documented use of nocturnal PAP after extubation and before the onset of POAF; and 2) follow-up documentation confirmed PAP use at least one night before hospital discharge.

Primary outcome

The primary outcome was time to incident POAF. We defined POAF as atrial fibrillation requiring either pharmacologic treatment or direct current cardioversion after initial extubation from cardiac surgery and before discharge from hospital. We determined the timing of POAF by reviewing physicians and nurses' notes, pharmacy records, procedural notes, electrocardiography (EKG) and telemetry strips. All cardiac surgery patients were on telemetry monitoring for their entire hospitalization.

Statistical analysis

We tested differences in demographic variables, comorbidities, and perioperative characteristics using t-tests for continuous variables and chi-square tests or Fisher's exact tests for categorical variables. All tests were two-tailed. We considered variables to be statistically significant if they attained a p value of <0.05.

We treated postoperative PAP treatment as a time dependent variable in a multivariate Cox regression model. Because we lacked data on intermittent postoperative PAP use, we assumed that PAP treatment continued until discharge once it started. The regression model included covariates that differed in bivariate analyses (p ≤ 0.1) or that had previously been identified as potential confounders. We checked the proportional hazard assumption with log-log plots. All statistical analyses were performed using SAS version 9.4 (SAS Institute, Cary, NC).

This retrospective cohort study was approved by our Institutional Review Board. The requirement to obtain individual consent was waived because the data were collected retrospectively.

Results

We reviewed a total of 284 patient records. After excluding 132 patients for various reasons (Fig. 1), there were 152 patients eligible for study. Exactly half of the 152 eligible patients (N = 76) received postoperative PAP treatment.

Home PAP use was a strong predictor for postoperative PAP treatment (Table 1). 62 patients (82%) among those who received postoperative PAP had used PAP at home preoperatively, compared with 17 patients (22%) among those who did not receive postoperative PAP. Compared with patients who did not receive postoperative PAP, patients who received postoperative PAP were younger, more likely to be male, had a significantly lower proportion of preoperative comorbidities including history of cerebrovascular events and myocardial infarction, and had a significantly longer cardiopulmonary bypass time and aortic cross-clamp time. As shown in Table 1, we observed no differences between the two groups in body mass index, previous atrial fibrillation, or postoperative day of extubation.

Among patients who received postoperative PAP treatment, 33 (43%) started treatment immediately on the day of cardiac surgery, and 55 patients (72%) started within the first day after surgery. The remaining patients started postoperative PAP on postoperative day 2 to day 10 (Fig. 2a).

Eighty-six patients (57%) developed POAF after cardiac surgery. The majority of POAF cases occurred in the 3-day period from postoperative day 2 to day 4, with a peak incidence on day 2. POAF occurred slightly later among patients who received postoperative PAP than that among those who did not, but the difference was not statistically significant (Fig. 2b).

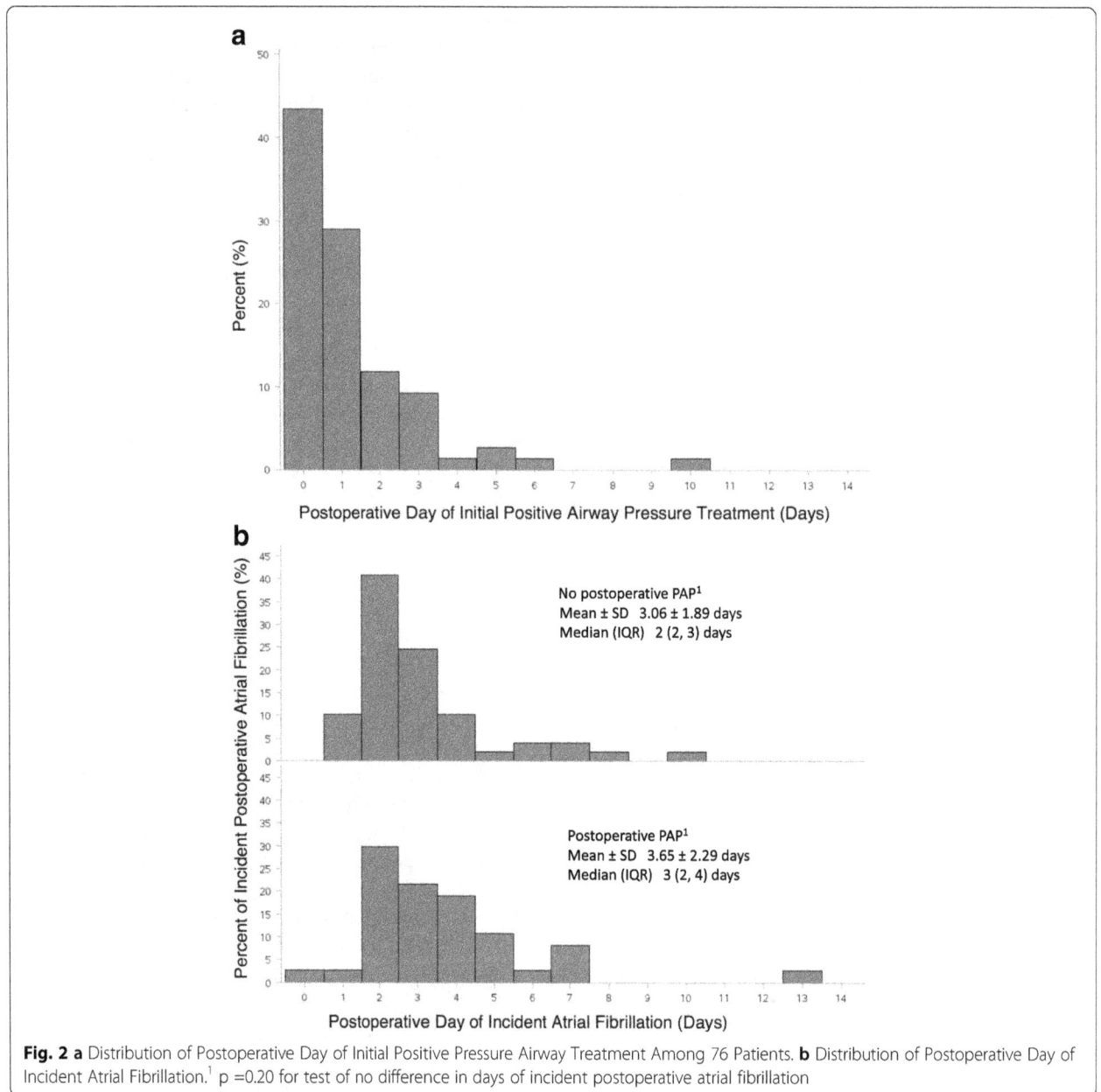

Fig. 2 a Distribution of Postoperative Day of Initial Positive Pressure Airway Treatment Among 76 Patients. **b** Distribution of Postoperative Day of Incident Atrial Fibrillation.[1] p =0.20 for test of no difference in days of incident postoperative atrial fibrillation

Figure 3 shows a forest plot of hazard ratios and 95% confidence intervals obtained from a multivariable Cox regression model. Thirty-seven (49%) of the 76 patients receiving postoperative PAP treatment developed POAF, compared with 49 (65%) of the 76 patients without postoperative PAP treatment. As seen in Fig. 3 and Table 2, analysis of time to incident POAF did not show an association between postoperative PAP treatment and POAF risk (adjusted hazard ratio: 0.93 [95% CI: 0.58 – 1.48]). In contrast, we observed a significant increase in POAF risk among older patients (adjusted hazard ratio for 10-year increase in age: 1.30 [95% CI: 1.04 – 1.61]) and those with a prior history of atrial fibrillation (adjusted hazard ratio: 2.34 [95% CI: 1.42 – 3.86]).

We did not find an effect of postoperative PAP treatment on other postoperative complications such as reintubation, ICU readmission, length of initial ICU stay or hospital stay (Table 3).

Discussion

POAF remains a common complication after cardiac surgery. Multiple risk factors have been identified, but few are modifiable. We hypothesized that PAP after cardiac surgery reduces the risk of POAF in patients with OSA.

OSA has been associated with increased risk of POAF after cardiac surgery. Several pathophysiologic mechanisms may contribute to the relationship between OSA and atrial fibrillation: sudden and repeated swings in intra-thoracic

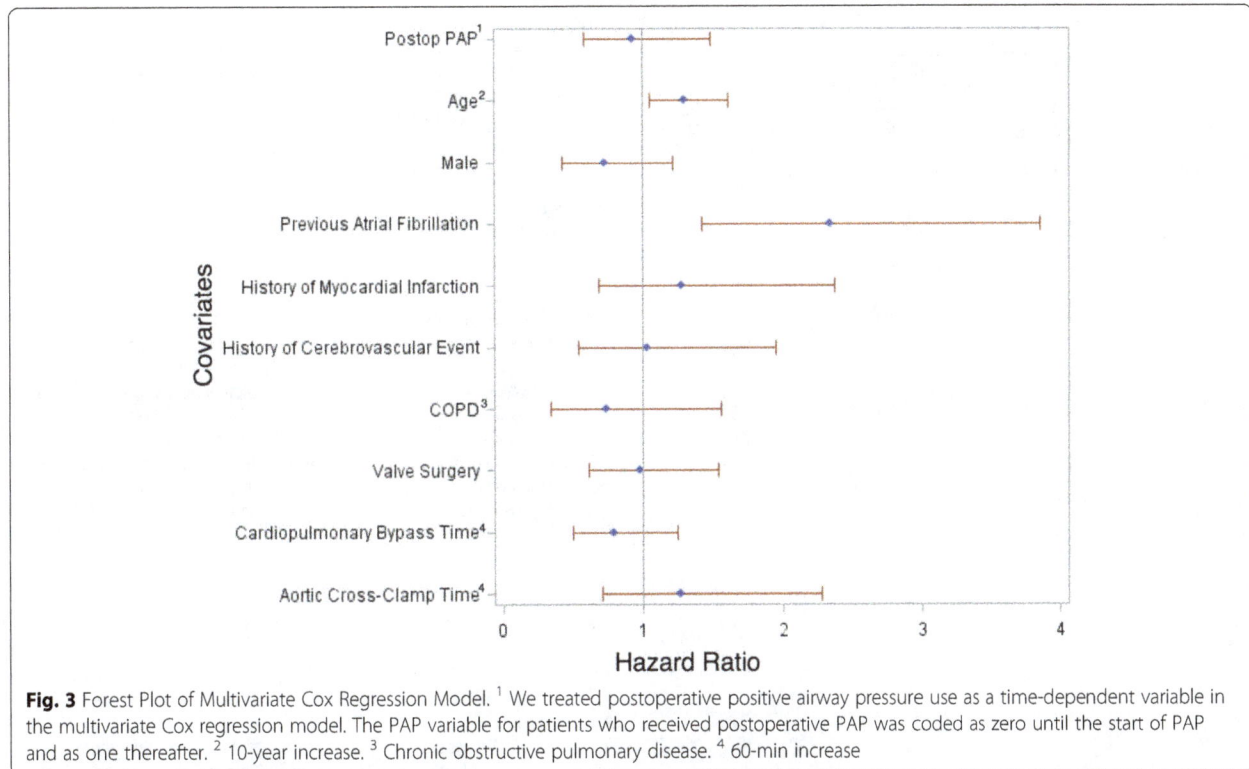

Fig. 3 Forest Plot of Multivariate Cox Regression Model. [1] We treated postoperative positive airway pressure use as a time-dependent variable in the multivariate Cox regression model. The PAP variable for patients who received postoperative PAP was coded as zero until the start of PAP and as one thereafter. [2] 10-year increase. [3] Chronic obstructive pulmonary disease. [4] 60-min increase

pressure, structural remodeling of the left atrium over time, systemic inflammation, and instability of autonomic tone associated with intermittent hypoxia or hypercapnia (Hohl et al. 2014; Orban et al. 2008; Neilan et al. 2013; Stevenson et al. 2010). In non-surgical OSA patients, PAP treatment reduces or abolishes hypopnea and apnea episodes, reverses cardiac remodeling, mitigates systemic inflammation and reduces atrial fibrillation recurrence risk in patients with prior atrial fibrillation history (Qureshi et al. 2015; Neilan et al. 2013; Xie et al. 2013). It follows, therefore, that PAP treatment after cardiac surgery may reduce the risk of POAF.

In this analysis, we did not find an association between postoperative PAP therapy and POAF risk. One concern is misclassification of postoperative PAP use. PAP use was determined by physicians or nurses' notes rather than objective device adherence data, which could lead to misclassification because nightly PAP use cannot be objectively confirmed. This misclassification may bias the association between postoperative PAP treatment and POAF risk towards null.

Unmeasured potential confounders are another concern. Patients who received post-operative PAP treatment and who did not differed in several baseline and perioperative characteristics such as previous history of myocardial infarction and length of aortic cross-clamp time (Table 1). Although we adjusted for all these measured potential confounders in the multivariate Cox regression model, the concern for unmeasured potential confounders remains. For example, perioperative medication use may differ between those who did or did not receive postoperative PAP therapy, and also be related to POAF risk (Mathew et al. 2004). Other limitations include the lack of OSA severity data and the high correlation between home and postoperative PAP use. This correlation complicates the determination of whether any reduction in POAF risk reflects home PAP use, postoperative PAP use, or both.

Nevertheless, we are unaware of previous studies exploring the effect of postoperative PAP administration on risk of POAF after cardiac surgery in OSA patients. Few studies have investigated the effect of perioperative (preoperative

Table 2 Risk of Postoperative Atrial Fibrillation (POAF) in Relation to Postoperative Positive Airway Pressure (PAP) Treatment

	No Postoperative PAP (N = 76)	Postoperative PAP (N = 76)	Unadjusted Hazard Ratio[a] (95% CI)	Adjusted Hazard Ratio[b] (95% CI)
POAF	49 (64.5%)	37 (48.7%)	0.81 (0.53 – 1.24)	0.93 (0.58 – 1.48)

[a]We treated postoperative PAP use as a time-dependent variable in the Cox regression model. The PAP variable for patients who received postoperative PAP was coded as zero until the start of PAP and as one thereafter

[b]Adjusted for age, gender, previous atrial fibrillation, history of cerebrovascular event, history of myocardial infarction, chronic obstructive pulmonary disease, surgery type, cardiopulmonary bypass time, and aortic cross-clamp time

Table 3 Other Postoperative Complications in Relation to Postoperative Positive Airway Pressure (PAP) Treatment

Outcomes Categorical Variables, N (%)	No Postoperative PAP (N = 76)	Postoperative PAP (N = 76)	Unadjusted Odds Ratio (95% CI)
In-Hospital Death	3 (4.0)	4 (5.3)	1.35 (0.29 – 6.26)
Code Blue while on Telemetry Floor	4 (5.3)	2 (2.6)	0.49 (0.09 –2.74)
Reinbutation	4 (5.3)	7 (9.2)	1.83 (0.51 – 6.52)
Tracheostomy	0	1 (1.3)	
PE and/or DVT[a]	4 (5.3)	5 (6.6)	1.27 (0.33 – 4.91)
Renal Replacement Therapy	5 (6.6)	4 (5.3)	0.79 (0.20 – 3.06)
ICU[b] Readmission	4 (5.3)	3 (4.0)	0.74 (0.16 – 3.42)
Cerebrovascular Event	4 (5.3)	2 (2.6)	0.49 (0.09 – 2.74)
Seizures	0	1 (1.3)	
Initial ICU Length of Stay[c] ≥ 4 days	27 (35.5)	31 (40.8)	1.25 (0.65 – 2.41)
Hospital Length of Stay ≥ 10 days	29 (38.2)	24 (31.6)	0.75 (0.38 – 1.46)
Length of Stay as Continuous Variable, Median (IQR)			
Initial ICU Length of Stay (days)	3 (2 – 5)	2 (2 – 4.5)	
Hospital Length of Stay (days)	8 (7 – 12)	8 (6 – 12.5)	

[a]Pulmonary embolus and/or deep vein thrombosis as indicated by radiographic (including ultrasound) or autopsy
[b]Intensive care unit
[c]The period between immediate postoperative care to discharge to telemetry unit, not including ICU readmission days

and/or postoperative) PAP treatment on other postoperative complications but with inconsistent results (Nagappa et al. 2015; Liao et al. 2013). Given the difficulty in reliably determining the postoperative PAP use, the only way to answer this question might be a prospective randomized trial with a clearly defined protocol.

Conclusions

This is the first study to examine the effect of postoperative PAP treatment on the risk of POAF after cardiac surgery in patients with OSA. We did not find a reduction in POAF occurrence after cardiac surgery in OSA patients given postoperative PAP. However, given the limitations of this study, postoperative PAP should continue to be recommended in OSA patients until future prospective randomized trials with more rigorous data collection can be performed to further clarify this issue.

Abbreviations
BPAP: Bilevel positive airway pressure; CABG: Coronary artery bypass grafting; CPAP: Continuous positive airway pressure; EKG: Electrocardiography; OSA: Obstructive sleep apnea; PAP: Positive airway pressure; POAF: Postoperative atrial fibrillation

Funding
No financial support for this research project.

Authors' contributions
FD contributed to the study design, data collection, statistical analysis, and manuscript drafting. JK-HW contributed to the conception and design of the study, acquisition of data for the work and intellectual discussion of the results. ASW had substantial contributions to the study design, interpretation of the results and critical revision of the work. CAK had substantial contributions to the study design, intellectual discussion for the content and critical revision of the work. In addition, all authors approved to publish the final version of the work and agreed to be accountable for all aspects of the work.

Competing interests
The authors' declare that they have no competing interests.

Author details
[1]Division of Sleep Medicine, Department of Psychiatry and Behavioral Sciences, Stanford Sleep Medicine Center, 450 Broadway Street, MC 5704, Pavilion C, 2nd Floor, Redwood City, CA 94063-5704, USA. [2]Department of Anesthesia, Palo Alto Veterans Affairs, Stanford, CA, USA. [3]Division of Epidemiology, Department of Health Research and Policy, School of Medicine, Stanford University, Stanford, CA, USA.

References
Ahlsson A, Fengsrud E, Bodin L, Englund A. Postoperative atrial fibrillation in patients undergoing aortocoronary bypass surgery carries an eightfold risk of future atrial fibrillation and a doubled cardiovascular mortality. Eur J Cardiothorac Surg. 2010;37:1353–9.
Hohl M, Linz B, Bohm M, Linz D. Obstructive sleep apnea and atrial arrhythmogenesis. Current cardiology reviews. 2014;10:362–8.
Horwich P, Buth KJ, Légaré J-F. New onset postoperative atrial fibrillation is associated with a long-term risk for stroke and death following cardiac surgery. J Card Surg. 2013;28:8–13.
LaPar DJ, Speir AM, Crosby IK, et al. Postoperative atrial fibrillation significantly increases mortality, hospital readmission, and hospital costs. Ann Thorac Surg. 2014;98:527–33. discussion 33.
Liao P, Luo Q, Elsaid H, Kang W, Shapiro CM, Chung F. Perioperative auto-titrated continuous positive airway pressure treatment in surgical patients with obstructive sleep apnea: a randomized controlled trial. Anesthesiology. 2013; 119:837–47.
Mathew JP, Fontes ML, Tudor IC, et al. A multicenter risk index for atrial fibrillation after cardiac surgery. JAMA. 2004;291:1720–9.
Nagappa M, Mokhlesi B, Wong J, Wong DT, Kaw R, Chung F. The effects of continuous positive airway pressure on postoperative outcomes in obstructive sleep apnea patients undergoing surgery: a systematic review and meta-analysis. Anesthesia & Analgesia. 2015;120:1013–23.
Neilan TG, Farhad H, Dodson JA, et al. Effect of sleep apnea and continuous positive airway pressure on cardiac structure and recurrence of atrial fibrillation. J Am Heart Assoc. 2013;2, e000421.
Orban M, Bruce CJ, Pressman GS, et al. Dynamic changes of left ventricular performance and left atrial volume induced by the mueller maneuver in healthy young adults and implications for obstructive sleep apnea, atrial fibrillation, and heart failure. American Journal of Cardiology. 2008;102:1557–61.
Phan K, Ha HSK, Phan S, Medi C, Thomas SP, Yan TD. New-onset atrial fibrillation following coronary bypass surgery predicts long-term mortality: a systematic review and meta-analysis. Eur J Cardiothorac Surg. 2015;48:817–24.

Effect of postoperative positive airway pressure on risk of postoperative atrial fibrillation after cardiac...

47

Qaddoura A, Kabali C, Drew D, et al. Obstructive sleep apnea as a predictor of atrial fibrillation after coronary artery bypass grafting: a systematic review and meta-analysis. Can J Cardiol. 2014;30:1516–22.

Qureshi WT, Nasir UB, Alqalyoobi S, et al. Meta-analysis of continuous positive airway pressure as a therapy of atrial fibrillation in obstructive sleep apnea. Am J Cardiol. 2015;116:1767–73.

Stepnowsky CJ, Moore PJ. Improving CPAP use by patients with the sleep apnoea/hypopnoea syndrome (SAHS). Sleep Med Rev. 2003;7:445–6.

Stevenson IH, Roberts-Thomson KC, Kistler PM, et al. Atrial electrophysiology is altered by acute hypercapnia but not hypoxemia: Implications for promotion of atrial fibrillation in pulmonary disease and sleep apnea. Heart Rhythm. 2010;7:1263–70.

Uchôa CHG, Danzi-Soares NJ, Nunes FS, et al. Impact of OSA on cardiovascular events after coronary artery bypass surgery. Chest. 2015;147:1352–60.

van Oosten EM, Hamilton A, Petsikas D, et al. Effect of preoperative obstructive sleep apnea on the frequency of atrial fibrillation after coronary artery bypass grafting. Am J Cardiol. 2014;113:919–23.

Wong JK, Maxwell BG, Kushida CA, et al. Obstructive sleep apnea is an independent predictor of postoperative atrial fibrillation in cardiac surgery. J Cardiothorac Vasc Anesth. 2015;29:1140–7.

Xie XM, Pan L, Ren DQ, Du CJ, Guo YZ. Effects of continuous positive airway pressure therapy on systemic inflammation in obstructive sleep apnea: A meta-analysis. Sleep Med. 2013;14:1139–50.

Yadava M, Hughey AB, Crawford TC. Postoperative atrial fibrillation: incidence, mechanisms, and clinical correlates. Cardiol Clin. 2014;32:627–36.

Zhao L-P, Kofidis T, Lim T-W, et al. Sleep apnea is associated with new-onset atrial fibrillation after coronary artery bypass grafting. J Crit Care. 2015;30: 1418. e1-5.

7

Sleep and mild cognitive impairment

Erin L. Cassidy-Eagle[1] and Allison Siebern[2*]

Abstract

Older adults frequently suffer from sleep disturbances. In addition, with increasing age such disturbances may accompany mild cognitive changes that are symptomatic of a range of neurodegenerative conditions. There is increasing evidence that sleep may represent a prodromal symptom, risk factor or agitator of further decline in cognitive functioning of the older adult. Current research is focused on understanding the impact that effective sleep treatments have on a range of psychological and cognitive variables.

Background

Given the challenges posed by changing life circumstances and the accumulation of threats to physical health in later life, it is no surprise that almost 40% of those age 65 and older report experiencing some form of sleep disruption and as many as 70% of older adults suffer from four or more comorbid illnesses (Foley et al. 2004). The U.S. population of those age 65 and older is currently estimated at 40 million and this population is projected to double in the next 30 years underscoring the importance of attention and further research on geriatric sleep and treatments for common disturbances.

There are age dependent changes that occur and involve changes in the continuity, depth, and distribution of sleep. Age in itself does not necessarily equate to sleep disturbance but rather the interplay between health and psychosocial status in conjunction with the developmental changes combine to impact an older adult's sleep. There is a shift towards advance phase sleep leading to earlier bedtimes and wake times that starts during middle age (Buysse et al. 2005). Additional developmental changes in sleep include an increase in sleep fragmentation related to increase in N1 sleep architecture, a lighter sleep stage, at the expense of a decrease in N3 deep sleep (Dijk & Czeisler 1995). In the sleep regulatory system, N3 sleep is related to an increase in homeostatic pressure that builds throughout the day and in younger adults leads to shorter sleep onset and deep sleep the first half of the night of sleep (Cajochen et al. 2006). Following adolescence we experience a progressive decline in our amount of deep sleep with each passing decade. For those 65 and older there is very little deep sleep, contributing to an increase in sleep latency, increased awakenings after sleep onset, and decrease in sleep efficiency.

These changes, in combination with decreases in daytime activity levels, declines in health status and an increase in prescriptions to treat emerging health issues, can ultimately result in significant sleep disruptions and daytime symptoms, as well as compensatory behaviors, such as daytime napping (Bliwise et al. 2005). The prevalence rate of sleep disorders in older adults, such as obstructive sleep apnea is estimated 7% in women and 18% in men, periodic limb movement disorder at 3%, restless legs syndrome at 8%, can impact the quality and quantity of sleep and leave the older adult at risk for the development of insomnia (Bixler et al. 1998; Ohayon & Roth 2002). Insomnia is the most common sleep disorder across the lifespan and is estimated to be 35–40% in those age 65 and older (Foley et al. 1999). Insomnia is associated with negative consequences including depressive symptoms, decreased quality of life, increase in healthcare utilization and daytime impairment (Foley et al. 2004; Hatoum et al. 1998). There is cross sectional evidence that insomnia is related to an increased risk for dementia (de Almondes et al. 2016). McKinnon, et al. (McKinnon et al. 2014) and colleagues have found that depression symptoms, impaired cognition, antidepressant use, alcohol consumption, in addition to age and education, were all significant predictors of poor sleep quality. Not only does poor sleep negatively impact one's quality of life, studies have revealed that older individuals with both long and short sleep duration have increased rates of all-cause mortality (da Silva et al. 2016).

* Correspondence: ecassidy@stanford.edu
[2]Sleep Health Integrative Program Fayetteville NC Veterans Affairs Medical Center, Stanford University School of Medicine, Stanford, CA, USA
Full list of author information is available at the end of the article

Mild cognitive impairment- what is it?

Mild cognitive impairment (MCI) is the transitional state between intact cognitive functioning and dementia. The most common diagnostic criteria was proposed by Petersen (Petersen 2004), and includes those with a decline in cognitive functioning, while controlling for their particular age and education level, combined with a relatively intact performance in activities of daily living. Further subtypes have also been delineated, to specify impairment that is primarily due to memory impairment (amnestic MCI; aMCI) and impairment in cognitive domains other than memory (nonamnestic MCI; naMCI) (Petersen 2004).

Rates of conversion from MCI to dementia is at about 10–15% per year (Petersen et al. 2001). Because the identification of those in this transitional stage (between normal cognition and mild cognitive impairment) can be difficult, clinical symptoms and biomarkers that characterize this stage, including a range of neuropsychiatric symptoms such as sleep disturbance, depression and apathy, may be helpful in identifying patients that may be at an increased risk for continued decline. Sleep disturbances are one of the most common neuropsychiatric symptoms and appear to signal individuals at greater risk of conversion to dementia. This is particularly relevant given the high prevalence of sleep issues in older adults with mild cognitive impairment, with studies detecting rates that range from 14 to 59% (Beaulieu-Bonneau & Hudon 2009), and some as high as 63% (McKinnon et al. 2014), who report experiencing poor sleep quality.

Relationship between sleep and cognitive functioning

Although some sleep parameters change with normal aging as stated above, such changes are more prevalent and severe in individuals suffering from cognitive impairment, including those with preclinical signs and symptoms and those with detectable impairment, such as MCI (Lyketsos et al. 2002; Muangpaisan et al. 2008; Ramakers et al. 2010), and there is growing evidence for a shared neurodegenerative etiology. Sleep disturbances in quality and quantity of sleep, as well as disruption of the sleep-wake rhythm, occur frequently in older adults with cognitive impairment and there is growing support for a bidirectional relationship (Guarnieri & Sorbi 2015). Studies looking at cognitive functioning have linked sleep disturbance prospectively to the emergence of cognitive deficits (Beaulieu-Bonneau & Hudon 2009), and have identified sleep issues as part of a prodromal syndrome of various neurodegenerative diseases (Postuma et al. 2009). Sleep disturbance may also represent an early marker or a risk factor for cognitive decline. For example, a study by Diem, et al. (Diem et al. 2016) found that lower sleep efficiency and longer sleep latencies in older women were associated with a 1.5 and 1.4 greater odds of developing MCI or dementia within five years. In addition, worsening sleep problems are often observed to occur in conjunction with deteriorating cognitive symptoms (Moe et al. 1995), raising the question of whether they each play a part in fueling the other.

Studies on sleep and cognitive functioning have concluded that there is a strong relationship between disturbed sleep and an increased risk for cognitive impairment and dementia (Lim et al. 2013). Contributing to this idea, alterations in sleep architecture have been found in those with MCI and appear to negatively impact memory consolidation (Westerberg et al. 2012), which is believed to contribute to declines in memory functioning. Further support for this hypothesis comes from a study that tested the impact of artificially improving slow-wave sleep in older adults to determine if it would improve their subsequent performance on memory tests, when compared to a sham control group. Initial findings have found that the use of transcranial current oscillating at a slow frequency in the treatment group during sleep resulted in an improved performance on memory tests before and after the sleep period (Westerberg et al. 2015).

Sleep has been found to have strong ties to changes in the brain associated with neurodegenerative diseases. A recent study by Varga, et al. (Varga et al. 2016) found higher levels of amyloid beta in the brain, the deposition of which remains a hallmark of Alzheimer's Disease (AD), which are associated with reduced and fragmented slow-wave sleep. Further, the daytime sleepiness and nighttime experience of parasomnias, such a rapid eye movement (REM) behavior disorder (RBD), observed in association with Lewy Body and Parkinson's related dementia, provide yet another example of disturbed sleep's connection to cognitive impairment. Naismith, et al. (Naismith et al. 2014) found that circadian misalignment, and specifically advanced timing of melatonin secretion, were evident in MCI patients and also associated with disturbed sleep and poor performance on memory tests.

Clinically, neuropsychiatric symptoms, also referred to as behavioral and psychological symptoms of dementia (BPSD), are more prevalent in individuals with MCI than their counterparts with normal cognition, specifically, depression, sleep disturbances and apathy (Kohler et al. 2016), and often impact individuals quality of life. A study by Yu, et al. (Yu et al. 2016) studied individuals with MCI and found that the sleep parameters measured (e.g., sleep latency, disturbances, duration and efficiency) were worse in those with MCI, even when analyses controlled for clinical levels of anxiety and depression.

Sleep plays a crucial role in learning and memory across the lifespan (Poe et al. 2010), and thus is it not surprising that it is also associated with the decline in cognitive functioning. Several prospective studies have linked several sleep disturbances to a range of cognitive deficits and impaired performance, including measures assessing areas such as memory, attention, executive functioning and problems solving skills [see excellent review of studies in Yaffe, et al. (Yaffe et al. 2014)]. It appears that this connection between sleep disturbance and MCI is strong, regardless of MCI subtype. Naismith, et al. (Naismith et al. 2010) looked at a small group of individuals with the nonamnestic subtype of MCI and found that objectively assessed disturbed sleep was associated with impaired attention and executive functioning, while increased arousals during rest were related to poorer nonverbal learning and problem solving.

Questions under study in this area

Assessing sleep in older adults could help in the identification of those at risk for cognitive decline. In addition, sleep may be a target that, when treated, could alter the trajectory of cognitive decline, thereby providing a relatively efficient and cost-effective treatment that would positively impact outcomes of a large number of patients.

It may also be that targeting other factors that impact sleep may ultimately impact cognitive functioning as well. For example, given the connection of depression and antidepressant use to sleep quality in MCI (McKinnon et al. 2014), researchers have made the case that treating depression may also have a broader impact on individual functioning.

Our research

One key question, under investigation by our group, is whether established treatments can be successfully used with individuals who have both impaired sleep and MCI. Due to concerns of polypharmacy, cognitive impairment effects, and risk of falls with the use of sleep medications in older adults the use of nonpharmacological treatments, specifically cognitive behavioral therapy for insomnia (CBT-I), is an effective and optimal treatment choice for those with late life insomnia. CBT-I treatment outcomes have not been shown to be age related and are comparable to younger and middle aged adults (Morin et al. 1994; Morin et al. 2006). Significant improvements with CBT-I treatment have been seen in sleep quality, time to sleep onset, time awake after sleep onset, and sleep efficiency for those 55 and older (Irwin et al. 2006). Older adults with insomnia found CBT-I to be a more acceptable form of treatment, have less side effects, more beneficial for daytime functioning, and long-term effectiveness over pharmacotherapy for insomnia (Morin et al. 1992).

A CBT-I treatment was disseminated by a clinical psychologist to older adults with insomnia *and* MCI in two residential care facilities for the elderly (RCFEs). The study involved a two-arm individual randomization to 6 sessions of CBT-I intervention or six sessions of active control nutrition class. It was hypothesized that those that received the CBT-I intervention would experience improvement in assessed sleep parameters and, secondarily, positive changes in their performance on cognitive testing.

Participants were 28 older adults (mean age, 89.36 years), meeting the key inclusion criteria of meeting diagnostic criteria for insomnia according to the DSM-IV (APA 1994), and the core clinical criteria for MCI used by healthcare workers without access to advanced imaging techniques (Albert et al. 2011) (i.e., subject memory complaints, preservation of independence in functional abilities, performance on at least one of the cognitive tests at 1.5SD below published age/educational matched normative means, and not demented). In addition to having a positive effect on subjective (i.e., Insomnia Severity Index ratings) and objective ratings of several sleep parameters (i.e., improved sleep latency, wake after sleep onset, and sleep efficiency), we also found a positive improvement in the treatment group on an outcome measure of executive functioning (D-KEF Color-Word Interference Test) (Cassidy-Eagle et al. 2015). Deficits in executive processes (e.g., planning, problem solving), memory and language functions are, more frequently observed in MCI and are particularly important to assess in light of their potential impact on treatment given the cognitive processing involved in CBT. Nonpharmacological interventions such as CBT-I may be beneficial for people with MCI. Further study of CBT-I in people with MCI is warranted. Such research should include pre- and post-intervention measures of cognitive functions. Targeting of sleep has the potential to have broad public health impact, including in people with MCI.

Future opportunities

Over the entire trajectory of cognitive decline, does sleep play a role in causing or exacerbating cognitive impairment and/or is it the result of cognitive decline? In addition to studies that will further elucidate the neuronal overlap and causal mechanisms in these conditions, more work in this area is needed as the results could be incredibly useful in designing effective, personalized treatments.

There are many possible targets for intervention that merit further study and consideration for their potential role in preventing or slowing cognitive decline experienced by older adults. Given the impact of various medications, non-pharmacological interventions are of great interest. Exercise, increased socialization, bright-light therapy, and CBT-I all show promise and merit additional study. Naismith, et al. (Naismith et al. 2014) and colleagues have called for more focused studies on the potential use of supplemental melatonin as a potentially effective treatment of sleep-wake disorders in those with MCI. Treating older patients with sleep apnea with continuous positive airway pressure (CPAP) devices could also slow down or delay further the deterioration in cognitive functioning observed in MCI and AD (Yaffe et al. 2011; Canessa & Ferini-Strambi 2011).

Access to effective treatments is also a growing concern that needs to be addressed. Sleep disturbances in older adults are commonly addressed by sleep specialists. Given the shortage of clinicians specializing in assessing and treating sleep difficulties, it is imperative that sleep be evaluated routinely in other clinical settings and that alternative implementation models, such as using sleep coaches (Alessi et al. 2016), be considered to reach more patients in need of effective treatments. Given the high prevalence of sleep disturbances, assessments need to be incorporated in regular health checks and referrals made for a thorough diagnostic workup when disturbances are reported, particularly given the evidence that it may represent a prodromal state of dementia. Future work also needs to include prospective studies that utilize both subjective and objective measures of sleep parameters, in order to confirm or challenge studies to date that support a relationship between self-reported sleep disturbances (e.g., sleep quality or quantity measures).

Conclusions

Although challenging, sleep represents a clear, easily identified and measured, modifiable risk factor that plays a significant role in neurodegenerative conditions and has the potential to significantly impact the consequences of several major public health problems.

Acknowledgements
Not applicable.

Funding
The research summarized in this manuscript, including the support needed to carry out the interventions and analyze the findings, was supported by Grant #2012-199 from the Retirement Research Foundation.

Authors' contributions
Both ECE and AS contributed to the conceptualization, writing and research summarized in this review/manuscript. Both authors read and approved the final manuscript.

Competing interests
The authors declare that they have no competing interests.

Author details
[1]Department of Psychiatry and Behavioral Sciences, Stanford University School of Medicine, Stanford, CA, USA. [2]Sleep Health Integrative Program Fayetteville NC Veterans Affairs Medical Center, Stanford University School of Medicine, Stanford, CA, USA.

References
Albert MS, DeKosky ST, Dickson D, et al. The diagnosis of mild cognitive impairment due to Alzheimer's disease: recommendations from the National Institute on Aging-Alzheimer's Association workgroups on diagnostic guidelines for Alzheimer's disease. Alzheimers Dement. 2011;7(3):270–9. doi:10.1016/j.jalz.2011.03.008 [published Online First: Epub Date].

Alessi C, Martin JL, Fiorentino L, et al. Cognitive behavioral therapy for insomnia in older veterans using nonclinician sleep coaches: randomized controlled trial. J Am Geriatr Soc. 2016;64(9):1830–8. doi:10.1111/jgs.14304 [published Online First: Epub Date].

APA APA. Diagnostic and statistical manual of mental of mental disorders, Fourth Edition (DSM-IV). Washington, D.C.: American Psychiatric Association; 1994.

Beaulieu-Bonneau S, Hudon C. Sleep disturbances in older adults with mild cognitive impairment. Int Psychogeriatr. 2009;21(4):654–66. doi:10.1017/S1041610209009120 [published Online First: Epub Date].

Bixler EO, Vgontzas AN, Ten Have T, Tyson K, Kales A. Effects of age on sleep apnea in men: I. Prevalence and severity. Am J Respir Crit Care Med. 1998;157(1):144–8. doi:10.1164/ajrccm.157.1.9706079 [published Online First: Epub Date].

Bliwise DL, Ansari FP, Straight LB, Parker KP. Age changes in timing and 24-hour distribution of self-reported sleep. Am J Geriatr Psychiatry. 2005;13(12):1077–82. doi:10.1176/appi.ajgp.13.12.1077 [published Online First: Epub Date].

Buysse DJ, Monk TH, Carrier J, Begley A. Circadian patterns of sleep, sleepiness, and performance in older and younger adults. Sleep. 2005;28(11):1365–76.

Cajochen C, Munch M, Knoblauch V, Blatter K, Wirz-Justice A. Age-related changes in the circadian and homeostatic regulation of human sleep. Chronobiol Int. 2006;23(1–2):461–74. doi:10.1080/07420520500545813 [published Online First: Epub Date].

Canessa N, Ferini-Strambi L. Sleep-disordered breathing and cognitive decline in older adults. JAMA. 2011;306(6):654–5. doi:10.1001/jama.2011.1124 [published Online First: Epub Date].

Cassidy-Eagle E, Siebern A, Unti L, Glassman J, O'Hara R. Treating insomnia in older adults with mild cognitive impairment in residential care settings. Seattle: Associated Professional Sleep Societies; 2015.

da Silva AA, de Mello RG, Schaan CW, Fuchs FD, Redline S, Fuchs SC. Sleep duration and mortality in the elderly: a systematic review with meta-analysis. BMJ Open. 2016;6(2):e008119. doi:10.1136/bmjopen-2015-008119 [published Online First: Epub Date].

de Almondes KM, Costa MV, Malloy-Diniz LF, Diniz BS. Insomnia and risk of dementia in older adults: systematic review and meta-analysis. J Psychiatr Res. 2016;77:109–15. doi:10.1016/j.jpsychires.2016.02.021 [published Online First: Epub Date].

Diem SJ, Blackwell TL, Stone KL, et al. Measures of sleep-wake patterns and risk of mild cognitive impairment or dementia in older women. Am J Geriatr Psychiatry. 2016;24(3):248–58. doi:10.1016/j.jagp.2015.12.002 [published Online First: Epub Date].

Dijk DJ, Czeisler CA. Contribution of the circadian pacemaker and the sleep homeostat to sleep propensity, sleep structure, electroencephalographic slow waves, and sleep spindle activity in humans. J Neurosci. 1995;15(5 Pt 1): 3526–38.

Foley DJ, Monjan A, Simonsick EM, Wallace RB, Blazer DG. Incidence and remission of insomnia among elderly adults: an epidemiologic study of 6,800 persons over three years. Sleep. 1999;22 Suppl 2:S366–72.

Foley D, Ancoli-Israel S, Britz P, Walsh J. Sleep disturbances and chronic disease in older adults: results of the 2003 National Sleep Foundation Sleep in America Survey. J Psychosom Res. 2004;56(5):497–502. doi:10.1016/j.jpsychores.2004.02.010. published Online First: Epub Date.

Guarnieri B, Sorbi S. Sleep and cognitive decline: a strong bidirectional relationship. It is time for specific recommendations on routine assessment and the management of sleep disorders in patients with mild cognitive impairment and dementia. Eur Neurol. 2015;74(1-2):43–8. doi:10.1159/000434629 [published Online First: Epub Date].

Hatoum HT, Kong SX, Kania CM, Wong JM, Mendelson WB. Insomnia, health-related quality of life and healthcare resource consumption. A study of managed-care organisation enrollees. Pharmacoeconomics. 1998;14(6): 629–37.

Irwin MR, Cole JC, Nicassio PM. Comparative meta-analysis of behavioral interventions for insomnia and their efficacy in middle-aged adults and in older adults 55+ years of age. Health Psychol. 2006;25(1):3–14. doi:10.1037/0278-6133.25.1.3 [published Online First: Epub Date].

Kohler CA, Magalhaes TF, Oliveira JM, et al. Neuropsychiatric disturbances in Mild Cognitive Impairment (MCI): a systematic review of population-based studies. Curr Alzheimer Res. 2016;13(10):1066–82.

Lim AS, Kowgier M, Yu L, Buchman AS, Bennett DA. Sleep fragmentation and the risk of incident Alzheimer's disease and cognitive decline in older persons. Sleep. 2013;36(7):1027–32. doi:10.5665/sleep.2802 [published Online First: Epub Date].

Lyketsos CG, Lopez O, Jones B, Fitzpatrick AL, Breitner J, DeKosky S. Prevalence of neuropsychiatric symptoms in dementia and mild cognitive impairment: results from the cardiovascular health study. JAMA. 2002;288(12):1475–83.

McKinnon A, Terpening Z, Hickie IB, et al. Prevalence and predictors of poor sleep quality in mild cognitive impairment. J Geriatr Psychiatry Neurol. 2014; 27(3):204–11. doi:10.1177/0891988714527516 [published Online First: Epub Date].

Moe KE, Vitiello MV, Larsen LH, Prinz PN. Symposium: cognitive processes and sleep disturbances: sleep/wake patterns in Alzheimer's disease: relationships with cognition and function. J Sleep Res. 1995;4(1):15–20.

Morin CM, Gaulier B, Barry T, Kowatch RA. Patients' acceptance of psychological and pharmacological therapies for insomnia. Sleep. 1992;15(4):302–5.

Morin CM, Culbert JP, Schwartz SM. Nonpharmacological interventions for insomnia: a meta-analysis of treatment efficacy. Am J Psychiatry. 1994;151(8): 1172–80. doi:10.1176/ajp.151.8.1172 [published Online First: Epub Date].

Morin CM, Bootzin RR, Buysse DJ, Edinger JD, Espie CA, Lichstein KL. Psychological and behavioral treatment of insomnia:update of the recent evidence (1998-2004). Sleep. 2006;29(11):1398–414.

Muangpaisan W, Intalapaporn S, Assantachai P. Neuropsychiatric symptoms in the community-based patients with mild cognitive impairment and the influence of demographic factors. Int J Geriatr Psychiatry. 2008;23(7):699–703. doi:10.1002/gps.1963 [published Online First: Epub Date].

Naismith SL, Rogers NL, Hickie IB, Mackenzie J, Norrie LM, Lewis SJ. Sleep well, think well: sleep-wake disturbance in mild cognitive impairment. J Geriatr Psychiatry Neurol. 2010;23(2):123–30. doi:10.1177/0891988710363710 [published Online First: Epub Date].

Naismith SL, Hickie IB, Terpening Z, et al. Circadian misalignment and sleep disruption in mild cognitive impairment. J Alzheimers Dis. 2014;38(4):857–66. doi:10.3233/JAD-131217 [published Online First: Epub Date].

Ohayon MM, Roth T. Prevalence of restless legs syndrome and periodic limb movement disorder in the general population. J Psychosom Res. 2002; 53(1):547–54.

Petersen RC. Mild cognitive impairment as a diagnostic entity. J Intern Med. 2004;256(3):183–94. doi:10.1111/j.1365-2796.2004.01388.x [published Online First: Epub Date].

Petersen RC, Doody R, Kurz A, et al. Current concepts in mild cognitive impairment. Arch Neurol. 2001;58(12):1985–92.

Poe GR, Walsh CM, Bjorness TE. Cognitive neuroscience of sleep. Prog Brain Res. 2010;185:1–19. doi:10.1016/B978-0-444-53702-7.00001-4 [published Online First: Epub Date].

Postuma RB, Gagnon JF, Vendette M, Fantini ML, Massicotte-Marquez J, Montplaisir J. Quantifying the risk of neurodegenerative disease in idiopathic REM sleep behavior disorder. Neurology. 2009;72(15):1296–300. doi:10.1212/01.wnl.0000340980.19702.6e [published Online First: Epub Date].

Ramakers IH, Visser PJ, Aalten P, Kester A, Jolles J, Verhey FR. Affective symptoms as predictors of Alzheimer's disease in subjects with mild cognitive impairment: a 10-year follow-up study. Psychol Med. 2010;40(7):1193–201. doi:10.1017/S0033291709991577 [published Online First: Epub Date].

Varga AW, Wohlleber ME, Gimenez S, et al. Reduced slow-wave sleep is associated with high cerebrospinal fluid Abeta42 levels in cognitively normal elderly. Sleep. 2016;39(11):2041–8.

Westerberg CE, Mander BA, Florczak SM, et al. Concurrent impairments in sleep and memory in amnestic mild cognitive impairment. J Int Neuropsychol Soc. 2012;18(3):490–500. doi:10.1017/S135561771200001X [published Online First: Epub Date].

Westerberg CE, Florczak SM, Weintraub S, et al. Memory improvement via slow-oscillatory stimulation during sleep in older adults. Neurobiol Aging. 2015; 36(9):2577–86. doi:10.1016/j.neurobiolaging.2015.05.014 [published Online First: Epub Date].

Yaffe K, Laffan AM, Harrison SL, et al. Sleep-disordered breathing, hypoxia, and risk of mild cognitive impairment and dementia in older women. JAMA. 2011;306(6): 613–9. doi:10.1001/jama.2011.1115 [published Online First: Epub Date].

Yaffe K, Falvey CM, Hoang T. Connections between sleep and cognition in older adults. Lancet Neurol. 2014;13(10):1017–28. doi:10.1016/S1474-4422(14)70172-3 [published Online First: Epub Date].

Yu J, Mahendran R, Rawtaer I, Kua EH, Feng L. Poor sleep quality is observed in mild cognitive impairment and is largely unrelated to depression and anxiety. Aging Ment Health. 2016;1–6. doi:10.1080/13607863.2016.1161007 [published Online First: Epub Date].

8

Distinct polysomnographic and ECG-spectrographic phenotypes embedded within obstructive sleep apnea

Robert Joseph Thomas[1]*, Chol Shin[2], Matt Travis Bianchi[3], Clete Kushida[4] and Chang-Ho Yun[5]

Abstract

Background: The primary metric extracted from the polysomnogram in patients with sleep apnea is the apnea-hypopnea index (or respiratory disturbance index) and its derivatives. Other phenomena of possible importance such as periods of stable breathing, features suggestive of high respiratory control loop gain, and sleep fragmentation phenotypes are not commonly generated in clinical practice or research. A broader phenotype designation can provide insights into biological processes, and possibly clinical therapy outcome effects.

Methods: The dataset used for this study was the archived baseline diagnostic polysomnograms from the Apnea Positive Pressure Long-term Efficacy Study (APPLES). The electrocardiogram (ECG)-derived cardiopulmonary coupling sleep spectrogram was computed from the polysomnogram. Sleep fragmentation phenotypes used thresholds of sleep efficiency (SE) $\leq$ 70%, non-rapid eye movement (NREM) sleep N1 $\geq$ 30%, wake after sleep onset (WASO) $\geq$ 60 min, and high frequency coupling (HFC) on the ECG-spectrogram $\leq$ 30%. Sleep consolidation phenotypes used thresholds of SE $\geq$ 90%, WASO $\leq$ 30 min, HFC $\geq$ 50% and N1 $\leq$ 10%. Multiple and logistic regression analysis explored cross-sectional associations with covariates and across phenotype categories. NREM vs. REM dominant apnea categories were identified when the NREM divided by REM respiratory disturbance index (RDI) was > 1.

Results: The data was binned first into mild, moderate, severe and extreme categories based on the respiratory disturbance index of < 10, 10–30, 30–60, and greater than 60, per hour of sleep. Using these criteria, 70, 394, 320 and 188 for polysomnogram, and 54, 296, 209 and 112 subjects for ECG-spectrogram analysis groups. All phenotypes were seen at all severity levels. There was a higher correlation of NREM-RDI with the amount of ECG-spectrogram narrow band coupling, vs. REM-RDI, 0.41 vs 0.14, respectively. NREM dominance was associated with male gender and higher mixed/central apnea indices. Absence of the ECG-spectrogram sleep consolidated phenotype was associated with an increased odds of being on antihypertensive medications, OR 2.65 [CI: 1.64–4.26], $p = $ < 0.001.

Conclusions: Distinct phenotypes are readily seen at all severities of sleep apnea, and can be identified from conventional polysomnography. The ECG-spectrogram analysis provides further phenotypic differentiation.

Keywords: Sleep apnea, Phenotypes, NREM-dominant, Sleep fragmentation, ECG-spectrogram, Cardiopulmonary coupling

* Correspondence: rthomas1@bidmc.harvard.edu
[1]Division of Pulmonary, Critical Care, and Sleep Medicine, Beth Israel Deaconess Medical Center, Boston, MA, USA
Full list of author information is available at the end of the article

Background

Traditional sleep apnea morphological categories include obstructive, central, and periodic breathing/Cheyne-Stokes respiration types. Conventionally, polysomnogram (PSG) recordings are scored using 30 s epochs, into wake, rapid eye movement (REM) and non-rapid eye movement (NREM) stages. Respiratory events may be dominant in NREM or REM sleep, and at times be equally severe in both states. These events can be short, as at high altitude (25 s or less), or long, as in congestive heart failure (often over 60 s). NREM stages are further characterized into grades, N1 through N3. Alternate methods of characterizing sleep include cyclic alternating pattern (CAP) of NREM sleep (Parrino et al. 2014), and cardiopulmonary coupling (high, low and very low frequency coupling of autonomic and respiratory drives, modulated by cortical delta power) (Thomas et al. 2014). Periods of stable breathing are usually associated with N3, and always associated with non-CAP and high frequency coupling.

The apnea-hypopnea index is the result of distinct interacting biological processes, all of which can contribute to the severity of clinical sleep apnea individually and collectively. These are high loop gain, low arousal threshold, airway collapsibility, and reduced negative pressure reflex response (Owens et al. 2015; Wellman et al. 2013; Eckert et al. 2013). A computational method to derive loop gain from routine PSG data was recently proposed, based on the concept that ventilatory fluctuations from apneas/hypopneas cause opposing changes in ventilatory drive according to the loop gain (Terrill et al. 2015). It would be more useful in clinical practice if there were features on the conventional PSG or metrics computed from PSG signals which differentiated phenotypes that could guide therapy. Specifically, a high loop gain phenotype may benefit from supplemental oxygen (Wellman et al. 2008), acetazolamide (Edwards et al. 2012), or hypocapnia minimization strategies, while sedatives could be an option in those who have low arousal thresholds in NREM sleep (Smales et al. 2015).

The conventional scoring criteria for central hypopnea strongly skews the events index to obstruction-most importantly, flow-limitation is frequently seen in periodic breathing, even at high altitude (Weiss et al. 2009), a quintessential model of high loop gain sleep apnea. High loop gain apnea is NREM dominant, regardless of the admixed obstructive features (Xie et al. 2011). Quantifying NREM vs. REM dominance may thus provide a pathophysiological phenotype. The oscillatory profile of respiratory oscillations or downstream respiration-driven or associated oscillations such as heart rate variability, blood pressure or even the electroencephalogram can be quantified (Maestri et al. 2010). We present use of a ECG-derived cardiopulmonary coupling analysis to detect high loop gain apnea independent of conventional scoring.

Respiration is stable during conventional slow wave sleep. The state of the cortical sleep network seems important (Thomas 2002). Increased genioglossus tone and increases in CO_2 occur during periods of stable breathing (Jordan et al. 2009), with overt hypoventilation and hypoxia if flow limitation is severe during stable breathing periods. Central sleep apnea, periodic breathing, and treatment-emergent/complex apnea are NREM sleep phenomena. Stable breathing periods have traditionally not been quantified-the focus has been on the various thresholds and associations to determine clinically significant apnea or hypopnea. We quantified stable breathing using the ECG-based cardiopulmonary coupling technique, as described below. Stable breathing periods in apnea patients will likely demonstrate increased upper airway resistance. Despite the strong link between stable breathing and stage N3, the relationship is not exclusive: specifically, most periods of stable breathing occur in stage N2, even in those patients with no scored N3 sleep.

It is a common clinical observation that some patients with sleep apnea have disproportionate sleep fragmentation, and some with severe apnea demonstrate relatively intact macro-architecture of sleep. We used a well characterized sleep apnea clinical trial dataset, the Apnea Positive Pressure Long-term Efficacy Study (APPLES) (Kushida et al. 2006), to determine if at every severity of sleep apnea, discernable sleep and sleep apnea phenotypes exist. We used conventional polysomnogram metrics complemented with an electrocardiogram (ECG)-based analysis that can detect periods of stable breathing (Thomas et al. 2005) and pathological respiratory chemoreflex activation (Thomas et al. 2007a).

Methods

Database

The APPLES data was obtained in Alice™ and European Data Format, the latter was used for ECG-spectrogram analysis. He study randomized just over 1000 subjects to continuous positive airway pressure (CPAP) or placebo CPAP. A total of 972 baseline diagnostic polysomnograms were obtained; a subset of the data was embargoed by the primary study for administrative reasons. The following subjective and objective measures of sleepiness, mood and cognition were available: Hamilton Depression Scale, Epworth Sleepiness Scale, Stanford Sleepiness Scale, Paced Auditory Serial Addition Test, Psychomotor Vigilance Test Median and Mean reaction times, Maintenance of Wakefulness Test, and Short Term Working Memory.

Polysomnogram scoring

Standard scoring was done based on pre-2007 criteria on the polysomnogram data, generating respiratory, arousal, and sleep stage indices. The respiratory disturbance index used in the APPLES is equivalent to the current hypopnea definition with a 3% oxygen desaturation and/or arousal (Berry, 2017). We combined stage III and IV as the equivalent of current stage N3 (slow wave sleep). In this paper, we use the current terminology and designations to keep with current terms used in publications, though stage N1 and N2 will show some differences, typically greater N1, if the data were re-scored. A breakdown of REM and NREM RDI was also available. The characteristics of the full study population have also been published (Kushida et al. 2006; Quan et al. 2011). NREM vs. REM dominance was computed as the ratio of NREM/REM RDI; a value > 1 was considered NREM dominance.

ECG-spectrogram analysis

The cardiopulmonary coupling (CPC) analysis (Figs. 1 and 2) of the ECG signal was performed as previously described in detail (Thomas et al. 2005). Briefly, heart rate variability and ECG-derived respiration (EDR; amplitude variations in the QRS complex due to shifts in the cardiac electrical axis relative to the electrodes during respiration and changes in thoracic impedance as the lungs fill and empty) are extracted from a single channel of ECG. Time series of normal-to-normal sinus (N-N) intervals and the time series of the EDR

associated with these NN intervals are then extracted from the original R-R (QRS to QRS) interval time series. Outliers due to false or missed R-wave detections are removed using a sliding window average filter with a window of 41 data points and rejection of central points lying outside 20% of the window average. The resulting NN interval series and its associated EDR are then resampled using cubic splines at 2 Hz. The cross-spectral power and coherence of these two signals are calculated over a 1024 sample (8.5 min) window using the Fast Fourier Transform applied to the 3 overlapping 512 sample sub-windows within the 1024 coherence window. The 1024 coherence window is then advanced by 256 samples (2.1 min) and the calculation repeated until the entire NN interval/EDR series is analyzed. For each 1024 window the product of the coherence and cross-spectral power is used to calculate the ratio of coherent cross power in the low frequency (0.01–0.1 Hz.) band to that in the high frequency (0.1–0.4 Hz.) band. The logarithm of the high to low frequency cardiopulmonary coupling ratio (log [HFC/LFC]) is then computed to yield a continuously varying measure of cardiopulmonary coupling. The graph of the amplitude of cardiopulmonary coupling at relevant frequencies (ordinate) vs. time (abscissa) provides a sleep spectrogram. Since the period of central apnea

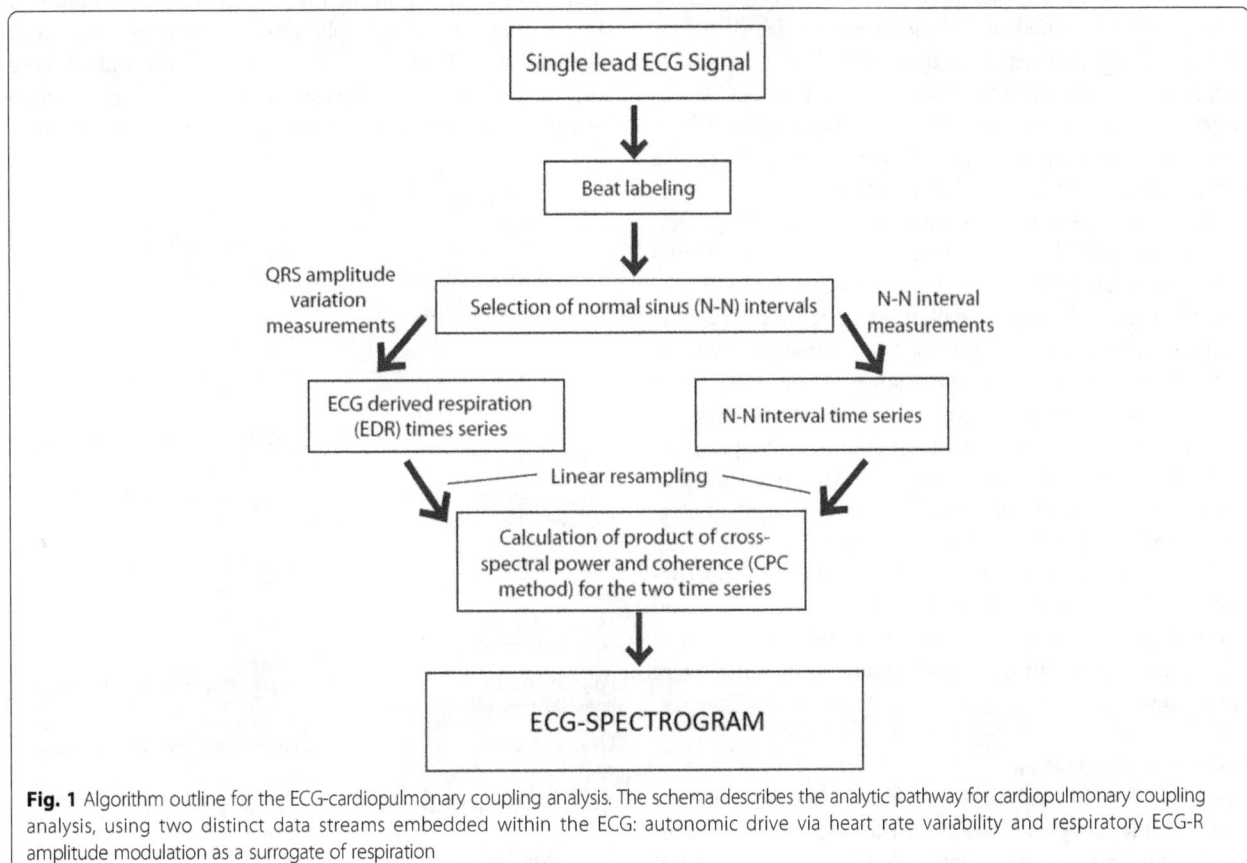

Fig. 1 Algorithm outline for the ECG-cardiopulmonary coupling analysis. The schema describes the analytic pathway for cardiopulmonary coupling analysis, using two distinct data streams embedded within the ECG: autonomic drive via heart rate variability and respiratory ECG-R amplitude modulation as a surrogate of respiration

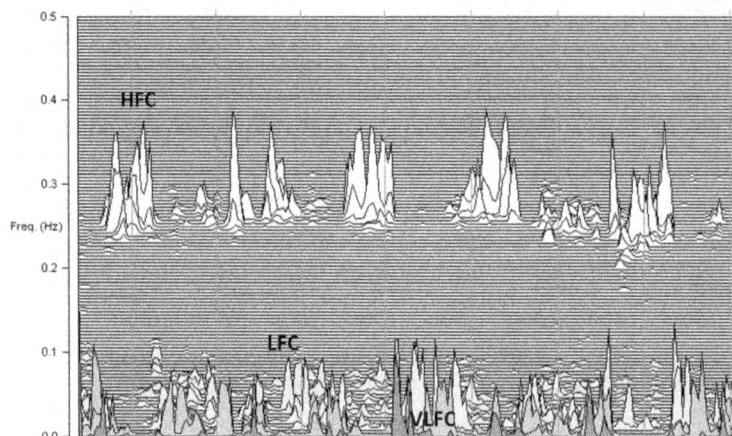

Fig. 2 Sample ECG-spectrogram. Note high, low and very low frequency coupling (HFC, LFC and VLFC respectively) and the clear separation in signal space of HFC from LFC/VLFC. HFC is the ECG-spectrogram signal biomarker of stable breathing and stable sleep. VLFC reflects REM or wake

can be as slow as 120 s or longer, we used the frequency band between 0.006 and 0.1 Hz to define narrow spectral band e-LFC (putative central sleep apnea, periodic breathing, or complex sleep apnea). We required (1) a minimum power in this band of 0.3 normalized units and (2) that the coupling frequency of each pair of consecutive measurements remains within 0.0059 Hz of each other over 5 consecutive sampling windows (totaling 17 continuous min). Periods of e-LFC not meeting these criteria were defined as broad spectral band e-LFC (putative pure obstructive sleep apnea). The amounts of broad and narrow spectral band coupling in e-LFC bands were then expressed as the percentage of windows detected in relation to the total sleep period. Thus, the narrow spectral band e-LFC identified periods with oscillations that have a single dominant coupling frequency, suggesting central sleep apnea or periodic breathing (Thomas et al. 2007a). The broad spectral band e-LFC identified periods with oscillations that have variable coupling frequencies, suggesting an alternative mechanism, which we posited was dominance of anatomic upper airway obstructive processes. As it takes 17 min of continuous narrow-band cardiopulmonary coupling to reach the detection threshold, we estimated that this would be approximately equal to an averaged central apnea index of 5/h of sleep, assuming 6 h of sleep and a periodic breathing cycle length of approximately 35 s. Finally, using the mean frequency and percentage of total sleep time in state, the LFC and e-LFC oscillation indices and mean cycle time were computed.

Phenotype designation

The data was binned first into mild, moderate, severe and extreme categories based on the respiratory disturbance index (respiratory events scored with a 3-s arousal

or 4% oxygen desaturation) of < 10, 10–30, 30–60, and greater than 60, per hour of sleep. These severity groups were chosen to capture a range from mild to most severe. For example, ≥ 60 could be considered "extreme", but would be subsumed otherwise if ≥ 30 only was used as a "severe" cut off. Phenotype percentages were based on 972 and 617 subjects for polysomnographic and spectrographic phenotyping, respectively. Table 1 lists the criteria for the phenotypes. Figure 3 shows that individual phenotypes may or may not coexist. The criteria for a sleep fragmentation phenotype was based on clinical reasonableness, as no formal criteria exist. On a polysomnogram, a "fragmentation

Table 1 Phenotype Definitions

Phenotype	Phenotype criteria
Polysomnogram chemoreflex	Central apnea index $\geq$ 5/h of sleep
Spectrogram chemoreflex	Presence of narrow band elevated low frequency coupling
Polysomnogram fragmentation—SE	Sleep efficiency $\leq$ 70% total sleep time
Polysomnogram fragmentation—N1	NREM N1 $\geq$ 30% total sleep time
Polysomnogram fragmentation—WASO	Wake after sleep onset $\geq$ 60 min
Spectrogram fragmentation	High frequency coupling $\leq$ 30% total sleep time
Polysomnogram consolidation—SE	Sleep efficiency $\geq$ 90% total sleep time
Polysomnogram consolidation—N1	NREM N1 $\leq$ 10% total sleep time
Polysomnogram consolidation—WASO	Wake after sleep onset $\leq$ 30 min
Spectrogram consolidation	High frequency coupling $\geq$ 50% total sleep time

SE sleep efficiency; *N1* NREM stage 1; *WASO* wake after sleep onset

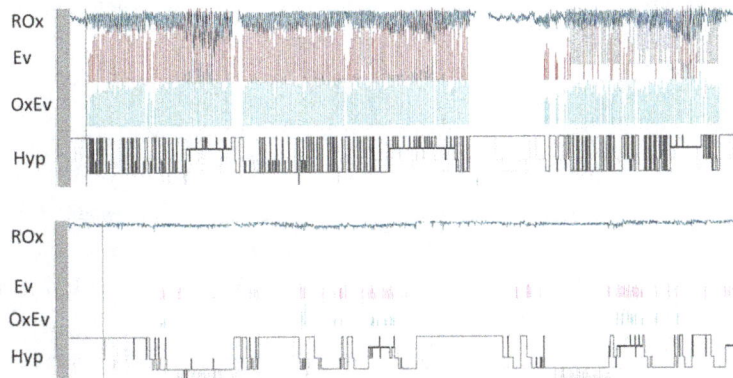

Fig. 3 Patterns of sleep fragmentation phenotype based on sleep efficiency. The upper hypnogram shows rapid sleep-wake transitions from severe sleep apnea, while the lower hypnogram shows nearly the same sleep efficiency but with consolidated periods of wake separated by consolidated periods of sleep. The % N1 is markedly increased in the patient with rapid transitions (44.2%). Thus, individual phenotypes can mix and match. ROx: raw oximetry. EV: respiratory events. OxEv: Oximetry desaturation events. Hyp: sleep stage hypnogram

phenotype" can be suggested by prolonged return to sleep following arousals/awakenings, low sleep efficiency (<70%), high N1, and high wake after sleep onset (Thomas 2014). There is too little N3 to be a useful discriminatory metric. We choose a high frequency coupling % of ≥ 50 and ≤ 30 as thresholds for consolidated and fragmented phenotypes, guided by data from healthy individuals (Thomas et al. 2005) and analysis of the Sleep Heart Health Study (Thomas et al. 2014; Thomas et al. 2009).

Statistical analysis

Summary measures were mean/standard deviations for continuous measures, and proportions for categorical measures. T-tests were used to assess differences between NREM and REM dominance ratios. Logistic Regression with adjustment for age, gender, BMI, ethnicity and overall RDI assessed Odds Ratios for different phenotypic categories, with the following predictor categories: central apnea index, presence/absence of narrow band coupling, and the ECG-spectrogram sleep fragmentation category. The full multiple regression model assessing associations of individual phenotypes adjusted for age, gender, ethnicity, body mass index and sleep apnea severity (RDI), and total sleep time for PSG-based metrics. Pearson's Correlation estimated relationships between ECG spectrogram and polysomnogram indices. Chi^2 test was used to assess significant differences of phenotypes across categories of apnea severity.

Results

Demographics and polysomnography

The demographic and polysomnographic characteristics of the subjects are described in Table 2, the 972 with polysomnogram and the 671 with ECG-spectrogram

analysis. There were no significant differences. Loss of ECG-spectrogram analysis occurred from the following reasons: 1) Movement artifact or gaps, including bathroom breaks, ≥ 10 min. Such dropouts made up the majority (86%) of lost data. 2) Signal drop out, e.g., displaced electrode. There were no significant differences between included and excluded subjects, in terms of demographics and clinical conditions such as hypertension and diabetes. Central sleep apnea, defined as CAI ≥ 5/h of sleep, was noted in 47/972 (5.1%) and 30/671 (4.5%), respectively.

ECG-spectrogram characteristics

Characteristics of the APPLES is described in Table 3. The mean cycle time calculated by the ECG spectrogram was just over 30 s. There was a higher correlation of NREM-RDI with the amount of narrow band coupling, vs. REM-RDI, 0.41 vs 0.14, respectively (Table 4).

Polysomnographic and spectrographic phenotypes

There were 70, 394, 320 and 188 subjects in the four categories of increasing severity (Tables 5 and 6). The corresponding sample size with the ECG-spectrogram was 54, 296, 209 and 112, respectively. The proportion of clinical phenotypes were different across severity in some but not all categories (Table 5). Specifically, the ECG-spectrogram categories did not show significant changes across severity, but the polysomnogram phenotype categories did. While no subject in the mild category had central sleep apnea, 8% did in the most severe category.

NREM vs. REM dominance

NREM dominance of sleep apnea was observed in 26.1% (242/671) of the cohort. The characteristics of the NREM vs. REM dominance groups are in Table 7. Notable features associated with NREM dominance are: 1)

Table 2 Polysomnographic and Demographic features

Demographics and Polysomnogram Metrics	Summary statistic (972) Mean ± SD	Summary statistic (671) Mean ± SD
Age	50.8 ± 12.9	50.2 ± 12.7 years
Gender	65.3% male	63.9% male
Race	70.2% white	71.7% white
Body Mass Index Kg/M²	31.8 ± 7.4	31 ± 7.1
Total sleep time (TST)	379.4 ± 66.6	385.1 ± 60.3
Sleep efficiency (% TST)	79 ± 12.6	80.1 ± 11.6%
Wake After Sleep Onset (minutes)	83.4 ± 51.8	78.3 ± 48.3
S1 (% TST)	18.3 ± 14.6	17.3 ± 13.1
S2 (% TST)	60.3 ± 13.4	60.9 ± 12.3
S3 (% TST)	2.7 ± 4.9	2.7 ± 4.9
S4 (% TST)	0.7 ± 2.4	0.7 ± 2.4
REM (% TST)	17.9 ± 7.1	18.2 ± 6.8
Arousal Index/hour of sleep	29 ± 21.7	27.6 ± 20.8
RDI/hour of sleep	38.8 ± 27.1	36.4 ± 26.1
Obstructive apnea index/ hour of sleep	16.9 ± 21.9	15.2 ± 20.2
Central apnea index/hour of sleep	1.1 ± 4.6	1.1 ± 4.9 (Median 0.1, 25th/75th percentile 0. 0.1)
Mixed apnea index/hour of sleep	1.5 ± 5.6	1.3 ± 4.8
Hypopnea index/hour of sleep	19.3 ± 13.2	18.9 ± 13
RDI-NREM/hour of sleep	37.4 ± 28.9	34.9 ± 27.9
RDI-REM/hour of sleep	43.2 ± 26.6	42.1 ± 26.5
Oxygen desaturation index/hour of sleep	25.5 ± 25.6	22.7 ± 24
Minimum saturation %	81 ± 9.1	81.7 ± 8.4
Time less than 85% saturation (minutes)	2.9 ± 8.2	2.4 ± 7.5
PLM/hour of sleep	6.4 ± 15.4	6 ± 15

RDI respiratory disturbance index; *REM* rapid eye movement; *NREM* non-rapid eye movement; *PLM* periodic limb movement

Table 3 ECG-spectrogram features in the APPLES

ECG-spectrogram metrics	Mean ± SD (n = 671)
High frequency coupling % TST	38.9 ± 22.3
High frequency coupling duration (minutes)	151.4 ± 92.7
Low frequency coupling % TST	43 ± 20.2
Low frequency coupling duration (minutes)	164.1 ± 82
Elevated low frequency coupling % TST	20.8 ± 17.9
Elevated low frequency coupling duration (minutes)	79.4 ± 69.3
Narrow band coupling % TST	3.4 ± 8.1
Narrow band coupling duration (minutes)	12.9 ± 31.4
Very low frequency coupling % TST	16.1 ± 7.3
Very low frequency coupling duration (minutes)	61 ± 28.2
CPC e-LFC index/hour of sleep	20.6 ± 19.3
CPC e-LFC cycle time (seconds)	30.4 ± 8.1
CPC LFC index/hour of sleep	52.4 ± 24.9
CPC LFC cycle time (seconds)	31 ± 8.4

TST total sleep time; *CPC* cardiopulmonary coupling; *LFC* low frequency coupling; *e-LFC* elevated-low frequency coupling

the following were the r values, all *p*: < 0.001: WASO-N1 (0.33), WASO-sleep efficiency (−0.93), and N1-sleep efficiency (−0.31). The categories of fragmentation or consolidation were related but also showed independence. After adjusting for age, gender, race, body mass index, total sleep time and sleep apnea severity, using logistic regression, the following were noted: 1) Sleep fragmentation: a) efficiency-N1: OR 1.89 [CI: 0.94–3.79], p: 0.072; b) efficiency-WASO: OR 4.19 [1.18–14.86], p: 0.027; c) N1-WASO: OR 2.18 [1.24–3.83], p: 0.007. 2) Sleep consolidation: a) efficiency-N1: OR 2.6 [CI: 1.68–4.03], *p*: < 0.001; b) efficiency-WASO: OR 50.19 [24.26–103.84], *p*: < 0.001; c) N1-WASO: OR 1.96 [0.97–3.05], p: 0.07.

In a multiple regression analysis adjusted for age, gender, ethnicity, body mass index and sleep apnea severity (RDI), age was a consistent positive predictor of sleep efficiency, wake after sleep onset and N1 fragmentation categories. Coefficient ± SE, p was 0.007 ± 0.001; *p*: < 0.001; 0.015 ± 0.001, *p*: < 0.001; and 0.004 ± 0.001, *p*: < 0.001, respectively. Male sex was predictive for N1 sleep fragmentation category; 0.06 ± 0.03, p: 0.020. Central apnea category was predicted by age (0.001 ± 0.001 per year, p: 0.024) and male sex (0.048 ± 0.016, p: 0.003).

In a logistic regression analysis (Table 9), the central apnea category increased the odds of ECG-spectrogram fragmentation phenotype, and reduced that of the N1 PSG consolidation phenotype. The presence of narrow band coupling increased the odds of the N1 and the ECG-spectrogram fragmentation phenotypes, while reducing the odds of the ECG-spectrogram consolidation phenotype. Finally, the ECG-spectrogram fragmentation phenotype increased the odds of the N1 fragmentation

male gender; 2) greater degrees of sleep fragmentation; 3) more severe sleep apnea; 4) higher central and mixed apnea indices. The presence of narrow band coupling predicted NREM dominance, Odds Ratio 1.56 [CI: 1.1–2.29, p: 0.021], adjusted for age, gender, ethnicity, body mass index and overall RDI. Table 8 shows the predictors of NREM dominance, which included sleep fragmentation (positively) and ECG-sleep consolidation (negatively), adjusted for age, gender, BMI, ethnicity, and overall RDI.

Predictors of phenotypes

Correlation between the measures of sleep fragmentation or consolidation are to be expected. In our sample,

Table 4 Correlation (r) of ECG-spectrogram and PSG respiratory indices

CPC metric	RDI	NREM-RDI	REM-RDI	CAI/hour of sleep	Desaturation Index/hour of sleep
LFC index	0.50 [p: 0.021	0.52 [p: 0.024]	0.20 [p: 0.043]	0.21 [p: 0.041]	0.44 (p: 0.001)
e-LFC index	0.56 [p: 0.02]	0.59 [p: 0.001]	0.22 [p: 0.041]	0.25 [p: 0.031]	0.50 [p: 0.001]
e-LFC$_{NB}$	0.39 [p: 0.021]	0.41 [p: 0.001]	0.14 [p: 0.071]	0.19 [p: 0.043]	0.36 P: [0.013]
LFC cycle time	−0.01 [p: 0.601]	−0.01 [p: 0.311]	0.01 [p: 0.212]	−0.01 [p: 0.311]	−0.02 [p: 0.511]
e-LFC cycle time	0.09 [p: 0.413]	0.09 [p: 0.211]	0.08 [p: 0.412]	0.02 [p: 0.121]	0.41 [p: 0.013]

LFC low frequency coupling; *e-LFC* elevated low frequency coupling; *RDI* respiratory disturbance index; *REM* rapid eye movement sleep; *NREM* non-rapid eye movement sleep; *CAI* central apnea index; *CPC* cardiopulmonary coupling

phenotype and reduced the odds of the N1 and WASO consolidation phenotypes.

Cycle time influences

The cycle time of LFC (30.4 ± 8.1) and e-LFC (31 ± 8.4) was not significantly different across various sleep fragmented or consolidated phenotypes, or NREM vs. REM dominance (the latter 31 ± 8.8 vs. 31 ± 8.2, p: 0.99). Those with narrow-band coupling had a shorter cycle time than those without, 27.5 ± 5.7 vs. 32.8 ± 8.8 s, *p*: < 0.001 for LFC, and 27.8 ± 6.8 vs. 32.6 ± 8.7 s, *p*: < 0.001, for e-LFC.

Phenotypes and clinical baseline covariates

The total Epworth Sleepiness Scale was modified by NREM vs. REM dominance: 9.2 ± 4.2 vs. 10.2 ± 4.3, *t*-test, p: 0.009. A multiple regression with adjustment for age, gender, body mass index, ethnicity, and total RDI remained significant: Beta Coefficient $-0.003 \pm$ SE 0.38, p: 0.009. Absence of the ECG-spectrogram sleep consolidated phenotype was associated with an increased odds of being on antihypertensive medications, OR 2.65 [CI: 1.64–4.26], *p*: < 0.001, adjusted for age, gender, BMI, total sleep time, and slow wave sleep (pre 2007 stages S3 + S4). The difference in high frequency coupling in those with and without the ECG-spectrogram consolidated phenotype was substantial and clinically meaningful, 50.7 ± 22.4 vs. $37.3 \pm 21.8\%$ total sleep time. Evening and morning systolic and diastolic blood pressures were, however, not significantly different. Other phenotypes at baseline including all cognitive measures did not show

Table 5 Polysomnographic and spectrographic metrics across apnea severity groups (mean ± SD)

Polysomnographic variable	Mild ($n = 70$)	Moderate ($n = 394$)	Severe ($n = 320$)	Extreme ($n = 188$)
Total Sleep Time (minutes)	386 ± 68	376 ± 64	388 ± 63	368 ± 74
Sleep efficiency % TST	80.9 ± 13.3	79 ± 12.8	80.1 ± 11.1	76.4 ± 14.2
Arousal index/hour of sleep	14.2 ± 10.4	19.8 ± 12.1	29 ± 15.3	53.9 ± 28.6
S1 % TST	11.4 ± 7.9	14 ± 8.4	18.1 ± 11.2	30.6 ± 22.5
S2 % TST	63.6 ± 8.4	62.6 ± 9.7	60.6 ± 11	53.7 ± 20.9
S3 + S4 % TST	5.5 ± 7.2	4 ± 6.7	3 ± 5.4	1.7 ± 4.3
REM % TST	19.4 ± 6.6	19.2 ± 6.5	18.2 ± 6.8	13.9 ± 7.2
RDI/hour of sleep	5.5 ± 2.7	19.1 ± 5.8	44 ± 8.7	83.6 ± 17.6
CAI/hour of sleep	0.8 ± 0.2	0.3 ± 1	1.2 ± 3	3.2 ± 9.3
Minimum SaO$_2$	87.7 ± 11.5	84.8 ± 5.1	79.7 ± 7.5	72.7 ± 10.6
ECG-spectrographic variable	$n = 54$	$n = 296$	$n = 209$	$n = 112$
HFC % TST	50.8 ± 19.6	44.5 ± 21	36.9 ± 20.8	22.1 ± 19.7
LFC % TST	29.4 ± 13.8	35.7 ± 16.2	45.6 ± 17.8	62.8 ± 21
e-LFC % TST	11.1 ± 10.1	15.3 ± 11.5	22.3 ± 16.2	37.3 ± 25.2
e-LFC$_{NB}$ % TST	0.02 ± 0.07	1.2 ± 2.7	3.8 ± 8.5	9.9 ± 13.3
VLFC % TST	17.6 ± 7.1	17.6 ± 7.4	15.2 ± 6.9	12.9 ± 6.9

WASO wake after sleep onset; *N1* stage 1 NREM sleep; *CAI* central apnea index; *S2-S4* pre-2007 NREM sleep stages; *HFC* high frequency coupling; *REM* rapid eye movement; *LFC* low frequency coupling; *VLFC* very low frequency coupling; *e-LCF* elevated-low frequency coupling; *e-LFC$_{NB}$* narrow band e-LFC

Table 6 Phenotypes across sleep apnea severity categories

Phenotype across apnea severity categories	Mild	Moderate	Severe	Extreme	Chi², p, for phenotypes across categories
Chemoreflex phenotype—PSG (CAI ≥ 5/hour of sleep)	0 (0%)	1 (0.25%)	13 (4.1%)	15 (8%)	44.86, <0.001
Chemoreflex phenotype—spectrogram (e-LFC$_{NB}$ present)	4 (7.4%)	70 (23.7%)	75 (23.4%)	67 (35.6%)	4.83, 0.19
Sleep fragmentation phenotype—sleep efficiency ≤ 70%	13 (18.6%)	82 (20.8%)	53 (16.6%)	48 (25.5%)	6.16, 0.10
Sleep fragmentation phenotype—N1 ≥ 30%	3 (4.3%)	24 (6.1%)	45 (14.1%)	76 (40.4%)	124.78, <0.001
Sleep fragmentation phenotype—WASO ≥ 60 min	38 (54.3%)	240 (60.9%)	196 (61.3%)	136 (72.3%)	10.42, 0.02
Sleep fragmentation phenotype—spectrogram (HFC ≤ 30%)	9 (16.7%)	75 (25.3%)	80 (38.3%)	79 (70.5%)	
Sleep consolidation phenotype—sleep efficiency ≥ 90%	22 (31.4%)	76 (19.3%)	55 (17.2%)	27 (14.4%)	9.89, 0.02
Sleep consolidation phenotype—N1 ≤ 10%	42 (60%)	157 (39.9%)	85 (26.6%)	33 (17.6%)	58.01, <0.001
Sleep consolidation phenotype—WASO ≤ 30 min	15 21.4%)	57 (14.5%)	34 (10.6%)	15 (8%)	11.08, 0.01
Sleep consolidation phenotype—spectrogram (HFC ≥ 50%)	28 (51.9%)	126 (42.6%)	61 (29.2%)	15 (12.3%)	2.46, 0.48

WASO wake after sleep onset; *N1* stage 1 NREM sleep; *CAI* central apnea index; *HFC* high frequency coupling; *LFC* low frequency coupling; *e-LFC$_{NB}$* narrow band e-LFC

Table 7 NREM vs. REM dominance: clinical and polysomnographic features

Demographics and Polysomnogram Metrics	NREM dominant (242)	REM dominant (429)	p
Age (years)	51.2 ± 13.9	49.6 ± 11.9	0.11
Gender (male %)	80.2	55.7	<0.001 (Chi²)
Race (white, %)	74.8	69.9	0.10
Body Mass Index Kg/M₂	30.6 ± 6.7	31.3 ± 7.3	0.25
Total sleep time (TST)	282.8 ± 64	386.4 ± 58.1	0.46
Sleep efficiency % TST	79.2 ± 12.2	80.7 ± 11.1	0.10
S1 % TST	21.7 ± 16.8	14.9 ± 10.1	<0.001
S2 % TST	58.3 ± 15.5	62.3 ± 9.8	<0.001
S3+ S4 % TST	2.1 ± 3.8	3.1 ± 5.3	0.005
REM	17.1 ± 6.7	18.9 ± 6.7	0.002
Arousal Index/hour of sleep	36.5 ± 26.1	22.6 ± 15.1	<0.001
RDI/hour of sleep	49.9 ± 29.9	28.8 ± 20.1	<0.001
Obstructive apnea index/hour of sleep	25 ± 15.4	9.6 ± 13.7	<0.001
Central apnea index/hour of sleep	2 ± 7.2	0.5 ± 2.1	<0.001
Mixed apnea index/hour of sleep	3 ± 7.4	0.4 ± 1.5	<0.001
Hypopnea index/hour of sleep	19.9 ± 14.5	18.3 ± 11.9	0.11
RDI-NREM/hour of sleep	52.9 ± 30.5	24.7 ± 20.3	<0.001
RDI-REM/hour of sleep	34.5 ± 25.3	46.5 ± 25.3	<0.001
Oxygen desaturation index/hour of sleep	34 ± 29.6	16.4 ± 17.2	<0.001
Minimum saturation	79.5 ± 10.3	82.9 ± 6.8	<0.001
Time less than 85% saturation (minutes)	4.8 ± 11.5	1 ± 2.6	<0.001
PLM/hour of sleep	5.8 ± 12.5	6.2 ± 16.2	0.77

All values mean and standard deviation, unless other specified
S1-S4 Pre-2007 NREM sleep stages; *RDI* respiratory disturbance index; *REM* rapid eye movement NREM: non-rapid eye movement; *PLM* periodic limb movement

Table 8 Predictors of NREM dominance

Phenotype	NREM dominance (OR), p
PSG SF—SE	1.16 [CI: 0.72–1.86], 0.527
PSG SF—N1	1.72 [CI: 1.01–2.93], 0.046*
PSG SF—WASO	0.90 [CI: 0.61–1.34], 0.614
ECG SF	1.53 [CI: 1.04–2.25], 0.029*
PSG SC—SE	0.92 [CI: 0.58–1.50], 0.758
PSG SC—N1	0.91 [CI: 0.61–1.35], 0.643
PSG SC—WASO	0.81 [CI: 0.47–1.43], 0.483
ECG SC	0.44 [CI: 0.29–0.67], <0.001*
Central sleep apnea +	1.96 [CI: 0.78–4.91], 0.152
e-LFC$_{NB}$ +	1.56 [CI: 1.07–2.29], 0.022

Adjusted for age, gender, body mass index, ethnicity, respiratory disturbance index
CI confidence intervals; *NREM* non-rapid eye movement sleep *PSG*: polysomnographic; *SE* sleep efficiency; *N1* NREM stage 1; *WASO* wake after sleep onset; *ECG* electrocardiogram-based analysis; *SC* sleep consolidation; *SF* sleep fragmentation; *e-LFC$_{NB}$* elevated-low frequency coupling narrow band
* Statistically significant

differences in clinical covariates. The evening systolic blood pressure was higher in the NREM-dominant group, 125.3 ± 14.7 vs. 122.6 ± 14.7 mm Hg, but was no longer significant after adjustment for age.

CPAP compliance

Use of CPAP during the last month of the 6-month trial was 4.2 ± 2.2 h, and 3.9 ± 2.1 h across the entire duration. The percentage of use of CPAP for 4 or more hours, average of all subjects, was $55 \pm 20\%$.

Mean compliance across the 6 months was lower in those with the sleep fragmentation-N1 group, 3.6 ± 2 vs. 4 ± 2.1 h. Other categories had no impact.

Discussion

The results of our analysis show that discernable phenotypes are present within what is otherwise considered generic obstructive sleep apnea. Fragmented and consolidated phenotypes are see at milder and more severe

extremes of obstructive sleep apnea, using both conventional and computed analysis of polysomnogram signals. Presumptive high loop gain phenotypes, central sleep apnea on polysomnography and narrow-band coupling on ECG-spectrogram, are associated with greater degrees of sleep fragmentation. Stage dominance, NREM vs. REM shows clear differences. Cycle time metrics provide further insight into pathological interactions that result in a final common output, that of an apnea-hypopnea index. Several aspects of extractable phenotypes provide novel insights into sleep apnea.

Periods of stable breathing during NREM sleep

Some clues to the nature of this phenomenon can be gained from the concept of NREM sleep bimodality. The first clue came from the description of CAP and non-CAP from Italian researchers in the mid 1980's (Terzano et al. 1985). CAP and non-CAP periods occur across NREM sleep. CAP occurs in N1 and parts of N2; non-CAP occurs in parts of N2 and most of N3 (Parrino et al. 2014). Subsequently, the autonomic and respiratory associations of CAP/non-CAP were described (Kara et al. 2003). Finally, the description of the cardiopulmonary coupling technique showed that NREM sleep has bimodal characteristics in health and disease. High frequency coupling is associated with high delta power, non-CAP EEG, stable breathing, strong sinus arrhythmia, and blood pressure dipping (Thomas et al. 2014). Low frequency coupling is associated with unstable breathing, cyclic variation in heart rate, CAP EEG, and blood pressure non-dipping. Thus, stable breathing periods reflect natural integrated network states of the brain. Benzodiazepines and related drugs increase non-CAP (Parrino et al. 1997; Terzano et al. 1995), and may be expected to increase stable breathing periods. Zolpidem increases blood pressure dipping (Huang et al. 2012), and could do so through the induction of stable NREM periods.

Table 9 Predictors of Primary Phenotypes

Phenotype	CAI (OR), p	e-LFC$_{NB}$ (OR), p	ECG SF (OR), p
PSG SF—SE	1.03 [CI: 0.41–2.62], 0.939	0.88 [CI: 0.56–1.37], 0.566	1.37 [CI: 0.90–1.12], 0.144
PSG SF—N1	1.70 [CI:0.71–4.09], 0.228	2.97 [CI:1.86–4.74], < 0.001*	1.95 [CI:1.22–3.13], 0.005*
PSG SF—WASO	1.07 [CI:0.46–2.48], 0.882	0.99 [CI:0.69–1.43], 0.975	1.34 [CI:0.93–1.93], 0.111
ECG SF	3.69 [CI:1.58–8.64], 0.003*	2.06 [CI:1.47–2.93], < 0.001*	
PSG SC—SE	0.51 [CI:0.14–1.78], 0.288	0.89 [CI:0.57–1.38], 0.593	0.72 [CI:0.46–1.13], 0.155
PSG SC—N1	0.26 [CI:0.08–0.87], 0.029*	0.64 [CI:0.44–0.92], 0.018	0.61 [CI:0.42–0.88], 0.009*
PSG SC—WASO	0.25 [CI:0.03–1.91], 0.182	1.01 [CI:0.61–1.69], 0.955	0.57 [CI:0.33–0.97], 0.040*
ECG SC	0.31 [CI:0.09–1.04], 0.057	0.28 [CI:0.18–0.43], < 0.001*	

CI confidence intervals; *PSG* polysomnogram; *ECG* electrocardiogram; *N1* NREM stage 1; *SF* sleep fragmentation; *WASO* wake after sleep onset; *SC* sleep consolidation; *SE* sleep efficiency; *CAI* central apnea index; *e-LFC$_{NB}$* elevated-low frequency coupling, narrow band
* Statistically significant

The proportion of stable breathing periods will impact the computed apnea-hypopnea index, as these periods do not contribute to the metric. Varying proportions of stable breathing on a night to night basis can contribute to night to night variability of the apnea-hypopnea index. The fact that even at the most severe end of the spectrum there are patients with consolidated sleep by any measure suggests that this is an individual trait.

NREM vs. REM dominance

In general, periodic breathing and hypocapnic central apnea does not occur in REM sleep (exception, a patient with congestive heart failure who demonstrates periodic breathing during wake state). NREM dominance is well described in idiopathic central sleep apnea (Quadri et al. 2009), periodic breathing associated with heart failure or stroke (Hanly et al. 1989), opiate-induced sleep apnea (Walker et al. 2007), and high altitude periodic breathing (Thomas et al. 2007b). NREM dominance is also a feature of complex apnea/treatment-emergent central sleep apnea, regardless of the exact definition used (Rao & Thomas 2013). In the APPLES data, NREM dominance was associated with greater severity of disease, male sex, and increased central/mixed apneas, even if less than the conventional threshold for central sleep apnea was used (which requires ≥ 50% of all events to be central). It is possible that NREM dominant obstructive sleep apnea reflects high loop gain (Rao & Thomas 2013; Stanchina et al. 2015), and is thus a recognizable phenotype from standard polysomnograms even without further computational analysis.

Accurate estimation of central sleep apnea from clinical polysomnograms

In the APPLES data, the amount of central apnea/presumed high loop gain features estimated by conventional features vs. ECG-spectrogram diverged markedly. The American Academy of Sleep Medicine (AASM) criteria defines a central apnea as an oronasal flow drop by > 90% of baseline, lasting 10 s, in the absence of inspiratory effort. (Iber & American Academy of Sleep Medicine 2007) A central hypopnea requires proportional and concordant flow and effort reduction and absence of snoring (except possibly at recovery) and flow-limitation. However, events both at sea level (often) and high altitude (always) in patients with positive pressure induced or amplified respiratory instability have short cycles that are less than 30 s. If 40 s is a requirement, then these short-cycle hypopnea events will be falsely characterized as obstructive. The International Classification of Sleep Disorders (ICSD)-3 specifies that these should make up ≥ 50% of all scored events, so substantial central events can still carry an obstructive summary label.

The scoring guidelines state that flow limitation excludes a "central hypopnea" in the scoring manual yet several lines of evidence argue strongly against this: a) at high-altitude, a pure chemoreflex form of sleep apnea, flow-limitation occurs frequently; b) studies using esophageal manometry and endoscopy show that pharyngeal airway narrowing and occlusion occur during central apneas in healthy individuals as well as in patients with heart failure. c) the airway can close during polysomnographic central apnea; (Badr 1996; Badr et al. 1995) d) central hypopneas demonstrate flow-limitation (Badr et al. 1995; Sankri-Tarbichi et al. 2009; Guilleminault et al. 1997; Dowdell et al. 1990). Despite the known presence of flow limitation and airway narrowing during both central and obstructive events (Dempsey et al. 2014), hypopnea scoring is biased towards obstructive disease (Rao & Thomas 2013; Eckert et al. 2007; Javaheri & Dempsey 2013).

The APPLES scoring did not include central hypopneas and thus likely underestimated high loop gain features. The ECG-spectrogram analysis showed that central/periodic breathing-type oscillations were present in nearly one third of the APPLES cohort, and that this signal biomarker was more closely associated with NREM than REM RDI. The shorter cycle time in the e-LFC$_{NB}$ group is consistent with short-cycle periodic breathing being associated with NREM dominant sleep apnea and high loop gain (Gilmartin et al. 2005).

A sleep fragmentation phenotype

A distinct sleep fragmentation phenotype was evident at all severities of obstructive sleep apnea. This result is generally consistent with the variability of arousal phenomena in sleep apnea, contributing to amplification of disease, especially in NREM sleep (Eckert & Younes 2014). While low arousal threshold is a measurable sleep apnea phenotype (Eckert et al. 2013), the return to sleep after arousal is probably just as important. Recovery from arousal is a continuous process of variable dynamics (Younes & Hanly 2016; Younes et al. 2015), and if delayed, the epoch will be scored as wake or N1/S1. If this phenotype is a trait, sedatives may have a role in management, similar to reducing the apnea-hypopnea index in NREM sleep in those with low arousal threshold (Smales et al. 2015). As no physiological sleep apnea trait estimates were performed in the APPLES, concordance or discordance of a low arousal vs. sleep fragmentation phenotype could not be determined. High N1 fragmentation phenotype was associated with reduced compliance.

A need for improved phenotyping

From a diagnostic standpoint, there is minimal relationship of the AHI with subjective or objective sleepiness measurements (Gottlieb et al. 1999; Eiseman et al. 2012). From a treatment standpoint, predicting paradoxical PAP response (complex apnea) is not reliably predicted standard metrics, but is predicted by CPC metrics (Thomas et al. 2007a). Diagnostic phenotyping is important for appropriate clinical case detection, epidemiology, and clinical trial planning purposes. Treatment phenotypes should reasonably focus on response to therapy, positive pressure or otherwise. Persistence of phenotypes or conversion of one phenotype to another can have clinical implications. For example, a fragmentation phenotype which persists may benefit from sedatives, cognitive behavioral therapy or re-looking at therapeutic precision, while a fragmentation to consolidated phenotype shift implies therapeutic success. Therapies can target driving phenotypes to more desirable ones, e.g., acetazolamide for a high loop gain/NREM-dominant phenotype (Edwards et al. 2012).

Phenotypes and clinical covariates

The slightly lower subjective sleepiness score in NREM dominant sleep apnea is largely in keeping with lesser degrees of subjective sleepiness in patients with strong respiratory chemoreflex activation. Heart rate variability and muscle sympathetic nerve activity are inversely related to subjective sleepiness in heart failure (Taranto Montemurro et al. 2012; Taranto Montemurro et al. 2014). The tight link of the respiratory chemoreflex and sympathetic centers in the brainstem is one plausible explanation-that these individuals have heightened sympathetic drive for a given degree of sleep apnea. Increased hypertension risk in those with reduced high frequency coupling, a signal biomarker of stable breathing and sleep, could reflect the impact of longer periods of stable breathing and the associated vagal dominance, even in those with sleep apnea, on overall blood pressure control.

The relative lack of impact of the various phenotypes on any measure of cognition was a surprise. This result may reflect the characteristics of the APPLES population which resulted in a negative result in the primary study (CPAP vs. placebo CPAP). The mechanisms which impair cognition and mood in sleep apnea are not well understood, and likely reflect an interaction of the stressor and individual resilience factors. Our result may also reflect our current inability to identify the factors associated with a certain apnea-hypopnea index which determines an adverse impact on brain function. The APPLES follow-up data we aim to analyze may provide additional clues.

Limitations of the analysis

The primary limitation of the presented analysis is that the impact of phenotypes on outcomes cannot be determined. The criteria for various phenotype categories were necessarily arbitrary but are "clinically reasonable". Moreover, if these patterns are maintained over time despite positive pressure therapy is important to know, and will need further follow-up analysis of the APPLES data. Body position effects were not quantified. Respiratory Effort Related Arousal events were not scored in the APPLES, and could alter some of our conclusions. Careful scoring of periodic breathing without the filter of flow limitation may provide higher estimates of loop gain than standard scoring. A more detailed analysis of compliance metrics across the 6 months, including differentiating sham vs. real CPAP, will be required to establish an impact of phenotypes described here.

Conclusions

Distinct phenotypes of fragmentation, consolidation, NREM vs. REM dominance, and high loop gain can be identified in the conventional polysomnogram, by both standard scoring and estimates of cardiopulmonary coupling. Baseline clinical characteristics including cognition were not impacted by the phenotypes. The impact of these phenotypes on treatment clinical outcomes require analysis and research.

Abbreviations
AASM: American Academy of Sleep Medicine; APPLES: Apnea Positive Pressure Long-term Efficacy Study; BMI: Body mass index; CAI: Central apnea index; CPAP: Continuous positive airway pressure; CPC: Cardiopulmonary coupling; CSR: Cheyne-Stokes respiration; ECG: Electrocardiogram; EEG: Electroencephalogram; HFC: High frequency coupling; LFC: Low frequency coupling; NREM: Non-rapid eye movement; PSG: Polysomnogram; RDI: Respiratory disturbance index; REM: rapid eye movement; SC: Sleep consolidation; SF: Sleep fragmentation; VLFC: Very low frequency coupling; WASO: Wake after sleep onset

Acknowledgments
Joseph Mietus, B.S, (deceased) developer of the original cardiopulmonary coupling software, and who performed some of the ECG analysis.
APPLES
Acknowledgment List
APPLES was funded by contract 5UO1-HL-068060 from the National Heart, Lung and Blood Institute. The APPLES pilot studies were supported by grants from the American Academy of Sleep Medicine and the Sleep Medicine Education and Research Foundation to Stanford University and by the National Institute of Neurological Disorders and Stroke (N44-NS-002394) to SAM Technology.
In addition, APPLES investigators gratefully recognize the vital input and support of Dr. Sylvan Green who died before the results of this trial were analyzed, but was instrumental in its design and conduct.
ADMINISTRATIVE CORE
Clete A. Kushida, M.D., Ph.D., Deborah A. Nichols, M.S., Eileen B. Leary, B.A., RPSGT, Pamela R. Hyde, M.A., Tyson H. Holmes, Ph.D., Daniel A. Bloch, Ph.D., William C. Dement, M.D., Ph.D.
DATA COORDINATING CENTER
Daniel A. Bloch, Ph.D., Tyson H. Holmes, Ph.D., Deborah A. Nichols, M.S., Rik Jadrnicek, Microflow, Ric Miller, Microflow, Usman Aijaz, M.S., Aamir Farooq, Ph.D., Darryl Thomander, Ph.D., Chia-Yu Cardell, RPSGT, Emily Kees, Michael E. Sorel, M.P.H., Oscar Carrillo, RPSGT, Tami Crabtree, M.S., Booil Jo, Ph.D., Ray Balise, Ph.D., Tracy Kuo, Ph.D.
CLINICAL COORDINATING CENTER
Clete A. Kushida, M.D., Ph.D., William C. Dement, M.D., Ph.D., Pamela R. Hyde, M.A., Rhonda M. Wong, B.A., Pete Silva, Max Hirshkowitz, Ph.D., Alan Gevins,

D.Sc., Gary Kay, Ph.D., Linda K. McEvoy, Ph.D., Cynthia S. Chan, B.S., Sylvan Green, M.D.

CLINICAL CENTERS

Stanford University
Christian Guilleminault, M.D., Eileen B. Leary, B.A., RPSGT, David Claman, M.D., Stephen Brooks, M.D., Julianne Blythe, P.A.-C, RPSGT, Jennifer Blair, B.A., Pam Simi, Ronelle Broussard, B.A., Emily Greenberg, M.P.H., Bethany Franklin, M.S., Amirah Khouzam, M.A., Sanjana Behari Black, B.S., RPSGT, Viola Arias, RPSGT, Romelyn Delos Santos, B.S., Tara Tanaka, Ph.D.

University of Arizona
Stuart F. Quan, M.D., James L. Goodwin, Ph.D., Wei Shen, M.D., Phillip Eichling, M.D., Rohit Budhiraja, M.D., Charles Wynstra, M.B.A., Cathy Ward, Colleen Dunn, B.S., Terry Smith, B.S., Dane Holderman, Michael Robinson, B.S., Osmara Molina, B.S., Aaron Ostrovsky, Jesus Wences, Sean Priefert, Julia Rogers, B.S., Megan Ruiter, B.S., Leslie Crosby, B.S., R.N.

St. Mary Medical Center
Richard D. Simon, Jr., M.D., Kevin Hurlburt, RPSGT, Michael Bernstein, M.D., Timothy Davidson, M.D., Jeannine Orock-Takele, RPSGT, Shelly Rubin, M.A., Phillip Smith, RPSGT, Erica Roth, RPSGT, Julie Flaa, RPSGT, Jennifer Blair, B.A., Jennifer Schwartz, B.A., Anna Simon, B.A., Amber Randall, B.A.

St. Luke's Hospital
James K. Walsh, Ph.D., Paula K. Schweitzer, Ph.D., Anup Katyal, M.D., Rhody Eisenstein, M.D., Stephen Feren, M.D., Nancy Cline, Dena Robertson, R.N., Sheri Compton, R.N., Susan Greene, Kara Griffin, M.S., Janine Hall, Ph.D.

Brigham and Women's Hospital
Daniel J. Gottlieb, M.D., M.P.H., David P. White, M.D., Denise Clarke, B.Sc., RPSGT, Kevin Moore, B.A., Grace Brown, B.A., Paige Hardy, M.S., Kerry Eudy, Ph.D., Lawrence Epstein, M.D., Sanjay Patel, M.D. *Sleep HealthCenters for the use of their clinical facilities to conduct this research

CONSULTANT TEAMS
Methodology Team: Daniel A. Bloch, Ph.D., Sylvan Green, M.D., Tyson H. Holmes, Ph.D., Maurice M. Ohayon, M.D., D. Sc., David White, M.D., Terry Young, Ph.D.
Sleep-Disordered Breathing Protocol Team: Christian Guilleminault, M.D., Stuart Quan, M.D., David White, M.D.
EEG/Neurocognitive Function Team: Jed Black, M.D., Alan Gevins, D.Sc., Max Hirshkowitz, Ph.D., Gary Kay, Ph.D., Tracy Kuo, Ph.D.
Mood and Sleepiness Assessment Team: Ruth Benca, M.D., Ph.D., William C. Dement, M.D., Ph.D., Karl Doghramji, M.D., Tracy Kuo, Ph.D., James K. Walsh, Ph.D.
Quality of Life Assessment Team: W. Ward Flemons, M.D., Robert M. Kaplan, Ph.D.
ASA-NC Team: Dean Beebe, Ph.D., Robert Heaton, Ph.D., Joel Kramer, Psy.D., Ronald Lazar, Ph.D., David Loewenstein, Ph.D., Frederick Schmitt, Ph.D.

NATIONAL HEART, LUNG, AND BLOOD INSTITUTE (NHLBI)
Michael J. Twery, Ph.D., Gail G. Weinmann, M.D., Colin O. Wu, Ph.D.

DATA AND SAFETY MONITORING BOARD (DSMB)
Seven-year term: Richard J. Martin, M.D. (Chair), David F. Dinges, Ph.D., Charles F. Emery, Ph.D., Susan M. Harding M.D., John M. Lachin, Sc.D., Phyllis C. Zee, Ph.D.
Other term: Xihong Lin, Ph.D. (2 years), Thomas H. Murray, Ph.D. (1 year)
INDUSTRY SUPPORT – Philips Respironics, Inc.

Funding
To Robert J. Thomas: RC1HL099749-01 (National Heart Lung Blood Institute, USA), Beth Israel Deaconess Medical Center Chief Academic Officer's Research Innovation Initiative
APPLES was funded by contract 5UO1-HL-068060 from the National Heart, Lung and Blood Institute. The
APPLES pilot studies were supported by grants from the American Academy of Sleep Medicine and the Sleep
Medicine Education and Research Foundation to Stanford University and by the National Institute of Neurological Disorders and Stroke (N44-NS-002394) to SAM Technology.
The funding bodies had no role in the design of the study and collection, analysis, and interpretation of data and in writing the manuscript.

Authors' contributions
RJT, MTB and CY conceptualized the analysis. RJT performed the analysis and wrote the manuscript draft. CK provided access to and interpretation assistance for the APPLES data. All authors contributed to revision of the manuscript draft. All authors read and approved the final manuscript.

Competing interests
RJT reports the following: 1) Patent and license for a method to use the ECG to phenotype sleep and sleep apnea; 2) Patent to treat central and complex sleep apnea using low concentration carbon dioxide; 3) Patent submitted and licensed software in an auto-CPAP, joint work with DeVilbiss-DRIVE' 4) General sleep medicine consulting with GLG Councils.
MTB reports the following: Funding from the Center for Integration of Medicine and Innovative Technology, the Milton Family Foundation, and currently receives funding from the Department of Neurology, the MGH-MIT Grand Challenge, and the American Sleep Medicine Foundation. He has a patent pending on a home sleep monitoring device. He has consulting and research agreements with MC10, Insomnisolv, and McKesson. He has provided expert testimony in sleep medicine.
The other authors have no declared conflicts of interest.

Author details
[1]Division of Pulmonary, Critical Care, and Sleep Medicine, Beth Israel Deaconess Medical Center, Boston, MA, USA. [2]Institute of Human Genomic Study, Department of Respiratory Internal Medicine, Korea University Ansan Hospital, Ansan, South Korea. [3]Division of Sleep Medicine, Department of Neurology, Massachusetts General Hospital, Boston, MA, USA. [4]Psychiatry and Behavioral Sciences, Stanford Center for Sleep Sciences and Medicine, Stanford University Medical Center, Redwood City, CA, USA. [5]Department of Neurology, Seoul National University Bundang Hospital, Seongnam, South Korea.

References
Badr MS. Effect of ventilatory drive on upper airway patency in humans during NREM sleep. Respir Physiol. 1996;103:1–10.

Badr MS, Toiber F, Skatrud JB, Dempsey J. Pharyngeal narrowing/occlusion during central sleep apnea. J Appl Physiol. 1995;78:1806–15.

Berry RB BR, Gamaldo CE, Harding SM, Lloyd RM, Marcus CL and Vaughn BV for the American, Academy of Sleep Medicine. The AASM Manual for the Scoring of Sleep and Associated Events: Rules, Terminology and Technical Specifications VwaoD, Illinois: American Academy of Sleep Medicine. 2017 Version 2.4.

Dempsey JA, Xie A, Patz DS, Wang D. Physiology in medicine: obstructive sleep apnea pathogenesis and treatment–considerations beyond airway anatomy. J Appl Physiol. 2014;116:3–12.

Dowdell WT, Javaheri S, McGinnis W. Cheyne-Stokes respiration presenting as sleep apnea syndrome. Clinical and polysomnographic features. Am Rev Respir Dis. 1990;141:871–9.

Eckert DJ, Younes MK. Arousal from sleep: implications for obstructive sleep apnea pathogenesis and treatment. J Appl Physiol (1985). 2014;116:302–13.

Eckert DJ, Jordan AS, Merchia P, Malhotra A. Central sleep apnea: Pathophysiology and treatment. Chest. 2007;131:595–607.

Eckert DJ, White DP, Jordan AS, Malhotra A, Wellman A. Defining phenotypic causes of obstructive sleep apnea. Identification of novel therapeutic targets. Am J Respir Crit Care Med. 2013;188:996–1004.

Edwards BA, Sands SA, Eckert DJ, et al. Acetazolamide improves loop gain but not the other physiological traits causing obstructive sleep apnoea. J Physiol. 2012;590:1199–211.

Eiseman NA, Westover MB, Mietus JE, Thomas RJ, Bianchi MT. Classification algorithms for predicting sleepiness and sleep apnea severity. J Sleep Res. 2012;21:101–12.

Gilmartin GS, Daly RW, Thomas RJ. Recognition and management of complex sleep-disordered breathing. Curr Opin Pulm Med. 2005;11:485–93.

Gottlieb DJ, Whitney CW, Bonekat WH, et al. Relation of sleepiness to respiratory disturbance index: the Sleep Heart Health Study. Am J Respir Crit Care Med. 1999;159:502–7.

Guilleminault C, Hill MH, Simmons FB, Powell N, Riley R, Stoohs R. Passive constriction of the upper airway during central apneas: fiberoptic and EMG investigations. Respir Physiol. 1997;108:11–22.

Hanly PJ, Millar TW, Steljes DG, Baert R, Frais MA, Kryger MH. Respiration and abnormal sleep in patients with congestive heart failure. Chest. 1989;96:480–8.

Huang Y, Mai W, Cai X, et al. The effect of zolpidem on sleep quality, stress status, and nondipping hypertension. Sleep Med. 2012;13:263–8.

Iber C, American Academy of Sleep Medicine. The AASM manual for the scoring of sleep and associated events: rules, terminology, and technical specifications. Westchester: American Academy of Sleep Medicine; 2007.

Javaheri S, Dempsey JA. Central sleep apnea. Compr Physiol. 2013;3:141–63.

Jordan AS, White DP, Lo YL, et al. Airway dilator muscle activity and lung volume during stable breathing in obstructive sleep apnea. Sleep. 2009;32:361–8.

Kara T, Narkiewicz K, Somers VK. Chemoreflexes–physiology and clinical implications. Acta Physiol Scand. 2003;177:377–84.

Kushida CA, Nichols DA, Quan SF, et al. The Apnea Positive Pressure Long-term Efficacy Study (APPLES): rationale, design, methods, and procedures. J Clin Sleep Med. 2006;2:288–300.

Maestri R, La Rovere MT, Robbi E, Pinna GD. Fluctuations of the fractal dimension of the electroencephalogram during periodic breathing in heart failure patients. J Comput Neurosci. 2010;28:557–65.

Owens RL, Edwards BA, Eckert DJ, et al. An integrative model of physiological traits can be used to predict obstructive sleep apnea and response to non positive airway pressure therapy. Sleep. 2015;38:961–70.

Parrino L, Boselli M, Spaggiari MC, Smerieri A, Terzano MG. Multidrug comparison (lorazepam, triazolam, zolpidem, and zopiclone) in situational insomnia: polysomnographic analysis by means of the cyclic alternating pattern. Clin Neuropharmacol. 1997;20:253–63.

Parrino L, Grassi A, Milioli G. Cyclic alternating pattern in polysomnography: what is it and what does it mean? Curr Opin Pulm Med. 2014;20:533–41.

Quadri S, Drake C, Hudgel DW. Improvement of idiopathic central sleep apnea with zolpidem. J Clin Sleep Med. 2009;5:122–9.

Quan SF, Chan CS, Dement WC, et al. The association between obstructive sleep apnea and neurocognitive performance–the Apnea Positive Pressure Long-term Efficacy Study (APPLES). Sleep. 2011;34:303–14B.

Rao H, Thomas RJ. Complex sleep apnea. Curr Treat Options Neurol. 2013;15:677–91.

Sankri-Tarbichi AG, Rowley JA, Badr MS. Expiratory pharyngeal narrowing during central hypocapnic hypopnea. Am J Respir Crit Care Med. 2009;179:313–9.

Smales ET, Edwards BA, Deyoung PN, et al. Trazodone effects on obstructive sleep apnea and non-rem arousal threshold. Ann Am Thorac Soc. 2015;12:758–64.

Stanchina M, Robinson K, Corrao W, Donat W, Sands S, Malhotra A. Clinical use of loop gain measures to determine continuous positive airway pressure efficacy in patients with complex sleep apnea. A pilot study. Ann Am Thorac Soc. 2015;12:1351–7.

Taranto Montemurro L, Floras JS, Millar PJ, et al. Inverse relationship of subjective daytime sleepiness to sympathetic activity in patients with heart failure and obstructive sleep apnea. Chest. 2012;142:1222–8.

Taranto Montemurro L, Floras JS, Picton P, et al. Relationship of heart rate variability to sleepiness in patients with obstructive sleep apnea with and without heart failure. J Clin Sleep Med. 2014;10:271–6.

Terrill PI, Edwards BA, Nemati S, et al. Quantifying the ventilatory control contribution to sleep apnoea using polysomnography. Eur Respir J. 2015;45:408–18.

Terzano MG, Mancia D, Salati MR, Costani G, Decembrino A, Parrino L. The cyclic alternating pattern as a physiologic component of normal NREM sleep. Sleep. 1985;8:137–45.

Terzano MG, Parrino L, Boselli M, Dell'Orso S, Moroni M, Spaggiari MC. Changes of cyclic alternating pattern (CAP) parameters in situational insomnia under brotizolam and triazolam. Psychopharmacology (Berl). 1995;120:237–43.

Thomas RJ. Cyclic alternating pattern and positive airway pressure titration. Sleep Med. 2002;3:315–22.

Thomas RJ. Alternative approaches to treatment of Central Sleep Apnea. Sleep Med Clin. 2014;9:87–104.

Thomas RJ, Mietus JE, Peng CK, Goldberger AL. An electrocardiogram-based technique to assess cardiopulmonary coupling during sleep. Sleep. 2005;28:1151–61.

Thomas RJ, Mietus JE, Peng CK, et al. Differentiating obstructive from central and complex sleep apnea using an automated electrocardiogram-based method. Sleep. 2007a;30:1756–69.

Thomas RJ, Tamisier R, Boucher J, et al. Nocturnal hypoxia exposure with simulated altitude for 14 days does not significantly alter working memory or vigilance in humans. Sleep. 2007b;30:1195–203.

Thomas RJ, Weiss MD, Mietus JE, Peng CK, Goldberger AL, Gottlieb DJ. Prevalent hypertension and stroke in the Sleep Heart Health Study: association with an ECG-derived spectrographic marker of cardiopulmonary coupling. Sleep. 2009;32:897–904.

Thomas RJ, Mietus JE, Peng CK, et al. Relationship between delta power and the electrocardiogram-derived cardiopulmonary spectrogram: possible implications for assessing the effectiveness of sleep. Sleep Med. 2014;15:125–31.

Walker JM, Farney RJ, Rhondeau SM, et al. Chronic opioid use is a risk factor for the development of central sleep apnea and ataxic breathing. J Clin Sleep Med. 2007;3:455–61.

Weiss MD, Tamisier R, Boucher J, et al. A pilot study of sleep, cognition, and respiration under 4 weeks of intermittent nocturnal hypoxia in adult humans. Sleep Med. 2009;10:739–45.

Wellman A, Malhotra A, Jordan AS, Stevenson KE, Gautam S, White DP. Effect of oxygen in obstructive sleep apnea: role of loop gain. Respir Physiol Neurobiol. 2008;162:144–51.

Wellman A, Edwards BA, Sands SA, et al. A simplified method for determining phenotypic traits in patients with obstructive sleep apnea. J Appl Physiol (1985). 2013;114:911–22.

Xie A, Bedekar A, Skatrud JB, Teodorescu M, Gong Y, Dempsey JA. The heterogeneity of obstructive sleep apnea (predominant obstructive vs pure obstructive apnea). Sleep. 2011;34:745–50.

Younes M, Hanly PJ. Immediate postarousal sleep dynamics: an important determinant of sleep stability in obstructive sleep apnea. J Appl Physiol (1985). 2016;120:801–8.

Younes M, Ostrowski M, Soiferman M, et al. Odds ratio product of sleep EEG as a continuous measure of sleep state. Sleep. 2015;38:641–54.

9

Can 6-minute walk test predict severity of obstructive sleep apnea syndrome?

Parisa Adimi Naghan[1], Oldooz Aloosh[2*] ⓘ, Hamze Ali Torang[3] and Majid Malekmohammad[3]

Abstract

Background: When considering the benefits of the 6-min walking test (6-MWT) in research fields and the need of treatment for moderate to severe obstructive sleep apnea (OSA) patients, research in this field is of great advantage and may have a significant role in therapeutic grounds.

Methods: This cross-sectional study was conducted on 47 patients with confirmed diagnosis of OSA in the National Research Institute of Tuberculosis and Lung Disease, Masih Daneshvari Hospital. The 6-MWT was performed the day after polysomnography. The correlation between the 6-MWT and paraclinical findings during polysomnography in OSA patients was investigated.

Results: In cases with moderate to severe OSA, the male sex displayed correlation with high PCO2. Ages of patients examined displayed reversed correlation with the distance in the 6-MWT by observing the O2 saturation (Sat) at the end of the 6-MWT, displaying direct correlation with the duration of O2 Sat <90% during sleep. The BMI also showed reversed correlation with the distance in the 6-MWT. Similarly, the severity of the OSA had reversed correlation with the expected distance in the test. However, patients with higher duration of O2 Sat <90% during sleep had a higher reduction in O2 Sat during and after the 6-MWT. Patients with higher duration of O2 Sat <90% during sleep also completed less overall distance in the 6-MWT (P values <0.05 for all).

Conclusion: It appears that the 6-MWT can be used in patients with OSA to predict severity of the desaturation in OSA beyond functional capacity. Also, it can help predict the severity of disease and assist in follow up of the OSA patients in terms of functional capacity and selection of the most appropriate treatment strategy to increase the physical ability of the patients.

Background

Obstructive Sleep Apnea (OSA) syndrome is a chronic disease affecting 9% of males and 4% of females. It most commonly affects middle-aged individuals (Al Lawati et al., 2009). It is considered a public health dilemma due to the significant association of its complications with cardiovascular morbidities and placing a major burden on health care costs (Wittmann & Rodenstein, 2004). OSA is the most common form of sleep disorder breathing, characterized by frequent obstruction of the upper airways, causing intermittent hypoxia and consequent cardiovascular, cerebral, and metabolic complications (Pusalavidyasagar & Iber, 2015).

The prevalence of OSA has significantly increased mainly due to the obesity epidemic worldwide.

The OSA is often associated with decreased functional status, and patients cannot tolerate physical activities. Such a limitation in physical and sport activities is related to several factors. Recurrent episodes of the upper airway obstruction, which is often accompanied by increased respiratory effort results in hypoxia and transient nocturnal hypercapnia. This leads to increases in the autonomic sympathetic activity causing arterial vasoconstriction, which is regarded as an abnormal response to exercise (Kaleth et al., 2007). Muscle dysfunction is another explanation for limited physical activity in OSA patients. Vanuxem et al. reported decreased metabolic energy of muscles in patients with OSA manifested as decreased serum level of lactate and delayed elimination of lactate from blood circulation (Vanuxem et al., 1997). On the other hand, due to strong association of OSA

---
* Correspondence: oldoozaloosh@yahoo.com
[2]Chronic Respiratory Diseases Research Center, National Research Institute of Tuberculosis and Lung Diseases (NRITLD), Shahid Beheshti University of Medical Sciences, Masih Daneshvari Hospital, Darabad Avenue, Shahid Bahonar roundabout, Tehran, Iran
Full list of author information is available at the end of the article

and obesity, weight gain decreases pulmonary compliance and subsequently the lung volume. This leads to increase in respiratory effort, which is another factor limiting physical activity (Alameri et al., 2010).

The Six-Minute Walk Test (6-MWT) is an affordable and simple test serving as a standard tool for assessing the physical and exercise activities of cardiovascular patients. 6-MWD(six_minute walk distance); the distance walked within 6 min is significantly correlated with maximum oxygen consumption. Moreover, the distance walked within 6 min is a predictor of morbidity and mortality and disease severity in patients with congestive heart failure (Cahalin et al., 1996; Roul et al., 1998), chronic obstructive pulmonary disease, pulmonary hypertension (Hoeper et al., 2000), and pulmonary interstitial diseases (Flaherty et al., 2006). In other words, the ability to walk reflects the ability to tolerate many daily activities by patients and can be regarded as an index of quality of life (Mulgrew et al., 2007; Singh et al., 2014; Holland et al., 2014).

In adults, OSA is diagnosed by polysmnography. However, this test requires over-night monitoring of patients which is costly and time consuming. Although this test can not be a substitute to the diagnostic test for obstructive sleep apnea, it can predict the patients at higher risk of significant reduction of arterial oxygen (severity of desaturation) at night can be highly valuable. If a patient who is found not to do well on the 6-MWT and history of high risk for OSA, should be referred to a sleep specialist for an overnight diagnostic sleep study, as this research study shows that most likely patients who do not do well on the 6-MWT will at least have moderate to severe obstructive sleep apnea.

Often patients are resistant to doing an overnight sleep study due to discomfort/fear of spending the night in an unknown environment. By doing a 6-MWT during the day the physician can further support concern for obstructive sleep apnea. This may convince the patient to be evaluated and treated for obstructive sleep apnea.

It seems that the 6-MWT may be one of the best candidates. In the present study, the correlation between desaturation during the 6-MWT and paraclinical findings during polysomnography in OSA patients is investigated. In other words, this study aimed to show the severity of OSA had reverse correlation with expected distance in moderate and severe OSA. The effect of nocturnal intermittent hypoxia (despite compensation) on physical activity of individuals.

Methods

Study design

This cross-sectional study was conducted on 47 patients with confirmed diagnosis of OSA in the National Research Institute of Tuberculosis and Lung Disease

(NRITLD), Masih Daneshvari Hospital (a referral hospital in Tehran, Iran) during 1 year period starting from August 2012 to June 2013. Written informed consent was obtained from all of the patients prior to their participation in the study. The study protocol was approved by the ethics committee of the Shahid Beheshti University of Medical Sciences and local scientific committees and it was conducted in compliance with the Declaration of Helsinki.

Eligibility

All patients were newly diagnosed with moderate or severe OSA (aged < 80 years, BMI <35 kg/m^2, height < 2 m). In addition, they had normal chest radiographs and spirometry results. The patients had no history of using continuous positive airway pressure (CPAP). The exclusion criteria were including: psychosomatic disorders, acute arthritis, concomitant pulmonary diseases, congestive heart failure, ischemic heart disease, neuromuscular disorders, bronchospasm, severely decreased O_2 saturation, contraindications for the 6-MWT [including unstable angina symptoms during the month preceding the test, resting heart rate > 120 bpm, systolic-blood-pressure (SBP) > 180 mmHg and/or diastolic-blood-pressure (DBP) ≥100 mmHg], chronic obstructive pulmonary disease and other pulmonary diseases.

Polysomnography

Diagnosis of OSA and its severity is determined based on the Apnea-Hypopnea Index (AHI) score suggested by the American Academy of Sleep Medicine guidelines (Richard et al., 2015). The degree of hypoxemia was also determined by a sleep study in the Sleep Disorders Center. The polysomnography consisted of an overnight study and video monitoring,Standard EEG by AASM protocol,muscle tone and leg movements by chin and leg electromyography, eye movements by electrooculography, heart rate by electrocardiography, and oxygen saturation by pulse oximetry. Thoracic and abdominal belts were used for chest and abdominal wall movements.

Snoring was assessed using a microphone. The polysomnogram was analyzed manually using AASM guideline with Philips Respironic (Alice) Device. The Desaturation Index (DI) is defined as the number of desaturation events per hour of sleep. The severity of OSA was then graded based on AHI in accordance with the American Academy of Sleep Medicine guidelines (Richard et al., 2015)as mild (5–15 AHI events/h), moderate (15–30 AHI events/h), or severe (>30 AHI events/h).

Obstructive apnea is defined as absence of airflow for more than 10 s in presence of continued respiratory effort. Hypopnea here is defined as a reduction in airflow by ≥30%, compared with baseline that lasted for more than 10 s, resulting in 3% decrease in oxygen saturation, or arousal. The AHI score is defined as the number of apnea and hypopnea episodes per hour of sleep and is calculated for the total sleep time. The OSA is defined according to the International Classification of Sleep Disorders (International Classification of Sleep Disorders, 2005).

The 6-MWT

The 6-MWT was performed the day after polysomnography. It was conducted outdoors along a seldom-traveled, flat, straight hospital corridor (40 m long) and between eight and 10 AM according to the American Thoracic Society (ATS) protocol (ATS statement, 2002). Subjects avoided vigorous exercise for 2 h prior to the test and advised to have light meal and wear comfortable clothing and appropriate shoes. 10 min before the onset of the 6-MWT, resting dyspnea, heart rate, and O_2-saturation were measured. All the tests were performed by the same technician trained according to the ATS guidelines.

At the end of the 6-MWT, the same data in addition to the distance walked during the 6-MWT (6-MWD) and the number of stops during the 6-MWT, were recorded. Also, the patients were asked to rate their level of perceived dyspnea (breathless) using the Borg scale (see Additional file 1).

A 6-MWT result below the lower limit of normal was considered as "clinically significant" and showed walk intolerance. Other 6-MWT definitions were as follows:

- Stopping during the 6-MWT was defined as a sign of walk intolerance.
- The difference in oxygen saturation > 4 points before and after the test, was regarded as "clinically significant desaturation".
- Any dyspnea at the end of the test scored between 5 to 10 (according to the Borg scale) was considered as "clinically significant" and regarded as walk intolerance.
- If the heart rate at the end of the 6-MWT was <60% compared to the baseline then it was regarded as chronotropic incompetence (Ben Saad et al., 2014).

Statistical analysis

Sample size was calculated according to the eq. (1):

$$n = z2\sigma2/d2 \tag{1}$$

where d = 0.3σ with 5% level of significance for alpha. The sample size was calculated to be 43 as such. To assess the differences in categorical variables between the two groups, the chi-square test or Fisher's exact test was used. The differences in quantitative variables between the two groups were evaluated using the Student's t-test,

ANOVA or non-parametric Mann-Whitney test. Passive smoking was referred to cigarette smoke breathed in by non-smokers from active smokers. Ex-smoker (or former smoker) was defined as a person who reported not smoking at one examination while he/she had reported smoking at the examination 4 years earlier (i.e., individuals who had quit for ≤4 years or not smoking for 2 or more consecutive examinations after an examination at which they had reported smoking). Non-smoker was defined as an individual who had smoked less than 100 cigarettes in his/her lifetime (Sari et al., 2016). Statistical analysis was performed using SPSS version 18 (SPSS Inc.; Chicago, IL, USA).

Results

Of 47 eligible patients, 33 (70.21%) were males and 14 (29.79%) were females. Male/Female ratio was 2/3. Demographic characteristics of the patients are summarized in Table 1.

Polysomnographic findings are presented in Table 2. Severe and moderate OSA were seen in 23.4% (n = 11) and 75.6%(n = 36) of patients, respectively.

Univariate analysis between age, sex, smoking status, and other variables and polysomnographic data revealed a significant correlation between age and DI (r = 0.456, P = 0.001).

Among the 6-MWT parameters in patients with OSA Only significant raise of heart beat before and after of 6-MWT (P = <0.001) was determined.

Table 3 presents differences between patients with moderate versus severe OSA after the 6-MWT. The 6-MWD in the severe OSA group (477.44 ± 275.65 m) was statistically similar (P = 0.173) to that in the moderate OSA group (555.45 ± 107.82 m). However, the percentage predicted by the 6-MWT for the severe OSA group (75.91 ± 36.45) was significantly shorter than that for the moderate group (92.4 ± 10.41 m, P = 0.020).

Table 1 Characteristics of the study group

Variable mean ± SD[a](range)	
Age (years)	54.4 ± 14.33(22–80)
Height(cm)[b]	165.7 ± 8.77(147–182)
Weight(Kg)[c]	91.9 ± 15.58(58–125)
BMI [d](Kg/m²)[e]	33.74 ± 6.23(22.5–50)
Smoking status	
Active smoker	8.5%(n = 4)
Passive smoker	6.4%(n = 3)
Ex-smoker	17%(n = 8)
Non-smoker	68.1%(n = 32)

Abbreviations: a SD: Standard deviation, b cm: Centimeter, c kg: Kilograms, d BMI: Body mass index,
e kg/m²: Kilograms per square meter

Table 2 Polysomnographic data of the patients with OSA

Variable mean ± SD[a]	Male	Female	Total	P value
AHI [b]	53.27 ± 29.62	47.42 ± 18.78	51.53 ± 26.78	0.422
Desaturation index(DI)	56.02 ± 25.95	63.9 ± 26.71	55.39 ± 25.91	0.804
PaCo$_2^c$	51.28 ± 5.35	46.46 ± 7.53	49.72 ± 6.46	0.025*
Time spent < 90% [d]	110.21 ± 97.25	138.95 ± 98.81	118.77 ± 97.54	0.391
Severe OSA[e]	24(72.7%)	12(85.7%)	36(76.7%)	0.464
Moderate OSA	9(27.3%)	2(14.3%)	11(23.4%)	

Abbreviations: a SD: Standard deviation, b AHI: Apnea hypopnea index, c $PaCo_2$: Partial pressure of carbon dioxide in atrial blood, d Time spent < 90% (%): Time (minute) spent during sleep with O_2saturation < 90%,e OSA: Obstructive sleep apnea
* Significant P value

For further evaluation, the association of each demographic and polysomnographic parameter with the 6-MWT results were examined. The distance walked by the OSA patients negatively correlated with age ($r = -0.391$, $P = 0.0130$) and time spent <90% ($r = -0.316$ $P = 0.031$) in polysomnographic test and positively with the BMI ($r = 0.516$, $P < 0.001$). In addition, BMI had a reverse correlation with SaO_2 at the end of the 6MWT($r = -0.0456$, $P = 0.001$). However, the 6-MWD did not correlate with sex, smoking status, or other polysomnographic variables. In addition, polysomnographic data with the 6-MWT results were correlated. There was a significant reverse correlation between time spent <90% and AHI during polysomnography with SaO_2% at the end of the 6-MWT ($r = -0.521$, $P < 0.001$ and $r = -0.312$, $P = 0.044$). Furthermore, there was a significant correlation between the time spent <90% during polysomnography and DI during the 6-MWT($r = -0.328$, $P = 0.013$, Fig. 1).

Discussion

To the best of the authors' knowledge, the current study is among the very few studies on OSA patients in Iran and in the Middle East. Affliction with OSA is associated with decreased functional capacity and drop in daily physical activities. Such disabilities increase with age and BMI. Drop in physical activities can adversely affect the general health and quality of life of the patients. A significant association was found between the percentage of the 6-MWD and the severity of OSA in the current study. This highlights the significance of early detection of the OSA patients and indicates the impact of early diagnosis on maintenance of physical activity in such patients. On the other hand, the significant association between the 6-MWD and polysomnographic parameters such as time spent <90% indicates the optimal efficacy of this test (which is simpler than polysomnography) for detection of patients at risk of nocturnal hypoxia. The role of nocturnal intermittent hypoxia in disability of patients and also as a possible cause of dyspnea can also be evaluated as such.

A previous study has reported an association between sex and the 6-MWD and showed that female patients with OSA walked a significantly shorter distance (Pływaczewski et al., 2008). However, in the current study, no association was found between sex and any of the 6-MWT or polysomnographic findings except for $PaCO_2$, which was significantly higher in males in polysomnography. Higher prevalence of OSA in males and higher $PaCO_2$ may indicate potentially higher susceptibility of males to develop OSA and that slight changes in $PaCO_2$ may cause significant changes in SaO_2 during sleep. Studies on the effect of sex on physical activity tolerance are scarce and further investigations are required in this respect.

Most of the patients with OSA are in mid-life age (Jennum & Riha, 2009), which may be due to several factors such as structural changes and fat deposition in the para-pharyngeal area and elongation of soft palate.

Table 3 6-MWT parameters in patients with moderate vs severe OSA

	Moderate OSA[a] group	Severe OSA group	P value
6-MWD[b], m[c] ± SD[d]	555.45 ± 107.82	477.44 ± 275.65	0.173
6-MWD (%)[f] ± SD	92.4% ± 10.41	75.91 ± 36.45	0.020
HR [g],beats/min(from base-line) ± SD	30.09 ± 16.86	27.83 ± 19.26	0.733
HR·beats/min after 6-MWT ± SD	101.27 ± 24.31	104.45 ± 29.88	0.753
SaO_2% [h] at end of 6-MWT ± SD	91 ± 4.97	90.22 ± 7.67	0.758
SaO_2% at end of 6-MWT from base line ±SD	2.09 ± 5.26	1 ± 5.99	0.596

Abbreviations: a OSA: obstructive sleep apnea, b 6-MWD: distance walked during the 6-MWT, c 6-MWD,m: is expressed in absolute (meter), d SD: Standard deviation, f 6-MWD: 6-MWD is as percentage predicted (%) values, g HR: Heart rate, h SaO_2: Oxygen saturation

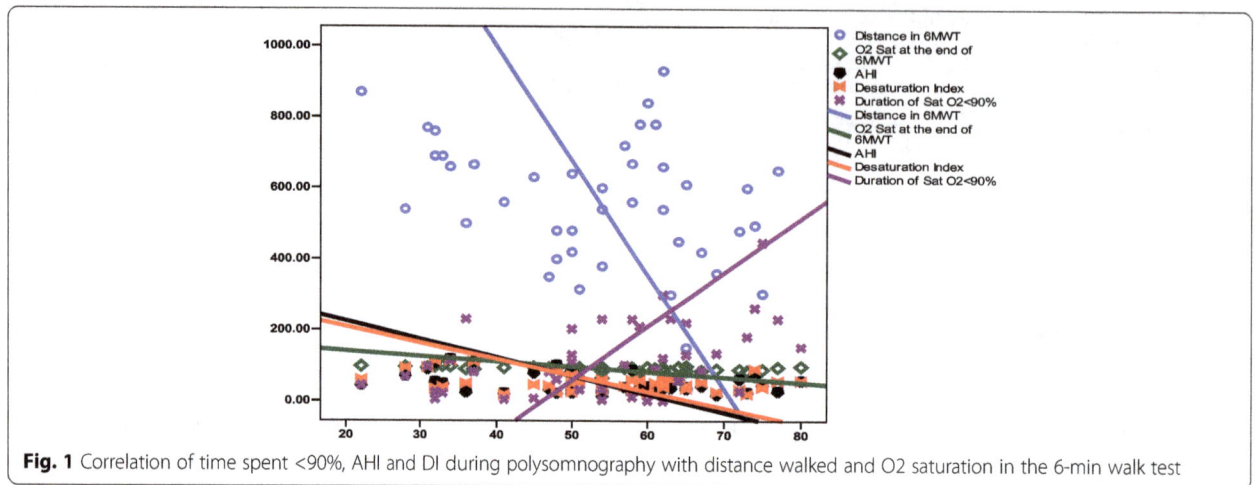

Fig. 1 Correlation of time spent <90%, AHI and DI during polysomnography with distance walked and O2 saturation in the 6-min walk test

These changes probably result in upper airway obstruction in the elderly (Eikermann et al., 2007). In the present study, an inverse correlation was found between age and the 6-MWD and oxygen saturation rate upon the completion of the test. On the other hand, age had a significant association with AHI and DI during polysomnography, indicating the possibility of nocturnal oxygen reduction and drop in daily physical activity with age. Thus, it seems that the 6-MWT can be highly efficient and applicable for detection of the elderly who carry the risk of OSA after rolling out other decreasing causes of capacity, but have yet to manifest its typical signs and symptoms.

Some researchers reported that is not a significant difference in dyspnea upon completion of the 6-MWT between those with OSA and healthy adults (Kaleth et al., 2007). However, this is a controversial topic since some other studies have demonstrated higher frequency of dyspnea upon completion of the 6-MWT in patients with OSA compared to others (Alameri et al., 2010). In the current study, approximately 80% of the patients had dyspnea upon completion of the 6-MWT; out of which, 30% had abnormal results with regard to the assessed parameters. This value was higher than that in studies reported by Pływaczewski et al. (18.5%) (Pływaczewski et al., 2008) and Ben Saad et al. (13%) (Ben Saad et al., 2015). Such a difference in the results of the studies may be due to the fact that Pływaczewski et al. (Pływaczewski et al., 2008) included patients with variable degrees of OSA, which can obviously affect the results. In the study by Ben Saad et al. (Ben Saad et al., 2015) patients were under treatment with CPAP; while the CPAP patients were excluded in the present study. Sample size and male/female ratio can also be responsible for the variability in the results of studies.

The 6-MWD in patients with severe OSA was significantly less than that in other patients, demonstrating the significant effect of disease severity on reduction of daily activities. It also shows that the patients who walk a shorter distance in the 6-MWT probably experience nocturnal apnea and hypoxia, which may be related to disease severity.

High BMI and obesity decrease functional capacity due to increased workload and decreased respiratory function and significantly affect the ability to perform physical activities. In the current study, higher BMI was associated with shorter 6-MWD, which is in agreement with the results of previous studies (Kaleth et al., 2007; Alameri et al., 2010; Pływaczewski et al., 2008). This finding suggests that weight control programs focusing on a healthy diet and regular exercise can significantly improve the performance of the patients.

Adults commonly experience a reduction in blood pressure and heart rate during sleep, which is probably due to the decreased activity of the autonomous system (sympathetic and parasympathetic) (Alameri et al., 2010). Interestingly, the opposite occurs in the OSA patients, and a significant increase in sympathetic tone during the nocturnal arousal episodes results in a significant increase in heart rate during sleep (Narkiewicz et al., 1998; Somers et al., 1993). The pattern of the heart rate response in the OSA patients is still a matter of controversy. Alameri et al. (Alameri et al., 2010) showed that, compared to healthy individuals, acceleration of heart rate is slower in the OSA patients and it takes longer for the heart rate to return back to normal after exercise and physical activity. In the current study, a significant increase in heart rate was noted after the conduction of the 6-MWT compared to baseline, which indicates the probable role of autonomous system dysregulation in the pathogenesis of OSA.

Furthermore, DI during the 6-MWT can provide us with valuable information about the desaturation caused by exercise and severity of the disease. The significant association of DI during the 6-MWT and time spent < 90% during polysomnographymay be attributed

Can 6-minute walk test predict severity of obstructive sleep apnea...

71

to the fact that decreased oxygen during sleep in patients with OSA can alter oxygen availability through alveolar capillaries in such a way to limit physical activities. Tachycardia or other arrhythmia during nocturnal hypoxemia can result in pulmonary arterial hypertension. These events can also explain nocturnal desaturation (Shepard et al., 1985; Coccagna & Lugaresi, 1978). By considering the fact that the reduction in arterial oxygen is correlated with the severity of the OSA, abnormal DI upon completion of the 6-MWT was expected in our patients, since they had moderate to severe OSA. The same results were reported in previous studies (Alameri et al., 2010; Ben Saad et al., 2015; Shepard et al., 1985; Coccagna & Lugaresi, 1978). This is particularly important as DI at the end of the 6-MWT can predict the level of nocturnal oxygen reduction in patients with OSA. This is useful in treatment planning and selection of treatment strategies. Casanova et al. demonstrated that in patients with chronic obstructive pulmonary disease, DI during the 6-MWT negatively affected the prognosis of patients. However, the accuracy of this finding in the OSA patients has not been yet tested (Casanova et al., 2008).

Significant correlation of arterial oxygen saturation, DI and AHI at the end of the 6-MWT with time spent <90% during polysomnography indicates that patients who have lower arterial oxygen saturation rate during daily activities experience greater and more significant changes in oxygenation at night. This further highlights the significance of the 6-MWT as a simple and efficient tool for assessment of the OSA patients. The 6-MWT is generally a screening tool for cardiac function and lower airway disease, but this study has shown that it can also be used to assess for an upper airway disease (i.e obstructive sleep apnea).

The present study had some limitations: First, there is not a control group. If a control group was present, possible significant differences between the test and control groups could have further confirmed the efficacy of the 6-MWT for early detection of patients with OSA or those at risk of developing OSA. The second limitation is that other factors limiting physical activities and subsequently the test results (such as muscle strength and psychological factors) were not taken into account.

Conclusion

In general, based on the above-mentioned findings, it appears that the 6-MWT can be used in patients with OSA to assess their physical ability and tolerance of activities. Also, it can help predict the severity of the disease and assist in selection of the most appropriate treatment strategy to increase the physical ability of the patients.

Acknowledgements
Not applicable.

Funding
There was no any providing funding. Authors paid all expenses including data collection, analysis and also writing by themselves.

Authors' contributions
Study conception and designs: PAN and MM had the main rule in this part. Acquisition of data: HAT collected data specially 6- MWT datasets, PAN and MM gathered PSGs' results and PAN also reported the PSG tests. Analysis and interpretation of data: Analysis and conclusion of data was done by OA and HAT. Drafting of manuscript: HAT and OA prepared initial manuscript. Critical revesion: PAN and OA wrote critical review. All authors reviewed the final article and approved the work.

Competing interests
The authors declare that they have no competing interests

Author details
[1]Clinical Tuberculosis and Epidemiology Research Center, National Research Institute of Tuberculosis and Lung Diseases (NRITLD), Shahid Beheshti University of Medical Sciences, Tehran, Iran. [2]Chronic Respiratory Diseases Research Center, National Research Institute of Tuberculosis and Lung Diseases (NRITLD), Shahid Beheshti University of Medical Sciences, Masih Daneshvari Hospital, Darabad Avenue, Shahid Bahonar roundabout, Tehran, Iran. [3]Tracheal Diseases Research Center, National Research Institute of Tuberculosis and Lung Diseases (NRITLD), Shahid Beheshti University of Medical Sciences, Tehran, Iran.

References
Al Lawati NM, Patel SR, Ayas NT. Epidemiology, risk factors, and consequences of obstructive sleep Apnea and short sleep duration. Prog Cardiovasc Dis. 2009; 51(4):285–93.

Alameri H, Al-Kabab Y, BaHammam A. Submaximal exercise in patients with severe obstructive sleep apnea. Sleep and Breathing. 2010;14(2):145–51.

ATS statement. Guidelines for the six-minute walk test. Am J Respir Crit Care Med. 2002;166:111e7.

Ben Saad H, Babba M, Boukamcha R, et al. Investigation of exclusive narghile smokers: deficiency and incapacity measured by spirometry and 6-minute walk test. Respir Care. 2014;59:1696e709.

Ben Saad H, Ben Hassen K, Ghannouchi I, Latiri I, Rouatbi S. 6-min walk-test data in severe obstructivesleep-apnea-hypopnea-syndrome (OSAHS) under continuous-positive-airway-pressure (CPAP) treatment. Respir Med. 2015;109: 642–55.

Cahalin LP, Mathier MA, Semigran MJ, Dec GW. DiSalvoTG. The six-minute walk test predicts peak oxygen uptake and survival in patients with advanced heart failure. Chest. 1996;110(2):325–32.

Casanova C, Cote C, Marin JM, et al. Distance and oxygen desaturation during the 6-min walk test as predictors of long-term mortality in patients with COPD. Chest. 2008;134:746–5.

Coccagna G, Lugaresi E. Arterial blood gases and pulmonary and systemic arterial pressure during sleep in chronic obstructive pulmonary disease. Sleep. 1978; 1:117–24.

Eikermann M, Jordan AS, Chamberlin NL, et al. The influence of aging on pharyngeal collapsibility during sleep. Chest. 2007;131:1702–9.

Flaherty KR, Andrei AC, Murray S, Fraley C, Colby TV, Travis WD, et al. Idiopathic pulmonary fibrosis: prognostic value of changes in physiology and six minute hall walk. Am J Respir Crit Care Med. 2006;174(7):803–9.

Hoeper MM, Schwarze M, Ehlerding S, Adler-Schuermeyer A, Spiekerkoetter E, Niedermeyer J, et al. Long-term treatment of primary pulmonary hypertension with aerosolized iloprost, a prostacyclin analogue. N Engl J Med. 2000;342(25):1866–70.

Holland AE, Spruit MA, Troosters T, et al. An official European Respiratory Society/ American Thoracic Society technical standard: field walking tests in chronic respiratory disease. Eur Respir J. 2014;44:1428–46.

International Classification of Sleep Disorders. Diagnostic & coding manual. 2nd ed. Westchester: American Academy of Sleep Medicine; 2005.

Jennum P, Riha RL. Epidemiology of sleep apnoea/hypopnoea syndrome and sleep-disordered breathing. Eur Respir J. 2009;33:907–14.

Kaleth AS, Chittenden TW, Hawkins BJ, Hargens TA, Guill SG, Zedalis D, et al. Unique cardiopulmonary exercise test responses in overweight middle-aged adults with obstructive sleep apnea. Sleep Med. 2007;8(2):160–8.

Mulgrew T, Ryan CF, Fleetham JA, et al. The impact of obstructive sleep apnea and daytime sleepiness on work limitation. Sleep Med. 2007;9:42–53.

Narkiewicz K, van de Borne PJ, Cooley RL, Dyken ME, Somers VK. Sympathetic activity in obese subjects with and without obstructive sleep apnea. Circulation. 1998;98(8):772–6.

Pływaczewski R, Stokłosa A, Bieleń P, Bednarek M, Czerniawska J, Jonczak L, Górecka D. Sliwiński six-minute walk test in obstructive sleep apnoea. Pneumonol Alergol Pol. 2008;76(2):75–82.

Pusalavidyasagar S, Iber C. Current medical concepts in obstructive sleep apnea. Oper Tech Otolaryngol Head Neck Surg. 2015;26(2):52–8.

Richard B, Charlene E, Susan M, Robin M, Carole L and Bradley V. The American Academy of sleep medicine the AASM manual for the scoring of sleep and associated events: rules, terminology and technical specifications,version 2. 2(2015).

Roul G, Germain P, Bareiss P. Does the 6-minute walk test predicts the prognosis in patients with NYHA class II or III chronic heart failure? Am Heart J. 1998; 136(3):449–57.

Sari AA, Rezaei S, Arab M, Majdzadeh R, Matin BK, Zandian H. Effects of smoking on cost of hospitalization and length of stay among patients with lung cancer in Iran: a hospital-based study. Asian Pac J Cancer Prev. 2016;17(9): 4421–6.

Shepard JW Jr, Garrison MW, Grither DA, Evans R, Schweitzer PK. Relationship of ventricular ectopy to nocturnal oxygen desaturation in patients with chronic obstructive pulmonary disease. Am J Med. 1985;78:28–34.

Singh SJ, Puhan MA, Andrianopoulos V, et al. An official systematic review of the European Respiratory Society/American Thoracic Society: measurement properties of field walking tests in chronic respiratory disease. Eur Respir J. 2014;44:1447–78.

Somers VK, Dyken ME, Mark AL, Abboud FM. Sympathetic-nerve activity during sleep in normal subjects. N Engl J Med. 1993;328(5):303–7.

Vanuxem D, Badier M, Guillot C, Delpierre S, Jahjah F, Vanuxem P. Impairment of muscle energy metabolism in patients with sleep apnoea syndrome. Respir Med. 1997;91(9):551–7.

Wittmann V, Rodenstein DO. Health care costs and the sleep apnea syndrome. Sleep Med Rev. 2004;8:269e79.

10

Yoga Nidra: An innovative approach for management of chronic insomnia- A case report

Karuna Datta[1], Manjari Tripathi[2] and Hruda Nanda Mallick[1*]

Abstract

Background: Chronic insomnia is a common sleep problem and there is a need to complement the existing treatment options. *Yoga nidra* practice is documented to be used for sleep by sages. Recently, *yoga nidra* has been used in patients of menstrual abnormalities, post- traumatic stress disorder, diabetes, anxiety and depression but little is known about its effect on sleep or sleep disorders. Although we find description of *yoga nidra* in literature, there is no scientific report of its application in sleep disorders. The objective of the study was to develop *yoga nidra* model in management of chronic insomnia patients. The model was developed using inputs from *yoga* school trained instructors of *yoga nidra*.

Case presentations: Patient 01: 60 years old widower with complaints of sleep maintenance insomnia since 20 years. He had worry at daytime regarding falling off to sleep which became even worse at bedtime. He had history of benign prostatic hypertrophy and had no history of any medications for sleep or any other disease. Patient 02: 78 years old male self-employed, company owner with complaints of sleep maintenance insomnia since 15 years. He felt quite energetic during the day due to the work requirement but in the evening started feeling anxious about sleep problem which worsened at bedtime. He was on tablet clonazepam 0.25 mg HS off and on since 1 year. After the baseline assessment, *yoga nidra* intervention was started followed by five supervised sessions after which the patients were instructed to practice *yoga nidra* daily on their own. Regular fortnightly follow ups were done till 4 weeks of start of *yoga nidra* intervention. Repeat PSG was offered in case patient volunteered. Sleep diary parameters were analysed using Friedman test and Wilcoxon Signed Ranks test. There was an improvement in sleep quality, insomnia severity, depression anxiety and stress scores after *yoga nidra*. The improvement remained even after 3 months of start of intervention. Repeat PSG in second patient showed an increase in N3 after 4 weeks of *yoga nidra* intervention.

Conclusion: *Yoga nidra* can be used as an important adjunct in management of chronic insomnia patients.

Keywords: *Yoga nidra*, Chronic insomnia, Intervention, *Yoga nidra* intervention model, Case report

Background

Chronic insomnia is a common sleep problem and is associated with increased morbidity and mortality (Taylor et al. 2007). Available treatment options include pharmacological and non-pharmacological approach. Studies have shown sleeping pill users at a greater mortality risk (Kripke et al. 2002) and though drugs like zolpidem have been found to be safe for short term use (Schutte-Rodin et al. 2008) but when taken for years these medications also produce unwanted side effects like sleep related eating disorders and sleep walking (Hoque and Chesson 2009) and even increased cancer risk (Kao et al. 2012).

Non pharmacological approach using cognitive behavioral therapy for insomnia (CBTI) is considered beneficial. CBTI though remains the first line of therapy for insomnia but is often underutilized (Schutte-Rodin et al. 2008). Underutilisation of CBTI is reported because of reasons which are both patient centred and system based issues. Patient related reasons include time and cost

* Correspondence: drhmallick@yahoo.com
[1]Department of Physiology, All India Institute of Medical Sciences, New Delhi, India
Full list of author information is available at the end of the article

involvement and limited availability of CBTI trained specialists being a major system based problem.

Complementary and alternative medicine in the form of Kundalini yoga (Khalsa 2004), Tai Chih Chi (Irwin et al. 2008), mindfulness meditation (Ong et al. 2014), acupuncture and Chinese herbal medicines have been tried in insomnia patients. There is a felt need to complement the existing gamut of treatment options for insomnia patients.

According to the ancient Indian scriptures, sages are known to sleep using *yoga nidra*. *Yoga Nidra* is derived from two Sanskrit words, 'Yoga' ('yuj' = yoke) meaning union or one pointed awareness and 'nidra' means sleep. *Yoga nidra* is derived from '*pratyahara*' of raja yoga and tantric practise of '*nyasa*'. In '*pratyahara*' mind and mental awareness are dissociated from the sensory channels. '*Nyasa*' means 'to place or to take the mind to that point'. *Yoga nidra* is documented as neither *nyasa* nor meditation as *yoga nidra* is done in supine position and unlike meditation which is an aware awake state, *yoga nidra* is considered as aware sleep state (Saraswati 1998). '*Nyasa*' is practised in sitting posture and involves the recitation of *mantras* in Sanskrit to experience different parts of the body which increases the scope of this practise beyond different cultures.

Yoga nidra was known to be practised by sages and it was passed on to their disciples traditionally. Swami Satyananda Saraswati, renowned teacher from Bihar School of Yoga, Munger, Bihar, India laid down the basics of learning *yoga nidra* in the form of a book. He described *yoga nidra* as a 'systematic method of inducing complete physical, mental and emotional relaxation and in this state the relaxation is achieved by turning inwards, away from outer experiences' (Saraswati 1998). It can be done following instructions from his book by a teacher or by a way of audio compact disc (CD).

Yoga nidra has been tried as a therapeutic option for many diseases. The relative ease of practise has made it an acceptable therapeutic option for many diseases. *Yoga nidra* has been used in patients of menstrual abnormalities (Rani et al. 2011), post- traumatic stress disorder (Stankovic 2011), diabetes (Amita et al. 2009), anxiety and depression (Rani et al. 2012) but little is known about its effect on sleep or sleep disorders.

Although we find description of *yoga nidra* in literature, there is no scientific report of its application in sleep disorders.

Since *yoga nidra* has been used as a therapeutic option with no documented side effects and it is mentioned related to sleep in scriptures, there was a felt need to develop this method as a model in management of chronic insomnia patients.

The objective of the study was to develop *yoga nidra* as a complementary model in management of chronic insomnia patients. Authors had asked for volunteers through advertisement placed at various OPDs. Two patients aged 60 and 78 years, who volunteered for the model of yoga nidra, are discussed. They were explained about the nature of study and informed consent was obtained. The study was approved by the Institutional ethical committee of All India Institute of Medical Sciences, New Delhi, India (reference number IESC/T-394/ 02.11.2012).

Case presentations

Diagnosed chronic insomnia patients came from sleep clinic out patients department (OPD) of MT[1], senior neurologist and certified sleep specialist. They were on treatment and were referred to KD[2] in case they volunteered to add *yoga nidra* intervention to the already prescribed treatment. An informed consent from the patient was taken.

Inclusion criteria

Patients following usual sleep wake schedule during the study period. Patients with morning circadian preference were included. Patients who were keen to volunteer for the study were included and they had a right to withdraw anytime during the study.

Exclusion criteria

Any patient who was likely to plan an intercontinental flight or was not able to follow usual sleep wake schedule during the study period. Patients with evening circadian preference were excluded from the study. Morningness Eveningness Scale (MES) (Horne and Ostberg 1976; Paine et al. 2006) was used to screen patients and only those patients with a morning preference were taken. This was done as the patients should have been most alert at the time of *yoga nidra* session which was in the morning from 0900 h to 1130 h making it important to exclude patients with delayed circadian rhythm. The scale also assess the time of the morning when they were most alert which helped in planning the *yoga nidra* sessions further. We included morning preference also because we did not want circadian rhythm as a confounding factor since the effect of *yoga nidra* on circadian rhythm is not known.

Patients

Two patients Patient 01 and 02 underwent the intervention using *yoga nidra* model.

Patient 01: 60 years old widower with complaints of not able to sleep after getting up at night since 20 years for more than 30 min and more than three times a week. Patient had worry at daytime regarding falling off to sleep which became even worse at bedtime. Patient had history of benign prostatic hypertrophy and had no history of any medications for sleep or any other disease.

Patient 02: 78 years old male self-employed, company owner with complaints of not able to sleep after getting awake at night for more than 30 min and more than three times a week since 15 years. He felt quite energetic during the day due to the work requirement but in the evening started feeling anxious about sleep problem which worsened at bedtime. He was on tablet clonazepam 0.25 mg HS off and on since 1 year.

Development of a model for using *yoga nidra* in insomnia patients

KD[2] visited Bihar School of Yoga, Munger and attended sessions of *yoga nidra* taken by teachers. Permission to use *yoga nidra* for chronic insomnia patients was taken. She had discussions with the teachers and doctor in the school. The teachers brought out the usual problems faced during conducting and also while doing the session oneself. KD[2] also did sessions herself under supervision while in ashram to get a hands-on feel of the session which would help planning for the patients subsequently. Planning of the session was done keeping the discussion in mind. The patients were taught using pre-recorded audio CD on *yoga nidra*© from the school which are easily available for sale.

The discussion brought out that a *yoga nidra* session every day for 3 to 4 days as done in short yoga programmes helps their subject to make them comfortable during the session. It was also pointed out that at times the instructions are not clear to all the subjects and might require elaboration on an individual basis. Keeping these points in mind five supervised sessions were planned continuously every day for 5 days. The method of doing *yoga nidra* involves seven steps namely – preparation, samkalpa (samkalpa = idea or notion formed in the heart or mind), body part awareness or rotation of consciousness, breath awareness, feeling and sensation, visualization and ending of practice (Saraswati 1998).

Planning of the Model included three basic parts

a) Assessment for readiness and voluntary participation
   Discussion with yoga teachers and doctor at the school brought out that the subject has to be ready for taking a session as it included voluntarily following the instructions without sleeping. It was suggested by the Bihar school of yoga teachers that the session should be carried out when the person is most alert to avoid sleep during the session. Since the sessions were done in the morning hours, we excluded patients with an evening circadian preference in the study.
   The patient was verbally informed that this method was novel and though has been tried in other diseases with no reported side effects but it was

essential to follow up closely for initial days requiring the patient to report daily for a minimum of 5 days initially and subsequently for follow ups. Since it required time, volunteering was an indirect measure of the commitment of the patient towards the management. The patient was free to withdraw from the study at any time of the intervention.
   The patient was then briefed about *yoga nidra*, its philosophy and available reports of its use as a therapeutic option. Then baseline assessment was completed and documented.

b) Supervised sessions
   Initial five daily supervised sessions at the time when they are most alert during daytime was planned. Each session takes approximately 30 min. Before the start of the session, the patient was instructed to make himself comfortable. Since, insomnia patients are sensitive to changes in their daily routine on sleep (basic premise for use of principles of sleep hygiene and education), intervention like *yoga nidra* is likely to affect sleep and hence the patients were kept under direct supervision of a certified sleep specialist. The constant supervision was maintained by KD at all times, initially by planning daily supervised sessions and the monitoring using sleep diary/development of any new symptoms specifically for potential side effects (Edinger et al. 2015) and informing about regular follow ups.

What to do during the session for the observer
The patient was not interrupted during the session. Signs of restlessness e.g. tossing and turning, moving hands, shutting eyes too tightly, not looking relaxed etc. were observed. Cues of whether the patient was following instructions were carefully noted e.g. When the instructor asked the subject to take a deep breath, or look down while keeping eyes closed, the observer made a note of whether the patient followed. In case the patient was found not following instructions or appeared restless, time of the practise was noted from the player and subsequently discussed after the session.

Discussion by the observer with the patient after the session

I. The patient was asked of the various phases of *yoga nidra* (as mentioned in 'Additional file 1') he felt he went through. This is extremely important as *yoga nidra* is considered very relaxing and might put an insomnia patient to sleep despite being the most alert time of the day for him. According to the experienced teachers usually there is 50% retention of the basic various phases by the second day of practise. The practising subjects on an average start remembering all the different phases by the end of the fourth day. We gave 5 days considering some insomnia patients might fall sleepy during the sessions. Then the patients were asked to practise the session at home every day.

II. Patients were now asked about the problem faced during the session. The noted time points by the observer where he felt the patient was not following were also discussed. In case any clarifications regarding the instructions were required they were provided so as to better the next session.

III. The patient was also encouraged to listen to the tape at home after the first supervised session and was instructed to write down instructions which were not clear to the patient. This was done to increase his compliance during the subsequent sessions. These points of the patient were discussed the next day before starting the next day session as advised by yoga school since it relieves anxiety of the patient.

IV. The entire session was then discussed with the patient as to how he feels it went, the patient was assured and instructed to follow the instructions as they were and not analyse or worry about them.

Yoga nidra intervention was done using a copyrighted pre-recorded *Yoga Nidra* audio CD approximately 27.2 min from Bihar School of Yoga, Munger, Bihar, India. Conduct of *yoga nidra* session was done in a sound proof room, with minimal ambient lighting during daytime. The subject was made to lie in the supine posture on a comfortable mattress. The entire session was done in *shavasana* (*shava* means "corpse" and *asana* means "posture"). The posture used for this asana is lying on the back, the arms and legs are kept at about 45° with the palms facing upwards. A soft pillow is optional to give maximum comfort to the patient while the entire session. This posture minimises the contact points especially between the limbs of the body. Brief outline of practise of doing *yoga nidra* and general instructions given to subjects is attached in 'Additional file 1' (Saraswati 1998).

Outcome measures

a) Sleep diary– Sleep diary was used by the patients to mark the daily activities. This could be filled on paper or on an excel sheet according to the patients choice.

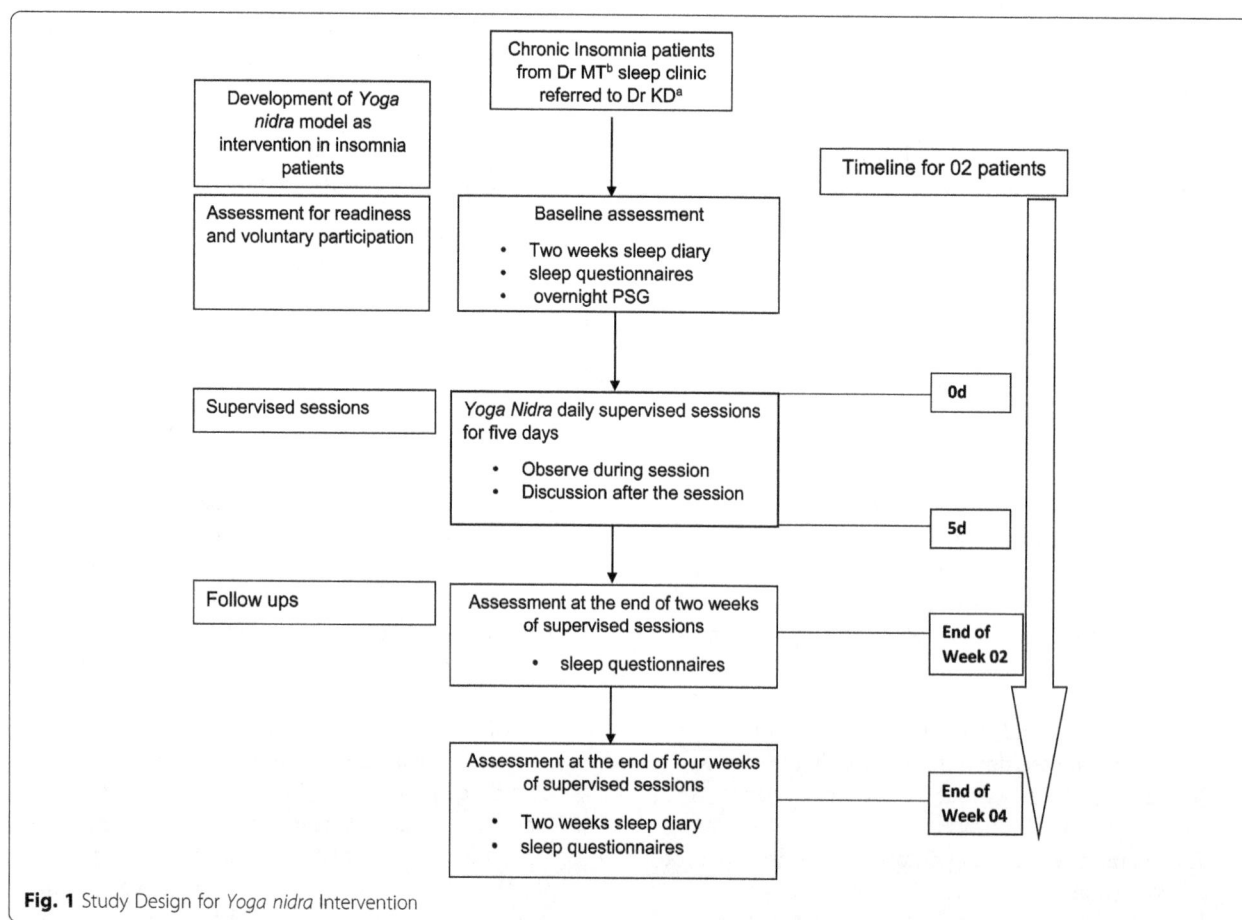

Fig. 1 Study Design for *Yoga nidra* Intervention

The diary was to be filled twice a day, once in the morning on getting up and then again at night just before bedtime. The individual fills in the details of time of lying in bed, approximate time required to fall asleep, wake up time, number of breaks in sleep and the approximate time that the individual feels that he was awake before falling off to sleep. Sleep quality on a scale of 10 was also reported in the diary along with other details of time of meals, exercise and time of *yoga nidra*. Parameters calculated using 2 weeks sleep diary were- Time in Bed (TIB): the total time the individual was lying in the bed i.e. the number of hours from the time of lying in bed to time of finally waking up; Sleep Onset Latency (SOL): the time initially spent in bed trying to sleep after lying in bed to sleep; Wake After Sleep Onset (WASO): time spent awake in bed after initially sleeping and before finally waking up; Total Sleep Time (TST): TST can be calculated by subtracting the SOL and WASO from TIB; Sleep Efficiency: calculated by the formula- (TST/TIB)

x100; Total Wake Duration (TWD): SOL + total time of sleep breaks. These parameters were calculated for each night for the patient. Day 01st to 14th represent baseline, 15th day represents the first day of *yoga nidra* intervention, 28th -41st was used for the data analysis i.e. when the patient came for fourth week follow up. Baseline sleep diary was a mandatory requirement as is considered an important tool in assessing sleep in an insomnia patient.

b) Sleep questionnaires- Pittsburgh Sleep Quality Index (PSQI) (Buysse et al. 1989), Insomnia Severity Index (ISI) (Morin et al. 2011), Depression Anxiety Stress Scale (DASS) (Lovibond and Lovibond 1995; Brown et al. 1997) Epworth Sleepiness Scale ("ESS © MW JOHNS 1990–1997. USED UNDER LICENSE") (Johns 1991) Pre Sleep Arousal Scale (PSAS) (Nicassio et al. 1985).

c) Digital polysomnography (PSG) - Overnight PSG was done using Somnomedics© PSG system, Germany with the standard montage. Electroencephalography (EEG), Electro-oculography

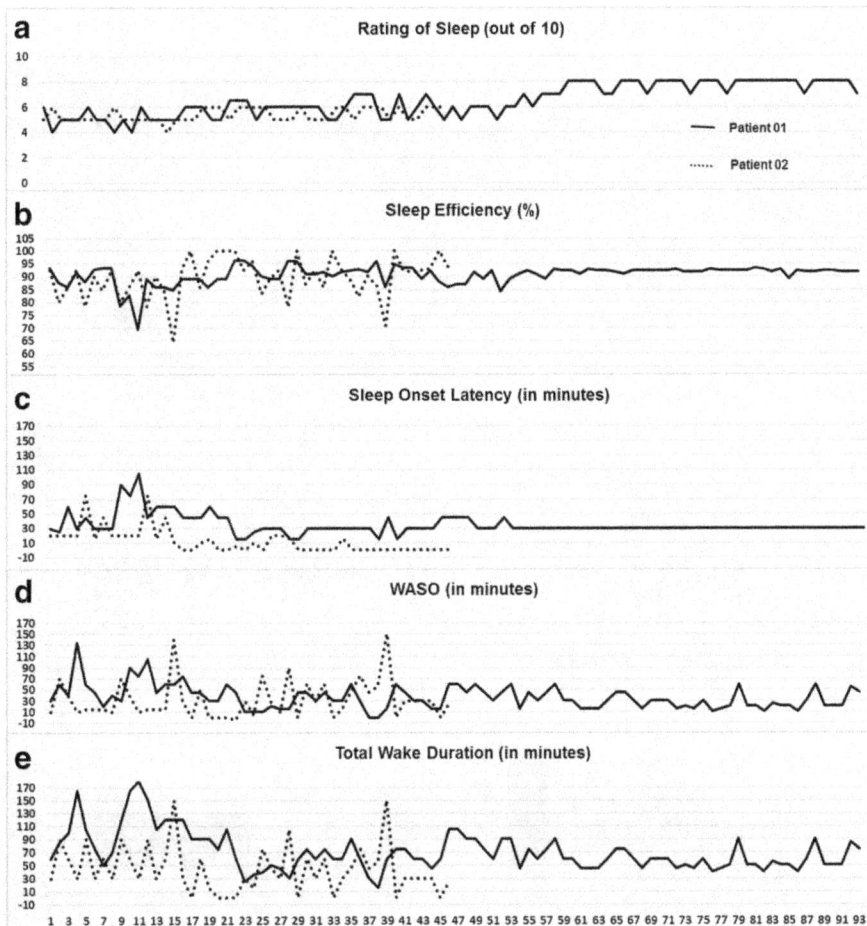

Fig. 2 a–e Sleep diary records of both patients

(EOG) and Electromyography (EMG) were sampled at 256 Hz. The low frequency and high frequency filter setting were EEG-0.3,35 Hz; EOG-0.3,35 Hz; EMG-10,256 Hz; EEG, EOG and EMG channels were placed along with pulse oximeter, RIP belts for thoracic and abdominal movements, Electrocardiography (ECG), oronasal pressure cannula and thermistor sensors according to American Association of Sleep Medicine (AASM) guidelines (Berry et al. 2014). Notch filter at 50 Hz was put and simultaneous video monitoring was done with the PSG device during the entire night. This was done in MT[1] sleep lab by technicians. The staging of the sleep was done using AASM criteria and relative percentages of various sleep stages were calculated. Parameters like TIB, TST, WASO, SPT, Sleep Period Time (TST+ WASO), SOL: Time from start of recording to first epoch of sleep and, REM Latency, SE = TSTx100/TBT were calculated. Various stages of rapid eye movement sleep (REM) and Non REM sleep (N1, N2, N3) were scored and calculated as percentage of TST and TIB.

Follow ups

Two fortnightly follow ups were considered mandatory for the patients after the start of *yoga nidra* intervention. During this study, patients were also instructed to meet MT[1] at least at the end of the month and at any time when the patient felt he deteriorated during this intervention.

Assessment of outcome measures

Primary outcome measures which were considered for improvement of patients were related to sleep and also improvement in daytime functioning (Edinger et al. 2015). These were sleep diary parameters -total sleep time, total wake duration, overall rating of sleep quality and Insomnia Severity Index for assessment of sleep. Day time functioning was evaluated by depression anxiety and stress scores during daytime using DASS and sleepiness during the day using "ESS © MW JOHNS 1990–1997 (Johns 1991). USED UNDER LICENSE". Pre sleep arousal scale was also used. From this scale a total score, somatic and cognitive score of pre sleep arousal were calculated. A reduction in these scores occurs with reduction in pre sleep arousal. An increase in insomnia severity index,

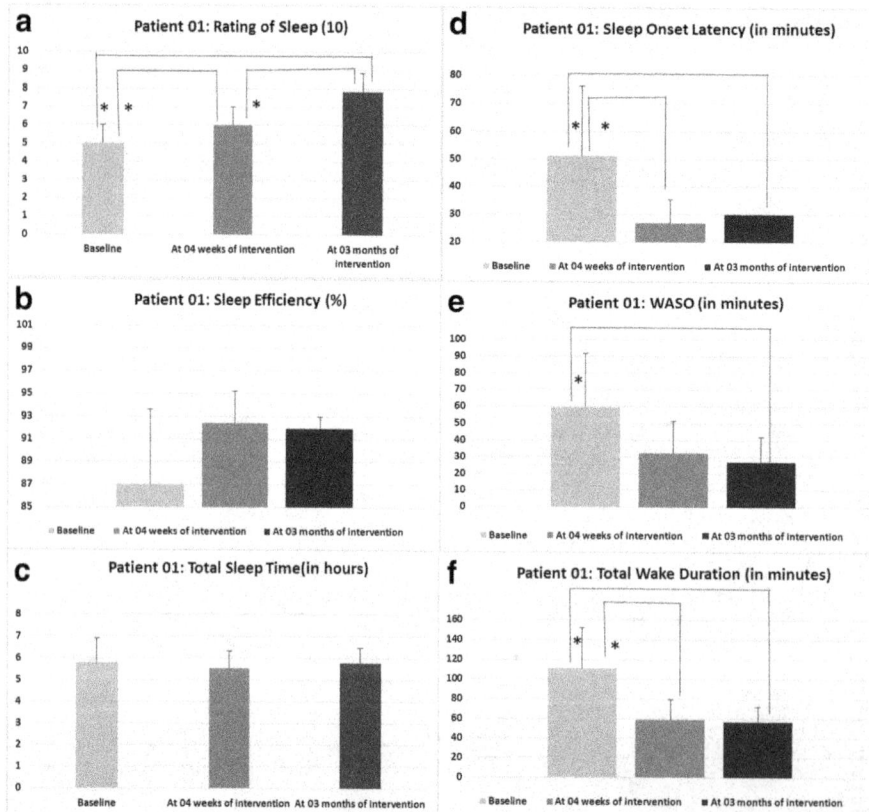

Fig. 3 a–f Sleep diary parameters of patient 01 showing various sleep wake parameters. *$p < 0.025$(using Wilcoxon Signed Rank test and adjusted Bonferroni correction $p < 0.05/2 = 0.025$)

ESS©MW JOHNS 1990–1997 (Johns 1991) and DASS shows increase in severity in insomnia, increase in daytime sleepiness and increase in depression, anxiety and stress scores respectively.

Study design consisting of first 2 weeks of baseline followed by intervention using supervised *yoga nidra* training is shown in timeline in Fig. 1.

Baseline assessment

After obtaining informed consent from the patient, as a baseline assessment apart from the 2 weeks sleep diary the patients had to fill sleep questionnaires ISI, "ESS (Johns 1991) © MW JOHNS 1990–1997. USED UNDER LICENSE", PSQI and pre sleep arousal scale. Patients also filled MES which was used to screen subjects and only those with morning preference were used for the study. Baseline PSG was done. This was done not only to assess insomnia but also to document presence of other sleep disorders.

Yoga nidra supervised sessions

Yoga nidra training was done using copyrighted CD. After 05 days of *yoga nidra* training under supervision, the patients were instructed to practice *yoga nidra* at home daily at a time when he was alert.

Assessment at the end of two weeks

PSQI, "ESS (Johns 1991) © MW JOHNS 1990–1997. USED UNDER LICENSE", ISI, and PSAS and patient were instructed to fill sleep diary for the next 14 days.

Assessment at the end of four weeks

Questionnaires like PSQI, "ESS (Johns 1991) © MW JOHNS 1990–1997. USED UNDER LICENSE", ISI, and PSAS were completed by the patient and 2 weeks sleep diary of the past 2 weeks was collected as assessed.

Outcomes

Sleep diaries for both the patients were analysed. Patient 01 filled the diary continuously till 93rd day i.e. 79th day after intervention (93-14 = 79) and patient 02 till 46th day i.e. 32nd day after starting intervention. Analysis of sleep diary was done as: baseline1-14; at 1 month-28–41 day and for patient 01 at 3 months as 79–93 day. Various sleep diary parameters are shown schematically for patient 01 and 02 in Fig. 2.

Sleep diary parameters of patient 01 showed significant changes in sleep onset latency (Friedman $\chi 2$ (2) = 12.606, $p < .005$), WASO (Friedman $\chi 2$ (2) = 7.370, $p < .05$), TWD (Friedman $\chi 2$ (2) = 16.618, $p < .005$) and rating of sleep on a scale of 0 to 10 (Friedman $\chi 2$ (2) = 23.192, $p < .0005$).

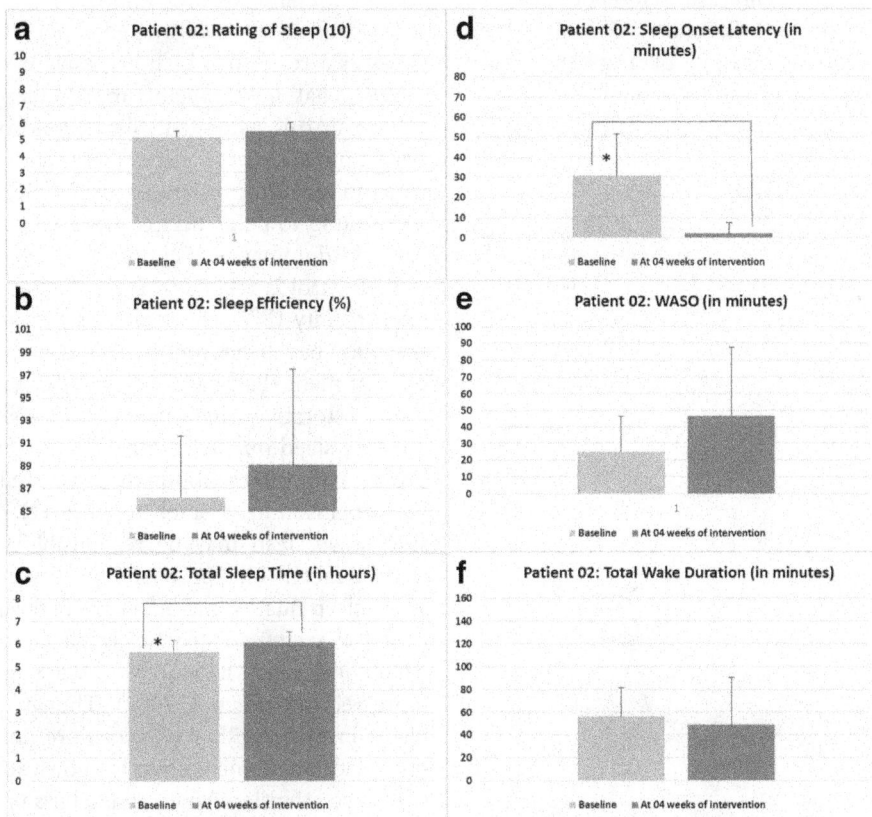

Fig. 4 a–f Sleep diary parameters of patient 02 showing various sleep wake parameters. *$p < 0.05$(using Wilcoxon Signed Rank test)

Table 1 Questionnaires of patient 01 during the intervention and at follow ups

Questionnaire	Patient 01				
	Baseline	Mid intervention after 14 days	After 04 weeks of intervention	Three months Post intervention	Six months Post intervention
Insomnia Severity Index	13	10	5	3	4
PSAS Total score	28	26	20	18	18
PSAS Total somatic score	8	8	8	8	8
PSAS Total Cognitive score	20	18	12	10	10
PSQI Total 0–21	8	–[a]	5	4	4
Depression of DASS	2	0	0	0	0
Anxiety of DASS	0	0	0	0	0
Stress of DASS	4	2	0	0	0
ESS[b]	13	10	5	3	3

[a]PSQI is filled keeping past 1 month in mind and hence was not collected at 14 days of intervention
[b] ESS (Johns 1991) © MW JOHNS 1990–1997. USED UNDER LICENSE

Results of post hoc tests are shown in Fig. 3. Sleep diary parameters of patient 02 are shown in Fig. 4. Significant improvement was found in SOL and TST as shown in the figure.

On regular visits patients were asked about the anxiety and worry regarding falling asleep. They reported an improvement in the problem. Our patients did not report any headaches, drowsiness, or any daytime symptom of excessive sleepiness. The ISI, DASS and PSAS scores were also noted. Questionnaireresults for both patients are shown in Tables 1 and 2. BaselinePSG data of both patients did not show association of any other sleep

Table 2 Questionnaires of patient 02 during the intervention and at follow ups

Questionnaire	Patient 02			
	Baseline	Mid intervention after 14 days	After 04 weeks of intervention	Three months Post intervention
Insomnia Severity Index	12	5	0	0
PSAS Total score	55	36	33	39
PSAS Total somatic score	15	11	11	13
PSAS Total Cognitive score	40	25	22	26
PSQI Total 0–21	11	–[a]	10	1
Depression of DASS	10	11	1	2
Anxiety of DASS	5	13	3	0
Stress of DASS	17	19	9	0
ESS[b]	4	6	6	3

[a]PSQI is filled keeping past 1 month in mind and hence was not collected at 14 days of intervention
[b] ESS (Johns 1991) © MW JOHNS 1990–1997. USED UNDER LICENSE

problem. The latencies and percentage of different stages is shown in Table 3 along with repeat PSG of Patient 01 who volunteered to undergo repeat PSG after 04 weeks of intervention.

Discussion and Conclusions

After *yoga nidra* intervention, we found significant changes in sleep parameters. In the first patient total sleep time did not change significantly though sleep onset latency and WASO improved significantly. In our study patients were instructed about sleep hygiene principles as a result of which excessive lying in bed was reduced. That may explain improvement in sleep onset latency in this patient. In the second patient both total sleep time and sleep onset latency showed improvement with no significant changes in WASO. *Yoga nidra* has been found to be associated with shift towards parasympathetic dominance (Markil et al. 2012). High cardiac vagal control is related to better subjective and objective sleep quality (Werner et al. 2015). Yoga practise in the morning has been found to increase parasympathetic drive at night (Patra and Telles 2010) causing sleep to be more restorative which may explain significant improvement in sleep quality ratings and WASO.N3% TST improved with intervention which is a reliable indicator in PSG in insomnia (Israel et al. 2012). This increase in slow wave sleep may be responsible for the improved sleep quality. The probable mechanisms which might affect sleep quality and subjectively feeling better may be linked to cognitive structuring effects of these practices which make the mental processing of external inputs more relaxed (Deepak 2002). Though probable mechanisms involved with *yoga nidra* are not clear at present but mindfulness meditation is known to target deficits in executive attention which characterise mood and anxiety (Ainsworth et al. 2013) and psychological symptoms (Smernoff et al. 2015). Reduction in sympathetic arousal

Table 3 PSG parameters of both patients

PSG Parameters	Patient 01		Patient 02
	Baseline	After 04 weeks of intervention	Baseline
TIB (min)	434	351	496
TST (min)	298	294	415
SPT (min)	421	337	477
SOL (min)	04	03	06
Sleep Efficiency (%)	68.6	83.8	83.6
WASO (min)	131	56	75
WASO/TST	0.44	0.19	0.18
ROL (min)	158	125	81
WAKE duration (min)	135	59	81
Wake % TIB	31.2	16.2	16.4
N1 duration (min)	101	79	45
N1 %TIB	23.3	22.6	9
N1 % TST	33.9	27	10.7
N2 duration (min)	112	79	309
N2 % TIB	25.7	39.7	62.2
N2 % TST	37.5	47.4	74.5
N3 duration (min)	61	139	1
N3 %TIB	13.9	39.7	0.2
N3 % TST	20.3	47.4	0.2
REM duration (min)	25	40	
REM %TIB	5.6	11.2	12.2
REM %TST	8.2	13.4	14.6

and reduced emotional states are the probable reasons for improvement in insomnia patients with mindfulness meditation (Ong et al. 2014; Morin et al. 1992; Ong et al. 2008; Ong et al. 2009; Martires and Zeidler 2015).

In our patients *yoga nidra* did not reduce total sleep time unlike a study on meditators where a reduced sleep need due to meditation was proposed (Kaul et al. 2010). *Yoga nidra* has been used in diseases and has been found to reduce perceived stress and anxiety (Rani et al. 2011; Stankovic 2011; Amita et al. 2009; Rani et al. 2012). In our patient we found improvement in depression and anxiety scores at 3 months of intervention. At 2 weeks patient 02 showed increased anxiety and stress and that may be attributable to his personal commitment of a business trip and his apprehension of doing *yoga nidra* which became better in subsequent trips. This is important to understand while planning this model that initial support is important during initial 3 to 4 weeks of intervention. Following the *yoga nidra* model planned for the patients there was no adverse effect reported but it is important that the intervention be given under supervision of a sleep practitioner because the changes seen in the patients need to be assessed and

monitored specially when an increased association to have anxiety, other somatic complaints like headaches, nausea is likely to be more in insomnia patients with mind body therapies including meditation (Jacobsen and Edinger 1982; Carlson and Nitz 1991).

This highlights the differences between patients and meditators and hence the medical supervision of these patients is extremely important.

Yoga nidra is easy to administer, relatively safe and does improve sleep in chronic insomnia. Another advantage of *yoga nidra* model is, that after the first five supervised sessions the patient is not dependant on the therapist, on the contrary he can do it all by himself in the comfort of his own house. This also gives confidence to the patient and alleviates his anxiety as seen in one of our patient. This may be one of the important factors for sustained improvement in anxiety and stress in both patients at 3 months of intervention.

The model developed for yoga nidra intervention can be used in chronic insomnia patients as an adjunct in management of chronic insomnia. Initial monitoring by a sleep physician should be done during 3 to 4 weeks of intervention. Though there are potential benefits of yoga nidra in insomnia patients, exact mechanism of yoga nidra is not yet clear. In our study both the volunteers were of elderly age group. Another limitation of our study is that in this case report there is a limited sample size (2 cases), so no firm conclusions can be drawn yet, until further studies are done on a larger number of patients. The efficacy of *yoga nidra* can be better understood in a randomised controlled trial in comparison to CBTI preferably in a younger age group.

Endnotes
[1]Second author: Dr Manjari Tripathi- MT
[2]First author: Dr Karuna Datta- KD

Abbreviations
AASM: American association of sleep medicine; CBTI: Cognitive behavioural therapy for insomnia; CD: Compact disc; DASS: Depression anxiety and stress scale; ECG: Electrocardiography; EEG: Electroencephalography; EMG: Electromyography; EOG: Electrooculography; ESS © MW JOHNS 1990–1997. USED UNDER LICENSE: Epworth sleepiness scale; ISI: Insomnia severity index; MES: Morningness eveningness scale; N1, 2, 3: Non REM stages as per AASM scoring criteria; OPD: Out patients department; PSAS: Pre sleep arousal scale; PSG: Polysomnography; PSQI: Pittsburgh sleep quality index; REM: Rapid eye movement; SOL: Sleep onset latency; SPT: Sleep period time; TIB: Time in bed; TST: Total sleep time; TWD: Total wake duration; WASO: Wake after sleep onset

Acknowledgements
The authors acknowledge the support of Bihar School of Yoga Munger, Bihar, India for providing valuable inputs, books, literature and blessings in

designing and completing the study. Authors are also thankful to the sleep technicians of MT sleep lab who conducted overnight polysomnography for the study. Authors thank MAPI trust for granting permission to use ESS "ESS contact information and permission to use: MAPIResearch Trust, Lyon, France. E-mail: PROinformation@mapi-trust.org – Internet: www.mapi-trust.org".

Funding

Funding for the study was provided from the department and Institute (All India Institute of Medical Sciences New Delhi, India) funds and resources. No separate funding agency was involved in the design of the study and collection, analysis, and interpretation of data and in writing the manuscript.

Authors' contributions

HM and MT helped KD design the study. Data collection was done by KD under guidance of MT. Analysis and interpretation of results and writing the manuscript was done by KD with guidance of HM and MT. All authors read and approved the final manuscript.

Competing interests

The authors declare that they have no competing interests.

Author details

[1]Department of Physiology, All India Institute of Medical Sciences, New Delhi, India. [2]Department of Neurology, All India Institute of Medical Sciences, New Delhi, India.

References

Ainsworth B, Eddershaw R, Meron D, Baldwin DS, Garner M. The effect of focused attention and open monitoring meditation on attention network function in healthy volunteers. Psychiatry Res. 2013;210:1226–31.

Amita S, Prabhakar S, Manoj I, Harminder S, Pavan T. Effect of yoga-nidra on blood glucose level in diabetic patients. Indian J Physiol Pharmacol. 2009;53:97–101.

Berry RB, Brooks R, Gamaldo CE, Harding SM, Lloyd RM, Marcus CL, Vaughn BV, for the American Academy of Sleep Medicine. The AASM Manual for the Scoring of Sleep and Associated Events: Rules, Terminology and Technical Specifications, Version 2.0.3. Darien: American Academy of Sleep Medicine; 2014. www.aasmnet.org.

Brown TA, Chorpita BF, Korotitsch W, Barlow DH. Psychometric properties of the depression anxiety stress scales (DASS) in clinical samples. Behav Res Ther. 1997;35:79–89.

Buysse DJ, Reynolds CF, Monk TH, Berman SR, Kupfer DJ. The Pittsburgh sleep quality index: a new instrument for psychiatric practice and research. Psychiatry Res. 1989;28:193–213.

Carlson CR, Nitz AJ. Negative side effects of self-regulation training: relaxation and the role of the professional in service delivery. Biofeedback Self-Regul. 1991;16:191–7.

Deepak KK. Neurophysiological mechanisms of induction of meditation: a hypothetico-deductive approach. Indian J Physiol Pharmacol. 2002;46:136–58.

Edinger JD, Buysse DJ, Deriy L, Germain A, Lewin DS, Ong JC, et al. Quality measures for the care of patients with insomnia. J Clin Sleep Med JCSM Off Publ Am Acad Sleep Med. 2015;11:311–34.

Hoque R, Chesson AL. Zolpidem-induced sleepwalking, sleep related eating disorder, and sleep-driving: fluorine-18-flourodeoxyglucose positron emission tomography analysis, and a literature review of other unexpected clinical effects of zolpidem. J Clin Sleep Med JCSM Off Publ Am Acad Sleep Med. 2009;5:471–6.

Horne JA, Ostberg O. A self-assessment questionnaire to determine morningness-eveningness in human circadian rhythms. Int J Chronobiol. 1976;4:97–110.

Irwin MR, Olmstead R, Motivala SJ. Improving sleep quality in older adults with moderate sleep complaints: a randomized controlled trial of Tai Chi Chih. Sleep. 2008;31:1001–8.

Israel B, Buysse DJ, Krafty RT, Begley A, Miewald J, Hall M. Short-term stability of sleep and heart rate variability in good sleepers and patients with insomnia: for some measures, one night is enough. Sleep. 2012;35:1285–91.

Jacobsen R, Edinger JD. Side effects of relaxation treatment. Am J Psychiatry. 1982;139:952–3.

Johns MW. A new method for measuring daytime sleepiness: the Epworth sleepiness scale. Sleep. 1991;14:540–5.

Kao C-H, Sun L-M, Liang J-A, Chang S-N, Sung F-C, Muo C-H. Relationship of zolpidem and cancer risk: a Taiwanese population-based cohort study. Mayo Clin Proc. 2012;87:430–6.

Kaul P, Passafiume J, Sargent CR, O'Hara BF. Meditation acutely improves psychomotor vigilance, and may decrease sleep need. Behav Brain Funct BBF. 2010;6:47.

Khalsa SBS. Treatment of chronic insomnia with yoga: a preliminary study with sleep-wake diaries. Appl Psychophysiol Biofeedback. 2004;29:269–78.

Kripke DF, Garfinkel L, Wingard DL, Klauber MR, Marler MR. Mortality associated with sleep duration and insomnia. Arch Gen Psychiatry. 2002;59:131–6.

Lovibond PF, Lovibond SH. The structure of negative emotional states: comparison of the depression anxiety stress scales (DASS) with the beck depression and anxiety inventories. Behav Res Ther. 1995;33:335–43.

Markil N, Whitehurst M, Jacobs PL, Zoeller RF. Yoga Nidra relaxation increases heart rate variability and is unaffected by a prior bout of Hatha yoga. J Altern Complement Med N Y N. 2012;18:953–8.

Martires J, Zeidler M. The value of mindfulness meditation in the treatment of insomnia. Curr Opin Pulm Med. 2015;21:547–52.

Morin CM, Gaulier B, Barry T, Kowatch RA. Patients' acceptance of psychological and pharmacological therapies for insomnia. Sleep. 1992;15:302–5.

Morin CM, Belleville G, Bélanger L, Ivers H. The Insomnia Severity Index: psychometric indicators to detect insomnia cases and evaluate treatment response. Sleep. 2011;34:601–8.

Nicassio PM, Mendlowitz DR, Fussell JJ, Petras L. The phenomenology of the pre-sleep state: the development of the pre-sleep arousal scale. Behav Res Ther. 1985;23:263–71.

Ong JC, Shapiro SL, Manber R. Combining mindfulness meditation with cognitive-behavior therapy for insomnia: a treatment-development study. Behav Ther. 2008;39:171–82.

Ong JC, Shapiro SL, Manber R. Mindfulness meditation and cognitive behavioral therapy for insomnia: a naturalistic 12-month follow-up. Explore N Y N. 2009; 5:30–6.

Ong JC, Manber R, Segal Z, Xia Y, Shapiro S, Wyatt JK. A randomized controlled trial of mindfulness meditation for chronic insomnia. Sleep. 2014;37: 1553–63.

Paine S-J, Gander PH, Travier N. The epidemiology of morningness/eveningness: influence of age, gender, ethnicity, and socioeconomic factors in adults (30-49 years). J Biol Rhythms. 2006;21:68–76.

Patra S, Telles S. Heart rate variability during sleep following the practice of cyclic meditation and supine rest. Appl Psychophysiol Biofeedback. 2010; 35:135–40.

Rani K, Tiwari S, Singh U, Agrawal G, Ghildiyal A, Srivastava N. Impact of Yoga Nidra on psychological general wellbeing in patients with menstrual irregularities: a randomized controlled trial. Int J Yoga. 2011;4:20–5.

Rani K, Tiwari S, Singh U, Singh I, Srivastava N. Yoga Nidra as a complementary treatment of anxiety and depressive symptoms in patients with menstrual disorder. Int J Yoga. 2012;5:52–6.

Saraswati S. Bihar School of Yoga. Yoga nidra. Munger: Yoga Publications Trust; 1998.

Schutte-Rodin S, Broch L, Buysse D, Dorsey C, Sateia M. Clinical guideline for the evaluation and management of chronic insomnia in adults. J Clin Sleep Med JCSM Off Publ Am Acad Sleep Med. 2008;4:487–504.

Smernoff E, Mitnik I, Kolodner K, Lev-Ari S. The effects of "The Work" meditation (Byron Katie) on psychological symptoms and quality of life–a pilot clinical study. Explore N Y N. 2015;11:24–31.

Stankovic L. Transforming trauma: a qualitative feasibility study of integrative restoration (iRest) yoga Nidra on combat-related post-traumatic stress disorder. Int J Yoga Ther. 2011;21:23–37.

Taylor DJ, Mallory LJ, Lichstein KL, Durrence HH, Riedel BW, Bush AJ. Comorbidity of chronic insomnia with medical problems. Sleep. 2007;30:213–8.

Werner GG, Ford BQ, Mauss IB, Schabus M, Blechert J, Wilhelm FH. High cardiac vagal control is related to better subjective and objective sleep quality. Biol Psychol. 2015;106:79–85.

11

Likelihood of obstructive sleep apnea in people living with HIV in Cameroon –preliminary findings

Andreas Ateke Njoh[1†], Eta Ngole Mbong[1,3*†], Valeri Oben Mbi[2], Michel Karngong Mengnjo[1], Leonard Njamnshi Nfor[1], Leonard Ngarka[1], Samuel Eric Chokote[1], Julius Yundze Fonsah[1], Samuel Kingue[1], Felicien Enyime Ntone[1] and Alfred Kongnyu Njamnshi[1†]

Abstract

Background: Obstructive Sleep Apnea (OSA) has been observed to be common among people living with HIV/AIDS (PLWHA). Sleep scales can be used to screen patients at increased "risk" of OSA who can benefit from polysomnography. This study therefore sought to generate preliminary data on this often unattended complication of HIV Infection in Cameroon.

Methods: A case control study carried out at the Yaoundé Central Hospital in which 82 participants were enrolled: 39 PLWHA age- and sex-matched with 43 controls. The Berlin sleep questionnaire was used to assess the likelihood of OSA in both groups.

Results: Participants were aged 20 to 59 years with a mean age of 34.27 ± 9.29 (35.72 ± 10.09 and 32.92 ± 8.41 respectively for cases and controls, $p = 0.180$). Cases (PLWHA) compared to controls had higher likelihood of OSA (43.6% versus 14.0%, AOR 3.93 95% CI 1.12–13.80 on adjusting for socioeconomic status, depression and smoking) as well as 10 times higher rates of daytime somnolence (23.1% versus 2.3%, $p = 0.005$). Significant differences were found between PLHWA at "risk" of OSA and those without only with regards to rate of compliance to Highly Active anti-Retroviral Therapy (HAART), and mean abdominal and waist circumferences.

Conclusions: The likelihood of obstructive sleep apnea (OSA) in PLHWA is higher than in HIV negative controls. Integration of screening for OSA in HIV/AIDS care with the aid of sleep scales would permit timely diagnosis and management and reduce the incidence of chronic cardiorespiratory co-morbidities in PLWHA.

Keywords: Obstructive sleep apnea, Persons living with HIV/AIDS, Sleep scales, HAART, Cameroon

Background

Obstructive sleep apnea (OSA), results from repeated episodes of upper airway obstruction during sleep caused by collapse of the pharyngeal airway (Somers et al. 2008). Alterations in upper airway anatomy as well as disturbances in neuromuscular control play an important role in the pathogenesis of OSA (McGinley et al. 2008; Isono et al. 1999; Smith et al. 1988; Gupta et al. 2010). The disease is characterized by periodic cessation of breathing during

sleep resulting in reduced blood oxygen levels, followed by brief arousal to reinitiate breathing (Taibi 2013). OSA is usually associated with obesity (Gupta et al. 2010; Resta et al. 2001) and the onset of sleep apnea frequently follows a marked increase in body weight (Smith et al. 1988). However, obesity alone is not essential for the development of OSA (Resta et al. 2001; Lo et al. 1998; Joy et al. 2008; Lo Re et al. 2006; Dorey-Stein et al. 2008; Epstein et al. 1995).

OSA has been observed by some authors to be common among persons living with HIV/AIDS (PLWHA) (Taibi 2013; Lo Re et al. 2006; Dorey-Stein et al. 2008; Epstein et al. 1995). In this group of persons, body composition abnormalities such as subcutaneous fat wasting, central fat accumulation (Brown et al. 2010), and adenotonsillar

* Correspondence: mbongeta@yahoo.fr
†Equal contributors
[1]Faculty of Medicine and Biomedical Sciences, University of Yaoundé 1, Yaoundé, Cameroon
[3]PC Great Soppo, P.O Box 547, Buea, Cameroon
Full list of author information is available at the end of the article

hypertrophy (Epstein et al. 1995) are common; partly due to the viral infection and Highly Active Anti-Retroviral Therapy (HAART) (Lo et al. 1998). Among non-obese PLWHA visceral fat has been found to be increased compared to HIV negative controls (Joy et al. 2008); fat accumulations are common along the cervical and dorsal regions of the bodies of PLWHA (Lo et al. 1998). Sleep scales can be used in clinical settings to screen patients likely to suffer from OSA who can be sent early to sleep laboratory for confirmatory polysomnography.

The impact of OSA on health cannot be over emphasized given the increased morbidity (Gupta et al. 2010) and mortality it is associated as a results of cardiovascular and metabolic complications in particular and impairment in quality of life in general (Somers et al. 2008; Brown et al. 2010; Kendzerska et al. 2014; Budhiraja and Quan 2005). Despite its known impact, data on this subtle but severe complication of HIV infection in Cameroon is inexistent.

It was therefore necessary to assess the "risk" of OSA among PLWHA in Cameroon in order to generate preliminary data from which initiatives to raise awareness and promote early diagnosis and management of OSA in this population can be started. This study sought therefore to study this often unattended-to complication of HIV Infection in Cameroon with the aid of the Berlin Questionnaire sleep scale, in a population of PLWHA compared with their HIV negative peers.

Methods

Study design

The study was a hospital-based case–control study conducted over a period of 8 months in 39 consenting PLWHA age- and sex-matched with 43 controls.

Study setting

The study was carried out in Yaoundé, the cosmopolitan capital city of Cameroon, specifically at the HIV/AIDS Treatment Centre and Neurology Service of the Yaoundé Central Hospital.

The Yaoundé Central Hospital is a government run tertiary health facility with a bustling HIV/AIDS outpatient department (the largest in the country), which serves PLWHA from Yaoundé and its environs. In addition, the Neurology Department of this hospital has a sleep laboratory that supports this kind of study.

Ethical approval was obtained from the review board of the Faculty of Medicine and Biomedical Sciences (FMBS) of the University of Yaoundé 1 and administrative clearance from the directorate of the Yaoundé Central Hospital. Information collected from study participants and patient files were coded and confidentially handled.

Study participants

Participants were adults aged 20 to 59 years (Khassawneh et al. 2009) with a confirmed HIV-positive serology (for cases) attending the HIV/AIDS Treatment Centre of the study site and clinically stable enough to participate in the study. Were excluded all PLWHA known to be obese (BMI ≥30 kg/m^2) prior to HIV diagnosis as well as pregnant women, demented patients, people with abnormal sleep-wake cycles due to night-shift work and all individuals who were on or had taken sleep inducing medications, or stimulants during the three months preceding the study.

Controls were selected from among other patients, care takers and others who visited the hospital and were confirmed HIV-negative at the time of the study.

Participants were contacted and recruited by the study investigators consecutively as they presented at the treatment center. The study objectives and procedures were explained to participants and informed consent obtained. A total of 82 participants were enrolled for the study.

Instruments

Socio-demographic and clinical data of study participants were collected through interviews with the aid of a pretested pre-structured questionnaire. Data collected included age (as at last birthday), sex, employment status, religion, monthly income bracket, highest level of formal education attained, cigarette smoking status, number of check-up and unwell visits to health care provider during the previous three months. PLWHA had their highly active antiretroviral treatment status, regimen and duration probed as well. All study participants benefitted from a complete physical examination with focus on neurological examination and anthropometric measurements.

The likelihood ("risk") of OSA was assessed with the aid of the Berlin Questionnaire and daytime sleepiness with the aid of the Epworth Sleepiness Scale (ESS). The *Berlin questionnaire* was designed to screen for sleep apnea in primary care population and stratifies patients into low or high "risk" (Netzer et al. 1999). It has high reliability (Cronbach α 0.86–0.92), and a high positive predictive value in identifying ambulatory OSA cases at high "risk" of sleep apnea (Netzer et al. 1999).

Study variables

HIV case: Confirmed by ELISA and dichotomized as positive or negative.

HIV serotype: Confirmed by laboratory analysis of blood samples of HIV positive cases; nominally grouped into HIV1, HIV 2, and HIV 1&2.

HIV clinical staging: Grouped into 4 clinical stages with respect to the WHO 2006 clinical staging algorithm (based on clinical signs and symptoms) (World Health

Organization 2007) and the CDC revised HIV classification algorithm (CDC 2014).

HAART use and regimen: Use of HAART was dichotomized as a yes or no as reported by the patient and confirmed by clinical records. Regimen type was nominally categorized.

Age at HIV diagnosis and disease duration: Age in years at which patient reported (confirmed by diagnosis report) he or she was diagnosed HIV positive from which *disease duration* was deducted after comparing with study date. The latter were expressed in years and

months respectively then categorized ordinally as shown on Table 2.

Number of routine visits to physician and number of unwell visits to physician during previous three months: As reported by study participants and confirmed by patient records. Assessed as continuous data and then ordinally categorized as shown on Table 2.

Compliance to HAART treatment during the previous month was assessed dichotomously as yes or no. Cases were considered compliant to HAART if they reported

Table 1 Socio-demographic characteristics of participants

	HIV status				2 sided sig. of difference	Entire study sample	
	Negative (Controls)		Positive (Cases)				
	N	%	n	%		N	%
N	43	52.4	39	47.6		82	100.0
Sex							
Male	19	44.2	13	33.3	0.314	32	39.0
Female	24	55.8	26	66.7		50	61.0
Age (years)							
Mean ± SD	32.92 ± 8.41		35.72 ± 10.09		0.180	34.27 ± 9.29	
20–29	16	37.2	14	35.9	0.541	30	36.6
30–39	16	37.2	11	28.2		27	32.9
≥40	11	25.6	14	35.9		25	30.5
Employment status							
Unemployed	12	27.9	11	28.1	0.003	23	28.0
Employed	31	72.1	28	71.8		59	72.0
Level of education							
Primary	9	20.9	7	17.9	0.005	16	19.5
Secondary	19	44.2	29	74.4		48	58.5
Tertiary	15	34.9	3	7.7		18	22.0
Marital status		0.0		0.0		0	0.0
Single	28	65.1	24	61.5	0.244	52	63.4
Married	15	34.9	12	30.8		27	32.9
Widow(er)	0	0.0	3	7.7		3	3.7
Socioeconomic status (SES)							
Low SES	23	53.5	19	48.7	0.911	42	51.2
Middle SES	19	44.2	19	48.7		38	46.3
High SES	1	2.3	1	2.6		2	2.4
Smokes							
Yes	2	4.7	1	2.6	1.00	3	3.7
No	41	95.3	38	97.4		79	96.3
Alcohol consumption							
Yes	19	44.2	22	56.4	0.269	41	50.0
No	24	55.8	17	43.6		41	50.0

not having missed taking prescribed HAART not more than 7 times in a month.

Risk of OSA: Dichotomized as "risk" or "no risk" of OSA based on responses to items on the Berlin questionnaire.

Daytime sleepiness: Ordinally categorized with respect to scores got on assessment with the Epworth sleep scale (ESS): score of 1–14 (restful sleep and no daytime sleepiness), score ≥15 (excessive daytime somnolence).

Data analyses

Data collected was entered into an excel sheet and uploaded for analyses unto version 20 of the Statistical Package for Social Sciences (SPSS 20). Continuous data are presented as means ± SD as well as ordinate categories, and non-continuous data as proportions (%). Strengths of associations between categorical variables are presented as odds ratios and the differences between

proportions determined with the aid of chi-squared tests (X^2). Differences between means of continuous variables between groups were done with the aid of t-tests. All test statistics are two-sided and considered statistically significant at $p < 0.05$.

Results

Socio-demographic characteristics of participants

A total of 82 participants were enrolled into the study (39 cases and 43 sex and age matched controls). Participants were as young as 20 and as old 59 years with a mean age of 34.27 years (SD 9.29). But for employment status and level of education, there was no significant difference between the socio-demographic characteristics of cases and controls (Table 1). More cases were unemployed than controls (5.1% versus 0.0%, $p = 0.003$) and fewer had attained tertiary levels of education (7.7% versus 34.9%, $p = 0.005$); Table1.

Table 2 Anthropometric and clinical characteristics of participants

| | HIV status | | | | 2 sided sig. of difference | Entire study sample | |
| | Negative (Controls) | | Positive (Cases) | | | | |
	N	%	n	%		N	%
BMI (kg/m^2)							
Mean ± SD	25.17 ± 4.34		25.23 ± 4.48		0.955	25.20 ± 4.38	
Underweight (<18.5)	1	2.3	1	2.6	0.928	2	2.5
Normal BMI (18.5–25.00)	25	58.1	21	55.3		46	56.8
Overweight (25.01–29.99)	10	23.3	11	28.9		21	25.9
Obese (≥30.00)	7	16.3	5	13.2		12	14.8
Weight gain (kg)	0.38 ± 5.20		−1.83 ± 6.10		0.104	−0.68 ± 5.72	
Neck circumference (cm)	36.53 ± 3.00		35.74 ± 4.70		0.360	36.16 ± 3.89	
Abdominal circumference (cm)	89.27 ± 12.80		86.30 ± 12.19		0.364	87.93 ± 12.52	
Waist circumference (cm)	86.28 ± 13.60		85.58 ± 11.98		0.808	85.95 ± 12.79	
Hip circumference (cm)	100.35 ± 13.80		100.05 ± 11.57		0.918	100.21 ± 12.73	
Waist Hip Ratio	0.86 ± 0.08		0.85 ± 0.06		0.712	0.86 ± 0.07	
Pulse (/min)							
Mean ± SD	74.29 ± 10.49		79.19 ± 16.57		0.086	76.46 ± 11.04	
Tachycardia	23	67.6	22	81.5	0.222	45	73.8
Normal	11	32.4	5	18.5		16	26.2
Blood pressure (mm/hg)							
Systolic (Mean ± SD)	119.51 ± 14.21		121.61 ± 17.77		0.561	120.47 ± 15.86	
Diastolic (Mean ± SD)	75.49 ± 10.27		75.42 ± 16.57		0.981	75.46 ± 13.42	
HBP							
Yes	6	14.0	8	22.2	0.338	14	17.7
No	37	86.0	28	77.8		65	82.3
Neurological examination							
Normal	43	100	36	92.3	0.103	79	96.3
Abnormal	0	0.0	3	7.7		3	3.7

Clinical and anthropometric assessments of participants

On clinical assessment (Table 2) anthropometric measurements, blood pressure and pulse were not significantly different between the two groups.

HIV disease characteristics and HAART

Almost a quarter (23.9%) of study cases were diagnosed positive with HIV at the age of under 25 years, three quarters (29; 76.2%) had lived with the disease for at least 6 months and two-thirds on HAART (24; 63.2%) of which half (54.1%) for at least 6 months (Table 3). 42.9% of cases on 1st line HAART were on a regimen with Efavirenz (Table 3).

HIV-AIDS disease history of cases and disease follow-up

Cases had a mean age of 32.26 ± 8.94 years and had been diagnosed HIV positive for more than three years (mean duration of 44.61 ± 50.12 months); Table 3. Two thirds (63.2%) were on HAART, mainly (92.1%) 1st line (Table 3).

Snoring habits and assessment of the "risk"/likelihood of OSA in cases and controls

Cases (PLWHA) compared to controls had higher rates of "risk" (moderate as well as high) of OSA (43.6% versus 14.0%, OR 4.77 95% CI 1.64–13.89 and AOR 3.93 95% CI 1.12–13.80 on adjusting for socioeconomic status, depression and smoking) and consequently had 10 times higher rates of daytime somnolence (Table 4).

HIV disease characteristics, and anthropometric and clinical parameters in PLWHA with and those without "risk" of OSA

With respect to OSA and HIV disease characteristics and management, cases with "risk" (moderate as well as high risk) of OSA differed significantly from those without, only with regards to compliance to HAART. The rate of compliance to HAART was higher in HIV cases with "risk" of OSA compared to HIV cases without (100.0% versus 60% respectively, $p = 0.034$); Table 5. With regards to anthropometry, significant differences were found with regards to abdominal and waist circumferences (Table 6).

Discussion

These preliminary findings are part of a study which sought to generate data on disordered sleep an often unattended complication of HIV Infection. Focus was on obstructive sleep apnea (OSA) whose likelihood was assessed with the aid of the Berlin Questionnaire sleep scale in people living with HIV/AIDS (PLWHA) compared to matched HIV negative controls.

Cases (PLWHA) compared to controls had higher "risk" (moderate as well as high) of OSA (43.6% versus 14.0%, $p = 0.003$ and AOR 3.98 95% CI 1.14–13.99 on adjusting for socioeconomic status, depression and

Table 3 HIV disease characteristics of the cases

	N	%
	39	47.6
Age at diagnosis (years)		
Mean ± SD	32.26 ± 8.94	
20–24	9	23.7
≥25	29	76.3
Disease duration since diagnosis		
Mean ± SD (months)	44.61 ± 50.12	
≤6 months	14	36.8
<6 months	24	63.2
CD4 count (count/mm³), Mean ± SD	410.92 ± 144.90	
<350	3	23.1
≥350	10	76.9
WHO disease stage		
Stage 1	26	68.4
Stage 2	3	7.9
Stage 3	7	18.4
Stage 4	2	5.3
CDC disease stage		
A1	11	78.6
A2	1	7.1
C1	1	7.1
C3	1	7.1
Routine check-ups in last 3 months		
Mean ± SD	1.00 ± 1.33	
None	20	54.1
At least 1	17	45.9
Patient on HAART		
No	14	36.8
Yes	24	63.2
Compliant to HAART		
Yes	17	70.8
No	7	29.2
HAART duration since onset		
Mean ± SD (months)	47.76 ± 44.71	
<6 months	4	23.5
≥6 months	13	76.5
HAART protocol type		
1st line	13	92.9
2nd line	1	7.1
HIV complications during 3 months preceeding study		
At least one	2	5.4
None	35	94.6
Presence of other concurrent disease		
At least one	5	13.5
None	32	86.5

Table 4 Snoring habits, and rates of 'risk' of OSA and daytime somnolence

	HIV status				2 sided sig. of difference	Entire study sample	
	Negative (Controls)		Positive (Cases)				
	N	%	n	%		N	%
N	43		39			82	
Snoring							
Yes	11	25.6	10	25.6	1.00	21	25.6
No	32	74.4	29	74.4		61	74.4
Risk of OSA							
No risk	37	86.0	22	56.4	0.003	59	72.0
Moderate Risk	6	14.0	12	30.8		18	22.0
High risk	0	0.0	5	12.8		5	6.0
Daytime somnolence							
Yes	1	2.3	9	23.1	0.005	10	12.2
No	42	97.7	30	76.9		72	87.8

OSA Obstructive Sleep Apnea

smoking); Table 4. These findings corroborate findings of other authors in other settings who demonstrated that compared with HIV negative controls, obstructive sleep apnea (OSA) is more common in PLWHA (Taibi 2013; Lo Re et al. 2006; Dorey-Stein et al. 2008; Epstein et al. 1995). In this group of persons, body composition abnormalities (Brown et al. 2010), and adenotonsillar hypertrophy (Epstein et al. 1995) are common; partly due to the viral infection and Highly Active Anti-Retroviral Therapy (HAART) (Lo et al. 1998).

The higher likelihood of OSA this study observed in PLWHA compared to their HIV negative peers was despite the fact that the former did not differ significantly from the latter (Table 2) with respect to aspects related to externally observable fat accumulation: BMI, neck, waist and abdominal circumferences and lipodystrophy known predisposing factors of OSA in HIV negative persons. With the aid of dual-energy X-ray absorptiometry and computed tomography, PLWHA without clinical evidence of lipodystrophy have been shown to have significantly greater percentage of total body fat in the trunk and significantly lower percent of body fat in the extremities compared to HIV negative controls (CDC 2014). These, physical examination misses.

Vgontzas AN and collaborators in 2000 (Kosmiski et al. 2003), demonstrated that sleep apnea patients had a significantly greater amount of visceral fat compared to obese controls and that indices of sleep disordered breathing (SDB) were positively correlated with visceral fat, and not with BMI, total and subcutaneous fat. Another author (Brown et al. 2010) however showed that BMI, waist circumference, and neck circumference have better predictive value for moderate-severe SDB in HIV uninfected men compared to HIV-

infected men, and had no value among HIV-infected men not receiving HAART. Among this latter group (HIV-infected men not on HAART), systemic inflammation is thought to contribute to the pathogenesis of SDB (Brown et al. 2010).

With respect to OSA and HIV disease characteristics and management, cases with "risk" of OSA in our study differed significantly from those without, only with regards to compliance to HAART (Table 5). Compliance to HAART favors fat redistribution in PLWHA: visceral as well as lipodystrophy (Lo Re et al. 2006; Kosmiski et al. 2003). Brigham and collaborators (McNicholas 2009) demonstrated that PLWHA not on HAART with moderate to severe OSA have high circulating levels of inflammatory markers especially TNF-alpha, compared to those with no-to-mild OSA after adjustment for age, race, smoking status, obstructive lung disease and BMI. Within this group, the association of high TNF-alpha concentrations with moderate-severe OSA was independent of CD4 cell count and viral load. Factors that reduce the inflammation associated with HIV infection such as HAART initially would reduce the occurrence of OSA in these patients. This improvement over time wanes due to fat redistribution secondary to HAART.

As was observed when compared with the HIV negative controls, HIV cases with "risk" of OSA did not show significant differences when compared HIV cases without risk of OSA with regards to mean BMI and neck circumferences (Table 6). Significant differences were however found between the two groups with respect to indices of abdominal obesity (waist and abdominal circumferences, Table 6). In the case of abdominal circumference, accumulation of fat in the abdominal wall may reduce respiratory effort and predispose to sleep apnea. Waist circumference on its

Table 5 "Risk" of OSA with respect to HIV disease characteristics

	OSA				2 sided sig. of difference	Entire HIV+ sample	
	No "risk" of OSA		"Risk" of OSA				
	N	%	N	%		N	%
HIV genotype							
HIV₁	8	42.1	5	31.3	0.679	13	37.1
HIV₂	1	5.3	2	12.5		3	8.6
HIV₁₊₂	0	0.0	1	6.3		1	2.9
Undetermined genotype	10	52.6	8	50.0		18	51.4
Age at diagnosis (years)							
Mean ± SD	34.55 ± 9.84		37.24 ± 10.51		0.416	34.27 ± 9.29	
20–24	6	28.6	3	17.6	0.425	9	23.7
≥25	15	71.4	14	82.4		29	76.3
Duration since diagnosis							
<= 6 months	8	38.1	6	35.3	0.717	14	36.8
>6 months	13	61.9	11	64.7		24	63.2
CD4 count (count/mm³)							
Mean ± SD	387.10 ± 150.58		490.33 ± 107.96		0.299	410.92 ± 144.90	
<350	3	30.0	0	0.0	0.528	3	23.1
≥350	7	70.0	3	100.0		10	76.9
WHO disease stage							
Stage 1	15	71.4	11	64.7	0.930	26	68.4
Stage 2	2	9.5	1	5.9		3	7.9
Stages 3–4	4	19.1	5	29.4		9	23.7
Routine check-ups in last 3 months							
None	10	50.0	10	58.8	0.591	20	54.1
At least 1	10	50.0	7	41.2		17	45.9
Patient on HAART							
Yes	8	38.1	6	35.3	1.00	14	36.8
No	13	61.9	11	64.7		24	63.2
HAART duration							
Mean ± SD	61.11 ± 51.59		32.75 ± 32.27		0.201	47.76 ± 44.71	
<6 months	2	22.2	2	25.0	1.00	4	23.5
≥6 months	7	77.8	6	75.0		13	76.5
HAART protocols		0.0				0	
1st line	8	100.0	5	83.3	0.429	13	92.9
2nd line	0	0.0	1	16.7		1	7.1
Compliance last 30 days							
Compliant	4	40.0	6	100.0	0.034ᵃ	10	62.5
Not complaint	6	60.0	0	0.0		6	37.5
Complications in last 3 months							
None	0	0.0	2	11.8	0.204	2	5.4
At least one	20	100.0	15	88.2		35	94.
Presence of other concurrent diseases							
At least one	2	10.0	3	17.6	0.644	5	13.5
None	18	90.0	14	82.4		32	86.5

[a]significant difference. *OSA* Obstructive Sleep Apnea

Table 6 Occurrence of snoring and means of anthropometric and blood pressure parameters in PLWHA cases with OSA compared to those without

Characteristic	OSA		2 sided sig. of difference	Entire HIV+ sample
	No risk of OSA	Risk of OSA		
Snores				
No	21 (95.5)	8 (47.1)	0.001	29 (74.4)
Yes	1 (4.5)	9 (52.9)		10 (25.6)
Means ± SD				
Neck circumference (cm)	35.05 ± 4.92	36.69 ± 4.35	0.294	35.74 ± 4.70
BMI (kg/m²)	24.54 ± 3.82	26.17 ± 5.24	0.273	25.23 ± 4.48
Abdominal circumference (cm)	81.80 ± 9.94	91.92 ± 12.80	*0.029*[a]	86.30 ± 12.19
Waist circumference (cm)	81.86 ± 12.38	90.69 ± 9.57	*0.023*[a]	85.58 ± 11.98
Waist hip ratio	0.84 ± 0.07	0.87 ± 0.04	0.114	0.85 ± 0.06
Systolic blood pressure (mm Hg)	123.30 ± 18.13	119.50 ± 17.66	0.532	121.61 ± 17.77
Diastolic blood pressure (mm Hg)	75.85 ± 15.63	74.88 ± 18.19	0.809	75.42 ± 16.57
Pulse (/min)	76.60 ± 12.09	82.42 ± 9.80	0.190	79.19 ± 16.57

[a]significant difference. *OSA* Obstructive Sleep Apnea, *PLWHA* Persons living with HIV/AIDS

part has not been shown to be a good surrogate marker of visceral obesity in PLWHA (Kapur et al. 1999). Further studies need to be done on the contribution of waist circumference in the occurrence of OSA in PLWHA.

Our study had some limitations. OSA was assessed with a questionnaire and was not confirmed with Polysomnography (PSG), the gold standard for the diagnosis of OSA. However, we used a standardized instrument (the Berlin Questionnaire) that has been validated and found to be reliable. Also, we did not clinically diagnose adenotonsillar hypertrophy known to play a role in the development of OSA in HIV positive persons (Epstein et al. 1995; McNicholas 2009). The study sample size as well as not all PLWHA having had a recent CD4 count at time of study as well as viral load limited comparisons with regards to disease progression and viral genotype.

Given the socio-economic burden of untreated OSA (Kapur et al. 1999), its association with HIV/AIDS (a pandemic most prevalent in sub-Saharan African settings like ours) and role of HAART (which more and more PLWHA in out setting now have access to) in HIV disease and OSA occurrence, it is relevant to integrate as part of care of PLWHA, routine screening to identify those at risk of OSA with the aid of sleep scales. Given the peculiarities of the pathophysiology OSA in PLWHA discussed above, unlike in HIV negative subjects, all PLWHA should be screened including those without obvious body fat changes and obesity and those not yet on HAART.

Early identification of the risk of OSA in PLWHA would go a long way to spur referrals for polysomnography, timely management and contribute to the reduction of the incidence of cardiorespiratory co-morbidities in HIV/AIDS, now a chronic condition in low resource settings like ours thanks to access to HAART. This however has to be supported by advocacy actions towards policy makers and duty bearers, for more sleep clinics to be set-up so as to ensure supply meets the increased demand which would be generated by raised awareness.

Conclusion

The "risk"/likelihood of obstructive sleep apnea (OSA) in people living with HIV/AIDS is higher than in HIV negative controls. Unlike HIV negative persons this risk appears not to be linked to externally obvious markers of obesity. Integration of screening for OSA with the aid of sleep scales (validated in our setting against gold standard polysomnography) in HIV/AIDS care will permit timely diagnosis and management which would go a long way to reduce the incidence of chronic cardiorespiratory co-morbidities in PLWHA.

Abbreviations
ESS: Epworth Sleepiness Scale; HAART: Highly Active Anti-Retroviral Therapy; PLWHA: People living with HIV/AIDS; PSQI: The Pittsburgh sleep quality index

Acknowledgments
Our gratitude to staff of the out-patients, neurology and Day Hospital (HIV/AIDS Treatment Center) of the Yaoundé Central Hospital for their contributions to data collection. Our thanks as well to the panel of professors of the Faculty of Medicine and Biomedical Sciences of the University of Yaoundé 1 who reviewed this work as part of the end-of-MD thesis exercise.

Funding
Not applicable.

Authors' contributions

AAN, AKN and ENM designed the study and collected study data. AAN and ENM did the data analyses. All authors reviewed the article drafts and approved the submitted version.

Competing interests

The authors declare that they have no competing interests.

Author details

[1]Faculty of Medicine and Biomedical Sciences, University of Yaoundé 1, Yaoundé, Cameroon. [2]ISEC Schools of Health Sciences, Yaoundé, Cameroon. [3]PC Great Soppo, P.O Box 547, Buea, Cameroon.

References

Brown TT, Patil SP, Jacobson LP, Margolick JB, Laffan AM, Godfrey RJ, et al. Anthropometry in the prediction of sleep disordered breathing in HIV-positive and HIV-negative men. Antivir Ther. 2010;15(4):651–9.

Budhiraja R, Quan SF. Sleep-disordered breathing and cardiovascular health. Curr Opin Pulm Med. 2005;11(6):501–6.

CDC. Revised surveillance case definition for HIV infection — United States, 2014: recommendations and reports. MMWR. 2014;63(RR03):1–10.

Dorey-Stein Z, Amorosa VK, Kostman JR, Lo Re 3rd V, Shannon RP. Severe weight gain, lipodystrophy, dyslipidemia, and obstructive sleep apnea in a human immunodeficiency virus-infected patient following highly active antiretroviral therapy. J Cardiometab Syndr. 2008;3(2):111–4.

Epstein LJ, Strollo Jr PJ, Donegan RB, Delmar J, Hendrix C, Westbrook PR. Obstructive sleep apnea in patients with human immunodeficiency virus (HIV) disease. Sleep. 1995;18(5):368–76.

Gupta RK, Chandra A, Verm AK, Kumar S. Obstructive sleep apnoea: a clinical review. J Assoc Physicians India. 2010;58:438–41.

Isono S, Tanaka A, Nishino T. Effects of tongue electrical stimulation on pharyngeal mechanics in anaesthetized patients with obstructive sleep apnoea. Eur Respir J. 1999;14(6):1258–65.

Joy T, Keogh HM, Hadigan C, Dolan SE, Fitch K, Liebau J, et al. Relation of body composition to body mass index in HIV-infected patients with metabolic abnormalities. J Acquir Immune Defic Syndr. 2008;47(2):174–84.

Kapur V, Blough DK, Sandblom RE, Hert R, de Maine JB, Sullivan SD, et al. The medical cost of undiagnosed sleep apnea. Sleep. 1999;22(6):749–55.

Kendzerska T, Gershon AS, Hawker G, Leung RS, Tomlinson G. Obstructive sleep apnea and risk of cardiovascular events and all-cause mortality: a decade-long historical cohort study. PLoS Med. 2014;11(2):e1001599.

Khassawneh B, Ghazzawi M, Khader Y, Alomari M, Amarin Z, Shahrour B, et al. Symptoms and risk of obstructive sleep apnea in primary care patients in Jordan. Sleep Breath. 2009;13(3):227–32.

Kosmiski L, Kuritzkes D, Hamilton J, Sharp T, Lichtenstien K, Hill J, et al. Fat distribution is altered in HIV-infected men without clinical evidence of the HIV lipodystrophy syndrome. HIV Med. 2003;4(3):235–40.

Lo JC, Mulligan K, Tai VW, Algren H, Schambelan M. "Buffalo hump" in men with HIV-1 infection. Lancet. 1998;351(9106):867–70.

Lo Re 3rd V, Schutte-Rodin S, Kostman JR. Obstructive sleep apnoea among HIV patients. Int J STD AIDS. 2006;17(9):614–20.

McGinley BM, Schwartz AR, Schneider H, Kirkness JP, Smith PL, Patil SP. Upper airway neuromuscular compensation during sleep is defective in obstructive sleep apnea. J Appl Physiol (1985). 2008;105(1):197–205.

McNicholas WT. Obstructive sleep apnea and inflammation. Prog Cardiovasc Dis. 2009;51(5):392–9.

Netzer NC, Stoohs RA, Netzer CM, Clark K, Strohl KP. Using the Berlin Questionnaire to identify patients at risk for the sleep apnea syndrome. Ann Intern Med. 1999;131(7):485–91.

Resta O, Foschino-Barbaro MP, Legari G, Talamo S, Bonfitto P, Palumbo A, et al. Sleep-related breathing disorders, loud snoring and excessive daytime sleepiness in obese subjects. Int J Obes Relat Metab Disord. 2001;25(5):669–75.

Smith PL, Wise RA, Gold AR, Schwartz AR, Permutt S. Upper airway pressure-flow relationships in obstructive sleep apnea. J Appl Physiol (1985). 1988;64(2):789–95.

Somers VK, White DP, Amin R, Abraham WT, Costa F, Culebras A, et al. Sleep apnea and cardiovascular disease: an American heart association/American college of cardiology foundation scientific statement from the American heart association council for high blood pressure research professional education committee, council on clinical cardiology, stroke council, and council on cardiovascular nursing. In collaboration with the national heart, lung, and blood institute national center on sleep disorders research (National Institutes of Health). Circulation. 2008;118(10):1080–111.

Taibi DM. Sleep disturbances in persons living with HIV. J Assoc Nurses AIDS Care. 2013;24(1 Suppl):S72–85.

World Health Organization. Case definition of HIV for surveillane and revised clinical staging and immunological classification of HIV-related diseases in adult and children. 2007. http://www.who.int/hiv/pub/guidelines/HIVstaging150307.pdf. Accessed 18 Sep 2016.

12

A circadian based inflammatory response – implications for respiratory disease and treatment

Maria Comas[1,2,5*] [iD], Christopher J. Gordon[1,7], Brian G. Oliver[2,3,8], Nicholas W. Stow[9], Gregory King[2,4,6,10], Pawan Sharma[2,3,8], Alaina J. Ammit[2,8], Ronald R. Grunstein[1,5] and Craig L. Phillips[1,2,6,10]

Abstract

Circadian clocks regulate the daily timing of many of our physiological, metabolic and biochemical functions. The immune system also displays circadian oscillations in immune cell count, synthesis and cytokine release, clock gene expression in cells and organs of the immune system as well as clock-controlled genes that regulate immune function. Circadian disruption leads to dysregulation of immune responses and inflammation which can further disrupt circadian rhythms. The response of organisms to immune challenges, such as allergic reactions also vary depending on time of the day, which can lead to detrimental responses particularly during the rest and early active periods. This review evaluates what is currently known in terms of circadian biology of immune response and the cross-talk between circadian and immune system. We discuss the circadian pattern of three respiratory-related inflammatory diseases, chronic obstructive pulmonary disease, allergic rhinitis and asthma. Increasing our knowledge on circadian patterns of immune responses and developing chronotherapeutic studies in inflammatory diseases with strong circadian patterns will lead to preventive measures as well as improved therapies focussing on the circadian rhythms of symptoms and the daily variation of the patients' responses to medication.

Keywords: Immune system, Circadian clock, COPD, Allergic rhinitis, Asthma

Introduction

Jürgen Aschoff traced back the interest in biological rhythms to the Greek poet Archilochus of Paros (ca. 680–640 BC) who wrote "recognize which rhythms govern man" (Aschoff 1974). More than 2500 years later biological rhythms are known to 'govern' many aspects in human behaviour, physiology, metabolism, disease symptoms and response to treatment in a rhythmic fashion with the circadian clock as time-keeper.

The circadian clock ensures that the processes it regulates recur every day at the most optimal times of the day for the functioning and survival of the organism in a coordinated manner (Dibner et al. 2010). Disturbance of circadian rhythms due to, for example, shift-work

(Kecklund and Axelsson 2016), circadian disorders or dysregulation of rhythmicity (McHill and Wright 2017; Morris et al. 2016; Kadono et al. 2016; Gamaldo et al. 2014; Dickerman et al. 2016) increase the morbidity risk of cardiovascular disease (Reutrakul and Knutson 2015), metabolic disease (Arble et al. 2010) and cancers (Levi and Schibler 2007). Recent work has shown that disruption of the circadian clock leads to dysregulation of immune responses which underlie the pathophysiological basis of disease, suggesting an important regulatory role of the circadian system. This relates to daily oscillations in the number of circulating innate and adaptive immune cells, cytokine and chemokine levels and expression of adhesion molecules that are integral components of the immune response (reviewed in (Labrecque and Cermakian 2015; Nakao 2014; Scheiermann et al. 2013; Cermakian et al. 2013; Cermakian et al. 2014)). Overall, multiple studies suggest that pro-inflammatory activity is elevated during rest and induces sleep whereas anti-inflammatory mediators are induced upon awakening and inhibit sleep (Bryant

* Correspondence: Maria.comassoberats@sydney.edu.au
[1]CIRUS, Centre for Sleep and Chronobiology, Woolcock Institute of Medical Research, University of Sydney, 431 Glebe Point Road, Glebe, Sydney, NSW 2037, Australia
[2]Woolcock Emphysema Centre, Woolcock Institute of Medical Research, University of Sydney, Sydney, NSW, Australia
Full list of author information is available at the end of the article

et al. 2004; Krueger 1990; Krueger et al. 2001; Kubota et al. 2001; Kubota et al. 2001; Kubota et al. 2001; Kushikata et al. 1999; Krueger 1987; Kubota et al. 2000). Interestingly, both symptom intensity and response to treatment of many illnesses, including autoimmune or inflammatory diseases, vary across the 24-h day (Smolensky et al. 2007; Smolensky et al. 2012; Buttgereit et al. 2015). For this reason, chronotherapy which entails optimal timing of administration of treatments for disease aims to ensure that effectiveness is maximized whilst any toxic side effects are minimised (Smolensky et al. 2016).

In the context of inflammation, it is crucial that we increase our understanding of the circadian patterns of immune responses and how they are regulated by the central and peripheral clocks to enable discovery of chronotherapeutic approaches for optimal timing of therapies and even preventive measures for inflammatory disease, allergies and infections. This descriptive review focuses on the relationship between circadian clocks and the immune system and inflammatory diseases and discusses the potential for developing new therapeutic approaches. We discuss the urgent need of bridging all the fundamental knowledge established in chronobiology with disease to develop novel translational strategies that take time of day into account.

How is entrainment achieved in circadian rhythms?

Periodic environmental changes in, for example, light intensity, temperature, food availability and predator pressure amongst many others have led to the evolution of biological clocks in most species (Daan 1981). Circadian clocks continue to oscillate in the absence of time cues but, in this scenario, their period is not equal to 24 h. Instead, they display rhythmicity characterized by their individual endogenous circadian period, τ, which is circa 24 h but not necessarily exactly 24 h. In the presence of an external synchronizer, called *Zeitgeber* (from German *Zeit* "time" and *Geber* "giver" (Aschoff 1951; Aschoff 1958)) with a period T, τ is adjusted daily to equal T (Pittendrigh 1981). In addition, a stable and distinctive phase angle difference between the *Zeitgeber* and the circadian clock results (Daan 2000; Hirschie Johnson et al. 2003). This process of synchronization of circadian clocks to the external *Zeitgebers* is called entrainment. For the purposes of this review, entrainment will refer to the central clock aligning to the external time cues, while synchronization will refer to the alignment of the central and peripheral clocks relative to each other.

The light-dark cycle due to the rotation of the Earth with a period T of 24 h is a very reliable signal organisms use to entrain circadian rhythms. Light is the most important *Zeitgeber* for many organisms (Pittendrigh 1981;

Daan 2000; Aschoff 1960; Beersma et al. 2009). The specific properties characterizing the light signal that will contribute to entraining the circadian clock of an organism, e.g. duration of light and dark signals (Comas et al. 2006; Comas et al. 2007), light intensity (Boulos 1995), spectral composition (Boulos 1995; Revell et al. 2005; van de Werken et al. 2013; Cajochen et al. 2005) or twilight duration (Comas and Hut 2009; Aschoff and Wever 1965; Boulos et al. 2002; Boulos and Macchi 2005; Roenneberg and Foster 1997), will determine the robustness of entrainment. Other time cues, particularly food availability, have been proven to be potent synchronizers as well (Dibner et al. 2010). In mammals, the suprachiasmatic nucleus (SCN) located in the hypothalamus at the base of the brain is the 'master circadian clock' that generates and regulates the body's circadian rhythms and synchronizes them to the environmental 24-h light-dark cycle.

In addition to the master clock, peripheral clocks are found in virtually all individual cells in the body where they coordinate cellular processes – most notably within organs and other tissues including spleen, lymph nodes and different cells of the immune system (e.g. macrophages, monocytes, neutrophils or natural killers) (Keller et al. 2009; Boivin et al. 2003; Bollinger et al. 2011). All peripheral clocks are synchronized daily and coordinated by the SCN via the hypothalamic pituitary adrenal (HPA) axis and the autonomic nervous system (ANS) (Dibner et al. 2010; Nader et al. 2010; Kalsbeek et al. 2012). Peripheral clocks can also be synchronized and even uncoupled from the SCN by, for example, food availability or temperature (Brown et al. 2002; Mistlberger and Marchant 1995; Damiola 2000; Stokkan et al. 2001; Comas et al. 2014). However, in mammals the SCN is the only component of the circadian system that receives light input to maintain circadian synchronization with other peripheral clocks (Bell-Pedersen et al. 2005) (Fig. 1).

A molecular circadian clock is ticking in each of our cells

The mammalian molecular clock machinery is present in virtually all cell types including immune cells (see reviews for detailed descriptions of the molecular clock machinery (Labrecque and Cermakian 2015; Papazyan et al. 2016; Herzog et al. 2017; Partch et al. 2014; Takahashi 2017; Stojkovic et al. 2014)). In brief, it is composed of a set of proteins that generate two interlocking auto-regulatory transcription-translation feedback loops (TTFLs) (Fig. 2). For clarity reasons, we will use italics when we refer to genes and capital letters when we refer to proteins throughout the text. The main loop is composed of a positive and a negative arm. Circadian Locomotor Output Cycles Kaput (CLOCK), or its paralog NPAS2(DeBruyne et al. 2006), and brain and

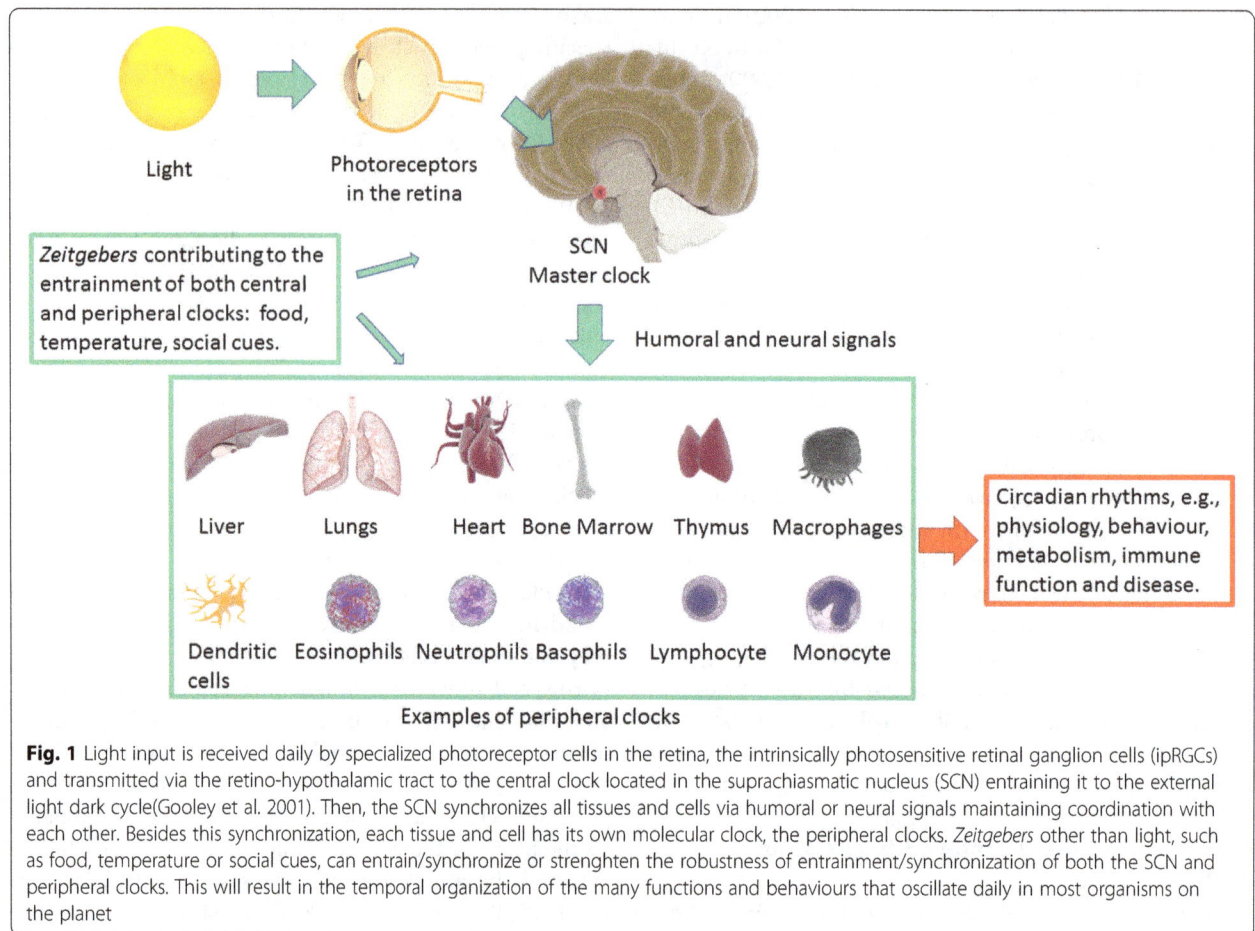

Fig. 1 Light input is received daily by specialized photoreceptor cells in the retina, the intrinsically photosensitive retinal ganglion cells (ipRGCs) and transmitted via the retino-hypothalamic tract to the central clock located in the suprachiasmatic nucleus (SCN) entraining it to the external light dark cycle(Gooley et al. 2001). Then, the SCN synchronizes all tissues and cells via humoral or neural signals maintaining coordination with each other. Besides this synchronization, each tissue and cell has its own molecular clock, the peripheral clocks. *Zeitgebers* other than light, such as food, temperature or social cues, can entrain/synchronize or strenghten the robustness of entrainment/synchronization of both the SCN and peripheral clocks. This will result in the temporal organization of the many functions and behaviours that oscillate daily in most organisms on the planet

muscle ARNT-like protein 1 (BMAL1) proteins are part of the positive arm of the loop. The CLOCK/BMAL1 heterodimer binds to E-box sequences in the promoters of the clock controlled genes regulating the timing of their expression around 24-h. CLOCK/BMAL1 also regulate the transcription of the negative components of the loop that will repress their own activity thereby closing the feedback loop, e.g., *Period* (*Per1, Per2, Per3*) and *Cryptochrome* (*Cry1, Cry2*). PER and CRY proteins heterodimerize and are phosphorylated by CASEIN KINASES 1 δ and ε (CK1δ and CK1ε) which targets them for translocating back into the nucleus where they directly bind to the BMAL1/CLOCK complex, disrupting it and repressing its actions. E3 ligase complexes will then target PER/CRY for ubiquitylation which will lead to degradation by the proteasome. As PER/CRY are degraded and their levels decline, repression of BMAL1/CLOCK will decrease and a new cycle will start. ROR-α and REV-ERB-α proteins conform a second adjoining loop binding to ROREs motifs found on the promoter of

Bmal1 activating or repressing its transcription respectively. What distinguishes the circadian clock feedback loop from any other feedback loops is that it takes about 24 h to be completed. This is achieved through, for example, protein phosphorylation, ubiquitylation, or SUMOylation that will tag proteins for e.g. trafficking or degradation creating delays in the 24 h feedback loops.

Importantly, the transcription of about 2-10% of mammalian genes, from different murine and human tissues or cells, are regulated by the molecular circadian clock (and these include genes related to immune response pathways as well as genes associated with inflammatory lung diseases (see examples and reviews (Partch et al. 2014; Logan and Sarkar 2012; Oishi et al. 2003; Sukumaran et al. 2011; Zhang et al. 2014a; Möller-Levet et al. 2013a; Akhtar 2002)). The percentage of proteins oscillating in mammalian tissues are as high as 20%(Mauvoisin et al. 2014; Reddy et al. 2006; Deery et al. 2009). This suggests that not only transcription but other mechanisms such as post-transcription, translation, post-translational

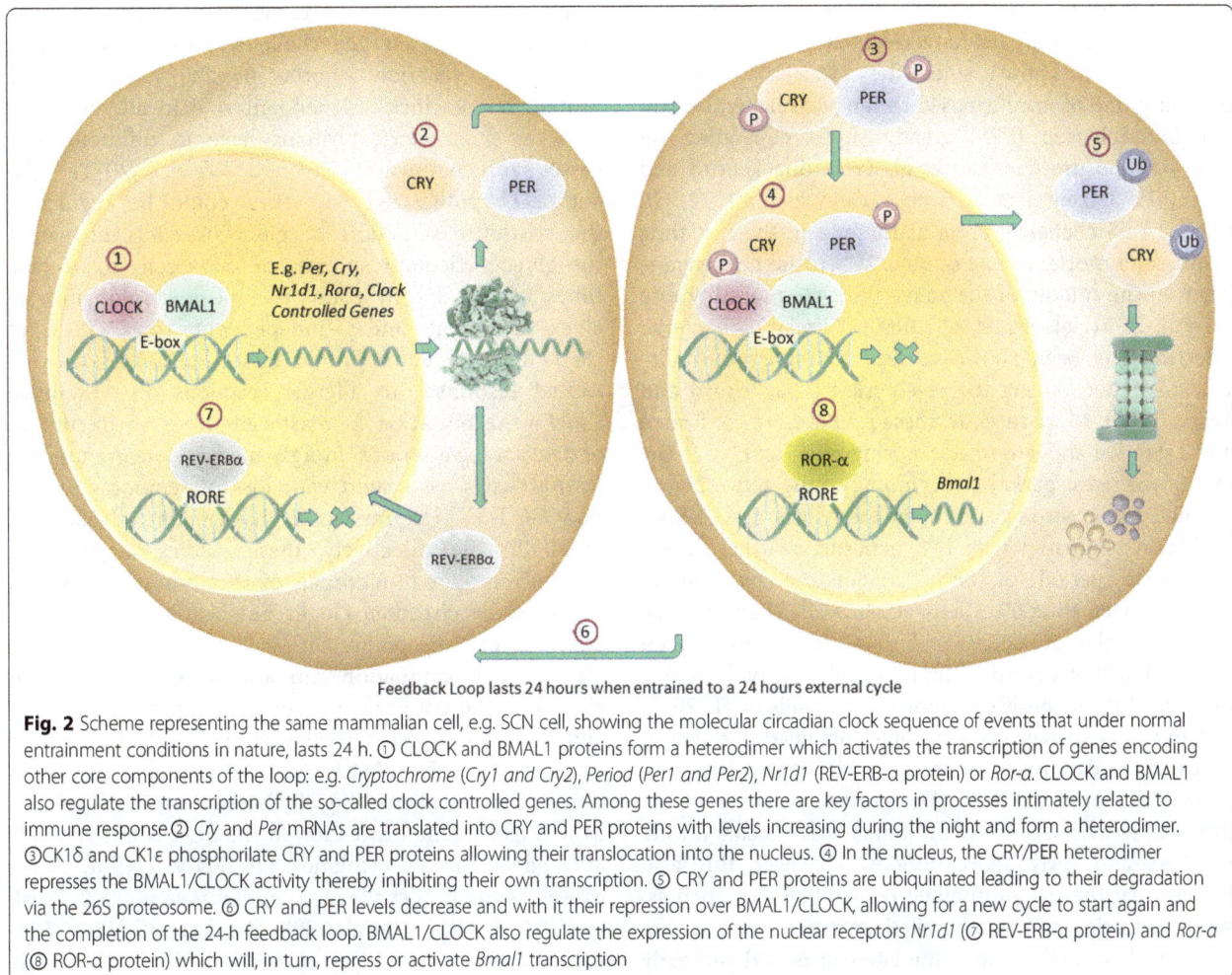

Feedback Loop lasts 24 hours when entrained to a 24 hours external cycle

Fig. 2 Scheme representing the same mammalian cell, e.g. SCN cell, showing the molecular circadian clock sequence of events that under normal entrainment conditions in nature, lasts 24 h. ① CLOCK and BMAL1 proteins form a heterodimer which activates the transcription of genes encoding other core components of the loop: e.g. *Cryptochrome* (*Cry1 and Cry2*), *Period* (*Per1 and Per2*), *Nr1d1* (REV-ERB-α protein) or *Ror-α*. CLOCK and BMAL1 also regulate the transcription of the so-called clock controlled genes. Among these genes there are key factors in processes intimately related to immune response.② *Cry* and *Per* mRNAs are translated into CRY and PER proteins with levels increasing during the night and form a heterodimer. ③CK1δ and CK1ε phosphorilate CRY and PER proteins allowing their translocation into the nucleus. ④ In the nucleus, the CRY/PER heterodimer represses the BMAL1/CLOCK activity thereby inhibiting their own transcription. ⑤ CRY and PER proteins are ubiquinated leading to their degradation via the 26S proteosome. ⑥ CRY and PER levels decrease and with it their repression over BMAL1/CLOCK, allowing for a new cycle to start again and the completion of the 24-h feedback loop. BMAL1/CLOCK also regulate the expression of the nuclear receptors *Nr1d1* (⑦ REV-ERB-α protein) and *Ror-α* (⑧ ROR-α protein) which will, in turn, repress or activate *Bmal1* transcription

modifications are oscillating or contributing to the circadian patterns of behaviour, physiology and metabolism.

There is a circadian variation in immune function

The immune system has as a primary function to protect against potentially harmful foreign bodies and disease. The innate component of the immune system comprises skin, all mucosal membranes, phagocytic cells (monocytes, neutrophils, eosinophils, macrophages and basophiles) and natural killer T-cells (NK). It is considered a first line of defence against foreign bodies and it also has a critical role in the activation and regulation of adaptive immunity (Iwasaki and Medzhitov 2015). This component is semi-specific, non-adaptable, non-plastic and has no 'memory'. In contrast, the adaptive component of immunity comprising B and T lymphocytes are adaptable, plastic and have 'memory'. Immune cells of both innate and adaptive immunity become activated and are recruited to sites of infection or injury in the process of inflammation (Riera Romo et al. 2016; Bennett et al. 2017; Ward and Rosenthal 2014). Although beneficial, this inflammatory response can become over expressed

leading to diseases and autoimmune disorders (Barnes 2008; Lien et al. 2012; Rose 2016).

Many cells and tissues of the immune system have been shown to have clocks that regulate many of their functions. In mammals, circadian clock genes oscillate in the spleen, lymph nodes, thymus, jejunum, macrophages, NK cells and CD4+ T cells (Keller et al. 2009; Bollinger et al. 2011; Alvarez and Sehgal 2005; Froy and Chapnik 2007; Arjona and Sarkar 2005; Arjona and Sarkar 2006). In fact, about 8% of the expressed genes in mice peritoneal macrophages show circadian variation, including genes involved in the regulation of pathogen recognition and cytokine secretion (Keller et al. 2009). A recent microarray study on the human blood transcriptome from sampled around the clock shows that the number of oscillating transcripts decreases and other genes are either up-, or down-regulated when subjects are sleep deprived, and genes associated with immune system amongst the most affected genes (Möller-Levet et al. 2013b). Whilst this suggests variations throughout the day in immune function, acute responses to infection or response to allergen exposure, future work is still needed to confirm a causal link between underlying rhythms in immunity and the clock mechanism and functional outcomes.

It has been known since the 1960s-70s that the mortality rate of mice exposed to the bacterial endotoxin lipopolysaccharide (LPS) greatly varies depending on time of exposure (Halberg et al. 1960; Shackelford and Feigin 1973; Feigin et al. 1969; Feigin et al. 1972). In mice, a LPS challenge given at the end of the rest time results in a mortality rate of 80%. When the challenge is given in the middle of the active time the mortality rate is only 20%(Halberg et al. 1960). Similarly, bacterial infection has been shown to lead to higher mortality when initiated during the rest period (Shackelford and Feigin 1973). More recently, these results were confirmed and extended showing that exposing mice to LPS at the end of their rest period or beginning of the active period resulted in a stronger cytokine response and NF-κB activation compared with LPS exposure starting during the active period or beginning of the rest period (Marpegan et al. 2009; Gibbs et al. 2012; Nguyen et al. 2013; Spengler et al. 2012). Similar results have been obtained in humans using the LPS challenge both in vivo injecting LPS to healthy volunteers (Alamili et al. 2014) and in vitro exposing blood samples obtained at different times of the day from volunteers to LPS (Petrovsky et al. 1998; Rahman et al. 2015). The greatest response of the immune system in terms of cytokine release occurs during the rest and early active periods. However, this also implies that the risk of immune-related illnesses, such as, sepsis, allergies and uncontrolled immune reactions are more likely to occur during the late rest period and early active period.

Allergic reactions are initiated with antigen specific IgE production and fixation of IgE to FcεRI receptors on mast cells and basophils (Stone et al. 2010). Importantly mast cells, eosinophils and basophils display circadian oscillations of clock gene expression as well as circadian gene expression and release of their mediators following IgE-mediated activation (Baumann et al. 2013; Wang et al. 2011; Ando et al. 2015; Baumann et al. 2015). Several recent studies have shown that the circadian clock regulated the daily rhythms in IgE/mast cell-mediated allergic reactions. For example, *Per2* mutant mice have a decreased sensitivity to the corticosteroid dexamethasone inhibition of the IgE-mediated degranulation in bone marrow-derived mast cells (Nakamura et al. 2011). Furthermore, anaphylactic reactions to an allergen challenge display a time of day dependent variation in wild-type mice which disappears in *Per2* mutant mice exhibiting a strong reaction at all times throughout the cycle (Nakamura et al. 2011). This could be due to the disrupted circadian clock that specifically results from the *Per2* mutation (Spoelstra et al. 2014; Albrecht et al. 2001; Chong et al. 2012; Xu et al. 2007)

compromising the mice's response to dexamethasone as well as to an allergen challenge and its consequent anaphylactic reaction. Another possibility is that PER2 protein has a clock-independent role in allergic reactions as most clock proteins have in different processes and pathways (Yu and Weaver 2011). The authors hypothesized that *Per2* could be regulating the rhythmic secretion of glucocorticoids or gating the glucocorticoid responses of mast cells to specific times of the day. It could also be a combination of clock-dependent and, –independent roles. Loss of clock function due to other factors also leads to disrupted responses to allergic reactions. For example, *Clock* gene mutation in mast cells leads to disruption of temporal variations in IgE mediated degranulation in mast cells associated with loss of temporal regulation of FcεRI expression and signalling (Nakamura et al. 2014). Collectively, these studies suggest that not only proper functioning of the immune system is regulated by circadian clocks but also allergies have a strong circadian component.

In turn, inflammation can also affect the circadian clock and the pathways it regulates such as metabolism and sleep-wake cycle (Bellet et al. 2013; Jewett and Krueger 2012; Lundkvist et al. 2002; Lundkvist et al. 2010). The circadian firing rhythms of the SCN neurons as well clock gene expression in the SCN is differentially affected by various cytokines, i.e. IFN-γ, TNF-α, IFN-α as well as the LPS challenge (Lundkvist et al. 2002; Kwak et al. 2008; Nygård et al. 2009; Okada et al. 2008). Furthermore, the effect of cytokines or LPS on clock gene expression in the SCN and peripheral clocks of rodents such as liver, heart or spleen, temperature or locomotor activity will vary depending on the time of day at which cytokines are administered (Duhart et al. 2013; Ohdo et al. 2001; Koyanagi and Ohdo 2002; Yamamura et al. 2010; Westfall et al. 2013; Marpegán et al. 2005; Leone et al. 2012; Boggio et al. 2003). Similarly in humans, LPS injection causes a suppression of clock genes e.g. *Clock, Cry1,2, Per1,2,3, Csnk1ε, Ror-α* and *Rev.-erb-α* in peripheral blood lymphocytes, neutrophils and monocytes (Haimovich et al. 2010).

Marpegan and colleagues suggested that immune responses may be acting as a synchronizing signal for the clock in a similar way to light that advances and delays circadian rhythms depending on time of day at which they administered (Marpegán et al. 2005). Immune responses could be acting as disrupting circadian clock signals instead. Chronic inflammation achieved by weekly injecting LPS to mice for 2 months leads to a decreased response of the SCN to light 7 days after the last LPS injection; however, the SCN response to light was restored 30 days after the last LPS injection (Palomba and Bentivoglio 2008).

As for potential mechanisms by which the immune system interacts with the molecular clock there are a few of studies so far. Cavadini and colleagues showed that TNF-α inhibits CLOCK-BMAL1 function by interfering with E-box mediated transcription leading to downregulation of expression of clock-controlled genes with E-boxes in their promotor (Cavadini et al. 2007). Petrzilka and colleagues extended this work and showed that TNF-α requires p38 mitogen-activated protein kinases (MAPK) and/or calcium signalling to upregulate expression of several core clock genes but it can downregulate *Dbp* (clock controlled gene) expression independently from p38 but requires calcium signalling (Petrzilka et al. 2009). And Bellet and co-workers showed that the RelB subunit of NF-kB interacts with BMAL1 protein and represses the circadian expression of *Dbp* (Bellet et al. 2012*)*. Overall, these studies provide clues to understand the cross-talk between the circadian and immune systems in inflammatory diseases. Further research should be directed at understanding the potential mechanisms by which the immune system gives time cues to the circadian system, both in health and in acute and in chronic inflammation.

The central clock regulates immune function

The central clock, located in the SCN, is thought to regulate aspects of immune responses. For instance, the SCN has been shown to regulate clock gene expression, oscillations in cytokines and cytosolic factors in NK cells and splenocytes in rats via the noradrenergic system (Logan et al. 2011). A lesion in the SCN leads to loss of the time of day dependence in passive systemic anaphylactic reaction in mice as well as loss of daily variations of cytokines (Nakamura et al. 2014). It has been shown that conditional ablation of *Bmal1* in T and B cells does not affect cell differentiation or their function suggesting a regulatory role of the central clock since circadian gating of IL-2 is preserved in *Bmal1*-deficient cells (Hemmers and Rudensky 2015).

The circadian regulation of the immune response is likely to be an integration of signals from the central clock and the peripheral clocks found in immune cells and organs as well as sites of infection. A very good example of this integration is the recent work by Gibbs and colleagues (Gibbs et al. 2014). They showed that the inflammatory response of the mouse lung to LPS has a daily rhythm peaking in the rest period which is regulated by both peripheral and central clocks. Thus, both the epithelial club cells (Clara) clock and the central clock through systemic glucocorticoid signals of adrenal origin, regulate the circadian oscillation of the CXCL5 chemokine which, in turn, drives the circadian

oscillation of neutrophil recruitment to the lung. Disruption of the central or Clara cell clocks, i.e. ablation of *Bmal1* in the Clara cells or adrenalectomy, leads to the disruption of circadian oscillation of CXCL5 and, in consequence, of the neutrophil recruitment to the lung. These experiments demonstrate the importance of central-peripheral clock interaction in mediating lung immune responses.

As for cortisol and melatonin, outputs of the central clock, control the circadian oscillation of the number of circulating T cells in humans (Dimitrov et al. 2009; Besedovsky et al. 2014). Melatonin regulates daily rhythms of core clock gene transcription factors, *Bmal1* and *Per1* expression in the spleen and a pinealectomy (the surgical removal of the pineal gland which produces melatonin) abolishes these rhythms (Prendergast et al. 2013). Melatonin is thought to have an immuno-modulatory role that can either be pro or anti-inflammatory however the mechanism is still unclear. Different studies showing the actions of endogenous and exogenous melatonin on the immune system have been reviewed elsewhere (Carrillo-Vico et al. 2005; Carrillo-Vico et al. 2013; Ren et al. 2017). Nevertheless it is worth mentioning the review by Carrillo-Vico and co-authors suggesting that melatonin may act as an immune buffer, whereby it may act as an immune stimulant under immune suppressive conditions and as an anti-inflammatory agent under conditions of exacerbated inflammation (Carrillo-Vico et al. 2013). If true, then interest in the potential for melatonin as a therapeutic with immune-modulatory properties will significantly increase in the future.

Peripheral clocks regulate immune function

Many cells and organs that are part of the immune system have been shown to display circadian oscillations in clock gene expression and function. Table 1 shows examples of immune system components displaying oscillations in number of cells and/or functionality. Toll-like receptors (TLRs) are proteins expressed on the surface of many cells and within endosomes and play a role in pathogen recognition and consequent activation of the innate immune system. The expression levels of TLRs display significant circadian oscillations in the mouse jejunum (Froy and Chapnik 2007). The levels of TLRs start to rise during the second part of the active phase and peak during the rest period which is probably when unwanted bacteria have reached the jejunum. Silver and colleagues demonstrated in mice that the expression of TLR9 in macrophages and B cells display circadian rhythmicity (Silver et al. 2012). The TLR9 circadian rhythm has functional consequences. For example, the time of day at which sepsis was experimentally induced in mice determines sepsis severity and mortality. This also coincides with the time of day when

Table 1 Examples of circadian rhythms in the immune system and the correspondent peaks and troughs of these oscillations

Organism	Oscillating component	Peak	Trough	Ref.
Mouse	Number of Ly6Chi monocyte in blood and spleen	ZT4-ZT8	ZT12-ZT24	(Nguyen et al. 2013)
Mouse	Circulating total leukocyte counts	ZT5	ZT13	(Scheiermann et al. 2012)
Mouse	Circulating HSCs and their progenitors	ZT5	ZT17	(Mendez-Ferrer et al. 2008)
Mouse	Number of LSK cells per ml of blood	ZT5	ZT13	(Mendez-Ferrer et al. 2008; Lucas et al. 2008)
Mouse	Activation of NF-κB	ZT6	ZT18	(Spengler et al. 2012)
Mouse	TNF-α and IL-6 secreted by spleens harvested around the clock and stimulated with LPS	CT8	CT20 (TNFα) CT16 (IL-6)	(Keller et al. 2009)
Mouse	Abundance of B cells and macrophages in the spleen	CT8	CT16	(Keller et al. 2009)
Mouse	Cytokine responses to LPS IL-1β, IL-6, MCP-1 and MIP1alpha	ZT11	ZT19	(Marpegan et al. 2009)
Mouse	TLR9 mRNA in macrophages	ZT11	ZT3	(Silver et al. 2012)
Mouse	Cytokine responses to LPS: IL-6, IL-12, CCL5, CXCL1 and CCL2	ZT12	ZT0	(Gibbs et al. 2012)
Mouse	Recruitment of leukocytes from the blood to tissues	ZT13	ZT5	(Scheiermann et al. 2012)
Mouse	ICAM1 protein abundance in muscle	ZT13	ZT5	(Scheiermann et al. 2012)
Mouse	Ccl2 mRNA abundance in cremasteric endothelial cells	ZT13	ZT1	(Scheiermann et al. 2012)
Mouse	CXCR4 expression in bone marrow LSK cells	ZT13	ZT5	(Lucas et al. 2008)
Mouse	TLR9 mRNA and protein abundance in the spleen	ZT19	ZT7	(Silver et al. 2012)
Mouse	Phagocytic activity of neutrophils	ZT20	ZT8	(Hriscu 2004)
Mouse	CXCL12 content in bone marrow extracellular fluids	ZT21	ZT9	(Mendez-Ferrer et al. 2008)
Human	Counts of peripheral monocytes	12:00 am	8:00 am	(Born et al. 1997)
Human	Counts of peripheral Lymphocytes, B-cells, T-cells, T-helper, T-suppressor	2:00 am-3:00 am	11:00 am	(Born et al. 1997)
Human	Circulating eosinophils	4:00 am	12:00 pm	(Haus and Smolensky 1999)
Human	Circulating lymphocytes	12:00 am-4:00 am	8:00 am	(Haus and Smolensky 1999)
Human	Counts of peripheral NK	11:00 am-6:00 pm	2:00 am	(Born et al. 1997)
Human	CD4+ T helper, CD8+ cytotoxic T cells: naïve, central memory, effector memory	1:31 pm-2:41 pm	2:00 pm	(Dimitrov et al. 2009)
Human	Effector CD8+ T cells	3:34 pm	3:00 am	(Dimitrov et al. 2009)
Human	Circulating monocytes	8:00 pm	8 am	(Haus and Smolensky 1999)
Human	HSC / progenitor cells in peripheral blood	8:00 pm	8:00 am	(Lucas et al. 2008)
Human	Circulating neutrophils	8:00 pm	8:00 am	(Haus and Smolensky 1999)

Note that in animal research, time of day does not correspond to "clock-time" but it is instead relative to the time of day at which lights are turned on and off in the animal facilities. Thus, ZT stands for *Zeitgeber* Time and ZT0 corresponds to the time of day when lights are turned-on and if mice are in a LD12:12 (12 h of light and 12 h of dark) ZT12 corresponds to time of day when lights are turned-off. If animals are in constant conditions (normally constant dark, but it could be constant light) then CT is used instead of ZT. CT stands for Circadian Time and CT0 corresponds to the time of day when animals start their resting time (as if lights were turned-on) and CT12 corresponds to the time of day when their activity time starts (as if lights were turned off). In the human studies that we have listed here, the authors provide "clock-times"

TLR9 inflammatory response is elevated, i.e. mid-dark period (Silver et al. 2012). Another example of circadian variation in innate immunity occurs in the spleen and NK cells of rats where transcripts of IFN-γ, granzyme B, perforin and TNF-α display circadian oscillations peaking at the end of the active phase and beginning of rest phase coinciding with the cytolytic activity of splenic NK cells (Arjona and Sarkar 2005; Arjona and Sarkar 2006; Arjona et al. 2004). Adaptive immune responses are also circadian regulated. The circadian clock in lymphocytes regulates their migration through lymph nodes which show a daily variation peaking at the beginning of the active phase in mice with a trough at the end of the active phase. Genetic disruption of T-cell clocks abolishes this rhythm (Druzd et al. 2017). The authors argue that the time of day of generation of the adaptive response as well as the numbers of cells present in the lymph node, are crucial in the regulation of the strength of the adaptive immune responses (Druzd et al. 2017; Moon et al. 2007). This idea is in agreement with Silver and colleagues work who showed that vaccinating mice with a TLR9 ligand as the adjuvant at the time of day when TLR9 was more responsive (active phase) led to an improved adaptive immune response 4 weeks later compared to animals vaccinated at other times (Silver et al. 2012).

It is interesting that the timing of peaks and troughs of function or number of immune cells do not necessarily coincide despite all components being part of the coordinated immune response. A plausible hypothesis to explain the function of differentially gating the timing of different immune system components may be to avoid an excessive simultaneous immune response to a threat that may prove detrimental for the organism (Man et al. 2016). On the other hand, hosts and parasites have evolved to exert selective pressure onto the other whilst the environment exerts pressure on both (Martinez-Bakker and Helm 2015). The host coordinate immune responses to times of day when exposure to threats are more likely to happen. Bacteria may, in turn, increase growth dependent on the host's circadian rhythms (Bellet et al. 2013). Bellet and colleagues infected mice with *Salmonella enterica serovar Typhimurium* at two timepoints, 4 h after beginning of active time and 4 h after resting time, and showed bacteria clearance 72 h after infection was greater 4 h after beginning of active time. The authors subsequently found that the antimicrobial peptide lipocalin-2 levels in the gut was higher during the day than during the night, which suppressed the growth of resident microbiota during the day. However, *Salmonella* is lipocalin-2 resistant allowing a window for Salmonella to increase outgrowth during the day when there is less competition with other microorganisms compared to night time (Bellet et al. 2013). Thus, despite the lack of proof that Salmonella has its own circadian clock it still takes advantage of circadian variations in levels of lipocalin-2 in its host.

In conclusion and as illustrated in Fig. 1, the coordination of the immune system oscillatory function is regulated at different levels, the master clock level as well as peripheral clock levels. This secures an optimization of the timing of the immune response around the clock so that it is most effective against threads to the organism and causes the least damage to the host organism. Dysregulation of the clock will cause disease as we will describe in the next section.

Dysregulation of the clock leads to a dysregulated immune response

Numerous experiments have shown that altering the period and/or amplitude of rhythm of the master clock in the SCN and/or peripheral clocks in organs such as the liver and lungs, result in dysregulation of the immune response. This has been demonstrated under conditions of shift- work where feeding/fasting and sleep/wake cycles are uncoupled from the master and peripheral clocks, with lesion of the SCN (which destroys the master clock), with

aging and with the generation of mutant mice or knock-out/knock-down mice for clock proteins involved in pro and anti-inflammatory responses.

Pro-inflammation

In rodents exposed to simulated shift-work with work and feeding during the day, which corresponds to their usual rest and fasting period, and inactivity and fasting at night (usual active feeding period), there is an uncoordinated inflammatory response to LPS challenge, resulting in elevated cytokine levels and increased mortality (Castanon-Cervantes et al. 2010; Adams et al. 2013; Guerrero-Vargas et al. 2015). Interestingly, if feeding time is restricted to the night time and normal active phase then the immune response is not dysregulated when undergoing LPS challenge. The TNF-α and IL-6 inflammatory cytokine levels remain at a similar level to control (ad libitum feeding and activity) rats. In contrast, when animals not subjected to simulated shift-work are restricted to feeding in the day time (the normal resting period), the immune response is also dysregulated with elevated TNF-α and IL-6 levels (Guerrero-Vargas et al. 2015). These data suggest that feeding is a stronger *Zeitgeber* than light in keeping the immune system synchronized and undisturbed. In this context, the gut microbiome is increasingly being implicated in playing a role in chronic inflammation. It has recently been proposed that a desynchronization between sleep, circadian and feeding/fasting cycles, such as that which occurs during shift-work, may promote alterations in gut microbiota leading to chronic inflammation (Reynolds et al. 2017). This research, however, is relatively new and requires further extensive examination (Phillips and Comas 2017). A different method to induce circadian disruption is by lesion of the SCN master clock (Moore and Eichler 1972; Stephan and Zucker 1972). Similar to simulated shift-work, bilateral lesions of the SCN in rats leads to a dysregulated immune response with significantly higher levels of cytokines after exposure to LPS compared to controls (Guerrero-Vargas et al. 2014). Aging has also been shown in rats to dysregulate the circadian clock by decreasing the amplitudes of oscillation of clock genes and cytokine mRNA. This in turn resulted in a chronic state of inflammation with loss of the inflammatory response to an LPS challenge (Fonken et al. 2016). Circadian disruption can also be induced by mutation or knocking down different clock genes. This has resulted in decreased levels of cytokines suggesting a pro-inflammatory role for these clock genes. For example, mutation or knocking down *Per2* resulted in decreased levels of granzyme B (Arjona and Sarkar 2006), perforin proteins (Arjona and Sarkar 2006), IFN-γ (Arjona and Sarkar 2006; Arjona and Dk 2006; Liu et al. 2006) and IL-1β (Liu et al. 2006). In accordance with these studies, *Per2* mutant mice are more resistant to the LPS challenge compared to wild types (Liu et al. 2006). A reduction of cytokine production (in response to the LPS challenge or *Salmonella Typhimurium* infection) is observed in macrophages from *Clock* mutant mice (Bellet et al. 2013). This is in agreement with the finding that CLOCK protein activates the NF-κB pathway leading to upregulation of cytokines (Spengler et al. 2012).

Anti-inflammation

When a different set of clock genes are compromised then inflammation increases suggesting that other clock proteins have *anti-inflammatory* roles. This has been shown with deletion of *Ror-α* in mice which leads to abnormal immune responses such as hyper responsive macrophages producing higher levels of cytokines in bronchoalveolar lavage fluids after LPS challenge (Sidman et al. 1962; Kopmels et al. 1990; Trenkner and Hoffmann 1966; Stapleton et al. 2005; Dzhagalov et al. 2004). Macrophages from *Rev.-erb-α*$^{-/-}$ mice and from LysM-*Bmal*$^{-/-}$ mice (mice that lack *Bmal1* in their macrophages, monocytes and neutrophils) show loss of circadian gating and constitutively elevated levels of IL-6 in response to the LPS challenge (Gibbs et al. 2012). Two more studies show the important role of BMAL1 protein in inflammation. *Bmal1*$^{-/-}$Lys-MCre mice are more susceptible to LPS challenge compared to wild type mice with decreased survival. Interestingly, deletion of MiR-155 which represses *Bmal1* leads to a reduced inflammatory response to the LPS challenge (Curtis et al. 2015). Thus, this work suggests that *Bmal1* has an important anti-inflammatory role which is relevant not only at the protein level but also at the miRNA regulation level. Knocking down or silencing *Cry1* and *Cry2* also leads to increased inflammation (Narasimamurthy et al. 2012; Hoffman et al. 2009). Whether we can assign definitive anti or pro-inflammatory roles to specific clock genes still requires more work. The effects observed so far for each clock protein may be cell-specific, immune function-specific (e.g. innate vs adaptive) or even species specific.

These studies highlight the need for further research exploring the mechanistic links between circadian clock function and inflammation. However, the available data does provide a framework for continuing translational research in chronotherapy to more effectively manage acute and chronic inflammation.

Circadian rhythms in respiratory inflammatory disease

It is quite clear that the stronger responses of the immune system occur from the second half of the rest time and the first hours of the activity time. Thus, in humans, immune responses are stronger in the second half of the night and early morning hours. These are the times when inflammation is exacerbated and symptoms and mortality rates are highest (Buttgereit et al. 2015; Smolensky et al. 2015). In parallel, timed therapies that decrease inflammation during the night and early morning hours has proven to be more successful than untimed therapy (Smolensky et al. 2007; Buttgereit et al. 2015; Smolensky et al. 2015). Below we discuss these concepts in the context of several common respiratory inflammatory diseases.

Chronic obstructive pulmonary disease

Chronic obstructive pulmonary disease (COPD), is the fourth highest cause of death globally (GOLD, 2016). Like other chronic diseases, it is largely caused by preventable risk factors (cigarette smoking and noxious air-borne particles). COPD is a systemic disease with significant extrapulmonary effects that contribute to morbidity and mortality. Its pulmonary component is characterised by airflow limitation which is not fully reversible and is usually progressive and associated with an abnormal inflammatory response of the lung to noxious particles or gases (GOLD, 2016). A patient suffering from COPD may have persistent inflammation, increased mucus secretion (chronic bronchitis) and narrowing and destruction of their small airways (small airways disease) and/ or they may have destruction of the lung alveoli resulting in emphysema. COPD symptoms vary throughout the day. While some patients report worsening of their symptoms (cough, shortness of breath and phlegm) in the early morning upon awakening, others complain of nocturnal symptoms, most commonly wheezing, shortness of breath and cough which also cause sleep disruption (Kessler et al. 2011; Price et al. 2013; Lange et al. 2014; Agusti et al. 2011; Stephenson et al. 2015; Jen et al. 2016; Partridge et al. 2009; Espinosa de los Monteros et al. 2012; Kuyucu et al. 2011; Kim et al. 2012; Decramer et al. 2013; Roche et al. 2013; Roche et al. 2013; Miravitlles et al. 2014; Tsai et al. 2007).

Lung cells have their own molecular circadian clocks that coordinate tissue-specific functions and responses to environmental stimuli (Sukumaran et al. 2011; Gibbs et al. 2009; Oishi et al. 1998). This results in circadian oscillations in many common lung function indices (e.g. forced vital capacity (FVC), forced expiratory volume in 1 s (FEV$_1$) and peak expiratory flow (Agusti et al. 2011; Spengler and Shea 2000)). These normal circadian oscillations in airway calibre may be partly responsible for nocturnal COPD exacerbations and worsening hypoxia (Agusti et al. 2011; Tsai et al. 2007) however, the impact appears to be much greater in asthmatics (Tsai et al. 2007; Brenner et al. 2001), perhaps because of airway hyperresponsiveness (the ability of airways to contract too much and too easily). Although the underlying basis of airway hyperresponsiveness is unknown, the excessive circadian variations in airway calibre could be due to changes in the contractile properties of airway smooth muscle, inflammation (Kraft et al. 1996), neural activity or changes in lung mechanics during sleep (Irvin et al. 2000). Given that several studies have found that critically ill COPD patients are more likely to die at night and that this is attributable to COPD exacerbations, there is a clear role of the clock in adverse outcomes (Tsai et al. 2007; Martin 1990; Petty 1988; McNicholas and Fitzgerald 1984; Tirlapur 1984; Kimura et al. 1998; Chaouat et al. 2001). Nevertheless early morning symptoms and night time symptoms remain one of the adverse outcomes of COPD, particularly in more severe cases (Partridge et al. 2009). Importantly, a recent study showed that COPD patients that report both or either nocturnal or early morning symptoms have poorer health compared with patients who do not have a worsening of symptoms at specific times of day (Stephenson et al. 2015). This could potentially be used as a biomarker of disease status and there is scope for developing chronotherapeutic approaches for these patients to cover the times of day with worsening symptoms. Very little is known about circadian changes in lung function or disease activity in COPD or why nocturnal symptoms are associated with poorer outcomes. Perhaps research in this area will translate to future clinical benefit.

Additionally, and in the context of this review, several studies have found a potential mechanism connecting disruption of lungs circadian clock, inflammation and COPD (Yao et al. 2015; Hwang et al. 2014; Rajendrasozhan et al. 2008). Importantly, levels of the deacetylase SIRT1 are reduced in COPD patients, as well as in smokers and in mice exposed to cigarette smoke (Yao et al. 2015; Hwang et al. 2014). Furthermore, SIRT1 regulates both central and peripheral circadian clocks (Masri and Sassone-Corsi 2014). A decrease in SIRT1 levels in COPD patients, smokers and mice exposed to cigarette smoke results in increased acetylation of BMAL1 leading to an increased BMAL1 protein degradation and, in consequence, to a molecular clock dysregulation and an increased inflammatory response is observed (Yao et al. 2015; Hwang et al. 2014). To confirm the role of BMAL1 in lung inflammation, Hwang and colleagues studied mice carrying a targeted deletion of *Bmal1* in lung epithelium and they observed that these mice also suffer from increased inflammatory response to cigarette smoke which is not reduced when mice are treated with a SIRT1 activator (Hwang et al. 2014). The authors concluded that both BMAL1 protein as well as its regulation by SIRT1 must have a key role in lung inflammation in COPD patients and smokers (Hwang et al. 2014).

Apart from cigarette smoke (Yao et al. 2015; Hwang et al. 2014; Vasu et al. 2009; Gebel et al. 2006), other environmental factors such as respiratory infections or even chronic jet-lag can lead to dysregulation of the lung circadian clock leading to increased lung inflammation. Sundar and co-workers showed mice with chronic exposure to cigarette smoke combined with infection of influenza A virus altered lung clock gene expression and increased lung inflammation as well as emphysema. The same experiment performed on *Bmal1* Knockout mice resulted in increased lung inflammation and pulmonary fibrosis (Sundar et al. 2015). Disruption of circadian rhythms in mice using a chronic jet-lag protocol for 4 weeks leads to disruption in lung physiology and lung clock gene expression (Hadden et al. 2012). Evidence from a study which investigated the effect of chronic exposure to real-life ambient air particles showed that pollution leads to circadian clock gene expression disruption in the lungs of rats as well as increased lung and systemic inflammation and oxidative stress (Song et al. 2017). These animals were housed in the Haidian district of Beijing which has characteristically high levels of polluted air due to heavy traffic.

The specific pathways regulated by the circadian clock that influence COPD are not clear yet. However, several recent publications have demonstrated that if the circadian clock controlled expression of genes is unregulated, it may lead to pulmonary disease. Disruption of the circadian clocks regulation of Nrf2 expression in mouse lungs leads to chronic pulmonary diseases including COPD, asthma, idiopathic pulmonary fibrosis and cancer (Pekovic-Vaughan et al. 2014). Sukumaran and co-workers showed in rats lungs that genes associated with COPD display circadian oscillations and that some of these oscillating genes are potential COPD drug targets i.e. Myristoylated Ala-rich PKC substrate (*Marcks*) and Adrenergic β2 receptor (*Adrb2*) (Sukumaran et al. 2011). Similarly, Zhang and colleagues listed drugs that are indicated to treat COPD and that target genes that oscillate (Zhang et al. 2014b). Disentangling the molecular pathways that contribute to emphysema and bronchitis in COPD patients regulated by the circadian clock will permit the development of novel chronotherapeutic approaches.

Allergic rhinitis

Allergic rhinitis (AR) is increasing worldwide with current prevalence rates of between 10% and 30%. The prevalence is particularly high in developed countries (Bousquet et al. 2008; Mullol et al. 2008). AR is an immune system-mediated upper airway hypersensitivity to environmental allergens. It is characterized by respiratory tissue inflammation, mucus gland hyperactivation and blood vessel dilation. In people suffering from AR, the allergen triggers early and late phase reactions that are mediated by a series of inflammatory cells and mediators. The early phase occurs immediately after allergen exposure and the late phase develops 8 to 12 h after allergen exposure. The most common symptoms of AR are sneezing, itching, rhinorrhoea, nasal congestion, and post-nasal drip. The symptoms of the late phase are similar to the early phase, but with more severe congestion (Stull et al. 2009; Hansen et al. 2004).

A daily rhythm in allergic symptoms has been known since the 1960s (Reinberg et al. 1963; Reinberg et al. 1969). Symptoms often intensify overnight and are worst upon wakening, displaying a "morning attack" (Smolensky et al. 2007; Smolensky et al. 2015; Long 2007; Gelfand 2004; Smolensky et al. 1995; Reinberg et al. 1988). Due to the time at which symptoms intensify, AR symptoms often disrupt sleep (Craig et al. 2008; González-Núñez et al. 2013; Santos et al. 2006). This may lead to daytime fatigue, interfering with daily activities, including the capability to work or study and overall quality of life (Stull et al. 2009; González-Núñez et al. 2013; Santos et al. 2006; Bousquet et al. 2013; Walker et al. 2007; de la Hoz et al. 2012; Blanc et al. 2001). Work and school absenteeism and decreased productivity at work due to AR are associated with substantial economic costs, ranging between 2 and 5 billion US dollars (Blaiss 2010; Lamb et al. 2006; Roger et al. 2016). Importantly, the upper airway obstruction that characterizes AR is a risk factor for sleep disordered breathing events, such as apnoeas, hypopneas and snoring in adults and children (Long 2007). AR patients have daily rhythms of salivary melatonin that have a decreased amplitude, baseline and peak levels, as well as lower amplitude of salivary cortisol daily rhythm and delayed peak compared to healthy controls (Fidan et al. 2013). The reason for the lower robustness of these rhythms is unknown but may be due to sleep disruption and/or as a consequence of inflammation. It is also unclear if these disrupted rhythms further worsen inflammation and allergy.

Mouse nasal mucosa has a functional circadian clock and its response to glucocorticoids is dependent on the time of day (Honma et al. 2015). This daily rhythm in hypersensitivity to allergens contributes to the daily rhythms observed in AR (Nakamura et al. 2011; Nakamura et al. 2014; Nakamura et al. 2014; Nakamura et al. 2016). For example in children exposed to an allergic challenge at 6 am, more nasal secretions are produced than when exposed at 3 pm (Aoyagi et al. 1999). Furthermore, the commonest allergen for patients suffering from AR is house dust mite. The greatest allergen challenge occurs from the bedding exposure to dust mite during time in bed during the night which coincides with the worst time for the circadian clock to deal with allergen challenge.

In the context of chronotherapy, Reinberg and colleagues tested whether H1 receptor antagonists were more effective at 7 am compared to 7 pm and found that evening administration was more effective (Reinberg 1997). Importantly, whilst corticosteroid nasal sprays have been shown to effectively treat allergic symptoms, they also interfere with the nasal circadian clock. From a mechanistic perspective, studies have shown that endogenous glucocorticoids regulate clock gene expression by binding directly onto the promoter of clock genes (*Per1, Per2 and Rev.-erb-α*) (Cheon et al. 2013; Yamamoto et al. 2005) and that administration of prednisolone induces *Per1* expression, affecting normal clock function (Fukuoka et al. 2005; Koyanagi et al. 2006). However, the disruption of clock function by prednisolone can be reduced, simply by changing the time of day at which it is administered (Koyanagi et al. 2006). Therefore, the questions arise, what is the best chronotherapeutic strategy to maximise treatment effectiveness? And does it have to minimally disrupt the nasal mucosa circadian clock? Based on their work in mice, Honma and colleagues proposed that the best time to administer intranasal corticosteroids to treat AR is when they disrupt the nasal clock least, which corresponds to early evening for humans (Honma et al. 2015). The authors argued that this timing corresponds to the same time at which aerosol corticosteroid is most efficient to treat asthma and that repeated disruption of circadian clocks leads to other health issues or worsens previous conditions (Honma et al. 2015). Nakamura's work, on the other hand, suggested that the best time to treat allergies was at the time the circadian clock was most susceptible to be disrupted, which is during the night in humans and during the day in mice (Nakamura et al. 2016). They showed that treating with dexamethasone at a time of day that resulted in increasing PER2 levels and reducing FcεRI signalling in mast cells or basophils resulted in suppression of IgE mediated allergic reactions in a mouse model of AR. Furthermore, dexamethasone did not decrease the allergic reactions in both *Clock*-mutated or *Per2*-mutated mast cells. They further hypothesized that reduction of FcεRI signalling depends on PER2 upregulation by glucocorticoids (Nakamura et al. 2016). Even though it appears as a very promising chronotherapeutic approach it is important to understand the long-term consequences of upregulating PER2 by glucocorticoids and thus disrupting the circadian clock in a chronic disease such as AR. Understanding the circadian patterns of allergic response and its regulation by the central and peripheral clocks, specifically in humans will enable discovery of preventive measures which utilise chronotherapy to treat AR patients.

Asthma

Asthma is a chronic inflammatory disease of the lungs that affects approximately 334 million people worldwide (Global

Asthma report, 2014). It is characterized classically by hypersensitivity to environmental antigens which leads to inflammation driven by IgE-dependent mechanisms, constriction and obstruction of the airways. However, nonallergic asthma phenotypes are also common. Asthma shares a lot of characteristics with allergic diseases, including genetic risk factors (Bousquet et al. 2000). Asthma episodes, as well as asthma exacerbations, are more prone to happen during the night and early morning compared to other times of the day both in adults and in children (Smolensky et al. 2007; Reinberg et al. 1988; Turner-Warwick 1988; Smolensky and D'Alonzo 1997; Hoskyns et al. 1995; Jarjour 1999; Bohadana et al. 2002; Litinski et al. 2009). One of the first studies involving 3000 asthma patients found that asthma episodes during washout from regular maintenance asthma treatment occurred 70-fold more frequently between 4 am and 5 am compared to 2 pm-3 pm (Dethlefsen and Repges 1985). Death from severe asthma attacks is also known to mostly occur during the night or early morning (Smolensky and D'Alonzo 1997; Cochrane and Clark 1975).These times coincide with the times at which lung function is reduced and inflammation and airway hyperreactivity is increased (Spengler and Shea 2000; Kraft et al. 1996; Jarjour 1999; Martin et al. 1991; Hetzel and Clark 1980; Gervais et al. 1977; Bonnet et al. 1991; Panzer et al. 2003; Kelly et al. 2004).

Studies with asthmatics using sleep deprivation protocols have shed some light on the partial contribution of sleep and of circadian variation to airway calibre and lung function. Ballard and colleagues studied pulmonary function in asthmatic patients during a sleep deprived night and a normal sleep night (Ballard et al. 1989). They observed that lower airway resistance increases during the night, regardless of whether asthmatic patients sleep or not, but the rate of increase is two-fold higher if patients are allowed to sleep compared to sleep deprivation, implying that sleep itself increases lower airway resistance. However, decrements in forced expired volume in 1 s (FEV_1) were not significantly different between the sleeping night and the sleep deprived night (Ballard et al. 1989). Using the same protocol, another group found that in asthmatics, nocturnal bronchoconstriction occurred both in the sleep and sleep-deprived nights but the morning values of peak expiratory flow (PEF) were higher after the awake night and the absolute and percentage falls in PEF were greater in the sleep night, suggesting the contribution of sleep to nocturnal bronchoconstriction (Catterall et al. 1986). Furthermore, the amplitude of PEF variation in asthmatics is greater compared to non-asthmatics, indicating an exaggeration of daily variation in airway calibre in asthmatics during the night (Hetzel and Clark

1980). However, the Hetzel study showed that sleep deprivation does not improve the overnight fall in PEF, suggesting that it is the circadian variation in pulmonary function, rather than sleep, causing the PEF fall in asthmatics (Hetzel and Clark 1979). The overnight decrease in PEF is related to greater severity of daytime asthma (Martin et al. 1990). Similarly, the time of day at which an asthmatic is undergoing an allergen challenge will have an impact in the chances of developing a late asthmatic response, being higher in the evening compared to the morning (Mohiuddin and Martin 1990).

Nocturnal worsening of asthma has also been associated with nocturnal increases in lung inflammation. For example, analysis of bronchoalveolar lavage fluid from asthmatic patients showed that patients with nocturnal asthma had higher leukocytes count, specifically eosinophils and neutrophils, at 4 am compared to 4 pm, whereas in asthmatic patients without nocturnal episodes, there was no difference between these two time-points. When comparing both groups of patients, there was a significant difference between them at 4 am but not at 4 pm (Martin et al. 1991). Therefore, day time leukocytes count were similar between groups but the difference was attributable to the number of immune cells found during the night. These results were confirmed in other studies with a comparable protocol looking at neutrophils, macrophages and CD4+ cells (Kraft et al. 1996; Kraft et al. 1999) as well as when comparing non-asthmatic controls to nocturnal asthmatic patients (Mackay et al. 1994; Oosterhoff et al. 1995). Another study also showed a higher blood concentration of eosinophils at 4 am compared to 4 pm in nocturnal asthmatics (Calhoun et al. 1992). Furthermore, the night fall in PEF was positively correlated with change in neutrophils and eosinophils, further indicating a relationship between nocturnal inflammation and decline of pulmonary function in nocturnal asthmatics (Martin et al. 1991). Another study investigated FEV_1 and sputum inflammatory cells in mild asthmatics at 4 pm and 7 am resulting in similar findings to the previous studies, that is, lower FEV_1 at 7 am with higher numbers of sputum inflammatory cells compared to 4 pm timepoint (Panzer et al. 2003).

Studies on bronchial hyperreactivity in asthmatic patients in the 1970s have also shown a clear daily variation. Gervais and colleagues exposed asthmatic patients to a bronchial challenge with house dust in an otherwise allergen-shielded room. They measured airway calibre using FEV_1 15 min after house dust inhalation at 8 am, 3 pm, 7 pm and 11 pm and showed that the strongest response occurred at 11 pm whilst the weakest response occurred at 8 am (Gervais et al. 1977). In addition, the effects of histamine and methacholine on airways responsiveness were tested on patients with mild asthma with night time symptoms at different times of the day and night. Airway hyperresponsiveness as measured by the dose required to cause a 20% decline in FEV1 ($PC_{20}FEV_1$) was greater when the challenges occurred in the middle of the night (3-5 am) compared with daytime (Bonnet et al. 1991). A recent review has confirmed that the circadian variation of bronchial hyperreactivity to different agents in asthma is more profound during the night, except to cold dry air, which shows a peak in the afternoon (Jarjour 1999). Interestingly, this review also found that the amplitude of circadian oscillation of airway hyperreactivity correlated with the amplitude of pulmonary function oscillation. The greater the decline of pulmonary function during the night in asthmatics, the greater the increase of night time airways hyperreactivity in asthmatic patients (Jarjour 1999).

The impairment of lung function at night and early morning also correlated with the expression of several core clock genes. A recent study by Ehlers and colleagues studied the expression pattern of multiple core clock genes in respiratory tract of mild/moderate and severe asthmatic patients (Ehlers et al. 2017). They found reduced expression in 6 core clock genes (including Bmal1 and Per2) and higher expression of Clock gene in asthmatics patients (mild-moderate and severe) when compared to controls. Similarly, another study found higher gene expression of Arntl2 (a paralog of Bmal1) and lower of Per2 in severe asthmatics when compared to mild asthmatics and healthy donors (Fajt et al. 2015). This suggests a relationship These findings are supported by a recent longitudinal study that demonstrated the association of insomnia and risk of developing asthma in approximately 18,000 participants (Brumpton et al. 2017).

In the context of treatment, similar to COPD, genes associated with asthma display circadian oscillation patterns of expression in rats lungs and some of these genes may represent asthma drug targets i.e. Selectin P (Selp), Adenosine A2a receptor (Adora2a), Hepatocyte growth factor (Hgf), Myristoylated Ala-rich PKC substrate (Marcks) and Adrenergic-2 receptor (Adrb2) (Sukumaran et al. 2011) using chronotherapy. Research on the circadian patterns of disease as well as on potential to use chronotherapy on both asthma and allergic rhinitis has been accumulating for decades (Smolensky et al. 2007). As always, more research needs to be undertaken in order to apply chronotherapy in asthma but it is one of the most promising diseases to take advantage of time of day to significantly improve therapeutic results.

Conclusion

In recent years, mounting evidence has demonstrated that the immune system displays circadian oscillations (see reviews (Labrecque and Cermakian 2015; Nakao 2014; Scheiermann et al. 2013; Cermakian et al. 2013; Cermakian et al. 2014)). Pro-inflammatory cytokines are elevated during rest time and anti-inflammatory cytokines are elevated during activity time. Organisms display stronger immune responses during the rest period and early active period as compared to other times of the day. Oscillations in immune function are observed in immune challenges (such as LPS challenge or bacterial infection) as well as in disease, including autoimmune and inflammatory diseases. Although the precise mechanism by which the circadian clocks regulate immune function are unclear, there is a clear role for both central and peripheral clocks in regulating the immune response. For example, the SCN regulates the recruitment of leukocytes to tissues and regulates clock gene expression in immune system tissues and cells as well as oscillations in cytokine production. Furthermore, immune function is also regulated through SCN-mediation of hormones (cortisol, melatonin). Peripheral clocks found in many cells and tissues, including those composing the immune system, also regulate circadian oscillations of immune functions. Overall, the interplay between circadian physiology and disease is complex and is further complicated by the bi-directional nature of these systems. Thus, not only does the circadian clock regulate immune function but inflammation will in turn affect the circadian clock and the pathways it regulates. Altogether, the interaction and inter-regulation of the circadian and immune systems seems to be directed at optimizing immune responses around the clock.

In respiratory diseases, signs and symptoms as well as severity show circadian variability across the 24-h cycle. Specifically, obstructive airways diseases and allergic rhinitis demonstrate increased inflammation and disease severity at night. Consequently, exposure to inflammatory insults at night also has greater effects. Altogether, evidence suggests that inflammatory diseases may be response to chronotherapy to improve disease control due to circadian clock control of symptoms and exacerbations. If medicine is evolving towards a more personalized approach this will certainly be an aspect to consider. Chronotherapy into clinical trials studies with existing and new drugs are needed to test whether outcomes can be improved in inflammatory diseases when therapy is administered at different times of day. Assessing circadian periodicity in humans in field studies are also required to understand the influence on patho-physiological processes and therapies. Overall, a better understanding of the circadian clock regulation of the immune system will improve the understanding of the pathophysiology of inflammatory disease and this could lead to development of more effective chronotherapeutic strategies.

Abbreviations

Adora2a: Adenosine A2a receptor; *Adrb2*: Adrenergic β2 receptor; ANS: Autonomic nervous system; AR: Allergic rhinitis; BMAL1: ARNT-like protein 1; CK: Casein Kinases; CLOCK: Circadian Locomotor Output Cycles Kaput; COPD: Chronic obstructive pulmonary disease; Cry: Cryptochrome; FEV_1: Forced expiratory volume in 1 s; FVC: Forced vital capacity; *Hgf*: Hepatocyte growth factor; HPA: Hypothalamic pituitary adrenal; LPS: Lipopolysaccharide; MAPK: p38 mitogen-activated protein Kinases; *Marcks*: Myristoylated Ala-rich PKC substrate; NK: Natural Killer T-cells; PEF: Peak expiratory volume; Per: Period; SCN: Suprachiasmatic nucleus; *Selp*: Selectin P; TLRs: Toll-like receptors; TTFLs: Transcription-translation feedback loops

Acknowledgments

The figures were done with the help of the library that can be downloaded from www.somersault1824.com.

Funding

Not applicable.

Authors' contributions

MC drafted and coordinated the completion of the manuscript, CP and CG improved the draft of the manuscript and drafted the conclusions, BO and PS improved the asthma section of the manuscript, AA and GK improved the COPD section of the manuscript and NS improved the allergic rhinitis section of the manuscript. All authors read and approved the final manuscript.

Competing interests

The authors declare that they have no competing interests.

Author details

[1]CIRUS, Centre for Sleep and Chronobiology, Woolcock Institute of Medical Research, University of Sydney, 431 Glebe Point Road, Glebe, Sydney, NSW 2037, Australia. [2]Woolcock Emphysema Centre, Woolcock Institute of Medical Research, University of Sydney, Sydney, NSW, Australia. [3]Respiratory Cellular and Molecular Biology, Woolcock Institute of Medical Research, University of Sydney, Sydney, NSW, Australia. [4]Physiology and Imaging Group, Woolcock Institute of Medical Research, University of Sydney, Sydney, NSW, Australia. [5]Central Clinical School, Faculty of Medicine, University of Sydney, Sydney, NSW, Australia. [6]Northern Clinical School, Faculty of Medicine, University of Sydney, Sydney, NSW, Australia. [7]Sydney Nursing School, University of Sydney, Sydney, NSW, Australia. [8]School of Life Sciences, Faculty of Science, and Centre for Health Technology, University of Technology Sydney, Sydney, NSW, Australia. [9]Department of Otolaryngology, Mona Vale Hospital, Sydney, NSW, Australia. [10]Department of Respiratory and Sleep Medicine, Royal North Shore Hospital, Sydney, NSW, Australia.

References

Adams KL, Castanon-Cervantes O, Evans JA, Davidson AJ. Environmental circadian disruption elevates the IL-6 response to lipopolysaccharide in blood. J Biol Rhythm. 2013;28:272–7.

Agusti A, Hedner J, Marin JM, Barbé F, Cazzola M, Rennard S. Night-time symptoms: a forgotten dimension of COPD. Eur Respir Rev. 2011;20:183–94.

Akhtar RA. Circadian cycling of the mouse liver transcriptome, as revealed by cDNA microarray, is driven by the suprachiasmatic nucleus. Curr Biol. 2002;12:540–50.

Alamili M, Bendtzen K, Lykkesfeldt J, Rosenberg J, Gögenur I. Pronounced inflammatory response to endotoxaemia during nighttime: a randomised cross-over trial. PLoS One. 2014;9:e87413.

Albrecht U, Zheng B, Larkin D, Sun ZS, Lee CC. mPer1 and mPer2 are essential for normal resetting of the circadian clock. J Biol Rhythm. 2001;16:100–4.

Alvarez JD, Sehgal A. The thymus is similar to the testis in its pattern of circadian clock gene expression. J Biol Rhythm. 2005;20:111–21.

Ando N, Nakamura Y, Ishimaru K, et al. Allergen-specific basophil reactivity exhibits daily variations in seasonal allergic rhinitis. Allergy. 2015;70:319–22.

Aoyagi M, Watanabe H, Sekine K, et al. Circadian variation in nasal reactivity in children with allergic rhinitis: correlation with the activity of eosinophils and basophilic cells. Int Arch Allergy Immunol. 1999;120:95–9.

Arble DM, Ramsey KM, Bass J, Turek FW. Circadian disruption and metabolic disease: findings from animal models. Best Pract Res Clin Endocrinol Metab. 2010;24:785–800.

Arjona A, Boyadjieva N, Sarkar DK. Circadian rhythms of granzyme B, perforin, IFN-γ, and NK cell cytolytic activity in the spleen: effects of chronic ethanol. J Immunol. 2004;172:2811–7.

Arjona A, Dk S. The circadian gene mPer2 regulates the daily rhythm of IFN-γ. J Interferon Cytokine Res. 2006;26:645–9.

Arjona A, Sarkar DK. Circadian oscillations of clock genes, cytolytic factors, and cytokines in rat NK cells. J Immunol. 2005;174:7618–24.

Arjona A, Sarkar DK. Evidence supporting a circadian control of natural killer cell function. Brain Behav Immun. 2006;20:469–76.

Aschoff J. Die 24-Stunden-Periodik der Maus unter konstanten Umgebungsbedingungen. Naturwissenschaften. 1951;38:506–7.

Aschoff J. Tierische Periodik unter dem Einfluß von Zeitgebern. Z Tierpsychol. 1958;15:1–30.

Aschoff J. Exogenous and endogenous components in circadian rhythms. Cold Spring Harb Symp Quant Biol. 1960;25:11–28.

Aschoff J. Speech after dinner. In: Aschoff J, Ceresa F, Halberg F (Eds) Chronobiological aspects of endocrinology chronobiologia 1974;1 (Suppl. 1):483–495.

Aschoff J, Wever R. Circadian rhythms of finches in light-dark cycles with interposed twilights. Comp Biochem Physiol. 1965;16:507–14.

Ballard RD, Saathoff MC, Patel DK, Kelly PL, Martin RJ. Effect of sleep on nocturnal bronchoconstriction and ventilatory patterns in asthmatics. J Appl Physiol. 1989;67:243–9.

Barnes PJ. Immunology of asthma and chronic obstructive pulmonary disease. Nat Rev Immunol. 2008;8:183–92.

Baumann A, Feilhauer K, Bischoff SC, Froy O, Lorentz A. IgE-dependent activation of human mast cells and fMLP-mediated activation of human eosinophils is controlled by the circadian clock. Mol Immunol. 2015;64:76–81.

Baumann A, Gönnenwein S, Bischoff SC, et al. The circadian clock is functional in eosinophils and mast cells. Immunology. 2013;140:465–74.

Beersma DGM, Comas M, Hut RA, Gordijn MCM, Rueger M, Daan S. The progression of circadian phase during light exposure in animals and humans. J Biol Rhythm. 2009;24:153–60.

Bellet MM, Deriu E, Liu JZ, et al. Circadian clock regulates the host response to salmonella. Proc Natl Acad Sci U S A. 2013;110:9897–902.

Bellet MM, Zocchi L, Sassone-Corsi P. The RelB subunit of NFκB acts as a negative regulator of circadian gene expression. Cell Cycle. 2012;11:3304–11.

Bell-Pedersen D, Cassone VM, Earnest DJ, et al. Circadian rhythms from multiple oscillators: lessons from diverse organisms. Nat Rev Genet. 2005;6:544–56.

Bennett KM, Rooijakkers SHM, Gorham RD. Let's tie the knot: marriage of complement and adaptive immunity in pathogen evasion, for better or worse. Front Microbiol. 2017;8:89.

Besedovsky L, Born J, Lange T. Endogenous glucocorticoid receptor signaling drives rhythmic changes in human T-cell subset numbers and the expression of the chemokine receptor CXCR4. FASEB J. 2014;28:67–75.

Blaiss MS. Allergic rhinitis: direct and indirect costs. Allergy Asthma Proc. 2010;31:375–80.

Blanc PD, Trupin L, Eisner M, et al. The work impact of asthma and rhinitis: findings from a population-based survey. J Clin Epidemiol. 2001;54:610–8.

Boggio VI, Castrillón PO, Perez Lloret S, et al. Cerebroventricular administration of interferon-gamma modifies locomotor activity in the golden hamster. Neurosignals. 2003;12:89–94.

Bohadana AB, Hannhart B, Teculescu DB. Nocturnal worsening of asthma and sleep-disordered breathing. J Asthma. 2002;39:85–100.

Boivin DB, James FO, Wu A, Cho-Park PF, Xiong H, Sun ZS. Circadian clock genes oscillate in human peripheral blood mononuclear cells. Blood. 2003;102:4143–5.

Bollinger T, Leutz A, Leliavski A, et al. Circadian clocks in mouse and human CD4 + T cells. PLoS One. 2011;6:e29801.

Bonnet R, Jorres R, Heitmann U, Magnussen H. Circadian rhythm in airway responsiveness and airway tone in patients with mild asthma. J Appl Physiol. 1991; 71:1598–605.

Born J, Lange T, Hansen K, Mölle M, Fehm HL. Effects of sleep and circadian rhythm on human circulating immune cells. J Immunol. 1997;158:4454–64.

Boulos Z. Wavelength dependence of light-induced phase shifts and period changes in hamsters. Physiol Behav. 1995;57:1025–33.

Boulos Z, Macchi MM. Season- and latitude-dependent effects of simulated twilights on circadian entrainment. J Biol Rhythm. 2005;20:132–44.

Boulos Z, Macchi MM, Terman M. Twilights widen the range of photic entrainment in hamsters. J Biol Rhythm. 2002;17:353–63.

Bousquet J, Jeffery P, Busse W, Johnson M, Vignola A. Asthma. From bronchoconstriction to airways inflammation and remodeling. Am J Respir Crit Care Med. 2000;161:1720–45.

Bousquet J, Khaltaev N, Cruz AA, et al. Allergic rhinitis and its impact on asthma (ARIA) 2008 update (in collaboration with the World Health Organization, GA(2)LEN and AllerGen). Allergy. 2008;63:8–160.

Bousquet PJ, Demoly P, Devillier P, Mesbah K, Bousquet J. Impact of allergic rhinitis symptoms on quality of life in primary care. Int Arch Allergy Immunol. 2013;160:393–400.

Brenner BE, Chavda KK, Karakurum MB, Karras DJ, Camargo CAJ. Circadian differences among 4,096 emergency department patients with acute asthma. Crit Care Med. 2001;29:1124–9.

Brown SA, Zumbrunn G, Fleury-Olela F, Preitner N, Schibler U. Rhythms of mammalian body temperature can sustain peripheral circadian clocks. Curr Biol. 2002;12:1574–83.

Brumpton B, Mai X-M, Langhammer A, Laugsand LE, Janszky I, Strand LB. Prospective study of insomnia and incident asthma in adults: the HUNT study. Eur Respir J. 2017;49(2):669.

Bryant PA, Trinder J, Curtis N. Sick and tired: does sleep have a vital role in the immune system? Nat Rev Immunol. 2004;4:457–67.

Buttgereit F, Smolen JS, Coogan AN, Cajochen C. Clocking in: chronobiology in rheumatoid arthritis. Nat Rev Rheumatol. 2015;11:349–56.

Cajochen C, Münch M, Kobialka S, et al. High sensitivity of human melatonin, alertness, thermoregulation, and heart rate to short wavelength light. J Clin Endocrinol Metab. 2005;90:1311–6.

Calhoun WJ, Bates ME, Schrader L, Sedgwick JB, Busse WW. Characteristics of peripheral blood Eosinophils in patients with nocturnal asthma. Am Rev Respir Dis. 1992;145:577–81.

Carrillo-Vico A, Guerrero JM, Lardone PJ, Reiter RJ. A review of the multiple actions of melatonin on the immune system. Endocrine. 2005; 27:189–200.

Carrillo-Vico A, Lardone P, Álvarez-Sánchez N, Rodríguez-Rodríguez A, Guerrero J. Melatonin: buffering the immune system. Int J Mol Sci. 2013;14:8638.

Castanon-Cervantes O, Wu M, Ehlen JC, et al. Disregulation of inflammatory responses by chronic circadian disruption. J Immunol (Baltimore, Md : 1950). 2010;185:5796–805.

Catterall JR, Rhind GB, Stewart IC, Whyte KF, Shapiro CM, Douglas NJ. Effect of sleep deprivation on overnight bronchoconstriction in nocturnal asthma. Thorax. 1986;41:676–80.

Cavadini G, Petrzilka S, Kohler P, et al. TNF-α suppresses the expression of clock genes by interfering with E-box-mediated transcription. Proc Natl Acad Sci U S A. 2007;104:12843–8.

Cermakian N, Lange T, Golombek D, et al. Crosstalk between the circadian clock circuitry and the immune system. Chronobiol Int. 2013;30:870–88.

Cermakian N, Westfall S, Kiessling S. Circadian clocks and inflammation: reciprocal regulation and shared mediators. Arch Immunol Ther Exp. 2014;62:303–18.

Chaouat A, Weitzenblum E, Kessler R, et al. Outcome of COPD patients with mild daytime hypoxaemia with or without sleep-related oxygen desaturation. Eur Respir J. 2001;17:848–55.

Cheon S, Park N, Cho S, Kim K. Glucocorticoid-mediated Period2 induction delays the phase of circadian rhythm. Nucleic Acids Res. 2013;41:6161–74.

Chong SYC, Ptáček LJ, Fu Y-H. Genetic insights on sleep schedules: this time, It's PERsonal. Trends Genet. 2012;28:598–605.

Cochrane GM, Clark JH. A survey of asthma mortality in patients between ages 35 and 64 in the greater London hospitals in 1971. Thorax. 1975;30:300–5.

Comas M, Beersma DGM, Spoelstra K, Daan S. Phase and period responses of the circadian system of mice (Mus Musculus) to light stimuli of different duration. J Biol Rhythm. 2006;21:362–72.

Comas M, Beersma DGM, Spoelstra K, Daan S. Circadian response reduction in light and response restoration in darkness: a "skeleton" light pulse PRC study in mice (Mus Musculus). J Biol Rhythm. 2007;22:432–44.

Comas M, Hut RA. Twilight and photoperiod affect behavioral entrainment in the house mouse (Mus Musculus). J Biol Rhythm. 2009;24:403–12.

Comas M, Kuropatwinski KK, Wrobel M, Toshkov I, Antoch MP. Daily rhythms are retained both in spontaneously developed sarcomas and in xenografts grown in immunocompromised SCID mice. Chronobiol Int. 2014;31:901–10.

Craig TJ, Ferguson BJ, Krouse JH. Sleep impairment in allergic rhinitis, rhinosinusitis, and nasal polyposis. Am J Otolaryngol. 2008;29:209–17.

Curtis AM, Fagundes CT, Yang G, et al. Circadian control of innate immunity in macrophages by miR-155 targeting Bmal1. Proc Natl Acad Sci. 2015;112:7231–6.

Daan S. Adaptive daily strategies in behavior. In: Aschoff J, editor. Biological rhythms. Boston: Springer US; 1981. p. 275–98.

Daan S. Colin Pittendrigh, Jürgen Aschoff, and the natural entrainment of circadian systems. J Biol Rhythm. 2000;15:195–207.

Damiola F. Restricted feeding uncouples circadian oscillators in peripheral tissues from the central pacemaker in the suprachiasmatic nucleus. Genes Dev. 2000;14:2950–61.

de la Hoz CB, Rodríguez M, Fraj J, Cerecedo I, Antolín-Amérigo D, Colás C. Allergic rhinitis and its impact on work productivity in primary care practice and a comparison with other common diseases: the cross-sectional study to evAluate work productivity in allergic rhinitis compared with other common dIseases (CAPRI) study. Am J Rhinol Allergy. 2012;26:390–4.

DeBruyne JP, Noton E, Lambert CM, Maywood ES, Weaver DR, Reppert SM. A CLOCKlock shock: mouse CLOCK is not required for circadian oscillator function. Neuron. 2006;50:465–77.

Decramer M, Brusselle G, Buffels J, et al. COPD awareness survey: do Belgian pulmonary physicians comply with the GOLD guidelines 2010? Acta Clin Belg. 2013;68:325–40.

Deery MJ, Maywood ES, Chesham JE, et al. Proteomic analysis reveals the role of synaptic vesicle cycling in sustaining the Suprachiasmatic circadian clock. Curr Biol. 2009;19:2031–6.

Dethlefsen U, Repges R. Ein neues Therapieprinzip bei nächtlichem Asthma. Med Klin. 1985;80:44–7.

Dibner C, Schibler U, Albrecht U. The mammalian circadian timing system: organization and coordination of central and peripheral clocks. Annu Rev Physiol. 2010;72:517–49.

Dickerman BA, Markt SC, Koskenvuo M, et al. Sleep disruption, chronotype, shift work, and prostate cancer risk and mortality: a 30-year prospective cohort study of Finnish twins. Cancer Causes Control. 2016;27:1361–70.

Dimitrov S, Benedict C, Heutling D, Westermann J, Born J, Lange T. Cortisol and epinephrine control opposing circadian rhythms in T cell subsets. Blood. 2009;113:5134–43.

Druzd D, Matveeva O, Ince L, et al. Lymphocyte circadian clocks control lymph node trafficking and adaptive immune responses. Immunity. 2017;46:120–32.

Duhart JM, Leone MJ, Paladino N, et al. Suprachiasmatic astrocytes modulate the circadian clock in response to TNF-α. J Immunol (Baltimore, Md : 1950). 2013; 191:4656–64. doi: 10.4049/jimmunol.1300450.

Dzhagalov I, Giguère V, He Y-W. Lymphocyte development and function in the absence of retinoic acid-related orphan receptor α. J Immunol. 2004;173:2952–9.

Ehlers A, Xie W, Agapov E, Brown S, Steinberg D, Tidwell R, Sajol G, Schutz R, Weaver R, Yu H, et al. BMAL1 links the circadian clock to viral airway pathology and asthma phenotypes. Mucosal Immunol. 2017. doi: 10.1038/mi.2017.24.

Espinosa de los Monteros MJ, Peña C, Soto Hurtado EJ, Jareño J, Miravitlles M. Variability of respiratory symptoms in severe COPD. Arch Bronconeumol. 2012;48:3–7.

Fajt ML, Tedrow JR, Milosevic J, Trudeau JB, Bleecker ER, Meyers DA, Erzurum SC, Gaston BM, Busse WW, Jarjour NN, Kaminski N, Wenzel SE. Circadian rhythm and clock gene expression are altered in asthmatic epithelium and bronchoalveolar lavage (BAL) cells. In: B93 Genetic Signatures of Asthma: Key to Endotypes, American Thoracic Society International Conference. Denver: 2015. p. A3628.

Feigin RD, Joaquin VHS, Haymond MW, Wyatt RG. Daily periodicity of susceptibility of mice to pneumococcal infection. Nature. 1969;224:379–80.

Feigin RD, Middelkamp JN, Reed C. Circadian rhythmicity in susceptibility of mice to sublethal Coxsackie B3 infection. Nature New Biology. 1972;240:57–8.

Fidan V, Alp HH, Gozeler M, Karaaslan O, Binay O, Cingi C. Variance of melatonin and cortisol rhythm in patients with allergic rhinitis. Am J Otolaryngol. 2013;34:416–9.

Fonken LK, Kitt MM, Gaudet AD, Barrientos RM, Watkins LR, Maier SF. Diminished circadian rhythms in hippocampal microglia may contribute to age-related neuroinflammatory sensitization. Neurobiol Aging. 2016;47:102–12.

Froy O, Chapnik N. Circadian oscillation of innate immunity components in mouse small intestine. Mol Immunol. 2007;44:1954–60.

Fukuoka Y, Burioka N, Takata M, et al. Glucocorticoid administration increases hPer1 mRNA levels in human peripheral blood mononuclear cells in vitro or in vivo. J Biol Rhythm. 2005;20:550–3.

Gamaldo CE, Chung Y, Kang YM, Salas RME. Tick–tock–tick–tock: the impact of circadian rhythm disorders on cardiovascular health and wellness. J Am Soc Hypertens. 2014;8:921–9.

Gebel S, Gerstmayer B, Kuhl P, Borlak J, Meurrens K, Müller T. The kinetics of transcriptomic changes induced by cigarette smoke in rat lungs reveals a specific program of defense, inflammation, and circadian clock gene expression. Toxicol Sci. 2006;93:422–31.

Gelfand EW. Inflammatory mediators in allergic rhinitis. J Allergy Clin Immunol. 2004;114:S135–S8.

Gervais P, Reinberg A, Gervais C, Smolensky M, DeFrance O. Twenty-four-hour rhythm in the bronchial hyperreactivity to house dust in asthmatics. J Allergy Clin Immunol. 1977;59:207–13.

Gibbs J, Ince L, Matthews L, et al. An epithelial circadian clock controls pulmonary inflammation and glucocorticoid action. Nat Med. 2014;20:919–26.

Gibbs JE, Beesley S, Plumb J, et al. Circadian timing in the lung; a specific role for bronchiolar epithelial cells. Endocrinology. 2009;150:268–76.

Gibbs JE, Blaikley J, Beesley S, et al. The nuclear receptor REV-ERBα mediates circadian regulation of innate immunity through selective regulation of inflammatory cytokines. Proc Natl Acad Sci U S A. 2012;109:582–7.

González-Núñez V, Valero AL, Mullol J. Impact of sleep as a specific marker of quality of life in allergic rhinitis. Curr Allergy Asthma Rep. 2013;13:131–41.

Gooley JJ, Lu J, Chou TC, Scammell TE, Saper CB. Melanopsin in cells of origin of the retinohypothalamic tract. Nat Neurosci. 2001;4:1165.

Guerrero-Vargas NN, Guzmán-Ruiz M, Fuentes R, et al. Shift work in rats results in increased inflammatory response after lipopolysaccharide administration. J Biol Rhythm. 2015;30:318–30.

Guerrero-Vargas NN, Salgado-Delgado R, Basualdo MC, et al. Reciprocal interaction between the suprachiasmatic nucleus and the immune system tunes down the inflammatory response to lipopolysaccharide. J Neuroimmunol. 2014;273:22–30.

Hadden H, Soldin SJ, Massaro D. Circadian disruption alters mouse lung clock gene expression and lung mechanics. J Appl Physiol. 2012;113:385–92.

Haimovich B, Calvano J, Haimovich AD, Calvano SE, Coyle SM, Lowry SF. In vivo endotoxin synchronizes and suppresses clock gene expression in human peripheral blood leukocytes. Crit Care Med. 2010;38:751–8.

Halberg F, Johnson EA, Brown BW, Bittner JJ. Susceptibility rhythm to E. coli endotoxin and bioassay. Proceedings of the Society of Experimental Biology and Medicine. 1960;103:142–4.

Hansen I, Klimek L, Mösges R, Hörmann K. Mediators of inflammation in the early and the late phase of allergic rhinitis. Curr Opin Allergy Clin Immunol. 2004;4:159–63.

Haus E, Smolensky MH. Biological rhythms in the immune system. Chronobiol Int. 1999;16:581–622.

Hemmers S, Rudensky AY. The cell-intrinsic circadian clock is dispensable for lymphocyte differentiation and function. Cell Rep. 2015;11:1339–49.

Herzog ED, Hermanstyne T, Smyllie NJ, Hastings MH. Regulating the Suprachiasmatic nucleus (SCN) circadian clockwork: interplay between cell-autonomous and circuit-level mechanisms. Cold Spring Harb Perspect Biol. 2017;9:a027706.

Hetzel MR, Clark TJ. Does sleep cause nocturnal asthma? Thorax. 1979;34:749–54.

Hetzel MR, Clark TJ. Comparison of normal and asthmatic circadian rhythms in peak expiratory flow rate. Thorax. 1980;35:732–8.

Hirschie Johnson C, Elliott JA, Foster R. Entrainment of circadian programs. Chronobiol Int. 2003;20:741–74.

Hoffman AE, Zheng T, Stevens RG, et al. Clock-cancer connection in non-Hodgkin's lymphoma: a genetic association study and pathway analysis of the circadian gene cryptochrome 2. Cancer Res. 2009;69:3605–13.

Honma A, Yamada Y, Nakamaru Y, Fukuda S, Honma K-i, Honma S. Glucocorticoids reset the nasal circadian clock in mice. Endocrinology. 2015;156:4302–11.

Hoskyns EW, Beardsmore CS, Simpson H. Chronic night cough and asthma severity in children with stable asthma. Eur J Pediatr. 1995; 154:320–5.

Hriscu ML. Circadian phagocytic activity of neutrophils and its modulation by light. J Appl Biomed. 2004;2:199–211.

Hwang J-W, Sundar IK, Yao H, Sellix MT, Rahman I. Circadian clock function is disrupted by environmental tobacco/cigarette smoke, leading to lung inflammation and injury via a SIRT1-BMAL1 pathway. FASEB J. 2014;28:176–94.

Irvin CG, Pak J, Martin RJ. Airway–parenchyma uncoupling in nocturnal asthma. Am J Respir Crit Care Med. 2000;161:50–6.

Iwasaki A, Medzhitov R. Control of adaptive immunity by the innate immune system. Nat Immunol. 2015;16:343–53.

Jarjour NN. Circadian variation in allergen and nonspecific bronchial responsiveness in asthma. Chronobiol Int. 1999;16:631–9.

Jen R, Li Y, Owens RL, Malhotra A. Sleep in chronic obstructive pulmonary disease: evidence gaps and challenges. Can Respir J. 2016;2016:7947198.

Jewett KA, Krueger JM. Humoral sleep regulation; Interleukin-1 and tumor necrosis factor. Vitam Horm. 2012;89:241–57.

Kadono M, Nakanishi N, Yamazaki M, Hasegawa G, Nakamura N, Fukui M. Various patterns of disrupted daily rest–activity rhythmicity associated with diabetes. J Sleep Res. 2016;25:426–37.

Kalsbeek A, van der Spek R, Lei J, Endert E, Buijs RM, Fliers E. Circadian rhythms in the hypothalamo–pituitary–adrenal (HPA) axis. Mol Cell Endocrinol. 2012;349:20–9.

Kecklund G, Axelsson J. Health consequences of shift work and insufficient sleep. BMJ. 2016;355:i5210.

Keller M, Mazuch J, Abraham U, et al. A circadian clock in macrophages controls inflammatory immune responses. Proc Natl Acad Sci U S A. 2009;106:21407–12.

Kelly EAB, Houtman JJ, Jarjour NN. Inflammatory changes associated with circadian variation in pulmonary function in subjects with mild asthma. Clin Exp Allergy. 2004;34:227–33.

Kessler R, Partridge MR, Miravitlles M, et al. Symptom variability in patients with severe COPD: a pan-European cross-sectional study. Eur Respir J. 2011;37:264–72.

Kim YJ, Lee BK, Jung CY, et al. Patient's perception of symptoms related to morning activity in chronic obstructive pulmonary disease: the SYMBOL study. Korean J Intern Med. 2012;27:426–35.

Kimura H, Suda A, Sakuma T, et al. Nocturnal oxyhemoglobin desaturation and prognosis in chronic obstructive pulmonary disease and late Sequelae of pulmonary tuberculosis. Intern Med. 1998;37:354–9.

Kopmels B, Wollman EE, Guastavino JM, Delhaye-Bouchaud N, Fradelizi D, Mariani J. Interleukin-1 hyperproduction by in vitro activated peripheral macrophages from Cerebellar mutant mice. J Neurochem. 1990;55:1980–5.

Koyanagi S, Ohdo S. Alteration of intrinsic biological rhythms during interferon treatment and its possible mechanism. Mol Pharmacol. 2002;62:1393–9.

Koyanagi S, Okazawa S, Kuramoto Y, et al. Chronic treatment with Prednisolone represses the circadian oscillation of clock gene expression in mouse peripheral tissues. Mol Endocrinol. 2006;20:573–83.

Kraft M, Djukanovic R, Wilson S, Holgate ST, Martin RJ. Alveolar tissue inflammation in asthma. Am J Respir Crit Care Med. 1996;154:1505–10.

Kraft M, Martin RJ, Wilson S, Djukanovic R, Holgate ST. Lymphocyte and Eosinophil influx into alveolar tissue in nocturnal asthma. Am J Respir Crit Care Med. 1999;159:228–34.

Krueger JM. Interferon alpha-2 enhances slow-wave sleep in rabbits. Int J Immunopharmacol. 1987;9:23–30.

Krueger JM. Somnogenic activity of immune response modifiers. Trends Pharmacol Sci. 1990;11:122–6.

Krueger JM, Obál F, Fang J, Kubota T, Taishi P. The role of cytokines in physiological sleep regulation. Ann N Y Acad Sci. 2001;933:211–21.

Kubota T, Brown RA, Fang J, Krueger JM. Interleukin-15 and interleukin-2 enhance non-REM sleep in rabbits. Am J Physiol Regul Integr Comp Physiol. 2001;281: R1004–R12.

Kubota T, Fang J, Brown RA, Krueger JM. Interleukin-18 promotes sleep in rabbits and rats. Am J Physiol Regul Integr Comp Physiol. 2001;281:R828–R38.

Kubota T, Fang J, Kushikata T, Krueger JM. Interleukin-13 and transforming growth factor-β1 inhibit spontaneous sleep in rabbits. Am J Physiol Regul Integr Comp Physiol. 2000;279:R786–R92.

Kubota T, Majde JA, Brown RA, Krueger JM. Tumor necrosis factor receptor fragment attenuates interferon-gamma-induced non-REM sleep in rabbits. J Neuroimmunol. 2001;119:192–8.

Kushikata T, Fang J, Krueger JM. Interleukin-10 inhibits spontaneous sleep in rabbits. J Interf Cytokine Res. 1999;19:1025–30.

Kuyucu T, Güçlü SZ, Saylan B, et al. A cross-sectional observational study to investigate daily symptom variability, effects of symptom on morning activities and therapeutic expectations of patients and physicians in COPD-SUNRISE study. Tüberküloz ve Toraks Dergisi. 2011;59:328–39.

Kwak Y, Lundkvist GB, Brask J, et al. Interferon-γ alters electrical activity and clock gene expression in suprachiasmatic nucleus neurons. J Biol Rhythm. 2008;23:150–9.

Labrecque N, Cermakian N. Circadian clocks in the immune system. J Biol Rhythm. 2015;30:277–90.

Lamb CE, Ratner PH, Johnson CE, et al. Economic impact of workplace productivity losses due to allergic rhinitis compared with select medical conditions in the United States from an employer perspective. Curr Med Res Opin. 2006;22:1203–10.

Lange P, Marott JL, Vestbo J, Nordestgaard BG. Prevalence of night-time dyspnoea in COPD and its implications for prognosis. Eur Respir J. 2014;43:1590–8.

Leone MJ, Marpegan L, Duhart JM, Golombek DA. Role of Proinflammatory cytokines on lipopolysaccharide-induced phase shifts in Locomotor activity circadian rhythm. Chronobiol Int. 2012;29:715–23.

Levi F, Schibler U. Circadian rhythms: mechanisms and therapeutic implications. Annu Rev Pharmacol Toxicol. 2007;47:593–628.

Lien C, Thibaut Van Z, Lara D, et al. Local inflammation in chronic upper airway disease. Curr Pharm Des. 2012;18:2336–46.

Litinski M, Scheer FAJL, Shea SA. Influence of the circadian system on disease severity. Sleep Med Clin. 2009;4:143–63.

Liu J, Mankani G, Shi X, et al. The circadian clock period 2 gene regulates gamma interferon production of NK cells in host response to lipopolysaccharide-induced endotoxic shock. Infect Immun. 2006;74:4750–6.

Logan RW, Arjona A, Sarkar DK. Role of sympathetic nervous system in the entrainment of circadian natural-killer cell function. Brain Behav Immun. 2011;25:101–9.

Logan RW, Sarkar DK. Circadian nature of immune function. Mol Cell Endocrinol. 2012;349:82–90.

Long AA. Findings from a 1000-patient internet-based survey assessing the impact of morning symptoms on individuals with allergic rhinitis. Clin Ther. 2007;29:342–51.

Lucas D, Battista M, Shi PA, Isola L, Frenette PS. Mobilized hematopoietic stem cell yield depends on species-specific circadian timing. Cell Stem Cell. 2008;3:364–6.

Lundkvist GB, Hill RH, Kristensson K. Disruption of circadian rhythms in synaptic activity of the Suprachiasmatic nuclei by African trypanosomes and cytokines. Neurobiol Dis. 2002;11:20–7.

Lundkvist GBS, Sellix MT, Nygård M, et al. Clock gene expression during chronic inflammation induced by infection with Trypanosoma brucei brucei in rats. J Biol Rhythm. 2010;25:92–102.

Mackay TW, Wallace WA, Howie SE, et al. Role of inflammation in nocturnal asthma. Thorax. 1994;49:257–62.

Man K, Loudon A, Chawla A. Immunity around the clock. Science. 2016;354:999–1003.

Marpegán L, Bekinschtein TA, Costas MA, Golombek DA. Circadian responses to endotoxin treatment in mice. J Neuroimmunol. 2005;160:102–9.

Marpegan L, Leone MJ, Katz ME, Sobrero PM, Bekinstein TA, Golombek DA. Diurnal variation in endotoxin-induced mortality in mice: correlation with proinflammatory factors. Chronobiol Int. 2009;26:1430–42.

Martin RJ. The sleep-related worsening of lower airways obstruction: understanding and intervention. Med Clin N Am. 1990;74:701–14.

Martin RJ, Cicutto LC, Ballard RD. Factors related to the nocturnal worsening of asthma. Am Rev Respir Dis. 1990;141:33–8.

Martin RJ, Cicutto LC, Smith HR, Ballard RD, Szefler SJ. Airways inflammation in nocturnal asthma. Am Rev Respir Dis. 1991;143:351–7.

Martinez-Bakker M, Helm B. The influence of biological rhythms on host–parasite interactions. Trends Ecol Evol. 2015;30:314–26.

Masri S, Sassone-Corsi P. Sirtuins and the circadian clock: bridging chromatin and metabolism. Sci Signal. 2014;7:re6-re.

Mauvoisin D, Wang J, Jouffe C, et al. Circadian clock-dependent and -independent rhythmic proteomes implement distinct diurnal functions in mouse liver. Proc Natl Acad Sci. 2014;111:167–72.

McHill AW, Wright KP. Role of sleep and circadian disruption on energy expenditure and in metabolic predisposition to human obesity and metabolic disease. Obes Rev. 2017;18:15–24.

McNicholas WT, Fitzgerald MX. Nocturnal deaths among patients with chronic bronchitis and emphysema. Br Med J (Clinical research ed). 1984;289:878.

Mendez-Ferrer S, Lucas D, Battista M, Frenette PS. Haematopoietic stem cell release is regulated by circadian oscillations. Nature. 2008;452:442–7.

Miravitlles M, Worth H, Soler Cataluña JJ, et al. Observational study to characterise 24-hour COPD symptoms and their relationship with patient-reported outcomes: results from the ASSESS study. Respir Res. 2014;15:122.

Mistlberger RE, Marchant EG. Computational and entrainment models of circadian food-anticipatory activity: evidence from non-24-hr feeding schedules. Behav Neurosci. 1995;109:790–8.

Mohiuddin AA, Martin RJ. Circadian basis of the late asthmatic response. Am Rev Respir Dis. 1990;142:1153–7.

Möller-Levet CS, Archer SN, Bucca G, et al. Effects of insufficient sleep on circadian rhythmicity and expression amplitude of the human blood transcriptome. Proc Natl Acad Sci. 2013a;110:E1132–E41.

Möller-Levet CS, Archer SN, Bucca G, et al. Effects of insufficient sleep on circadian rhythmicity and expression amplitude of the human blood transcriptome. Proc Natl Acad Sci U S A. 2013b;110:E1132–41.

Moon JJ, Chu HH, Pepper M, et al. Naive CD4(+) T cell frequency varies for different epitopes and predicts repertoire diversity and response magnitude. Immunity. 2007;27:203–13.

Moore RY, Eichler VB. Loss of a circadian adrenal corticosterone rhythm following suprachiasmatic lesions in the rat. Brain Res. 1972;42:201–6.

Morris CJ, Purvis TE, Hu K, Scheer FAJL. Circadian misalignment increases cardiovascular disease risk factors in humans. Proc Natl Acad Sci U S A. 2016; 113:E1402–E11.

Mullol J, Valero A, Alobid I, et al. Allergic rhinitis and its impact on asthma update (ARIA 2008).The perspective from Spain. J Investig Allergol Clin Immunol. 2008;18:327–34.

Nader N, Chrousos GP, Kino T. Interactions of the circadian CLOCK system and the HPA axis. Trends Endocrinol Metab. 2010;21:277–86.

Nakamura Y, Harama D, Shimokawa N, et al. Circadian clock gene Period2 regulates a time-of-day–dependent variation in cutaneous anaphylactic reaction. J Allergy Clin Immunol. 2011;127:1038-45.e3.

Nakamura Y, Ishimaru K, Tahara Y, Shibata S, Nakao A. Disruption of the suprachiasmatic nucleus blunts a time of day-dependent variation in systemic anaphylactic reaction in mice. J Immunol Res. 2014;2014:474217.

Nakamura Y, Nakano N, Ishimaru K, et al. Circadian regulation of allergic reactions by the mast cell clock in mice. J Allergy Clin Immunol. 2014;133:568-75.e12.

Nakamura Y, Nakano N, Ishimaru K, et al. Inhibition of IgE-mediated allergic reactions by pharmacologically targeting the circadian clock. J Allergy Clin Immunol. 2016;137:1226–35.

Nakao A. Temporal regulation of cytokines by the circadian clock. J Immunol Res. 2014;2014:4.

Narasimamurthy R, Hatori M, Nayak SK, Liu F, Panda S, Verma IM. Circadian clock protein cryptochrome regulates the expression of proinflammatory cytokines. Proc Natl Acad Sci U S A. 2012;109:12662–7.

Nguyen KD, Fentress SJ, Qiu Y, Yun K, Cox JS, Chawla A. Circadian gene Bmal1 regulates diurnal oscillations of Ly6C(hi) inflammatory monocytes. Science (New York, NY). 2013;341:1483–810. doi: 10.1126/science.1240636.

Nygård M, Lundkvist GB, Hill RH, Kristensson K. Rapid nitric oxide-dependent effects of tumor necrosis factor-α on suprachiasmatic nuclei neuronal activity. Neuroreport. 2009;20:213–7.

Ohdo S, Koyanagi S, Suyama H, Higuchi S, Aramaki H. Changing the dosing schedule minimizes the disruptive effects of interferon on clock function. Nat Med. 2001;7:356–60.

Oishi K, Miyazaki K, Kadota K, et al. Genome-wide expression analysis of mouse liver reveals CLOCK-regulated circadian output genes. J Biol Chem. 2003;278:41519–27.

Oishi K, Sakamoto K, Okada T, Nagase T, Ishida N. Antiphase circadian expression between BMAL1 and period homologue mRNA in the Suprachiasmatic nucleus and peripheral tissues of rats. Biochem Biophys Res Commun. 1998;253:199–203.

Okada K, Yano M, Doki Y, et al. Injection of LPS causes transient suppression of biological clock genes in rats. J Surg Res. 2008;145:5–12.

Oosterhoff Y, Kauffman HF, Rutgers B, Zijlstra FJ, Koëter GH, Postma DS. Inflammatory cell number and mediators in bronchoalveolar lavage fluid and peripheral blood in subjects with asthma with increased nocturnal airways narrowing. J Allergy Clin Immunol. 1995;96:219–29.

Palomba M, Bentivoglio M. Chronic inflammation affects the photic response of the suprachiasmatic nucleus. J Neuroimmunol. 2008;193:24–7.

Panzer SE, Dodge AM, Kelly EAB, Jarjour NN. Circadian variation of sputum inflammatory cells in mild asthma. J Allergy Clin Immunol. 2003;111:308–12.

Papazyan R, Zhang Y, Lazar MA. Genetic and epigenomic mechanisms of mammalian circadian transcription. Nat Struct Mol Biol. 2016;23:1045–52.

Partch CL, Green CB, Takahashi JS. Molecular architecture of the mammalian circadian clock. Trends Cell Biol. 2014;24:90–9.

Partridge MR, Karlsson N, Small IR. Patient insight into the impact of chronic obstructive pulmonary disease in the morning: an internet survey. Curr Med Res Opin. 2009;25:2043–8.

Pekovic-Vaughan V, Gibbs J, Yoshitane H, et al. The circadian clock regulates rhythmic activation of the NRF2/glutathione-mediated antioxidant defense pathway to modulate pulmonary fibrosis. Genes Dev. 2014;28:548–60.

Petrovsky N, McNair P, Harrison LC. Diurnal rhythms of pro-inflammatory cytokines: regulation by plasma cortisol and therapeutic implications. Cytokine. 1998;10:307–12.

Petrzilka S, Taraborrelli C, Cavadini G, Fontana A, Birchler T. Clock gene modulation by TNF-α depends on calcium and p38 MAP Kinase signaling. J Biol Rhythm. 2009;24:283–94.

Petty TL. Circadian variations in chronic asthma and chronic obstructive pulmonary disease. Am J Med. 1988;85:21–3.

Phillips CL, Comas M. Is a "gut full" of bad bugs driving metabolic disease in shift workers? Sleep Med Rev. 2017;34:1–2.

Pittendrigh CS. Circadian systems: entrainment. In: Aschoff J, editor. Handbook of behavioural neurobiology, biological rhythms; 1981.

Prendergast BJ, Cable EJ, Patel PN, et al. Impaired leukocyte trafficking and skin inflammatory responses in hamsters lacking a functional circadian system. Brain Behav Immun. 2013;32:94–104.

Price D, Small M, Milligan G, Higgins V, Gil EG, Estruch J. Impact of night-time symptoms in COPD: a real-world study in five European countries. Int J Chron Obstruct Pulmon Dis. 2013;8:595–603.

Rahman SA, Castanon-Cervantes O, Scheer FAJL, et al. Endogenous circadian regulation of pro-inflammatory cytokines and chemokines in the presence of bacterial lipopolysaccharide in humans. Brain Behav Immun. 2015;47:4–13.

Rajendrasozhan S, Yang S-R, Kinnula VL, Rahman I. SIRT1, an antiinflammatory and antiaging protein, is decreased in lungs of patients with chronic obstructive pulmonary disease. Am J Respir Crit Care Med. 2008;177:861–70.

Reddy AB, Karp NA, Maywood ES, et al. Circadian orchestration of the hepatic proteome. Curr Biol. 2006;16:1107–15.

Reinberg A, Gervais P, Levi F, Smolensky M, Del Cerro L, Ugolini C. Circadian and circannual rhythms of allergic rhinitis: an epidemiologic study involving chronobiologic methods. J Allergy Clin Immunol. 1988;81:51–62.

Reinberg A, Ghata J, Sidi E. Nocturnal asthma attacks: their relationship to the circadian adrenal cycle. J Allergy. 1963;34:323–30.

Reinberg A, Zagula-Mally Z, Ghata J, Halberg F. Circadian reactivity rhythm of human skin to house dust, penicillin, and histamine. J Allergy. 1969;44:292–306.

Reinberg AE. Chronopharmacology of H1-receptor antagonists: experimental and clinical aspects (allergic diseases). In: Redfern PH, Lemmer B, editors. Physiology and pharmacology of biological rhythms. Berlin, Heidelberg: Springer Berlin Heidelberg; 1997. p. 589–606.

Ren W, Liu G, Chen S, et al. Melatonin signaling in T cells: functions and applications. J Pineal Res. 2017;62:e12394–n/a.

Reutrakul S, Knutson KL. Consequences of circadian disruption on Cardiometabolic health. Sleep Med Clin. 2015;10:455–68.

Revell VL, Arendt J, Terman M, Skene DJ. Short-wavelength sensitivity of the human circadian system to phase-advancing light. J Biol Rhythm. 2005;20:270–2.

Reynolds AC, Paterson JL, Ferguson SA, Stanley D, Wright KP Jr, Dawson D. The shift work and health research agenda: considering changes in gut microbiota as a pathway linking shift work, sleep loss and circadian misalignment, and metabolic disease. Sleep Med Rev. 2017;34:3–9.

Riera Romo M, Pérez-Martínez D, Castillo FC. Innate immunity in vertebrates: an overview. Immunology. 2016;148:125–39.

Roche N, Chavannes NH, Miravitlles M. COPD symptoms in the morning: impact, evaluation and management. Respir Res. 2013;14:112.

Roche N, Small M, Broomfield S, Higgins V, Pollard R. Real World COPD: association of morning symptoms with clinical and patient reported outcomes. J Chron Obstruct Pulmon Dis. 2013;10:679–86.

Roenneberg T, Foster RG. Twilight times: light and the circadian system. Photochem Photobiol. 1997;66:549–61.

Roger A, Arcalá Campillo E, Torres MC, et al. Reduced work/academic performance and quality of life in patients with allergic rhinitis and impact of allergen immunotherapy. Allergy, Asthma Clin Immunol. 2016;12:40.

Rose NR. Prediction and prevention of autoimmune disease in the 21st century: a review and preview. Am J Epidemiol. 2016;183:403–6.

Santos CB, Pratt EL, Hanks C, McCann J, Craig TJ. Allergic rhinitis and its effect on sleep, fatigue, and daytime somnolence. Ann Allergy Asthma Immunol. 2006;97:579–87.

Scheiermann C, Kunisaki Y, Frenette PS. Circadian control of the immune system. Nat Rev Immunol. 2013;13:190–8.

Scheiermann C, Kunisaki Y, Lucas D, et al. Adrenergic nerves govern circadian leukocyte recruitment to tissues. Immunity. 2012;37:290–301.

Shackelford PG, Feigin RD. Periodicity of susceptibility to pneumococcal infection: influence of light and adrenocortical secretions. Science. 1973;182:285–7.

Sidman RL, Lane PW, Dickie MM. Staggerer, a new mutation in the mouse affecting the cerebellum. Science. 1962;137:610–2.

Silver AC, Arjona A, Walker WE, Fikrig E. The circadian clock controls toll-like receptor 9-mediated innate and adaptive immunity. Immunity. 2012;36:251–61.

Smolensky MH, D'Alonzo GE. Progress in the chronotherapy of nocturnal asthma. In: Redfern PH, Lemmer B, editors. Physiology and pharmacology of biological rhythms. Berlin, Heidelberg: Springer Berlin Heidelberg; 1997. p. 205–49.

Smolensky MH, Hermida RC, Reinberg A, Sackett-Lundeen L, Portaluppi F. Circadian disruption: new clinical perspective of disease pathology and basis for chronotherapeutic intervention. Chronobiol Int. 2016;33:1101–19.

Smolensky MH, Lemmer B, Reinberg AE. Chronobiology and chronotherapy of allergic rhinitis and bronchial asthma. Adv Drug Deliv Rev. 2007;59:852–82.

Smolensky MH, Portaluppi F, Manfredini R, et al. Diurnal and twenty-four hour patterning of human diseases: cardiac, vascular, and respiratory diseases, conditions, and syndromes. Sleep Med Rev. 2015;21:3–11.

Smolensky MH, Reinberg A, Labrecque G. Twenty-four hour pattern in symptom intensity of viral and allergic rhinitis: treatment implications. J Allergy Clin Immunol. 1995;95:1084–96.

Smolensky MH, Siegel RA, Haus E, Hermida R, Portaluppi F. Biological rhythms, drug delivery, and chronotherapeutics. In: Siepmann J, Siegel RA, Rathbone MJ, editors. Fundamentals and applications of controlled release drug delivery. Boston: Springer US; 2012. p. 359–443.

Song P, Li Z, Li X, et al. Transcriptome profiling of the lungs reveals molecular clock genes expression changes after chronic exposure to ambient air particles. Int J Environ Res Public Health. 2017;14:90.

Spengler CM, Shea SA. Endogenous circadian rhythm of pulmonary function in healthy humans. Am J Respir Crit Care Med. 2000;162:1038–46.

Spengler ML, Kuropatwinski KK, Comas M, et al. Core circadian protein CLOCK is a positive regulator of NF-κB–mediated transcription. Proc Natl Acad Sci U S A. 2012;109:E2457–E65.

Spoelstra K, Comas M, Daan S. Compression of daily activity time in mice lacking functional per or cry genes. Chronobiol Int. 2014;31:645–54.

Stapleton CM, Jaradat M, Dixon D, et al. Enhanced susceptibility of staggerer (RORαsg/sg) mice to lipopolysaccharide-induced lung inflammation. Am J Physiol Lung Cell Mol Physiol. 2005;289:L144–L52.

Stephan FK, Zucker I. Circadian rhythms in drinking behavior and Locomotor activity of rats are eliminated by hypothalamic lesions. Proc Natl Acad Sci U S A. 1972;69:1583–6.

Stephenson JJ, Cai Q, Mocarski M, Tan H, Doshi JA, Sullivan SD. Impact and factors associated with nighttime and early morning symptoms among patients with chronic obstructive pulmonary disease. Int J Chron Obstruct Pulmon Dis. 2015;10:577–86.

Stojkovic K, Wing SS, Cermakian N. A central role for ubiquitination within a circadian clock protein modification code. Front Mol Neurosci. 2014;7:69.

Stokkan K-A, Yamazaki S, Tei H, Sakaki Y, Menaker M. Entrainment of the circadian clock in the liver by feeding. Science. 2001;291:490–3.

Stone KD, Prussin C, Metcalfe DD. IgE, mast cells, basophils, and eosinophils. J Allergy Clin Immunol. 2010;125:S73–80.

Stull DE, Schaefer M, Crespi S, Sandor DW. Relative strength of relationships of nasal congestion and ocular symptoms with sleep, mood and productivity. Curr Med Res Opin. 2009;25:1785–92.

Sukumaran S, Jusko WJ, DuBois DC, Almon RR. Light-dark oscillations in the lung transcriptome: implications for lung homeostasis, repair, metabolism, disease, and drug action. J Appl Physiol. 2011;110:1732–47.

Sundar IK, Ahmad T, Yao H, et al. Influenza a virus-dependent remodeling of pulmonary clock function in a mouse model of COPD. Sci Rep. 2015;4:9927.

Takahashi JS. Transcriptional architecture of the mammalian circadian clock. Nat Rev Genet. 2017;18:164–79.

Tirlapur VG. Nocturnal deaths among patients with chronic bronchitis and emphysema. Br Med J (Clinical research ed). 1984;289:1540.

Trenkner E, Hoffmann MK. Defective development of the thymus and immunological abnormalities in the neurological mouse mutation "Staggerer" the. J Neurosci. 1966;6:1733–7.

Tsai CL, Brenner BE, Camargo CA. Circadian-rhythm differences among emergency department patients with chronic obstructive pulmonary disease exacerbation. Chronobiol Int. 2007;24:699–713.

Turner-Warwick M. Epidemiology of nocturnal asthma. Am J Med. 1988;85:6–8.

van de Werken M, Giménez MC, de Vries B, Beersma DGM, Gordijn MCM. Short-wavelength attenuated polychromatic white light during work at night: limited melatonin suppression without substantial decline of alertness. Chronobiol Int. 2013;30:843–54.

Vasu VT, Cross CE, Gohil K. Nr1d1, an important circadian pathway regulatory gene, is suppressed by cigarette smoke in Murine lungs. Integr Cancer Ther. 2009;8:321–8.

Walker S, Khan-Wasti S, Fletcher M, Cullinan P, Harris J, Sheikh A. Seasonal allergic rhinitis is associated with a detrimental effect on examination performance in United Kingdom teenagers: case-control study. J Allergy Clin Immunol. 2007;120:381–7.

Wang X, Reece SP, Van Scott MR, Brown JM. A circadian clock in murine bone marrow-derived mast cells modulates IgE-dependent activation in vitro. Brain Behav Immun. 2011;25:127–34.

Ward AE, Rosenthal BM. Evolutionary responses of innate immunity to adaptive immunity. Infect Genet Evol. 2014;21:492–6.

Westfall S, Aguilar-Valles A, Mongrain V, Luheshi GN, Cermakian N. Time-dependent effects of localized inflammation on peripheral clock gene expression in rats. PLoS One. 2013;8:e59808.

Xu Y, Toh KL, Jones CR, Shin J-Y, Fu YH, Ptáček LJ. Modeling of a human circadian mutation yields novel insights into clock regulation by PER2. Cell. 2007;128:59–70.

Yamamoto T, Nakahata Y, Tanaka M, et al. Acute physical stress elevates mouse Period1 mRNA expression in mouse peripheral tissues via a Glucocorticoid-responsive element. J Biol Chem. 2005;280:42036–43.

Yamamura Y, Yano I, Kudo T, Shibata S. Time-dependent inhibitory effect of lipopolysaccharide injection on Per1 and Per2 gene expression in the mouse heart and liver. Chronobiol Int. 2010;27:213–32.

Yao H, Sundar IK, Huang Y, et al. Disruption of sirtuin 1–mediated control of circadian molecular clock and inflammation in chronic obstructive pulmonary disease. Am J Respir Cell Mol Biol. 2015;53:782–92.

Yu EA, Weaver DR. Disrupting the circadian clock: gene-specific effects on aging, cancer, and other phenotypes. Aging. 2011;3:479–93.

Zhang R, Lahens NF, Ballance HI, Hughes ME, Hogenesch JB. A circadian gene expression atlas in mammals: implications for biology and medicine. Proc Natl Acad Sci. 2014a;111:16219–24.

Zhang R, Lahens NF, Ballance HI, Hughes ME, Hogenesch JB. A circadian gene expression atlas in mammals: implications for biology and medicine. Proc Natl Acad Sci U S A. 2014b;111:16219–24.

13

Comparison of self-reported scales and structured interviews for the assessment of depression in an urban male working population in Japan

Tomiko Kadotani[1,2], Hiroshi Kadotani[1,3*] [iD], Honami Arai[3,4], Masanori Takami[3,4], Hiroyasu Ito[3], Masahiro Matsuo[4] and Naoto Yamada[4]

Abstract

Background: The present study aimed to analyze the association among depression, sleep quality, and quality of life using the Japanese version of the Structured Clinical Interview for DSM-IV Axis I Disorders Non-Patient Edition (SCID-I/NP), and to compare these findings with those obtained using self-reported scales, in an urban male working population in Japan.

Methods: The present study included 324 middle-aged participants (43.8 ± 8.37 years) (participation rate: 69.5%). The Japanese version of the SCID-I/NP was administered by a single physician. Self-reported scales, including the Zung Self-Rating Depression Scale (SDS), Epworth Sleepiness Scale (ESS), Pittsburgh Sleep Quality Assessment (PSQI), and 36-item Short-Form Health Survey (SF-36) were used to assess depression, sleepiness, sleep quality, and quality of life, respectively. Participants were then divided into a major depressive disorder (MDD) and control group based on the results of structured interviews, following which self-reported scale scores were compared between the two groups.

Results: A total of 24 participants met criteria for MDD based on responses during structured interviews (current: 4; past: 20). Patients with MDD did not report feeling sleepier than those without psychiatric disorders (controls) (ESS: $P = 0.184$), although they experienced slightly poorer sleep quality (PSQI: $P = 0.052$). In addition, participants of the MDD group exhibited lower SF-36 subscale scores for general health ($P = 0.002$), vitality ($P < 0.001$), social functioning ($P < 0.001$), role emotional ($P = 0.004$), and mental health ($P < 0.001$) domains, and higher SDS scores ($P = 0.038$) compared to controls. The area under the receiver (AUC) operating characteristic curve for the detection of MDD was 0.631 and 0.706 for the SDS and mental health subscales, respectively.

Conclusions: Our findings indicate that patients with MDD exhibit slightly poorer sleep quality and significantly poorer quality of life compared to controls, and that the SF-36 may be used as an alternative to the SDS to screen for depression in an urban male working population in Japan.

Keywords: Depression, Structured interview, Quality of life, ROC curve, Sleep

* Correspondence: kadotanisleep@gmail.com
[1]Horizontal Medical Research Organization, Graduate School of Medicine, Kyoto University, Yoshida-Konoe-cho, Sakyo-ku, Kyoto 606-8501, Japan
[3]Department of Sleep and Behavioral Sciences, Shiga University of Medical Science, Seta Tsukinowa-cho, Otsu City, Shiga 520-2192, Japan
Full list of author information is available at the end of the article

Background

Psychiatric disorders are highly prevalent and contribute substantially to the total burden on the general population (Murray et al. 2010). In particular, the Global Burden of disease report cites depressive disorders as a leading cause of burden (Ferrari et al. 2013), with more than 30,000 suicides committed in Japan alone between 1998 and 2011 (Ministry of Health et al. 2016). In 2005, the total cost due to depression among adults in Japan was estimated to be 2 trillion yen (164 trillion USD) (Sado et al. 2011). Thus, adequate diagnosis remains a priority for mental health researchers and professionals.

The Structured Clinical Interview for DSM-IV Axis I Disorders (SCID-I) (First et al. 2002) is a semi-structured instrument that allows for evaluation of the most common mental health problems and has been used as a reference in epidemiological studies (Kessler et al. 2004; Pez et al. 2010). In Japan, the SCID-I has been used to diagnose depression in pregnant patients (Yoshida et al. 2001) and patients with cancer (Akechi et al. 2004), and to verify psychiatric diagnoses in case-control studies (Tsuchiya et al. 2005). However, the SCID-I Non-Patient Edition (SCID-I/NP) (First et al. 2002) requires a trained physician and is time-consuming to administer, which may not be suitable for screening in large populations. Thus, few Japanese studies have utilized structured interviews in non-clinical settings, instead relying on self-reported questionnaires for the assessment of psychiatric/affective disorders. However, no studies to date have compared self-reported scores and SCID-I/NP results in a non-clinical Japanese population.

Suicidal ideation represents a severe symptom of depression that disproportionately affects Japanese men: Since 1998, $70.6 \pm 0.01\%$ of suicide victims in Japan have been male (Ministry of Health et al. 2016). Suicide attempts are not only a severe health problem, but also contribute substantially to the economic burden (Kadotani et al. 2014). Previous studies have further indicated that the severity of depression is associated with symptoms such as insomnia, daytime sleepiness, short sleep duration, and a reduction in productivity at work, even among undiagnosed individuals (Jha et al. 2016; Penninx et al. 2008; Plante et al. 2016; Baglioni et al. 2011; Nakada et al. 2015). Therefore, in the present study, we aimed to analyze the association among depression, sleep quality, and quality of life using the Japanese version of the SCID-I/NP (First et al. 2002), and to compare these findings with those obtained using self-reported scales, in an urban male working population in Japan in order to determine the most effective instrument for screening for depression.

Methods

Participants

The present study included participants enrolled in an ongoing sleep and health epidemiological study (Nakayama-Ashida et al. 2008; Kadotani et al. 2011). A cross-sectional survey was conducted in a group of 476 male employees at a wholesale company in Osaka, Japan, from January 26, 2004, to December 19, 2005. Ten participants were excluded because they changed their workplace during the survey. Thus, 466 male employees were invited to participate in our survey, and 396 answered the baseline questionnaire (85.0%). Of the total number of respondents, 324 underwent face-to-face SCID-I/NP interviews (participants), while 72 answered the baseline questionnaire but did not participate in the interview (non-participants). Sleep-wake cycle schedules were obtained using 7-day sleep logs with coincident wrist actigraphy (Actiwatch AW-Light: Mini-Mitter, Bend, Ore.), which was recorded using one-minute bins and analyzed by Actiware-Sleep ver. 3.4 (Mini-Mitter Co. Inc., Bend, Ore.). The weekday sleep debt was calculated as the difference in sleep duration between weekdays and weekends as estimated via actigraphy.

Structured interviews

All interviews were performed by a single physician, while another physician reviewed the results item by item. The clinical editions of the SCID-I and SCID-I/NP contain the same items, with the exception of those related to psychosis (First et al. 2002). Simple, brief items are used to screen for psychosis in the SCID-I/NP (First et al. 2002). Questions related to current or past depression were asked separately. Participants whose answers were positive for at least one of the two screening questions for depression were asked further questions about their specific depressive symptoms. Participants with more than five out of nine symptoms or those currently receiving treatment with antidepressants were classified into a current major depressive disorder (MDD) group, while those with past MDD diagnoses or who had been previously treated with antidepressants were classified into a past MDD group.

Questionnaires

The Zung Self-Rating Depression Scale (SDS) contains 20 items (Zung et al. 1965). Scores of ≤ 39, 40–49, and ≥ 50 on the Japanese SDS indicate no, mild, and moderate-to-severe depressive symptoms, respectively (Fukuda and Kobayashi 1983).

The Medical Outcomes Study 36-Item Short Form Health Survey (SF-36) has been widely utilized to assess health-related quality of life (QOL) (McHorney et al. 1993). The SF-36 contains 36 items across eight subscales: physical functioning (PF), role limitations due to physical health (role-physical: RP), bodily pain (BP), general health perceptions (general health: GH), vitality (VT), social functioning (SF), role limitations due to emotional problems (role emotional: RE), and mental health (MH). For each subscale, a score ranging from 0 (worst) to 100 (best) is calculated and standardized to have a mean of 50 and a standard deviation of 10.

The Epworth Sleepiness Scale (ESS) (Johns 1991) and the Pittsburgh Sleep Quality Index (PSQI) (Buysse et al. 1989) were used to assess sleepiness and sleep quality, respectively. Participants with ESS scores of >10 and those with PSQI global scores of >5 were classified as having sleepiness and sleep problems, respectively.

We used Japanese translations of the SCID-I/NP (First et al. 2002), SDS (Fukuda and Kobayashi 1983), ESS (Takegami et al. 2009), and PSQI (Doi et al. 2000), and

the Japanese version 2 of the SF-36 (Fukuhara et al. 1998).

Statistical analysis

Categorical data are presented as proportions, while continuous data are presented as means and standard deviations. T-tests were used to compare differences in continuous data between participants and non-participants. Group proportions were compared using the chi-square test. Receiver operating characteristic (ROC) curve analysis was performed to compare the screening performance of the questionnaires. Pairwise comparisons of ROC curves were performed by calculating the standard error of the area under the curve (AUC) and difference between the two AUCs. Statistical analyses were performed using MedCalc version 16.8.4 (MedCalc Software, Mariakerke,

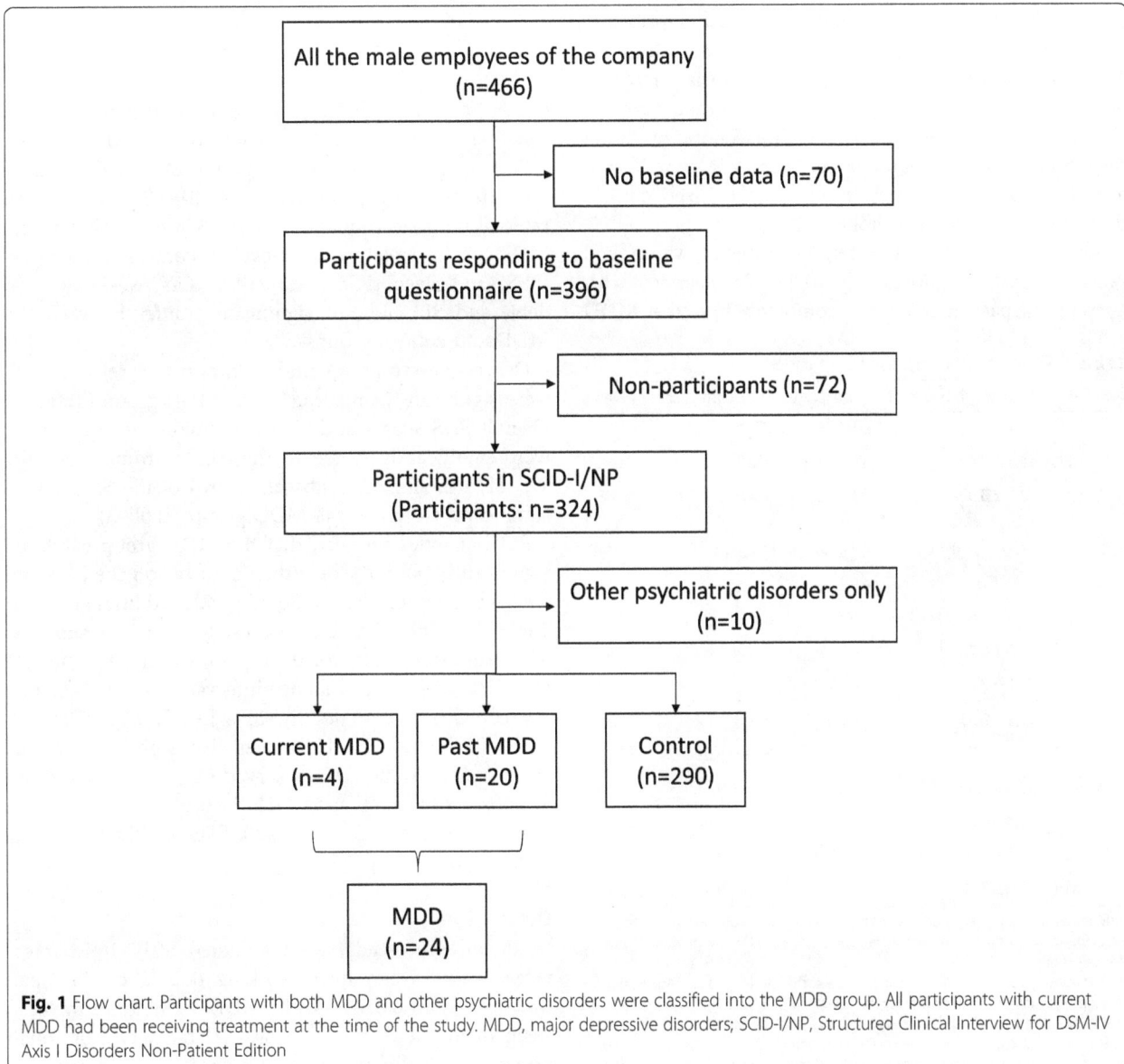

Fig. 1 Flow chart. Participants with both MDD and other psychiatric disorders were classified into the MDD group. All participants with current MDD had been receiving treatment at the time of the study. MDD, major depressive disorders; SCID-I/NP, Structured Clinical Interview for DSM-IV Axis I Disorders Non-Patient Edition

Belgium). Results with $P < 0.05$ were considered statistically significant.

Results

A total of 85.0% (396/466) and 69.5% (324/466) of all male employees at the company responded to the baseline questionnaire and the SCID-I/NP, respectively (Fig. 1). No statistical differences between the participants and non-participants were observed with respect to age, body mass index, ESS, total sleep time (TST), or SF-36 subscale scores (Table 1).

Four participants had current MDD, all of whom had been receiving treatment at the time of the study. Twenty participants had received past diagnoses of MDD (Table 2). Six participants answered positively to the screening question related to dysthymic disorder, although they were diagnosed with different affective disorders: Of the four participants with past depression, one answered positively to the screening questions for MDD but did not meet the diagnostic criteria for MDD, and one was diagnosed with bipolar I disorder. None of the participants were diagnosed with psychotic or eating disorders. Thirteen participants were diagnosed with anxiety disorders (panic disorder, 1; generalized anxiety disorder, 2; specific phobia, 7; social phobia, 2; obsessive–compulsive disorder, 1), three of whom had received past diagnoses of MDD. Participants with current or past MDD were combined into the MDD

Table 2 Prevalence of psychiatric disorders

Disorder	n (%)
Schizophrenia and other psychotic disorders	0 (0)
Affective disorders	
Major depressive disorder (current)	4 (1.23)
Major depressive disorder (past)	20 (6.17)
Bipolar disorders	1 (0.31)
Other mood disorders	0 (0)
Anxiety disorders	
Panic disorder	1 (0.31)
Generalized anxiety disorder	2 (0.62)
Specific phobia	7 (2.16)
Social phobia	2 (0.62)
Obsessive-compulsive disorder	1(0.31)
Other anxiety disorders	0 (0)
Eating disorders	0 (0)

group ($n = 24$), while those without psychiatric disorders were classified into the control group ($n = 290$) (Fig. 1).

Participants of the MDD group exhibited a slight impairment in sleep quality (Table 3). PSQI scores and rates of poor sleep quality (PSQI > 5) were higher in the MDD group, relative to those of controls. Sleepiness (ESS) and sleep time parameters (TST, weekday sleep debt, and SL) did not significantly differ between the MDD and control groups.

Depressive symptoms and mental health-related QOL were significantly impaired in the MDD group (Table 3). Overall SDS scores and SDS depression category scores were significantly worse in the MDD group. The GH, VT, SF, RE, and MH subscale scores of the SF-36 were significantly lower in the MDD group (Table 3).

ROC analyses revealed that the MDD group exhibited significantly poorer scores than controls on the SDS and five subscales of the SF-36 (Fig. 2) (Additional file 1: Table S1). The AUC was highest for the MH subscale. The diagnostic ability for depression was fair for the MH [AUC: 0.712 (95% confidence interval (CI): 0.658–0.761), $P = 0.0001$] and poor for the SDS [AUC: 0.631 (95% CI: 0.574–0.686), $P = 0.0319$] scales. No significant difference in AUC values was observed between SDS and SF-36 subscale scores (SDS vs. GH: $P = 0.3465$, SDS vs. VT: $P = 0.3103$, SDS vs. SF: $P = 0.8470$, SDS vs. RE: $P = 0.3036$, SDS vs. MH: $P = 0.0975$).

Discussion

In the present study, we conducted SCID-I/NP interviews in an urban male working population in Japan ($n = 324$). Participants with MDD exhibited impaired sleep quality and mental health-related QOL, although no significant differences in sleepiness or sleep duration

Table 1 Characteristics of study population

Variable	Total eligible sample	Participants	Non-participants	P-value
n	396	324	72	
Age, years	44.2 ± 8.42	43.8 ± 8.37	45.7 ± 8.56	0.089
BMI, kg/m²	23.6 ± 3.03	23.7 ± 3.07	23.2 ± 2.85	0.208
ESS	8.0 ± 4.3	8.1 ± 4.3	7.6 ± 4.4	0.305
PSQI	4.7 ± 2.0	4.8 ± 2.0	4.2 ± 1.9	0.011
TST, hour	5.9 ± 0.86	5.9 ± 0.85	6.0 ± 0.89	0.748
SF-36 PF	53.8 ± 6.28	53.8 ± 6.41	54.0 ± 5.69	0.746
RP	52.1 ± 7.80	52.3 ± 7.30	51.2 ± 9.71	0.332
BP	51.4 ± 9.63	51.4 ± 7.27	51.5 ± 11.2	0.893
GH	51.2 ± 8.88	51.0 ± 9.05	52.1 ± 8.07	0.341
VT	50.5 ± 8.54	50.2 ± 8.24	52.0 ± 9.71	0.110
SF	52.7 ± 8.00	52.8 ± 7.78	52.3 ± 8.97	0.620
RE	51.7 ± 7.90	51.5 ± 7.76	52.1 ± 8.54	0.567
MH	50.6 ± 8.90	50.6 ± 8.76	51.0 ± 9.57	0.715

Independent t-tests were performed to compare continuous data between participants and non-participants. The total sleep time (TST) was obtained from the questionnaire

PSQI Pittsburgh Sleep Quality Index, ESS Epworth sleepiness scale; Medical Outcomes Study 36-item Health Survey (SF-36), PF physical functioning, RP role limitations due to physical health (role-physical); BP, bodily pain, GH general health perceptions, VT vitality, SF social functioning, RE role limitations due to emotional problems (role-emotional); and MH mental health

Table 3 Sleep, depression, and quality of life in participants with major depressive disorders (MDD) and controls

		MDD	Control	p-value
n		24	290	
Age	(years)	41.3 ± 6.98	44.2 ± 8.41	0.109
BMI	(kg/m²)	23.1 ± 2.94	23.7 ± 3.03	0.344
PSQI		5.58 ± 2.28	4.76. ± 1.97	0.052
	>5 (n, %)	12, 50.0%	84, 29.5%	0.037
ESS		9.26 ± 4.65	8.06 ± 4.19	0.184
	>10 (n, %)	9, 37.5%	75, 26.7%	0.256
TST (questionnaire)	(hr)	5.93 ± 0.57	5.90 ± 0.87	0.882
TST (actigraphy)	(hr)	5.15 ± 0.87	5.22 ± 0.80	0.690
Weekday sleep debt (Actigraphy)	(hr)	1.06 ± 1.78	0.80 ± 1.36	0.401
SL (actigraphy)	(min)	15.3 ± 9.45	15.4 ± 16.4	0.970
SDS		38.8 ± 6.25	36.1 ± 6.26	0.038
	≤39	12	200	0.020
	40-49	11	70	
	≥50	1	5	
SF-36	PF	53.4 ± 5.19	53.8 ± 6.57	0.746
	RP	51.3 ± 6.89	52.5 ± 7.24	0.423
	BP	48.5 ± 9.54	51.6 ± 9.23	0.107
	GH	45.4 ± 9.27	51.4 ± 8.90	0.002
	VT	44.6 ± 8.85	50.7 ± 7.90	<0.001
	SF	46.7 ± 13.0	53.4 ± 6.64	<0.001
	RE	47.4 ± 7.89	52.0 ± 7.44	0.004
	MH	44.7 ± 8.50	51.3 ± 8.31	<0.001

Data were compared between participants without psychiatric disorders (control) and those with current and past MDD using independent t-tests and chi-square tests. Five, 9, 15, and four participants did not answer the PSQI, ESS, SDS, and SF-36, respectively. Actigraphy data from 12 participants were missing. Total sleep time (TST) was obtained from the questionnaires and via actigraphy. Sleep latency (SL) and weekday sleep debt were estimated from the actigraphy data. The weekday sleep debt was calculated as the TST on weekends minus the TST on weekdays
PSQI Pittsburgh Sleep Quality Index, ESS Epworth sleepiness scale, Medical Outcomes Study 36-item Health Survey (SF-36), PF physical functioning, RP role limitations due to physical health (role-physical), BP bodily pain, GH general health perceptions, VT vitality, SF social functioning, RE role limitations due to emotional problems (role-emotional); and MH mental health

parameters were observed between the MDD and control groups. In our ROC analysis, the MH score had the highest AUC among the GH, VT, SF, RE, MH, and SDS scores, suggesting that MH may be a good alternative to the SDS to screen for depression in a Japanese working male population.

Previous studies have reported a strong association among sleep problems, insomnia, and depression (Ferrari et al. 2013). In accordance with these findings, we observed impaired sleep quality in participants with MDD. Surprisingly, however, we observed no association among depression, sleepiness, and sleep duration parameters (TST, SL, weekday sleep debt) (Table 3). Although

this finding may have been due to our small sample size, is it also possible that treatment parameters influenced our results, as all participants with MDD were receiving treatment at the time of the study.

In our ROC analysis, GH, VT, SF, RE, MH of SF-36 exhibited slightly higher AUC and lower p-values than SDS. Previous studies have reported that negatively worded items in the SDS do not adequately screen for depression in the Japanese population (Umegaki et al. 2016). However, the SF-36 also contains negatively worded items, suggesting that factors other than negative wording are responsible for this difference. The SF-36 utilizes norm-based scoring, in which the scale and component summary scores have a mean of 50 and standard deviation of 10 in the general population (McHorney et al. 1993). This norm-based scoring system may be beneficial for detecting changes in non-clinical settings, in which most participants are likely to score near the norm. Furthermore, we observed no significant differences in AUCs between scores on the SDS and these SF-36 subscales. Thus, these findings indicate that the SF-36 can be used as an alternative to the SDS to screen for depression.

The company setting of the present study may represent an ideal site for data collection, providing a sufficient number of full-time, non-shift-working male employees working in the same industry and with the same employer, which allowed us to control for work environment factors such as occupational participation, employment sector, and employment policies (Kadotani et al. 2011).

Only a few psychiatric epidemiological studies have been conducted in the general Japanese population. Although some non-clinical studies have used the Composite International Diagnostic Interview (CIDI) (Kawakami et al. 2005), to our knowledge, previous Japanese studies utilizing the SCID-I were performed in clinical settings only. We used the SCID-I/NP in a Japanese working population. Among the 324 total participants, four (1.2%) and 20 (6.2%) had current and past diagnoses of MDD, respectively, while 13 (4.0%) had anxiety disorders. Furthermore, we observed no evidence of psychotic or eating disorders among participants of the present study, and that all patients with current MDD were undergoing treatment at the time of the study. As reported previously, the prevalence of affective and anxiety disorders is lower in Japan than in Western countries (Demyttenaere et al. 2004).

The present study possesses some limitations of note. Our target population was not representative of the Japanese population in general, but was specific to the working male population in a Japanese urban area. Furthermore, individuals with severe MDD or psychotic disorders could not attend work and thus could not

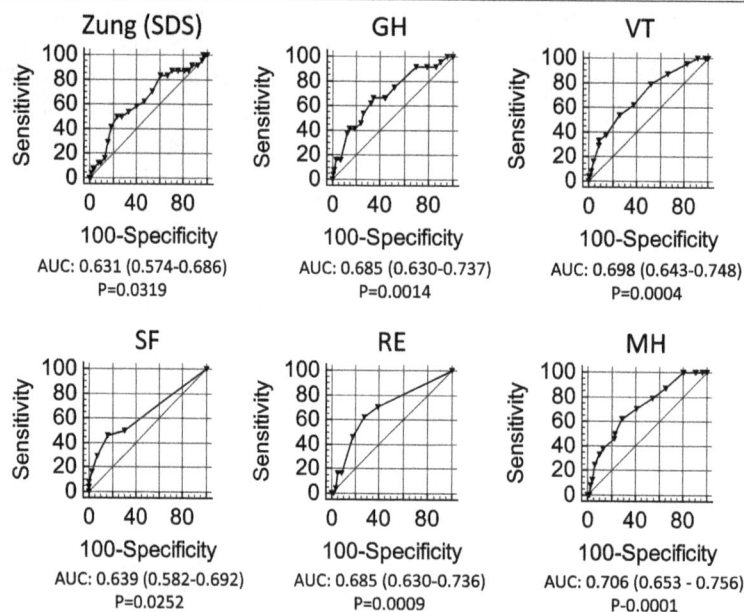

Fig. 2 Receiver operator characteristic (ROC) curves for the detection of MDD. The area under the ROC curve (AUC) is presented with 95% confidence intervals and p-values (Area = 0.5). SDS, Zung Self-Rating Depression Scale; Medical Outcomes Study 36-item Health Survey (SF-36) subscales: GH, general health perceptions (general health); VT, vitality; SF, social functioning; RE, role limitations due to emotional problems (role emotional); and MH, mental health

participate in this study, which may have resulted in a lower prevalence of both disorders. Nevertheless, we had a high participation rate of 69.5% (324/466). This survey was a part of a sleep and health epidemiological study; thus, participants with better sleep quality (lower PSQI scores) may have been reluctant to participate. However, TST was similar in participants and non-participants (Table 1). Thus, our study sample did not appear to have a self-selection bias, and our estimate of prevalence may well represent that of the entire participant population (i.e., all male employees of this company in the Osaka prefecture) (Kadotani et al. 2011).

Conclusions

In the present study, participants with MDD exhibited slightly poorer sleep quality and significantly poorer QOL than those without. Our findings further indicate that the SF-36, especially the MH subscale, may be used as an alternative to the SDS for the screening of depression in the working Japanese male population.

Abbreviations

AUC: Area under the receiver; BP: Bodily pain; ESS: Epworth sleepiness scale; GH: General health perceptions (general health); MDD: Major depressive disorder; MH: Mental health; PF: Physical functioning; PSQI: Pittsburgh sleep quality assessment; QOL: Quality of life; RE: Role limitations due to emotional problems (role emotional); ROC: Receiver operating characteristic; RP: Role limitations due to physical health (role-physical); SCID-I/NP: Structured clinical interview for DSM-IV axis I disorders/non-patient edition; SDS: Zung self-rating depression scale; SF: Social functioning; SF-36: Medical outcomes study 36-item short form health survey; SL: Sleep latency; TST: Total sleep time; VT: Vitality

Acknowledgments

We express gratitude to the participants, their families, and the company for which they worked. We would like to thank Editage (www.editage.jp) for English language editing. We would like to thank Y. Nakayama-Ashida, M. Takegami, K. Chin, K. Sumi, T. Nakamura, K. Takahashi, T. Wakamura, S. Horita, Y. Oka, I. Minami, and S. Fukuhara for data collection.

Funding

The present study was supported by the Special Coordination Funds for Promoting Science and Technology; a Grant-in-Aid for Scientific Research (KAKENHI)(23591672, 26507006); Grants-in-Aid from the Ministry of Health, Labor, and Welfare, Japan (H22-Nanchi-Ippan-008); and research grants from PRESTO JST, the Suzuken Memorial Foundation, the Takeda Science Foundation, the Mitsui Life Social Welfare Foundation, the Chiyoda Kenko Kaihatsu Jigyodan Foundation, the Health Science Center Foundation; and an Intramural Research Grant (23-3, 26-2) for Neurological and Psychiatric Disorders from NCNP.

Authors' contributions

HK conceived of and designed the study, and drafted the manuscript. TK and HK were responsible for data collection. HK conducted the statistical analyses and interpreted the data. HI assisted in the drafting of the manuscript. HA, MT, MM, and NY commented on drafts of the manuscript and assisted with interpretation of data. All authors read and approved the final manuscript.

Competing interests

The authors declare that they have no competing interests.

Comparison of self-reported scales and structured interviews for the assessment of depression...

117

Author details

[1]Horizontal Medical Research Organization, Graduate School of Medicine, Kyoto University, Yoshida-Konoe-cho, Sakyo-ku, Kyoto 606-8501, Japan. [2]Department of Pediatrics, Takatsuki General Hospital, 1-3-13 Kosobe-cho, Takatsuki, Osaka 569-1192, Japan. [3]Department of Sleep and Behavioral Sciences, Shiga University of Medical Science, Seta Tsukinowa-cho, Otsu City, Shiga 520-2192, Japan. [4]Department of Psychiatry, Shiga University of Medical Science, Seta Tsukinowa-cho, Otsu City, Shiga 520-2192, Japan.

References

Akechi T, Okuyama T, Sugawara Y, Nakano T, Shima Y, Uchitomi Y. Major depression, adjustment disorders, and post-traumatic stress disorder in terminally ill cancer patients: associated and predictive factors. J Clin Oncol. 2004;22(10):1957–65.

Baglioni C, Battagliese G, Feige B, Spiegelhalder K, Nissen C, Voderholzer U, et al. Insomnia as a predictor of depression: a meta-analytic evaluation of longitudinal epidemiological studies. J Affect Disord. 2011;135:10–9.

Buysse DJ, Reynolds 3rd CF, Monk TH, Berman SR, Kupfer DJ. The Pittsburg sleep quality index: a new instrument for psychiatric practice and research. Psychiatry Res. 1989;28:193–213.

Demyttenaere K, Bruffaerts R, Posada-Villa J, Gasquet I, Kovess V, Lepine JP, et al. Prevalence, severity, and unmet need for treatment of mental disorders in the World Health Organization World Mental Health Surveys. JAMA. 2004;291:2581–90.

Doi Y, Minowa M, Uchiyama M, Okawa M, Kim K, Shibui K, et al. Psychometric assessment of subjective sleep quality using the Japanese version of the Pittsburgh Sleep Quality Index (PSQI-J) in psychiatric disordered and control subjects. Psychiatry Res. 2000;97:165–72.

Ferrari AJ, Charlson FJ, Norman RE, Patten SB, Freedman G, Murray CJ, et al. Burden of depressive disorders by country, sex, age, and year: findings from the global burden of disease study 2010. PLoS Med. 2013;10:e1001547.

First MB, Spitzer RL, Gibbon M, Williams JBW. Structured clinical interview for DSM-IV-TR axis I disorders, research version, non-patient edition. (SCID-I/NP). New York: Biometrics Research, New York State Psychiatric Institute; 2002. (Japanese translation by S Takahashi, T Kitamura and S Okano).

Fukuda K, Kobayashi S. Manual of self-rating depression scale. Sankyo-bo: Tokyo; 1983.

Fukuhara S, Bito S, Green J, Hsiao A, Kurokawa K. Translation, adaptation, and validation of the SF-36 Health Survey for use in Japan. J Clin Epidemiol. 1998;51:1037–44.

Jha MK, Minhajuddin A, Greer TL, Carmody T, Rush AJ, Trivedi MH. Early improvement in work productivity predicts future clinical course in depressed outpatients: findings from the CO-MED trial. Am J Psychiatry. 2016;173:1196–204.

Johns MW. A new method for measuring daytime sleepiness: the Epworth sleepiness scale. Sleep. 1991;14:540–5.

Kadotani H, Nakayama AY, Nagai Y. Durability, safety, ease of use and reliability of a type-3 portable monitor and a sheet-style type-4 portable monitor. Sleep Biol Rhythms. 2011;9:86–94.

Kadotani H, Nagai Y, Sozu T. Railway suicide attempts are associated with amount of sunlight in recent days. J Affect Disord. 2014;152–4:162–8.

Kawakami N, Takeshima T, Ono Y, Uda H, Hata Y, Nakane Y, et al. Twelve-month prevalence, severity, and treatment of common mental disorders in communities in Japan: preliminary finding from the World Mental Health Japan Survey 2002–2003. Psychiatry Clin Neurosci. 2005;59:441–52.

Kessler RC, Abelson J, Demler O, Escobar JI, Gibbon M, Guyer ME, et al. Clinical calibration of DSM-IV diagnoses in the World Mental Health (WMH) version of the World Health Organization (WHO) Composite International Diagnostic Interview (WMHCIDI). Int J Methods Psychiatr Res. 2004;13(2):122–39.

McHorney CA, Ware Jr JE, Raczek AE. The MOS 36-Item Short-Form Health Survey (SF-36): II. Psychometric and clinical tests of validity in measuring physical and mental health constructs. Med Care. 1993;31:247–63.

Ministry of Health, Labor and Welfare, Japan. Counter-suicide White Paper in 2016. http://www.mhlw.go.jp/wp/hakusyo/jisatsu/16/. Accessed 10 Oct 2016. (In Japanese).

Murray CJ, Vos T, Lozano R, Naghavi M, Flaxman AD, Michaud C, et al. Disability-adjusted life years (DALYs) for 291 diseases and injuries in 21 regions, 1990–2010: a systematic analysis for the global burden of disease study. Lancet. 2010;380:2197–223.

Nakada Y, Murakami J, Kadotani H, Matsuo M, Itou H, Yamada N. A cross-sectional study on working hours, sleep duration and depressive symptoms in Japanese shift workers. J Oral Sleep Med. 2015;1:133–9.

Nakayama-Ashida Y, Takegami M, Chin K, Sumi K, Nakamura T, Takahashi K, et al. Sleep-disordered breathing in the usual lifestyle setting as detected with home monitoring in a population of working men in Japan. Sleep. 2008;31:419–25.

Penninx BW, Beekman AT, Smit JH, Zitman FG, Nolen WA, Spinhoven P, et al. The Netherlands Study of Depression and Anxiety (NESDA): rationale, objectives and methods. Int J Methods Psychiatr Res. 2008;17:121–40.

Pez O, Gilbert F, Bitfoi A, Carta MG, Jordanova V, Garcia-Mahia C, et al. Validity across translations of short survey psychiatric diagnostic instruments: CIDI-SF and CIS-R versus SCID-I/NP in four European countries. Soc Psychiatry Psychiatr Epidemiol. 2010;45(12):1149–59. doi:10.1007/s00127-009-0158-6.

Plante DT, Finn LA, Hagen EW, Mignot E, Peppard PE. Subjective and objective measures of hypersomnolence demonstrate divergent associations with depression among participants in the Wisconsin sleep cohort study. J Clin Sleep Med. 2016;12:571–8.

Sado M, Yamauchi K, Kawakami N, Ono Y, Furukawa TA, Tsuchiya M, et al. Cost of depression among adults in Japan in 2005. Psychiatry Clin Neurosci. 2011;65:442–50.

Takegami M, Suzukamo Y, Wakita T, Noguchi H, Chin K, Kadotani H, et al. Development of a Japanese version of the Epworth Sleepiness Scale (JESS) based on item response theory. Sleep Med. 2009;10:556–65.

Tsuchiya KJ, Takagai S, Kawai M, Matsumoto H, Nakamura K, Minabe Y, et al. Advanced paternal age associated with an elevated risk for schizophrenia in offspring in a Japanese population. Schizophr Res. 2005;76(2–3):337–42.

Umegaki Y, Todo N. Psychometric Properties of the Japanese CES-D, SDS, and PHQ-9 Depression Scales in University Students. Psychol Assess. 2016. doi.org/10.1037/pas0000351.

Yoshida K, Yamashita H, Ueda M, Tashiro N. Postnatal depression in Japanese mothers and the reconsideration of 'Satogaeri bunben'. Pediatr Int. 2001;43(2):189–93.

Zung WW, Richards CB, Short MJ. Self-rating depression scale in an outpatient clinic: further validation of the SDS. Arch Gen Psychiatry. 1965;13:508–15.

14

The case for using digital EEG analysis in clinical sleep medicine

Magdy Younes[1,2] ⓘD

Abstract

Evaluation of sleep in clinical polysomnograms continues to rely almost exclusively on visual scoring that implements rules proposed by Rechtschaffen and Kales nearly 50 years ago. Apart from its cost and time-consuming nature, visual scoring has limitations including: A) Sleep depth, which is a continuous variable, is treated as if it changes in a stepwise fashion from light (stage 1), to intermediate (stage 2) to deep (stage 3). B) Even with this limited scale, there is considerable inter-scorer variability, particularly in scoring stages 1 and 3 of non-REM sleep, thereby adding uncertainty to %time spent in these stages as a reliable metric for evaluating sleep depth. C) Limitation in scoring some of EEG features, including 1) arousal intensity, 2) extent of Alpha intrusion and 3) frequency, and characteristics of sleep spindles and K complexes. Digital analysis can solve these problems but producing a reliable system has been a challenge. In this review I begin with recent advances in digital scoring of sleep according to the Rechtschaffen and Kales rules and conclude that this technology has progressed enough to make it possible to obtain reliable, reproducible scoring, comparable in accuracy to scoring by highly experienced technologists, with minimal editing. This is followed by description of several new metrics that can be obtained if digital scoring systems were to be used routinely in clinical studies. The scientific evidence supporting the potential of these metrics to positively impact sleep medicine practice and the wide range of such metrics in patients studied in the sleep laboratory are highlighted.

Keywords: Sleep depth, Arousal intensity, Alpha intrusion, Sleep spindles, K Complexes, Odds ratio product, ORP, Michele sleep scoring

Background

The polysomnogram (PSG) is the cornerstone of investigations in clinical sleep medicine. Interpretation of sleep in these studies is based primarily on the scoring rules introduced by Rechtschaffen and Kales (R&K) almost 50 years ago (Rechtschaffen and Kales 1968). In 1996, Kubicki et al. lamented the fact that, up to then, digital analysis of PSGs was focused on implementing the R&K rules more efficiently and not on exploring the microstructure of sleep which, they argued, could provide clinically important information (Kubicki and Herrmann 1996). In the intervening 20 years, advances in digital technology have revolutionized almost every aspect of our lives. Yet, the only benefit to sleep studies from this digital revolution has been conversion of data format

from ink on paper to fancy digital displays. It is true that we now need much less space to store data, less time to retrieve patient information and the ability to store data on digital media, and change the montage and filters after data collection. But, the medically-helpful information we get has hardly changed. We still divide non-REM sleep into three distinct stages, consider arousals as simply present or absent, and we see all kinds of differences between patients' EEGs that might well explain the patient's problems, but we have no idea what they mean. R&K rules were introduced when visual scoring was the only way to make any sense of the massive data generated from sleep studies. It was not feasible then to propose visual criteria for defining more than a few sleep stages, to ask technologists to count spindles or alpha bursts or characterize their durations and intensity...etc. We have learned from basic science that differences in these features may mean something, but because we don't get this information in clinical studies we can't

Correspondence: mkyounes@shaw.ca
[1]Sleep Disorders Centre, Misericordia Health Centre, Winnipeg, Canada
[2]YRT Ltd, Winnipeg, MB, Canada

determine the clinical utility of measuring them. And, since we don't have proof that measuring these differences will impact patient care, why should we change how we score clinical studies? A catch 22!

Over the past four decades several dozen systems were proposed for digital sleep scoring and some of these have been validated for clinical use. There is, however, extreme resistance to the use of such systems in clinical practice. The usual excuse is that they are not reliable enough and require much human editing, thereby defeating their primary purpose of economy, speed and consistency. In this review I am hoping to make a strong case for using digital analysis of the EEG routinely in clinical studies. This case is based on two main arguments:

1) Criticism of digital systems' ability to reproduce R&K staging is no longer justified.
2) Even if full manual editing is still insisted upon, and the economy achieved by digital scoring according to R&K is not large, including digital scoring routinely in clinical studies would make it possible to easily obtain potentially valuable information that is not possible to obtain with visual scoring.

Although the evidence provided below in support of these arguments is primarily from my own work (Malhotra et al. 2013; Azarbarzin et al. 2014; Younes et al. 2015a; Azarbarzin et al. 2015; Younes et al. 2015b; Younes and Hanly 2016; Younes et al. 2015c; Meza et al. 2016; Younes et al. 2016; Younes and Hanly PJ 2016; Amatoury et al. In Press; Younes) (I found no other relevant work), such evidence can be produced by anyone who is involved in digital scoring, and the additional information I generated in my own system can be

generated by other systems. My intention is to simply encourage the use of digital scoring systems in clinical practice, regardless of which system is used. Availability of digital EEG analysis in every PSG system would greatly facilitate the introduction, testing and utilization of specialized information on microstructure. My own results are simply used here to illustrate some of what might be achieved with digital analysis.

Comparison between manual and automatic scoring of sleep according to Rechtschaffen and Kales

The inconsistent results and time-consuming, expensive nature of manual sleep staging are well recognized. For this reason, numerous attempts have been made to automate this process (See Penzel et al. (Penzel et al. 2007) and Lajnef et al. (Lajnef et al. 2015a) for a listing of various automatic systems proposed). Of the several dozen systems tried so far three have shown enough promise to be used in clinical studies and are commercially available (Malhotra et al. 2013; Younes et al. 2015b; Pittman et al. 2004; Anderer et al. 2005; Punjabi et al. 2015). Agreement between these systems and expert scorers for sleep variables is similar to agreement found between two scorers (Malhotra et al. 2013; Younes et al. 2015b; Younes et al. 2015c; Younes et al. 2016; Pittman et al. 2004; Anderer et al. 2005; Punjabi et al. 2015). One of these systems (Michele Sleep Scoring, MSS, YRT Ltd, Winnipeg, Canada) has received the most evaluation and its results (Younes et al. 2015b; Younes et al. 2015c; Younes et al. 2016) are shown in Table 1 in juxtaposition to reported agreement between two expert technologists. The data reported by

Table 1 Agreement between MSS and manual scoring compared to agreement between two scorers

Variable	ICCs MSS vs. Manual scoring			ICCs Between two scorers		
	Malhotra et al.[a]	Younes et al.[b]	Younes et al.[c]	Within site[a] Mean (range)	Between sites[a] Mean (95% CI)	From other sources[d]
Total sleep time	0.87	0.96	0.92	0.89(0.78–0.98)	0.87 (0.85–0.89)	
Sleep Efficiency	0.74	0.84	0.76	0.80 (0.69–0.96)	0.77 (0.73–0.80)	
Non-REM stage 1	0.56	0.65	0.63	0.62(0.39–0.80)	0.44 (0.39–0.49)	
Non-REM stage 2	0.84	0.85	0.80	0.75(0.49–0.90)	0.61 (0.57–0.66)	
Non-REM stage 3	0.47	0.65	0.74	0.56(0.27–0.83)	0.40 (0.35–0.45)	
REM Sleep	0.64	0.85	0.84	0.78(0.64–0.92)	0.69 (0.64–0.72)	
Sleep onset latency		0.72	0.76			0.30–1.00
REM onset latency	0.55	0.77	0.65	0.67(0.32–0.90)	0.55 (0.50–0.59)	
#Arousals-REM sleep	0.39			0.55(0.28–0.88)	0.52 (0.47–0.57)	
#Arousals-non REM sleep	0.83			0.59(0.24–0.75)	0.58 (0.53–0.62)	
Arousal/awakening Index		0.75	0.72			0.09–0.85

ICC intraclass correlation coefficient, CI confidence interval, MSS Michele sleep scoring, REM rapid-eye-movement sleep; [a]From (Malhotra et al. 2013); [b]From (Younes et al. 2015b); [c]From (Younes et al. 2015c); [d]Compiled from (Danker-Hopfe et al. 2004), (Pittman et al. 2004). (Magalang et al. 2013), and (Zhang et al. 2015)

Malhotra et al. (Malhotra et al. 2013) is used as the primary source for this information because each PSG was scored by 10 technologists from five academic centers and because the same scoring guidelines were used by MSS and technologists. Furthermore, their results, reported in Table 1, are representative of earlier reports (Pittman et al. 2004; Anderer et al. 2005; Ferri et al. 1989; Norman et al. 2000; Collop 2002; Danker-Hopfe et al. 2004; Magalang et al. 2013). Where information was missing in Malhotra's study, reference values were compiled from other sources (Pittman et al. 2004; Danker-Hopfe et al. 2004; Magalang et al. 2013; Zhang et al. 2015).

Table 1 shows that agreement between *unedited* MSS and the average of 10 scorers (leftmost column) is well within the range of ICCs observed for comparisons between two scorers in the same institution (fourth column) or between scorers in different institutions (fifth column) and exceeds the average between-site ICCs in several sleep variables. In two subsequent validation studies (second and third columns, Table 1), utilizing a newer version of MSS, agreement of unedited MSS scores with manual scoring (one scorer) was also within the range of agreement reported by Malhotra et al. (Malhotra et al. 2013) for comparison between two scorers (Table 1). In another study in which 5-stage epoch-by-epoch comparisons were made between MSS scores and the scores of two academic technologists, MSS scores agreed with the scoring of one or both scorers in 87% of epochs (Younes et al. 2016). The comparable figures in the literature range from 68.0% to 82.6% (Pittman et al. 2004; Anderer et al. 2005; Norman et al. 2000; Danker-Hopfe et al. 2004; Rosenberg and Van Hout 2013). In the same study (Younes et al. 2016) each PSG was scored seven times, three times by each of two technologists and once by a third technologist. A true scoring error was defined as one that was not assigned in any of the other sessions. The number of errors made by any of the technologists in a single session averaged 13 epochs/PSG. The corresponding number for the unedited Auto score was 23 epochs/PSG, a clinically insignificant difference of 10 epochs/PSG (<2% of epochs), even without editing.

Notwithstanding these good results, there has been tremendous resistance to using any of the three validated systems in clinical laboratories. As judged from my experience with our own system (MSS) the main reason for this resistance is that Auto-scoring differs from manual scoring by local technologists in many epochs. This necessitates editing. Because the location of epochs with scoring differences cannot be predicted, all epochs need to be reviewed. There is little saving in time or expense.

In a recent informal evaluation in our laboratory, we found that technologists spend between 30 and 120 min editing files scored by MSS. How can it be necessary to edit so much when it has been proven through rigorous studies (Malhotra et al. 2013; Younes et al. 2015b; Younes et al. 2015c; Younes et al. 2016) that, *without editing*, the summary results are not that different from manual scoring? To investigate this issue, we introduced an algorithm in MSS that recorded all editing actions taken and the time spent on editing. Technologists fully edited the automatic scoring of 42 PSGs (Younes et al. 2015b). Intraclass correlation coefficients (ICCs) for agreement between manual and auto-scoring *before editing* were 0.94 for TST, 0.76 for SE, 0.87 for stage W, 0.63 for N1, 0.81 for N2, 0.55 for N3, and 0.86 for REM sleep. Notwithstanding the fact that these ICCs were well within the range seen between expert scorers (Pittman et al. 2004; Anderer et al. 2005; Ferri et al. 1989; Norman et al. 2000; Collop 2002; Danker-Hopfe et al. 2004; Magalang et al. 2013; Zhang et al. 2015) the technologists performed an average 90 ± 47 changes/file to the automatic sleep stage (Younes et al. 2015b). These changes were often in opposite directions and involved many types of changes such that the net effect on duration of any sleep stage was clinically insignificant except in a few patients. Having found that the vast majority of editing changes are of little clinical consequence (e.g. changing TST from 360 to 350 min, or REM time from 35 to 45 min), we introduced a feature in MSS (Editing Helper) that scans the summary results looking for potential errors that, in our judgement, may influence clinical management (Younes et al. 2015b). These potentially significant errors included very early sleep or REM onset, too much awake time, N3 time or REM time, too little REM time...etc. The technologists were then asked to edit the automatic scoring of 102 full PSGs, once doing a full edit and once following only the suggestions of the Editing Helper. This group included 49 patients with sleep apnea, 12 patients with periodic limb movements >15 hr^{-1}, 14 patients with insomnia and 27 patients with no pathology. The Helper issued an average of 2.5 ± 1.2 suggestions per file (Younes et al. 2015b). Editing time was reduced from 59 ± 26 to 6 ± 7 min while the ICCs for comparisons between manual and the abbreviated editing were not different from the ICCs for manual vs. full edit comparisons (0.87 ± 0.08 vs. 0.89 ± 0.09) (Younes et al. 2015b).

In a more recent study (Younes and Hanly PJ 2016) epoch by epoch agreement in 5-stage sleep scoring between two senior technologists was 78.9% (kappa statistic = 71.1%). When the scoring of each technologist was independently edited based on features calculated within MSS (odds-ratio-product (Younes et al. 2015a), spindles, K complexes, delta wave duration), % agreement increased to 96.5% (kappa statistic = 95.1%). ICCs for comparisons between the edited and original manually determined times in different stages were excellent and well within the accepted range for agreement between two expert scorers (Younes and Hanly PJ 2016). Thus, using the features generated by MSS to edit the manual scores essentially eliminated inter-observer variability while the edited score was in acceptable agreement with the original scoring of both technologists. This shows that the features extracted by MSS to stage sleep are a good compromise between the scoring of these features by two expert technologists.

It is not clear what more evidence is needed to convince decision makers that digital systems currently exist that can save a lot of time and money while producing consistent reliable results. A paradox exists in this regard. As illustrated by the numerous studies reporting on inter-observer scoring variability (Pittman et al. 2004; Anderer et al. 2005; Norman et al. 2000; Danker-Hopfe et al. 2004; Rosenberg and Van Hout 2013) the most one can expect between two experts scoring sleep in the same PSGs is agreement in 85% of epochs. This means that it is acceptable to have 120 disagreements between two humans in a typical 800-epoch PSG. Yet, any difference between the automatic score and the scoring of the local physician/technologist is unacceptable! This paradox has two fundamental underpinnings. First, numerous very poor digital systems were previously introduced and failed miserably. This resulted in a general mistrust of automatic systems. Second, decisions to implement, or not, a new digital scoring system are made by a local expert, or by an administrator who relies on local experts. When evaluating the new system, the local expert will inevitably find differences between his/her scoring and the Auto-score. Human nature causes one to trust his/her own scoring over that of another system, regardless of how many validation studies were published, and the decision will almost invariably be against the digital system. It follows that use of automatic scoring will only become commonplace if payers or regulatory bodies encourage/promote its use, with obvious stipulations as to what is an acceptable automatic system and the editing required. The problem with regulatory bodies is that they also rely on experts, most of whom have, for the reasons mentioned above, already decided that automatic scoring is inaccurate. This impasse will remain as the main barrier to moving sleep staging into the 21st century.

Enhancements to conventional sleep scoring
Assessment of sleep depth and quality
Insomnia and non-restorative sleep, are very common in the general population (Ohayon and Reynolds 2009; Ohayon 2005) and in patients with cognitive and psychiatric disorders (Nissen et al. 2006; Riemann and Voderholzer 2003; Baglioni et al. 2010). Sleep studies in such patients

sometimes reveal organic disorders such as sleep apnea or a movement disorder. However, in many cases, sleep studies provide no explanation for the patient's complaint. Management of such patients is problematic. This is not a trivial issue since there is increasing evidence that poor sleep is a risk factor for cognitive impairment (Nissen et al. 2006; Altena et al. 2008), mood disorders (Riemann and Voderholzer 2003; Baglioni et al. 2010), weight gain (Patel and Hu 2008; Spiegel et al. 2009), diabetes (Nilsson et al. 2004; Mallon et al. 2005), and increased overall mortality (Gallicchio and Kalesan 2009; Cappuccio et al. 2010).

A normal sleep study in the face of sleep complaints may indicate either that the complaint represents a perception problem or that the criteria currently used to evaluate sleep quality are not sensitive enough to identify poor sleep. There are reasons to believe the latter proposition and that, as suggested by Jackson et al. (Jackson and Bruck 2012), analysis of sleep microstructure may provide a fruitful alternative for uncovering differences during sleep in these individuals:

A) *Sleep Depth is Not Adequately Described by the Conventional R&K Stages*: Figure 1 shows 6 epochs representing progression of EEG (C3/A2) from full wakefulness (Panel A), to deep sleep (stage N3, panel F). In panel B the dense beta activity seen in panel A disappeared and a sleep pattern appeared in the middle of the epoch (horizontal bar). Despite the marked difference in appearance between epochs A and B, epoch B continued to be staged awake because the alpha pattern occupied > 15 s (Berry et al. 2012). A little later, the sleep pattern extended for 18 s (panel C). This epoch is now staged N1 even though it is much closer in appearance to panel B than panel B is to panel A. The same pattern continued in the next epoch but a spindle appeared (panel D). The stage is now N2, even though the EEG looks very similar to that in panel C (staged N1) and panel B (staged awake). In panel E, the EEG is substantially different from that of panel D and much closer to the EEG in panel F (staged N3). Yet, it is still staged N2 because delta wave duration did not reach 6 s (Berry et al. 2012). This figure illustrates that: a) unlike the stepwise progression of R&K, sleep progresses gradually from full wakefulness to deep sleep, and b) the same stage may include a wide range of sleep depths. Clearly, 4 h of N2 with a D pattern, cannot be equated with 4 h of N2 consisting primarily of pattern E.

Apart from the above consideration, scoring of stages N1 and N3 is subject to much inter-rater variability (Malhotra et al. 2013; Anderer et al. 2005; Punjabi et al. 2015; Ferri et al. 1989; Norman et al. 2000; Collop 2002; Danker-Hopfe et al. 2004; Magalang et al. 2013; Zhang et al. 2015; Rosenberg and Van Hout 2013). In a recent study in which each epoch was scored manually three

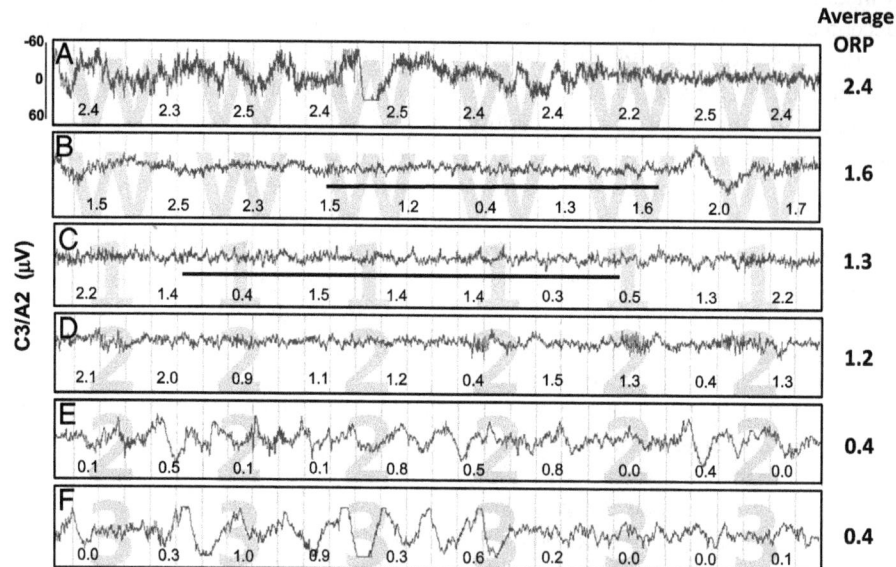

Fig. 1 Tracings showing progression from full wakefulness to deep sleep. Both tracings **a** and **b** were staged awake despite their substantially different visual appearance and the presence of a 12-second period of sleep in **b** (*horizontal line*; 15 s of sleep are required to score sleep). Although its pattern is substantially similar to that of tracing **b**, tracing **c** was scored asleep (stage 1) because the sleep pattern lasted 18 s (*horizontal line*). Tracings **d** and **e** were both scored stage 2 even though the pattern in **d** is very similar to stage 1 (**c**), but a spindle appeared, while the pattern in **e** is very similar to delta sleep (**f**) but the duration of delta waves was just shy of 6 s. The numbers within each tracing are the 3-second odds-ratio-product (ORP) values and the number to the right of each tracing is the 30-second ORP average. Note the marked difference in ORP distribution within the two awake tracings and the transient reduction in ORP during the brief sleep in tracing **b**. ORP values are quite different between the two stage 2 epochs with ORP in tracing **d** being close to that in tracing **c** while ORP in tracing **e** being similar to that of tracing **f**. C3/A2, electroencephalogram. ORP reflects the visual appearance of the EEG. Adapted from (Younes et al. 2015a)

times by two senior technologists and once by another senior technologist (i.e. 7 scores for each epoch) the likelihood of an epoch scored N1 by any technologist being scored N1 in all other six scores was only 9.7% (Younes and Hanly PJ 2016). The corresponding likelihood for an epoch scored N3 by at least one scorer was 24%. Given this uncertainty about the scores of two of the three non-REM stages, it is difficult to have much confidence in using the fractions of time spent in each of these stages as indices of sleep quality/depth.

B) Conventional Indices of Sleep Quality are Difficult to Interpret: Sleep quality is conventionally evaluated by a number of variables that include sleep onset latency (SOL), sleep efficiency (SE), times spent in different non-REM stages, and extent of sleep disruption (e.g. arousal and awakening index (A/AW index) and wake after sleep onset (WASO)). The normal range for each of these variables is very wide so that it is difficult to conclude that a person's sleep is poor unless one of these variables is grossly abnormal. Furthermore, in comparing two groups of patients, or the same patients in two conditions, the differences are often contradictory, for example SE may be better (higher) but N1% and/or A/AW index may be worse. Since the units of measurement of these indices are different (%, rate, minutes) the contradictory changes cannot be integrated into a unitary

index that describes the net difference in sleep quality between the two groups/interventions.

It is clearly impractical to visually divide sleep into many more stages than the current ones or to visually assign a number to overall sleep quality. Digital analysis is required. The first step in staging sleep by MSS is to generate an index called odds-ratio-product (ORP). ORP is the probability of 3-second EEG segments falling in epochs staged awake by a consensus of expert technologists (Younes et al. 2015a). Each 3-second segment is subjected to fast Fourier analysis to generate the power in four frequency bands; delta (0.33–2.33 Hz), theta (2.66–6.33 Hz), alpha/sigma (7.33–14 Hz), and beta (14.33 to 35.0 Hz). The power in each band is assigned a rank (0 to 9) depending on where it lies within the entire range of powers (in the relevant band) observed in >400,000 artifact-free 3-second segments collected from clinical PSGs (many with severe sleep fragmentation). Each 3-second segment is then assigned a four-digit number (bin number), consisting of the four ranks in succession, resulting in 10,000 possible spectral patterns. For example bin number 9549 describes a segment with very high delta power, average theta power, average alpha power and very high beta power. Figure 2 shows several examples of 3-second EEG tracings with their bin numbers.

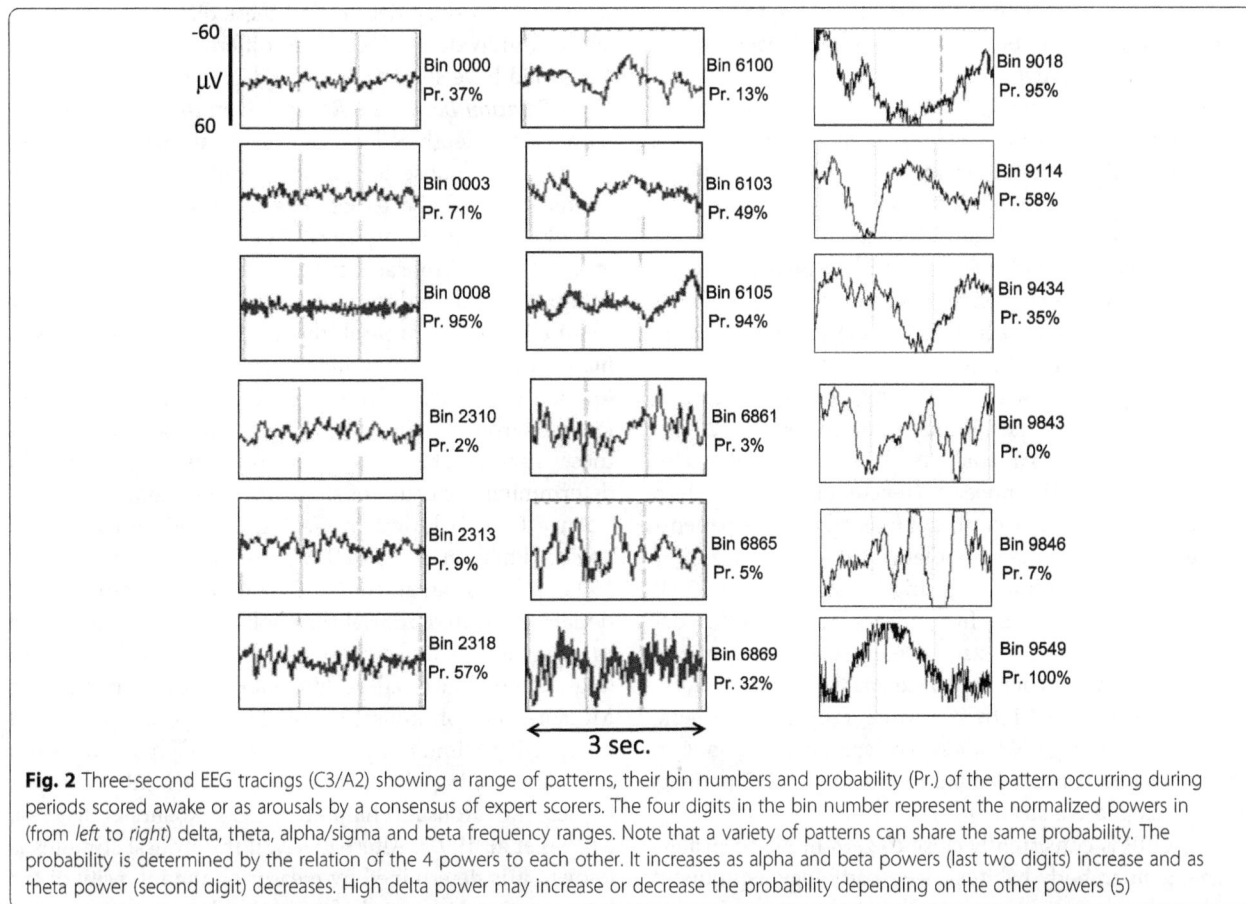

Fig. 2 Three-second EEG tracings (C3/A2) showing a range of patterns, their bin numbers and probability (Pr.) of the pattern occurring during periods scored awake or as arousals by a consensus of expert scorers. The four digits in the bin number represent the normalized powers in (from *left* to *right*) delta, theta, alpha/sigma and beta frequency ranges. Note that a variety of patterns can share the same probability. The probability is determined by the relation of the 4 powers to each other. It increases as alpha and beta powers (last two digits) increase and as theta power (second digit) decreases. High delta power may increase or decrease the probability depending on the other powers (5)

A look-up table is consulted to determine the probability of each of the 10,000 patterns occurring in 30-second epochs scored awake or during an event scored as an arousal. This table was constructed from the results of manual scoring, by three very senior technologists, of the same PSGs containing the 3-second segments used to generate the 10,000 bin numbers. This table indicates that a segment with, for example, a bin number of 9549 was never seen except during arousals or in epochs staged awake (i.e. probability is 100%, Fig. 2). On the other hand, the table indicates that only 7% of segments with bin number 9846 are seen during wakefulness or arousals; the probability is 7% (Fig. 2). The 0 to 100 probability values were all divided by 40 (% awake time in the development PSGs) to generate the ORP. Thus, an ORP of 2.5 indicates a pattern that only occurs during wakefulness or in arousals, an ORP of 1.25 indicates a pattern with an equal probability of occurring during wakefulness or sleep and an ORP of 0 never occurs during wakefulness or in arousals.

The average of the 10 ORP values in each 30s epoch is the primary variable used in MSS to determine whether the patient is almost certainly awake (ORP >2.0), almost certainly asleep (ORP < 1.0) or is in an intermediate state

(ORP 1.0–2.0) (Younes et al. 2015a). Epochs with intermediate values are staged awake or asleep based on a number of ancillary features. As indicated earlier, this staging system has proved quite accurate (Malhotra et al. 2013; Younes et al. 2015b; Younes et al. 2015c; Younes et al. 2016; Younes and Hanly PJ 2016). However, other than its utility in distinguishing wakefulness from sleep, ORP proved to be a good continuous measure of sleep depth, as indicated by the following observations (Younes et al. 2015a):

(A) *Relation between ORP and conventional sleep stages*: Figure 1 shows that average ORP in the 30s epochs decreased progressively as stage moved from full wakefulness (panel A) to deep sleep (panel F). Reflecting what the eye sees, there is little change in average ORP as stage moved from a "dozing" awake state (panel B) through stage 1 (Panel C) and early stage 2 (panel D) while there was a large drop in ORP within stage 2 as the pattern changed from one that resembles stage 1 (panel D) to a pattern that resembles stage 3 (panel E). Spindles are a traditional marker of stage 2 (Rechtschaffen and Kales 1968; Berry et al. 2012). However, spindles are present throughout stage 2, regardless of whether the background EEG pattern is close to that of stage 1 or stage 3, and there is no evidence that the first appearance of a spindle (or K complex) on an EEG background of stage 1 represents a major shift in sleep depth.

Figure 3 shows average ORP in all epochs scored in each of the conventional stages in individual patients. The data in this table are from 317 patients used in five different studies in two sleep centers ((Younes et al. 2015a; Younes et al. 2015c; Meza et al. 2016; Younes) and one internal study). These studies included males and females with a very wide range of age and body habitus. Studies 1, 2 and 4 included some patients with no sleep pathology and with insomnia but the majority had different degrees of sleep apnea and, to a lesser extent, PLMs (Younes et al. 2015a; Younes et al. 2015c; Younes). The internal Study (study 3) included exclusively patients with moderate/severe obstructive sleep apnea. Study 5 (Meza et al. 2016) included 30 patients with excessive daytime somnolence (Epworth scale 15 ± 3) and no sleep pathology during the nocturnal PSG. It can be seen that in all five studies average ORP decreased progressively as stage progressed from awake to N3 but that within each stage, except N3, values in individual patients varied over a wide range. The lowest values were in stage N3 where average ORP was <0.4 in all studies and it exceeded 0.6 in only 12 of 252 patients who developed N3 sleep.

That ORP is consistently close to zero in N3 regardless of age, gender, body habitus, sleep pathology, equipment used or the sleep center where the study was performed (Fig. 3), is of particular importance since it indicates that when the patient is in the deepest sleep by current criteria, ORP is always near zero. This supports the notion that differences in ORP within other stages reflect

differences in sleep depth. Had these differences been related to individual or technical differences ORP in stage N3 would have shown the same degree of variability.

(B) *Relation between ORP and Arousability*: By its very name, sleep depth reflects the ease with which the brain arouses in response to arousal stimuli (arousability); the lighter sleep is, the easier it is to arouse from a given stimulus (Philip et al. 1994; Roehrs et al. 1994; Berry et al. 1998). Arousal occurs when the intensity of a spontaneous or induced stimulus exceeds the intensity required to cause arousal; the arousal threshold. Thus, a high arousal/awakening index could indicate a generally low arousal threshold (light sleep), a high frequency of intense arousal stimuli, or both. Distinction between these two mechanisms is of obvious importance in determining the cause of sleep fragmentation.

Since ORP is lowest in N3 (Fig. 2) and arousability is lowest (Philip et al. 1994; Roehrs et al. 1994; Berry et al. 1998), it can be assumed that ORP correlates with conventionally measured arousal threshold. However, we wanted to determine if differences in ORP within lighter stages (Figs. 1 and 2) also reflect different degrees of arousability. Measurement of arousal threshold is typically performed by applying stimuli (e.g. sound) with different intensities and determining the minimum stimulus intensity that causes EEG arousal (Philip et al. 1994; Roehrs et al. 1994; Martin et al. 1997). Alternatively, if the arousal stimulus is known, it is determined by measuring the intensity of the known stimulus just before arousal (e.g. determining arousal threshold in OSA by measuring pharyngeal pressure just before arousal (Berry and Gleeson 1997)). Neither approach can be used to determine arousal threshold for spontaneous unknown stimuli. Furthermore,

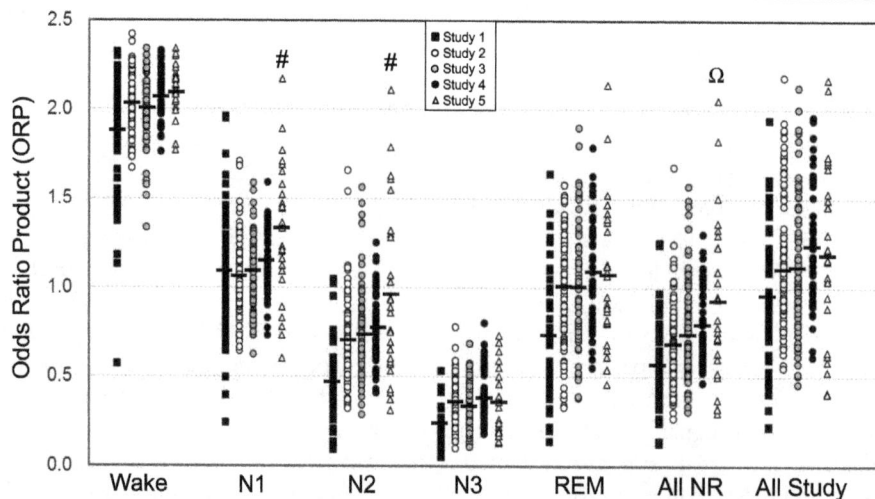

Fig. 3 Odds-ratio-product (ORP) in different conventional sleep stages compiled from five different studies. Each dot is the average ORP in all epochs staged as a given stage in one patient. N1-N3, stages 1–3 of non-rapid-eye-movement (NR) sleep. [#], significantly higher than in all other studies; [Ω], significantly higher than studies 1–3. Study 1, from (Younes et al. 2015a). Study 2, from (Younes et al. 2015c). Study 3, internally acquired validation data in 79 patients with moderate/severe obstructive sleep apnea. Study 4, from (Younes). Study 5, from (Meza et al. 2016)

with the first approach, multiple stimulus intensities need to be applied to determine the minimum intensity at which arousal occurs and the sequence needs to be repeated several times during stable sleep to allow for the spontaneous changes in threshold (Philip et al. 1994; Roehrs et al. 1994). Thus, much time of relatively stable sleep is required to determine a single arousal threshold value that represents the average threshold over the period of testing. Accordingly, current approaches cannot be used to determine the instantaneous arousal threshold or the arousal threshold for stimuli responsible for spontaneous arousals.

We used a completely different approach to determine the relation between instantaneous ORP and arousability (Younes et al. 2015a). The approach is based on the reasonable expectations that: a) the brain receives constantly sensory information from all parts of the body, b) the peripheral sensory information is independent of sleep depth, and c) these peripheral inputs include stimuli of different intensities. When the brain is more arousable, more of these spontaneous inputs will exceed the threshold for arousal, resulting in a higher probability for arousals to occur. All 30-second epochs in non-REM sleep were sorted by their ORP value and the total ORP range (0–2.5) was divided into 10 equal mini-ranges, 0.25 each. For each mini-range we determined the likelihood of an arousal/awakening to occur in the following 30-second epoch (arousability index). We pooled the results of 58 patients with assorted sleep disorders in order to filter out inter-individual differences in the range of intrinsic stimulus intensities. There was a near perfect correlation between current ORP and the arousability index (Fig. 4) (Younes et al. 2015a). This figure indicates that when ORP is, for example, 0.5 and the spontaneous sensory stimuli of the patient are comparable in frequency and

intensity to the average of all 58 patients used, the patient is expected to have an arousal every $\approx$ 5 epochs (20% probability), or an arousal index of 24 hr^{-1}. On the other hand, at an ORP of 1.5 the probability of developing an arousal in the next epoch is $\approx$ 44%, corresponding to an arousal index of 53 hr^{-1}. Clearly, if spontaneous arousal stimuli in a patient are weaker or less frequent than the average in the patients studied here the arousal index is expected to be less than the value predicted from this relation, and vice versa. This can be used to determine whether excessive sleep fragmentation is the result of increased arousability (high ORP) or excessive spontaneous stimuli (see *Potential Clinical Utility of ORP*, below).

The relation shown in Fig. 4 confirms that current ORP reflects the ease with which the brain can be aroused, and can therefore be used as a measure of arousability. It has advantages over conventional arousal threshold determination in that: a) No intervention is required. Therefore, it can be determined in clinical studies. b) Arousability can be determined on an epoch-by-epoch basis making it possible to examine dynamic changes in this important variable.

As may be expected from the data of Fig. 4, there was a strong correlation between average ORP in different sleep stages and the arousal/awakening index in different patients (Younes et al. 2015a). However, it was not clear whether a high average ORP was responsible for the high A/AW index or the converse; average ORP is high because there is more sleep fragmentation. Taking advantage of the newfound ability to measure instantaneous arousability using ORP, in a subsequent study we determined the dynamics of sleep recovery following arousals (Younes and Hanly 2016). We found that patients differ markedly in how quickly sleep deepens following an arousal (Fig. 5a). In all patients ORP increases during arousal and there is a step decrease in ORP at the end of arousal. However, patients differ in the ORP level at the end of this step decrease (about 9 s after the end of arousal) (Fig. 5a). Average ORP at 9 s following arousal (ORP-9) ranged from 0.23 (very deep sleep) to 1.74 (mean ± SD: 0.70 ± 0.32). When ORP-9 was high (e.g. patient X, Fig. 5a) ORP decreased gradually over a few minutes and, given time without arousal, deep sleep could be reached. There was a very strong correlation between ORP-9 and average ORP in non-REM sleep (Fig. 6). In multiple regression analysis to determine the main correlates with average non-REM ORP (ORP_{NR}), ORP-9 and A/AW index emerged as the only significant correlates, accounting for 83% of the variability in ORP_{NR} (Younes and Hanly 2016). The mechanism by which A/AW index influences average ORP_{NR} is illustrated in Fig. 5b. Thus, the more frequent the arousals, the less time is available for ORP to decrease before the next arousal resets ORP back to ORP-9.

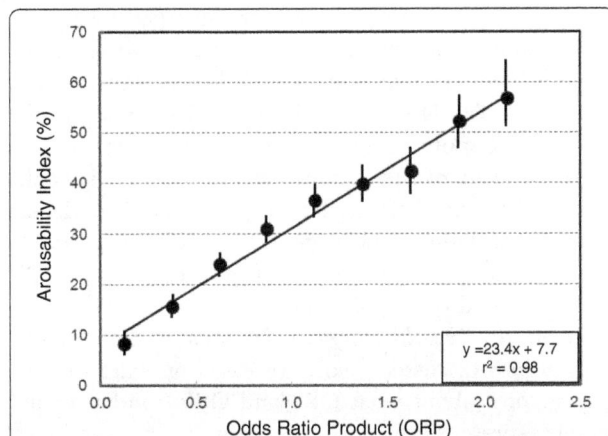

Fig. 4 Relationship between average ORP in current 30-second epochs and the likelihood of an arousal or awakening occurring in the next 30-second epoch (Arousability Index). Vertical bars are the confidence interval of the probability. From (Younes et al. 2015a)

The plot shows:
y = 23.4x + 7.7
$r^2 = 0.98$

Y-axis: Arousability Index (%)
X-axis: Odds Ratio Product (ORP)

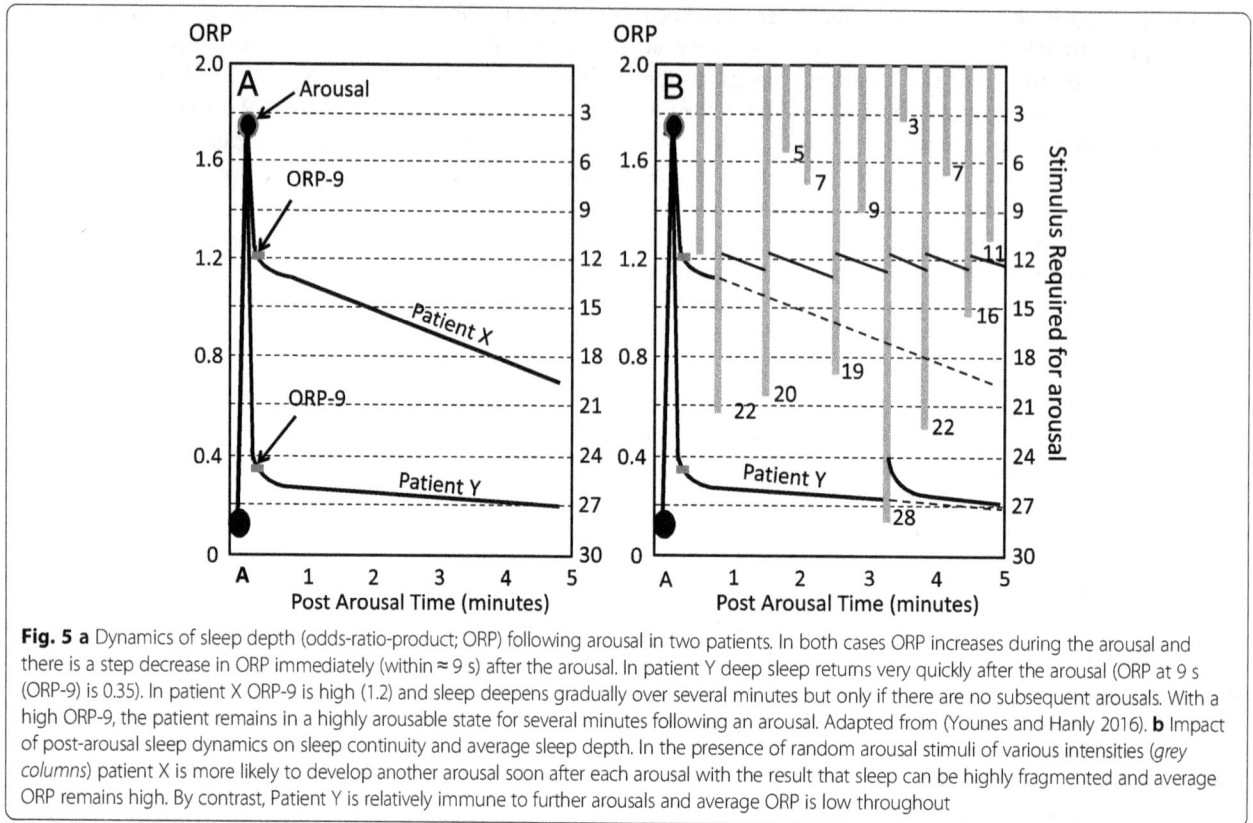

Fig. 5 a Dynamics of sleep depth (odds-ratio-product; ORP) following arousal in two patients. In both cases ORP increases during the arousal and there is a step decrease in ORP immediately (within ≈ 9 s) after the arousal. In patient Y deep sleep returns very quickly after the arousal (ORP at 9 s (ORP-9) is 0.35). In patient X ORP-9 is high (1.2) and sleep deepens gradually over several minutes but only if there are no subsequent arousals. With a high ORP-9, the patient remains in a highly arousable state for several minutes following an arousal. Adapted from (Younes and Hanly 2016). **b** Impact of post-arousal sleep dynamics on sleep continuity and average sleep depth. In the presence of random arousal stimuli of various intensities (*grey columns*) patient X is more likely to develop another arousal soon after each arousal with the result that sleep can be highly fragmented and average ORP remains high. By contrast, Patient Y is relatively immune to further arousals and average ORP is low throughout

It is interesting to note that ORP-9 was independent of age, gender, body habitus or the sleep disorder (Younes and Hanly 2016). Furthermore, ORP-9 was not affected when patients with severe OSA were placed on CPAP despite reductions in A/AW index and in average ORP. Thus, ORP-9 is likely a trait.

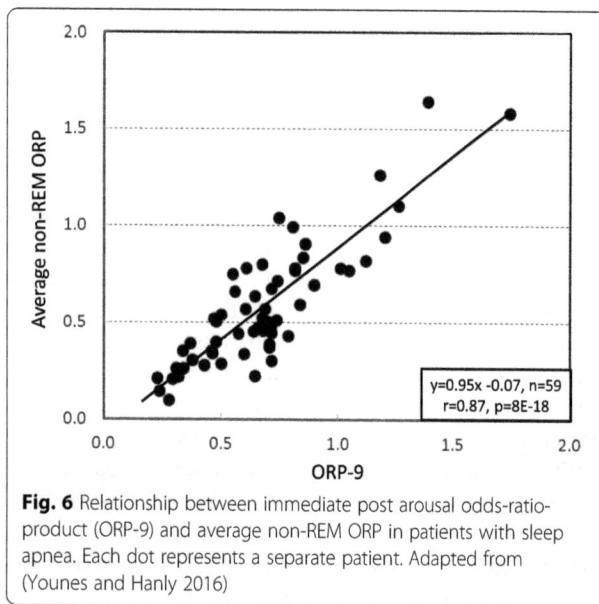

Fig. 6 Relationship between immediate post arousal odds-ratio-product (ORP-9) and average non-REM ORP in patients with sleep apnea. Each dot represents a separate patient. Adapted from (Younes and Hanly 2016)

In summary, average ORP during non-REM sleep is largely determined by the speed with which sleep deepens following arousals. When these dynamics are fast (low ORP-9), the patient returns to deep sleep very quickly and is resistant to all but very intense stimuli. Arousals will be infrequent and the patient remains in deep sleep (patient Y, Fig. 5b). However, when ORP-9 is high, the patient may or not progress to deep sleep depending on the frequency and intensity of arousal stimuli. In the presence of relatively frequent/strong stimuli these patients are more likely to sustain severe sleep fragmentation and to remain in light sleep throughout (patient X, Fig. 5b). It is well known that some healthy subjects are more prone to sleep disruption in the face of stress than others (Bonnet and Arand 2003; Drake et al. 2004) and that this trait may be inherited (Drake et al. 2008; Bonnet and Arand 2010; Heath et al. 1990). Post-arousal sleep dynamics may provide the basis for these inter-individual differences.

Potential Clinical Utility of ORP: Most of the potential applications discussed below are based on what we currently know about what ORP and ORP-9 indicate, and simply represent ideas for future research that can be facilitated by inclusion of ORP in clinical sleep reports:

a) Investigation of Primary Insomnia: Availability of ORP during periods staged awake may help distinguish patients who are wide awake during these periods (Fig. 1a) from those who develop frequent mini-sleep periods but fail to progress to sustained sleep (e.g. Fig. 1b). Furthermore, it is now well established that a hyperarousal state exists in some patients with primary insomnia (Bonnet and Arand 2010; Riemann et al. 2010). The EEG representation of the hyperarousal state is an increase in power in the beta frequency range during sleep (Freedman 1986; Krystal et al. 2002; Perlis et al. 2001; Buysse et al. 2008). ORP is extremely sensitive to relative EEG beta power (Younes et al. 2015a). Accordingly, ORP during non-REM sleep should be elevated in patients with the hyperarousal state. It is possible that the etiology in patients who are wide awake during awake periods and develop high quality sleep when they sleep is related to lifestyle issues and these patients may be better candidates for cognitive behavioral therapy, whereas in those who fail to progress to deep sleep the problem is in central sleep control or excessive arousal stimuli from some source. The last two possibilities can be distinguished by ORP-9.

b) Investigation of paradoxical insomnia: Previous studies identified microstructure abnormalities in patients with paradoxical insomnia (Krystal et al. 2002; Perlis et al. 2001; Parrino et al. 2009). All reported abnormalities (increased beta activity (Perlis et al. 2001), decreased delta and increased alpha/beta activity (Buysse et al. 2008), and cyclic alternating pattern (Parrino et al. 2009)) result in a higher ORP during non-REM sleep (Younes et al. 2015a). Thus, having ORP$_{NR}$ available in clinical studies may help identify patients with abnormal sleep quality from those in whom the problem is in perception of sleep. Furthermore, in a recent study (Meza et al. 2016) in which we measured ORP during multiple sleep latency tests (MSLTs) and correlated ORP values with probability of sleep being perceived after each nap we identified patients who failed to perceive sleep despite reaching ORP levels that were followed by sleep perception in the vast majority of patients. Thus, measurement of ORP and post-nap sleep perception during MSLTs may help identify patients with a central perception abnormality.

c) Investigation of patients with idiopathic hypersomnia and non-restorative sleep: These symptoms may be related to poor quality sleep or a need to sleep longer than the patient is sleeping. As indicated earlier, sleep may be of poor quality (e.g. Fig. 1d) even though the patient spends a normal amount of time in stage N2. Knowledge of ORP in stage N2 may help identify those in whom the problem is poor sleep quality. In a recent study (Meza et al. 2016), we found that patients with excessive somnolence (Epworth scale 15.2 ± 3.0) and

normal nocturnal sleep had, on average, significantly higher ORP values during non-REM sleep (Study #5, Fig. 2).

d) Evaluation of the impact of an intervention on sleep quality: A number of interventions are commonly used to improve sleep quality in patients with sleep disorders including mechanical devices (CPAP, mandibular devices) for respiratory sleep disorders and medications for insomnia, depression and nonrestorative sleep. As indicated above, conventional indices of sleep quality are not sensitive enough for this purpose and are often difficult to interpret. ORP may be suited for this purpose.

e) Enhancements to the multiple sleep latency test (MSLT) (Meza et al. 2016): Despite the fact that MSLTs are resource intensive, expensive and inconvenient to the patient the clinical utility of this test is very limited. Except for the occasional confirmation of narcolepsy, the only information gained is average sleep onset latency (SOL). A short SOL does not necessarily confirm pathologic somnolence since the range is extremely wide in asymptomatic subjects (Levine et al. 1988; Drake et al. 2010). Furthermore, a short SOL simply means that the patient managed to develop 15 s of light sleep (Berry et al. 2012) in no more than one epoch under conditions that are highly conducive to sleep. In many patients sleep does not progress beyond this extremely light phase (Meza et al. 2016). In a recent examination of 150 naps in 30 patients with excessive somnolence SOL was <5 min in 47 naps (21 patients). Of these, ORP decreased below 1.0 in only 13 naps (9 patients) and below 0.5 in only two naps in one patient (Meza et al. 2016). This indicates that within a given SOL there are gradations of objective sleepiness. Although, on average, patients with a SOL <5 min are at greater risk of motor vehicle accidents than those with SOL >10 min (Drake et al. 2010), the risk in an individual patient is difficult to assess from SOL; the difference in accident risk between the two groups was barely significant despite the fact that the study involved >600 patients followed for 10 years (Drake et al. 2010). It is possible that including the times at which different ORP values are reached may provide a better assessment of accident risk in individual patients (Meza et al. 2016).

f) Real time applications: ORP can be calculated very quickly and a monitor that outputs ORP in real time (every 3 s and/or as a moving average) has become available (Younes et al. 2016). Such information may be useful in monitoring depth of sedation in intensive care units. As well, ORP may be useful in detecting periods of intermittent dozing during activities that require vigilance (e.g. compare Fig. 1a and b).

Assessment of arousal intensity

The visual scoring of arousals involves a binary decision; present or not (Berry et al. 2012). Yet, visually, arousals vary greatly in intensity and duration (Fig. 7). These differences may have clinical implications. In one study in patients with OSA there was a strong correlation between intensity and the magnitude of post-event ventilatory overshoot, suggesting that arousal intensity promotes recurrence of the obstructive events (Younes 2004). It is clearly not practical to expect technologists to assign a visual scale to every arousal, and such a scale would be highly subjective. More recently, a method was developed for digital assessment of arousal intensity on a scale of 1 to 9 (Azarbarzin et al. 2014). Figure 7 shows examples of arousals with different digital scales. There was a linear relation in all patients between arousal scale and heart rate response to arousals (Azarbarzin et al. 2014). Interestingly, both the average arousal intensity and the slope of the relation between intensity and the increase in heart rate varied considerably among subjects (Azarbarzin et al. 2014). Arousal scale was also found to correlate with the magnitude of pharyngeal dilator muscles' response to arousal (Amatoury et al. 2016).

It is possible that differences in arousal intensity between subjects may explain why some patients develop more daytime symptoms than others for the same degree of sleep fragmentation. It is also possible that the heart rate response to arousal may be predictive for development of cardiovascular complications in patients with sleep fragmentation. Availability of this information in clinical sleep studies would facilitate investigation of these possibilities.

Assessment of alpha intrusion (alpha-delta sleep)

Intrusion of alpha activity in non-REM sleep is frequently present in patients with fibromyalgia, chronic fatigue and non-restorative sleep (Anch et al. 1991; Branco et al. 1994; Moldofsky et al. 1975; Olsen et al. 2013), arthritis (Mahowald et al. 1989), insomnia (Martinez et al. 2010; Riedner et al. 2016) and depression (Hauri and Hawkins 1973; Jaimchariyatam et al. 2011). Although it may be seen in asymptomatic subjects (Scheuler et al. 1983; Horne and Shackell 1991), its prevalence and extent are clearly greater in these disorders such that a clinical association is well established. Whether alpha intrusion causes the patient's complaints, is a consequence of disruptive stimuli, or both is not clear (Riedner et al. 2016; Pivik and Harman 1995; Stone et al. 2008). Large studies are needed to identify its clinical significance.

Visual quantification of the alpha intrusions in routine sleep studies is impractical. Utilization of this potentially useful marker in clinical practice has been hampered by the need for digital analysis and lack of quantitative guidelines for its identification and quantification. In order to generate ORP, our clinical sleep scoring program performs spectral analysis on consecutive 3-second

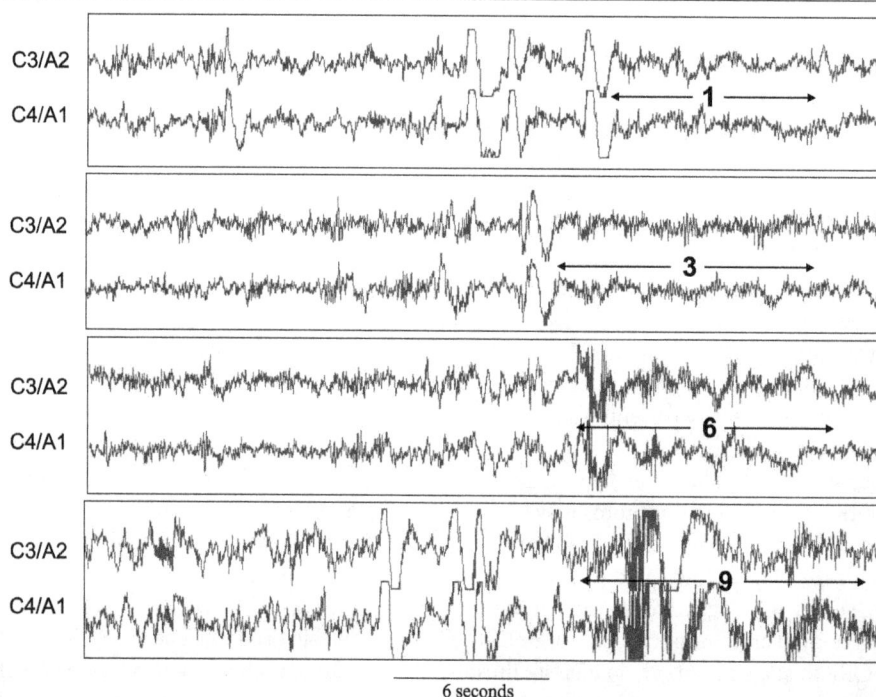

Fig. 7 Examples of arousal with different intensity scales in the same patient. C3/A2 and C4/A1 are central electroencephalograms. From (Azarbarzin et al. 2014)

epochs throughout the PSG and calculates power in different EEG frequency ranges including the alpha range (Younes et al. 2015a). By comparing the 3-second alpha power with the corresponding visual appearance of the EEG we established a threshold of 30 μV^2 for what one can confidently score as alpha intrusion. The fraction of 3-second epochs with ORP <1.0 (i.e. patient is clearly asleep) that meet this threshold is reported as the alpha intrusion index. The alpha intrusion index was evaluated in 448 PSGs scored by MSS. In 60% of patients the index was <1% while it was >5% in 15% of patients and >20% in 4% of patients. This information is presented not to suggest that the threshold for scoring alpha intrusion should be the same as used here. The criteria can obviously be changed with experience or by consensus. Rather, it is presented to show that if clinical PSGs are routinely subjected to digital analysis such an index, regardless of what criteria are used to measure it, can be painlessly obtained in a limitless number of studies, making it possible to identify its clinical significance easily and inexpensively.

Assessment of sleep spindles and K complexes

Sleep spindles have been extensively investigated in research studies (recently reviewed by Clawson et al. (Clawson et al. 2016)). It is clear that spindles are involved in learning and memory (Clemens et al. 2006; Cox et al. 2014; Yotsumoto et al. 2009) and their characteristics are correlated with intelligence and cognitive ability (Geiger et al. 2011; Fogel et al. 2007; Schabus et al. 2006). They are greatly reduced in developmental abnormalities in children (Ellingson and Peters 1980; Selvitellia et al. 2009; Godbout et al. 2000; Limoges et al. 2005), in adult schizophrenia (Ferrarelli et al. 2007; Ferrarelli et al. 2010; Manoach et al. 2010; Manoach et al. 2014) and in patients with Parkinson's disease with dementia (Latreille et al. 2015). Spindle density, duration and amplitude decrease with age but the rate of decline is not the same in all subjects (Nicolas et al. 2001; Crowley et al. 2002; Guazzelli et al. 1986; Wei et al. 1999; Principe and Smith 1982). There is a correlation between age-related decline in spindle activity and decline in cognitive functioning (Peters et al. 2008; Mander et al. 2014). Sleep disruption by sleep-related disorders (e.g. sleep apnea,) is frequently associated with cognitive impairment. It is not known whether cognitive impairment resulting from sleep fragmentation, per se, is also associated with reduced spindle activity. Availability of information about spindle characteristics during clinical studies before and after correction of the sleep fragmentation would make it possible to easily address this issue. Furthermore, should it become evident that cognitive impairment due to sleep disruption, per se, is not associated with reduced spindle activity, or is not reversible if

present, it will be clear that reduction of spindle activity is at least a marker for the presence of a neurodegenerative process.

Likewise, K complexes (Rechtschaffen and Kales 1968; Loomis et al. 1939) have been extensively investigated (see (Halasz 2005) (Halasz 2005) and Halasz (Halász 2015), for reviews). K complexes can be routinely evoked by experimental stimuli (e.g. noise or airway obstruction) but also occur spontaneously during stages N2 and N3 of non-REM sleep. Because of the similarity between K complexes and some of the delta waves encountered in deep sleep it is possible that some spontaneous complexes represent preliminary appearance of deeper sleep (De Gennaro et al. 2000). However, because the delta waves of deep sleep have no consistent pattern, it is reasonable to assume that a high frequency of slow waves with a consistent K complex appearance reflects a high frequency of naturally occurring noxious stimuli. Knowledge of the frequency of K complexes may therefore be helpful in identifying the presence of excessive subthreshold arousal stimuli that may contribute to the patient's complaints. Excessive K complexes in the absence of a clear cause in the PSG (e.g. sleep disordered breathing, PLMs) may prompt a search for, and correction of, other somatic or environmental sources of arousal stimuli.

In the current visual scoring of clinical studies spindles and K complexes are used exclusively to identify stage N2 (Berry et al. 2012). There is no consideration of spindle characteristics or frequency of K complexes. Accordingly, such potentially useful information is not captured. A number of digital methods for identifying and characterizing spindles (Ferrarelli et al. 2007; Martin et al. 2013; Wamsley et al. 2012; Mölle et al. 2002; Bódizs et al. 2009; Wendt et al. 2012; Devuyst et al. 2010; Lajnef et al. 2015b; Ray et al. 2015) and K complexes (Bremer et al. 1970; Krohne et al. 2014; Richard and Lengelle 1998; Bankman et al. 1992; Parekh et al. 2015) have been proposed and used in research studies but none has been adapted to clinical studies. Although there is agreement on the visual appearance of these events (Berry et al. 2012), there is no agreement on how to define them in quantitative terms. This and the considerable inter-scorer variability in visual scoring of these events (Warby et al. 2014; Wendt et al. 2015) have made it difficult to arrive at the "optimal" digital approach. In the opinion of this writer, it is preferable to begin using any reasonable approach, and refine it later if necessary, than wait for a consensus that has been elusive for over 50 years. Once such an approach becomes routinely available, its results in normal people can be established, making it possible to determine when a patient's value is abnormal.

As indicated earlier, there are three validated commercial systems for digital sleep scoring (Morpheus, somnolyzer, MSS). Since all three are capable of breaking down non-REM sleep into its three stages, all include algorithms for spindle and K complex detection. There is no information regarding these algorithms in Morpheus or Somnolyzer. The algorithms in MSS have proven robust enough such that when spindles and K complexes identified by this system were used to edit (overrule) the manual scoring of non-REM sleep N1/N2 discrepancies between scorers decreased from 42 ± 36 epochs/PSG to 10 ± 10 epochs/PSG (Younes and Hanly PJ. Minimizing Interrater Variability in Staging Sleep by Use of Computer-Derived Features. J Clin Sleep Med 2016). The algorithms used by MSS to identify spindles and K complexes have been described before (Younes and Hanly PJ 2016). In addition to calculating the frequency of the two events in stage N2, the software also determines average spindle duration and power. In 316 PSGs scored by MSS, average spindle density over all N2 time in each central derivation (C3/M2, C4/M1) ranged 0.2 to 8.9 min^{-1} in different subjects and K complex density ranged from 0.09 to 0.84 min^{-1}. Average spindle duration ranged from 1.05 to 1.7 s and average spindle power ranged from 1.9 to 117.0 μV^2. These values are presented here to show that there is a wide range in all these characteristics within the clinical sleep population, which likely reflects clinical/pathological differences between patients, and also to show the ease with which a large amount of such information can be obtained if digital identification of these characteristics becomes a routine component of EEG analysis.

Conclusion

It is argued that the technology of digital sleep scoring has progressed enough to make it possible to obtain reliable, reproducible scoring, comparable in accuracy to that of highly trained technologists, with minimal editing. At the same time, it has become clear that inter-rater variability in scoring sleep is sufficiently serious as to raise doubt about the validity of R&K's N1 to N3 stages as a measure of sleep depth. Apart from elimination of variability in conventional sleep assessment between scorers, and reduction in cost, inclusion of digital scoring in the routine analysis of clinical PSGs would make it possible to obtain information that is not possible to obtain with visual scoring. These include providing in each patient a continuous index of sleep depth, and quantitative estimates of arousal intensity, alpha intrusion, and characteristics of spindles and K complexes. Although the clinical utility of these indices has not yet been proven, there is sufficient information from scientific investigations that they might well explain some complaints/disorders that are currently not explained after conventional scoring. Widespread availability of this additional information at no cost and with no intervention would greatly facilitate research into the clinical utility of these indices.

Acknowledgements

The author acknowledges the contributions of all YRT employees, without whose work none of the new technologies could have been developed, and of the many collaborators in the research studies which evaluated these technologies (see references (Malhotra et al. 2013; Azarbarzin et al. 2014; Younes et al. 2015a; Azarbarzin et al. 2015; Younes et al. 2015b; Younes and Hanly 2016; Younes et al. 2015c; Meza et al. 2016; Younes et al. 2016; Younes and Hanly PJ 2016; Amatoury et al. 2016; Younes et al. J Clin Sleep Med. In Press.

Funding

Not Applicable.

Authors' contributions

The author was the sole contributor to this review.

Authors' information

MY (MD, FRCPC, PhD) is distinguished professor emeritus at the University of Manitoba.

Competing interests

MY is the owner of YRT Ltd, the company that developed the scoring system (MSS) and associated algorithms. A patent is pending for the ORP depth of sleep index.

Ethics approval and consent to participate

No new experimental recordings were generated for this review. All data provided here that were generated in the author's laboratory was: a) already published (see relevant publications for ethics approval), b) in submitted manuscripts (reference (Younes)) describing studies approved by the Research Ethics Board of the University of Manitoba, c) obtained from previously recorded PSGs used in published studies, or d) clinical PSGs obtained at the Misericordia Sleep Center and scored by MSS (MSS is an approved scoring system by FDA and Health Canada). Patients undergoing clinical sleep studies at our center sign/decline to sign a consent form allowing the use of their anonymized results in research. Only data from patients who agreed to the use of their data was included here.

References

Altena A, van der Werf YD, Strijers RL, Van Someren EJ. Sleep loss affects vigilance: effects of chronic insomnia and sleep therapy. J Sleep Res. 2008;17: 335–43.

Amatoury J, Azarbarzin A, Younes M, Jordan AS, Wellman A, Eckert DJ. Arousal Intensity is a Distinct Pathophysiological Trait in Obstructive Sleep Apnea. Sleep. 2016;39:2091–100.

Anch AM, Lue FA, MacLean AW, Moldofsky H. Sleep physiology and psychological aspects of the fibrositis (fibromyalgia) syndrome. Can J Psychol. 1991;45:179–84.

Anderer P, Gruber G, Parapatics S, Woertz M, Miazhynskaia T, Klosch G, et al. An E-health solution for automatic sleep classification according to rechtschaffen and kales: validation study of the somnolyzer 24 x 7 utilizing the siesta database. Neuropsychobiology. 2005;51:115–33.

Azarbarzin A, Ostrowski M, Hanly P, Younes M. Relationship between arousal intensity and heart rate response to arousal. Sleep. 2014;37:645–53.

Azarbarzin A, Ostrowski M, Keenan B, Younes M, Kuna S. Arousal responses during overnight polysomhography and their reproducibility in healthy young adults. Sleep. 2015;38:1313–21.

Baglioni C, Spiegelhalder K, Lombardo C, Riemann D. Sleep and emotions: focus on insomnia. Sleep Med Rev. 2010;14:227–38.

Bankman IN, Sigillito VG, Wise RA, Smith PL. Feature-based detection of the K-complex wave in the human electroencephalogram using neural networks. IEEE Trans Biomed Eng. 1992;39:1305–10.

Berry RB, Gleeson K. Respiratory arousal from sleep: mechanisms and significance. Sleep. 1997;20:654–75.

Berry RB, Asyali MA, McNellis MI, Khoo MC. Within-night variation in respiratory effort preceding apnea termination and EEG delta power in sleep apnea. J Appl Physiol (1985). 1998;85:1434–41.

Berry RB, Budhiraja R, Gottlieb DJ, Gozal D, Iber C, Kapur VK. Rules for scoring respiratory events in sleep: update of the 2007 AASM manual for the scoring of sleep and associated events. J Clin Sleep Med. 2012;8:597–619.

Bódizs R, Körmendi J, Rigó P, Lázár AS. The individual adjustment method of sleep spindle analysis: methodological improvements and roots in the fingerprint paradigm. J Neurosci Methods. 2009;178:205–13.

Bonnet MH, Arand DL. Situational insomnia: consistency, predictors, and outcomes. Sleep. 2003;26:1029–36.

Bonnet MH, Arand DL. Hyperarousal and insomnia: state of the science. Sleep Med Rev. 2010;14:9–15.

Branco J, Atalaia A, Paiva T. Sleep cycles and alpha-delta sleep in fibromyalgia syndrome. J Rheumatol. 1994;21:1113–7.

Bremer G, Smith JR, Karacan I. Automatic detection of the K-complex in sleep electroencephalograms. IEEE Trans Biomed Eng. 1970;17:314–23.

Buysse DJ, Germain A, Hall ML, et al. EEG spectral analysis in primary insomnia: NREM period effects and sex differences. Sleep. 2008;31:1673–82.

Cappuccio FP, D'Elia L, Strazzullo P, Miller MA. Sleep duration and all-cause mortality: a systematic review and meta-analysis of prospective studies. Sleep. 2010;33:585–92.

Clawson BC, Durkin J, Aton SJ. Form and function of sleep spindles across the lifespan. Neural Plast. 2016;2016:6936381. doi:10.1155/2016/6936381. Epub 2016 Apr 14.

Clemens Z, Fabo D, Hal'asz P. Twenty-four hours retention of visuospatial memory correlates with the number of parietal sleep spindles. Neurosci Lett. 2006;403:52–6.

Collop NA. Scoring variability between polysomnography technologists in different sleep laboratories. Sleep Med. 2002;3:43–7.

Cox R, Hofman WF, de Boer M, Talamini LM. Local sleep spindle modulations in relation to specific memory cues. NeuroImage. 2014;99:103–10.

Crowley K, Trinder J, Kim Y, Carrington M, Colrain IM. The effects of normal aging on sleep spindle and K-complex production. Clin Neurophysiol. 2002;113:1615–22.

Danker-Hopfe H, Kunz D, Gruber G, Klösch G, Lorenzo JL, Himanen SL, et al. Interrater reliability between scorers from eight European sleep laboratories in subjects with different sleep disorders. J Sleep Res. 2004;13:63–9.

De Gennaro L, Ferrara M, Bertini M. The spontaneous K-complex during stage 2 sleep: is it the 'forerunner' of delta waves? Neurosci Lett. 2000;291:41–3.

Devuyst S, Dutoit T, Stenuit P, Kerkhofs M. Automatic K-complexes detection in sleep EEG recordings using likelihood thresholds. Conf Proc IEEE Eng Med Biol Soc. 2010;2010:4658–61.

Drake C, Richardson G, Roehrs T, Scofield H, Roth T. Vulnerability to stress-related sleep disturbance and hyperarousal. Sleep. 2004;27:285–91.

Drake CL, Scofield H, Roth T. Vulnerability to insomnia: the role of familial aggregation. Sleep Med. 2008;9:297–302.

Drake C, Roehrs T, Breslau N, Johnson E, Jefferson C, Scofield H, et al. The 10-year risk of verified motor vehicle crashes in relation to physiologic sleepiness. Sleep. 2010;33:745–52.

Ellingson RJ, Peters JF. Development of EEG and daytime sleep patterns in trisomy-21 infants during the first year of life: longitudinal observations. Electroencephalogr Clin Neurophysiol. 1980;50:457–66.

Ferrarelli F, Huber R, Peterson MJ, Massimini M, Murphy M, Riedner BA, et al. Reduced sleep spindle activity in schizophrenia patients. Am J Psychiatry. 2007;164:483–92.

Ferrarelli F, Peterson MJ, Sarasso S, Riedner BA, Murphy MJ, Benca RM, et al. Thalamic dysfunction in schizophrenia suggested by whole-night deficits in slow and fast spindles. Am J Psychiatry. 2010;167:1339–48.

Ferri R, Ferri P, Colognola RM, Petrella MA, Musumeci SA, Bergonzi P. Comparison between the results of an automatic and a visual scoring of sleep EEG recordings. Sleep. 1989;12:354–62.

Fogel SM, Nader R, Cote KA, Smith CT. Sleep spindles and learning potential. Behav Neurosci. 2007;12:1–10.

Freedman RR. EEG power spectra in sleep-onset insomnia. Electroencephalogr Clin Neurophysiol. 1986;63:408–13.

Gallicchio L, Kalesan B. Sleep duration and mortality: a systematic review and meta-analysis. J Sleep Res. 2009;18:148–58.

Geiger A, Huber R, Kurth S, Ringli M, Jenni OG, Achermann P. The sleep EEG as a marker of intellectual ability in school age children. Sleep. 2011;34:181–89.

Godbout R, Bergeron C, Limoges E, Stip E, Mottron L. A laboratory study of sleep in Asperger's syndrome. Neuroreport. 2000;11:127–30.

Guazzelli M, Feinberg I, Aminoff M, Fein G, Floyd TC, Maggini C. Sleep spindles in normal elderly: comparison with young adult patterns and relation to nocturnal awakening, cognitive function and brain atrophy. Electroencephalogr Clin Neurophysiol. 1986;63:526–39.

Halasz P. K-complex, a reactive EEG graphoelement of NREM sleep: an old chap in a new garment. Sleep Med Rev. 2005;9:391–412.

Halász P. The K-complex as a special reactive sleep slow wave - a theoretical update. Sleep Med Rev. 2015;29:34–40.

Hauri P, Hawkins DR. Alpha-delta sleep. Electroencephalogr Clin Neurophysiol. 1973;34:233–7.

Heath AC, Kendler KS, Eaves LJ, Martin NG. Evidence for genetic influences on sleep disturbance and sleep pattern in twins. Sleep. 1990;13:318–35.

Horne JA, Shackell BS. Alpha-like EEG activity in non-REM sleep and the fibromyalgia (fibrositis) syndrome. Electroencephalogr Clin Neurophysiol. 1991;79:271–6.

Jackson ML, Bruck D. Sleep abnormalities in chronic fatigue syndrome/myalgic encephalomyelitis: a review. J Clin Sleep Med. 2012;8:719–28.

Jaimchariyatam N, Rodriguez CL, Budur K. Prevalence and correlates of alpha-delta sleep in major depressive disorders. Innov Clin Neurosci. 2011;8:35–49.

Krohne LK, Hansen RB, Christensen JA, Sorensen HB, Jennum P. Detection of K-complexes based on the wavelet transform. Conf Proc IEEE Eng Med Biol Soc. 2014;2014:5450–3.

Krystal AD, Edinger JD, Wohlgemuth WK, Marsh GR. NREM sleep EEG frequency spectral correlates of sleep complaints in primary insomnia subtypes. Sleep. 2002;25:630–40.

Kubicki S, Herrmann WM. The future of computer-assisted investigation of the polysomnogram: sleep microstructure. J Clin Neurophysiol. 1996;13:285–94.

Lajnef T, Chaibi S, Ruby P, Aguera PE, Eichenlaub JB, Samet M, et al. Learning machines and sleeping brains: automatic sleep stage classification using decision-tree multi-class support vector machines. J Neurosci Methods. 2015a;250:94–105.

Lajnef T, Chaibi S, Eichenlaub JB, Ruby PM, Aguera PE, Samet M, et al. Sleep spindle and K-complex detection using tunable Q-factor wavelet transform and morphological component analysis. Front Hum Neurosci. 2015b;9:414.

Latreille V, Carrier J, Lafortune M, Postuma RB, Bertrand JA, Panisset M, et al. Sleep spindles in Parkinson's disease may predict the development of dementia. Neurobiol Aging. 2015;36:1083–90.

Levine B, Roehrs T, Zorick F, Roth T. Daytime sleepiness in young adults. Sleep. 1988;11:39–46.

Limoges E, Mottron L, Bolduc C, Berthiaume C, Godbout R. Atypical sleep architecture and the autism phenotype. Brain. 2005;128:1049–61.

Loomis AL, Harvey EN, Hobart GA. Distribution of disturbance-patterns in the human electroencephalogram, with special reference to sleep. J Neurophysiol. 1939;2:413–30.

Magalang UJ, Chen NH, Cistulli PA, Fedson AC, Gíslason T, Hillman D, et al. Agreement in the scoring of respiratory events and sleep among international sleep centers. Sleep. 2013;36:591–6.

Mahowald MW, Mahowald ML, Bundlie SR, Ytterberg SR. Sleep fragmentation in rheumatoid arthritis. Arthritis Rheum. 1989;32:974–83.

Malhotra A, Younes M, Kuna ST, Benca R, Kushida CA, Walsh J, et al. Performance of an automated polysomnography scoring system versus computer-assisted manual scoring. Sleep. 2013;36:573–82.

Mallon L, Broman JE, Hetta J. High incidence of diabetes in men with sleep complaints or short sleep duration. Diabetes Care. 2005;28:2762–7.

Mander BA, Rao V, Lu B, Saletin JM, Ancoli-Israel S, Jagust WJ, Walker MP. Impaired prefrontal sleep spindle regulation of hippocampal-dependent learning in older adults. Cereb Cortex. 2014;24:3301–9.

Manoach DS, Thakkar KN, Stroynowski E, Ely A, McKinley SK, Wamsley E, et al. Reduced overnight consolidation of procedural learning in chronic medicated schizophrenia is related to specific sleep stages. J Psychiatr Res. 2010;44:112–20.

Manoach DS, Demanuele C, Wamsley EJ EJ, Vangel M, Montrose DM, Miewald J, et al. Sleep spindle deficits in antipsychotic-naïve early course schizophrenia and in non-psychotic first-degree relatives. Front Hum Neurosci. 2014;8:762. doi:10.3389/fnhum.2014.00762.eCollection2014.

Martin SE, Wraith PK, Deary IJ, Douglas NJ. The effect of nonvisible sleep fragmentation on daytime function. Am J Respir Crit Care Med. 1997;155:1596–601.

Martin N, Lafortune N, Godbout J, Barakat M, Robillard R, Poirier G, et al. Topography of age-related changes in sleep spindles. Neurobiol Aging. 2013;34:468–76.

Martinez D, Breitenbach TC, Lenz MDCS. Light sleep and sleep time misperception - relationship to alpha-delta sleep. Clin Neurophysiol. 2010;121:704–11.

Meza S, Giannouli E, Younes M. Enhancements to the multiple sleep latency test. Nat Sci Sleep. 2016;8:145–58.

Moldofsky H, Scarisbrick P, England R, Smythe H. Musculosketal symptoms and non-REM sleep disturbance in patients with "fibrositis syndrome" and healthy subjects. Psychosom Med. 1975;37:341–51.

Mölle M, Marshall L, Gais S, Born J. Grouping of spindle activity during slow oscillations in human non-rapid eye movement sleep. J Neurosci. 2002;22:10941–7.

Nicolas A, Petit D, Rompré S, Montplaisir J. Sleep spindle characteristics in healthy subjects of different age groups. Clin Neurophysiol. 2001;112:521–7.

Nilsson PM, Rööst M, Engström G, Hedblad B, Berglund G. Incidence of diabetes in middle-aged men is related to sleep disturbances. Diabetes Care. 2004;27:2464–69.

Nissen C, Kloepfer C, Nofzinger EA, Feige B, Voderholzer U, Riemann D. Impaired sleep-related memory consolidation in primary insomnia. Sleep. 2006;29:1068–73.

Norman RG, Pal I, Stewart C, Walsleben JA, Rapoport DM. Interobserver agreement among sleep scorers from different centers in a large dataset. Sleep. 2000;23:901–8.

Ohayon MM. Prevalence and correlates of nonrestorative sleep complaints. Arch Intern Med. 2005;165:35–41.

Ohayon M, Reynolds III CF. Epidemiological and clinical relevance of insomnia diagnoses algorithms according to the DSM-IV and the international classification of sleep disorders (ICSD). Sleep Med. 2009;10:952–60.

Olsen MN, Sherry DD, Boyne K, McCue R, Gallagher PR, Brooks LJ. Relationship between sleep and pain in adolescents with juvenile primary fibromyalgia syndrome. Sleep. 2013;36:509–16.

Parekh A, Selesnick IW, Rapoport DM, Ayappa I. Detection of K-complexes and sleep spindles (DETOKS) using sparse optimization. J Neurosci Methods. 2015;251:37–46.

Parrino L, Milioli G, De Paolis F, Grassi A, Terzano MG. Paradoxical insomnia: the role of CAP and arousals in sleep misperception. Sleep Med. 2009;10:1139–45.

Patel S, Hu FB. Short sleep duration and weight gain: a systematic review. Obesity. 2008;16:643–53.

Penzel T, Hirshkowitz M, Harsh J, Chervin RD, Butkov N, Kryger M, et al. Digital analysis and technical specifications. J Clin Sleep Med. 2007;3:109–20.

Perlis ML, Smith MT, Andrews PJ, Orff H, Giles DE. Beta/Gamma EEG activity in patients with primary and secondary insomnia and good sleeper controls. Sleep. 2001;24:110–7.

Peters KR, Rockwood K, Black SE, Hogan DB, Gauthier SG, Loy-English I, et al. Neuropsychiatric symptom clusters and functional disability in cognitively-impaired-not-demented individuals. Am J Geriatr Psychiatry. 2008;16:136–44.

Philip P, Stoohs R, Guilleminault C. Sleep fragmentation in normals: a model for sleepiness associated with upper airway resistance syndrome. Sleep. 1994;17:242–7.

Pittman SD, MacDonald MM, Fogel RB, Malhotra A, Todros K, Levy B, et al. Assessment of automated scoring of polysomnographic recordings in a population with suspected sleepdisordered breathing. Sleep. 2004;27:1394–403.

Pivik RT, Harman K. A reconceptualization of EEG alpha activity as an index of arousal during sleep: all alpha activity is not equal. J Sleep Res. 1995;4:131–37.

Principe JC, Smith JR. Sleep spindle characteristics as a function of age. Sleep. 1982;5:73–84.

Punjabi NM, Shifa N, Doffner G, Patil S, Pien G, Aurora RN. Computerassisted automated scoring of polysomnograms using the somnolyzer system. Sleep. 2015;38:1555–66.

Ray LB, Sockeel S, Soon M, Bore A, Myhr A, Stojanoski B, et al. Expert and crowd-sourced validation of an individualized sleep spindle detection method employing complex demodulation and individualized normalization. Front Hum Neurosci. 2015;9:507.

Rechtschaffen A, Kales A. A manual of standardized terminology, techniques and scoring system for sleep stages of human subjects. Washington, DC: National Institute of Health, Publ. 204, US Government Printing Office; 1968.

Richard C, Lengelle R. Joint time and time-frequency optimal detection of K-complexes in sleep EEG. Comput Biomed Res. 1998;31:209–29.

Riedner BA, Goldstein MR, Plante DT, Rumble ME, Ferrarelli F, Tononi G, et al. Regional patterns of elevated alpha and high-frequency electroencephalographic activity during nonrapid eye movement sleep in chronic insomnia: a pilot study. Sleep. 2016;39:801–12.

Riemann D, Voderholzer U. Primary insomnia: a risk factor to develop depression? J Affect Disorders. 2003;76:255–59.

Riemann D, Spiegelhalder K, Feige B, Voderholzer U, Berger M, Perlis M, et al. The hyperarousal model of insomnia: a review of the concept and its evidence. Sleep Med Rev. 2010;14:19–31.

Roehrs T, Merlotti L, Petrucelli N, Stepanski E, Roth T. Experimental sleep fragmentation. Sleep. 1994;17:438–43.

Rosenberg RS, Van Hout S. The American academy of sleep medicine interscorer reliability program: sleep stage scoring. J Clin Sleep Med. 2013;9:81–7.

Schabus M, Hodlmoser KH, Gruber G, Sauter C, Anderer P, Klösch G, et al. Sleep spindle-related activity in the human EEG and its relation to general cognitive and learning abilities. Eur J Neurosci. 2006;23:1738–46.

Scheuler W, Stinshoff D, Kubicki S. The alpha-sleep pattern. Differentiation from other sleep patterns and effect of hypnotics. Neuropsychobiology. 1983;10:183–9.

Selvitellia MF, Krishnamurthya KB, Herzog AG, Schomer DL, Chang BS. Sleep spindle alterations in patients with malformations of cortical development. Brain Dev. 2009;31:163–8.

Spiegel K, Tasali E, Leproult R, Van Cauter E. Effects of poor and short sleep on glucose metabolism and obesity risk. Nat Rev Endocr. 2009;5:253–61.

Stone KC, Taylor DJ, McCrae CS, Kalsekar A, Lichstein KL. Nonrestorative sleep. Sleep Med Rev. 2008;12:275–88.

Wamsley EJ, Tucker MA, Shinn AK, Ono KE, McKinley SK, Ely AV, et al. Reduced sleep spindles and spindle coherence in schizophrenia: mechanisms of impaired memory consolidation? Biol Psychiatry. 2012;71:154–61.

Warby SC, Wendt SL, Welinder P, Munk EG, Carrillo O, Sorensen HB, et al. Sleep-spindle detection: crowdsourcing and evaluating performance of experts, non-experts and automated methods. Nat Methods. 2014;11:385–92.

Wei HG, Riel E, Czeisler CA, Dijk DJ. Attenuated amplitude of circadian and sleep-dependent modulation of electroencephalographic sleep spindle characteristics in elderly human subjects. Neurosci Lett. 1999;260:29–32.

Wendt SL, Christensen JA, Kempfner J, Leonthin HL, Jennum P, Sorensen HB. Validation of a novel automatic sleep spindle detector with high performance during sleep in middle aged subjects. Conf Proc IEEE Eng Med Biol Soc. 2012;2012:4250–3.

Wendt SL, Welinder P, Sorensen HB, Peppard PE, Jennum P, Perona P, et al. Inter-expert and intra-expert reliability in sleep spindle scoring. Clin Neurophysiol. 2015;126:1548–56.

Yotsumoto Y, Sasaki Y, Chan P, Vasios CE, Bonmassar G, Ito N, et al. Location-specific cortical activation changes during sleep after training for perceptual learning. Curr Biol. 2009;19:1278–82.

Younes M. Role of arousals in the pathogenesis of obstructive sleep apnea. Amer J Respir Crit Care Med. 2004;169:623–33.

Younes M, Soiferman M, Thompson W, Giannouli E. Performance of a New Portable Wireless Sleep Monitor. J Clin Sleep Med. 2016. Acceptable for Publication with 2016 Oct 20.

Younes M, Hanly PJ. Immediate post-arousal sleep dynamics: an important determinant of sleep stability in obstructive sleep apnea. J Appl Physiol. 2016;120:801–8.

Younes M, Hanly PJ. Minimizing Interrater Variability in Staging Sleep by Use of Computer-Derived Features. J Clin Sleep Med. 2016. [Epub ahead of print].

Younes M, Ostrowski M, Soiferman M, Younes H, Younes M, Raneri J, Hanly P. Odds ratio product of sleep EEG as a continuous measure of sleep state. Sleep. 2015a;28:641–54.

Younes M, Thompson W, Leslie C, Egan T, Giannouli E. Utility of technologist editing of polysomnography scoring performed by a validated automatic system. Ann Am Thorac Soc. 2015b;12:1206–18.

Younes M, Younes M, Giannouli E. Accuracy of automatic polysomnography scoring using frontal electrodes. J Clin Sleep Med. 2015c;12:735–46.

Younes M, Raneri J, Hanly P. Staging sleep in polysomnograms: analysis of inter-scorer variability. J Clin Sleep Med. 2016;12:885–94.

Zhang X, Dong X, Kantelhardt JW, Li J, Zhao L, Garcia C, et al. Process and outcome for international reliability in sleep scoring. Sleep Breath. 2015;19:191–5.

15

Rapid Eye Movement (REM) rebound on initial exposure to CPAP therapy: a systematic review and meta-analysis

Gaurav Nigam[1*], Macario Camacho[2] and Muhammad Riaz[3]

Abstract

Objective: Rapid Eye Movement (REM) rebound is a polysomnographic phenomenon where a substantial increase in REM sleep is noted in patients with untreated obstructive sleep apnea (OSA) when first undergoing continuous positive airway pressure (CPAP) titration. The objectives of this study are to determine: 1) the percentage of patients experiencing REM rebound during CPAP titrations, 2) to quantify the relative increase in REM sleep duration and 3) to identify if there are patient variables associated with REM rebound.

Methods: Four databases (including PubMed/Medline) were systematically searched through March 12, 2017.

Results: Four hundred sixty-seven articles were screened, 58 were reviewed in full-text form and 14 studies met the criteria for inclusion in this review. Eleven of the fourteen studies noted a statistically significant increase in amount of REM sleep during the titration night, compared to baseline sleep study. Pre- and post-CPAP REM sleep duration percentage means ± standard deviations (M ± SD) in 1119 patients increased from 13.8 ± 8.2% to 20.0 ± 10.1%; random effects modeling demonstrated a mean difference of 7.86 (%) [95% CI 5.01, 10.70], p-value <0.00001, corresponding to a 57% relative increase in REM sleep duration. The standardized mean difference (SMD) is 0.90 [95% CI 0.59, 1.22], representing a large magnitude of effect.

Conclusions: In studies reporting REM rebound, the REM sleep duration increased by 57% during the first CPAP titration night compared to the baseline sleep study. The prevalence of REM rebound varied between 23 and 46%. A low amount of REM sleep on the diagnostic PSG predicted REM rebound.

Keywords: REM rebound, Continuous positive airway pressure, Cortical arousal, Adherence, Obstructive sleep apnea, Sleep hypnogram

Background

The hypnogram obtained during a sleep study in a patient with untreated obstructive sleep apnea (OSA) has certain distinct features. The majority of them have fragmented sleep architecture with limited amounts of Rapid Eye Movement (REM) and slow wave sleep. Historically, the sleep fragmentation has been attributed to the preponderance of arousals that are temporally associated with respiratory events in patients with untreated OSA (Remmers et al. 1978). Early experimental studies of selective sleep deprivation have demonstrated that stage REM sleep is highly susceptible to eradication by repetitive arousals, more so than stage slow wave sleep (Agnew et al. 1967). This might suggest that REM sleep is more frequently abolished by untreated OSA, as compared to slow wave sleep.

When first exposed to continuous positive airway pressure (CPAP), certain favorable changes occur in the sleep architecture. CPAP therapy leads to a reduction in the arousal index, sleep stage shifts and non-rapid eye movement (NREM) stage 1 (Loredo et al. 2006). Consequently, sleep becomes more consolidated with an increase in the duration of REM sleep compared to the diagnostic study. REM rebound (Brillante et al. 2012; Koo et al. 2012; Kushida et al. 2011; Yaegashi et al. 2009; Osuna et al. 2008; Drake et al. 2003; Verma et al. 2001; Randerath et al. 2001; Parrino et al. 2000; Yamashiro and

* Correspondence: dr.nigamgaurav@gmail.com
[1]Clay County Hospital, 911 Stacy Burk Drive, Flora, IL 62839, USA
Full list of author information is available at the end of the article

Kryger 1995; Lamphere et al. 1989; Aldrich et al. 1989; Issa and Sullivan 1986; Collard et al. 1996) is the polysomnographic phenomenon of substantial increase in duration of REM sleep in a patient with untreated OSA when first undergoing CPAP titration. Similarly, some patients may exhibit an increase in the duration of slow wave sleep called slow wave sleep rebound (Brillante et al. 2012; Osuna et al. 2008; Verma et al. 2001).

REM rebound on the first night of CPAP use has multiple clinical implications. Clinically, patients exhibiting REM rebound have reported better sleep quality on CPAP titration night than on nights with untreated OSA (Osuna et al. 2008). In new CPAP users early CPAP adherence was found to be higher in patients exhibiting significant REM rebound during CPAP titration night (Koo et al. 2012). Currently, there are no consensus guidelines as to how much increase in duration of REM sleep in the titration night over the baseline sleep study (or baseline portion of a split night study) qualifies as REM rebound. The primary objective of this study was to determine if there is a statistically significant increase in percentage of REM sleep during CPAP titration as compared to baseline polysomnogram (PSG), in patients undergoing CPAP titration after being diagnosed with OSA. Secondary objectives were to quantify the relative increase in REM sleep duration and to predict polysomnographic factors associated with REM rebound. In order to meet the objectives of this review, a systematic review of the literature was performed to identify studies reporting REM rebound on the CPAP titration night as compared to the baseline sleep study night, and the quantitative data was used to determine the percent increase in REM sleep duration using a meta-analysis with random effects modeling.

Methods

The Preferred Reporting Items for Systematic Reviews and Meta-Analyses (PRISMA) statement checklist was used to report the findings of this systematic review (Fig. 1). Two authors (GN and MR) conducted a systematic search of electronic databases that included PubMed, Medline, Scopus, Web of Science and Cochrane Library from inception through March 12, 2017.

Protocol

The Tripler Army Medical Center Department of Clinical Investigation approved the protocol for this meta-analysis (Protocol TAMC 16N14).

Search strategy

The search included Medical Subject Headings (MeSH) terms, key words, and phrases in combinations to obviate missing articles due to the use of select terminology in the different databases. To make the search thorough,

hand searches of the reference lists of relevant articles were performed in order to identify other pertinent articles. Also, meticulous grey literature and Google Scholar searches were performed to identify relevant publications that could have been missed during the electronic database search. Search was restricted to English language articles only. An example of a PubMed search is: (((("Continuous Positive Airway Pressure"[Mesh] AND "Sleep, REM"[Mesh] OR ("Continuous Positive Airway Pressure"[Mesh] AND "Sleep, REM"[Mesh]) AND "Sleep Apnea, Obstructive"[Mesh], Increase* in REM sleep AND CPAP*, rapid eye movement sleep [tiab] AND CPAP [tiab]))) All articles were reviewed which discussed REM rebound in patients with OSA. Articles meeting the inclusion criteria were included in the systematic review.

Inclusion criteria using **PICOS** were: 1) *Patients:* those diagnosed with OSA, 2) *Intervention:* CPAP therapy, 3) *Comparison:* a) studies assessing amount of increase in REM sleep during CPAP titration as compared to amount of REM sleep in baseline PSG, b) and/or studies discussing slow-wave sleep rebound in addition to REM rebound, and c) studies looking for correlation between sleep quality or CPAP adherence and REM rebound, 4) *Outcomes:* the REM sleep duration differences on CPAP therapy during the titration night compared to the baseline PSG, and 5) *Study design:* randomized controlled trials, prospective and retrospective cohort studies, and case series. Exclusion criteria included: 1) Studies on sleep-disordered breathing (SDB) which exclusively discussed slow-wave sleep rebound, 2) Home sleep apnea studies with no electrooculography (EEG) and electromyography (EMG) monitoring capability, and 3) Individual case reports, editorials, review articles, and meeting abstracts.

Statistical analysis

Statistical evaluation was performed using Review Manager (REVMAN) Software version 5.3. The pre- and post-CPAP REM percentage, standard deviations (SD), mean differences (MD), 95% confidence intervals (CI) and p-values were calculated using the IBM Statistical Package for Social Sciences (SPSS) software. Combined mean differences and 95% CI were calculated only for studies reporting means and SD. The null hypothesis for the study was that there is no difference in percentages of REM sleep rebound between baseline PSG versus titration study and in order to test this hypothesis the data was analyzed using post minus pre CPAP therapy outcome data. A random effects modeling was utilized and the overall effect size estimation was performed by calculating the standardized mean difference (SMD). Cohen's guidelines were used to determine the magnitude of the effect size, and the SMD cutoff values were:

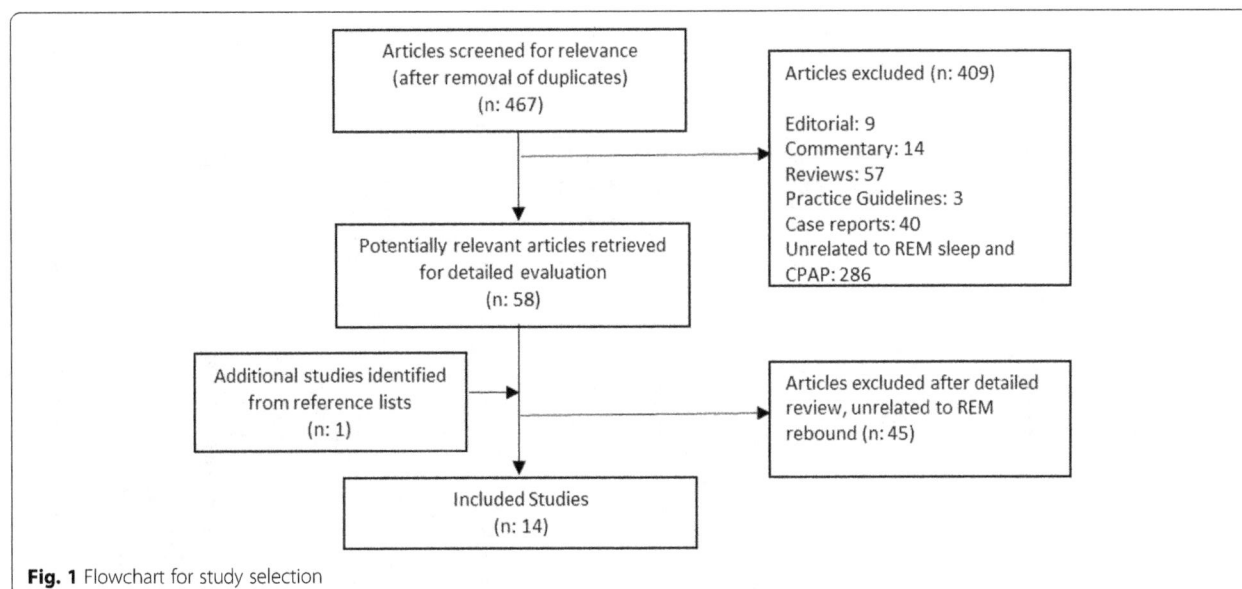

Fig. 1 Flowchart for study selection

small = 0.2, medium = 0.5 and large = 0.8 (Cohen 1988). Heterogeneity was defined as a REVMAN Q-statistic value of ≤0.10 (Lau et al. 1997), and the REVMAN I^2 value cutoffs for inconsistency were 25% = low inconsistency, 50% = moderate inconsistency and 75% = high inconsistency (Higgins et al. 2003). The risk of bias was assessed (as recommended by the Cochrane Collaboration) by assessment of the funnel plots if there are at least ten studies in the variable of interest.

Results

Four hundred sixty-seven articles were screened, 58 were evaluated in full-text form, and 14 studies met the established criteria (Brillante et al. 2012; Koo et al. 2012; Kushida et al. 2011; Yaegashi et al. 2009; Osuna et al. 2008; Drake et al. 2003; Verma et al. 2001; Randerath et al. 2001; Parrino et al. 2000; Yamashiro and Kryger 1995; Lamphere et al. 1989; Aldrich et al. 1989; Issa and Sullivan 1986; Collard et al. 1996). Eleven of the 14 studies noted a statistically significant increase in amount of REM sleep during the titration night, compared to the baseline sleep study. Overall, data was reported for 1119 patients, with an average age 53.7 ± 12.6 years and body mass index (BMI) 34.6 ± 11.2 kg/m² (Table 1). Patients with all severities of OSA were included with the highest mean apnea-hypopnea index (AHI) being 72.9 ± 21.5 in the Lamphere et al. study. All studies showed a predominance of male subjects, and they made up 66% (Osuna et al.) to 95% (Collard et al.) of the patient population being studied.

Of the 14 studies meeting inclusion criteria, only three studies (Brillante, Koo and Osuna et al. studies) defined what they considered as REM rebound. The remaining studies provided some measure of increase in REM sleep

during titration night compared to baseline sleep study. Most studies reported REM rebound in percentage increase in REM sleep duration when comparing titration to baseline sleep study except two studies (Aldrich et al. and Parrino et al.) where the relative increase in REM sleep was reported only in minutes. On an average, percentage of REM sleep in diagnostic PSG varied from 6.7 ± 9.3% in Koo et al. study to 18.4 ± 2.0% in Issa et al. study. During the titration study, 11 of the 14 studies noted a statistically significant increase in amount of REM sleep compared to baseline sleep study, with two studies (Koo and Kushida et al.) not mentioning the statistically significant status. One study (Randerath et al.) reported that the increase was not statistically significant. REM sleep percentages during titration study varied between 17.1 ± 7.4 in Randerath et al. study to 30.6 ± 2.0 in Issa et al. study.

In studies reporting statistically significant increase in the percentage of REM sleep, the percentage of increase varied on average from 1.5% in Brillante et al. study to 14.1% in Yamashiro et al. study (Fig. 2). Although Koo et al. study reported an even higher increase in the average percentage of REM sleep at 16.6% (compared to Yamashiro study reporting an increase of 14.1%) it was not stated whether this increase was statistically significant, when considering all patients. Incidentally, the two studies with highest percentage increase in REM sleep duration during CPAP titration also represented the only split night studies of this review.

As mentioned previously, three studies (Brillante, Koo and Osuna et al. studies) selected specific percentage cut-off values to define REM rebound. This was determined using a statistical prediction model used by the individual studies. Defining REM rebound as 20% or

Table 1 Demographic Characteristics along with Pre- and Post- CPAP means, standard deviations, mean differences, and confidence intervals for REM rebound percentage

Author, year	Study type	Definition of REM rebound	Number	Age, years	BMI, Kg/m²	Pre-CPAP REM %	Post-CPAP REM%	MD (95% CI)	P-value
Brillante et al. 2012	Retrospective	20% or more increase in % REM sleep on titration night when compared to baseline PSG	335	54.0 ± 13.9	33.3 ± 7.3	16.9 ± 7.8	18.4 ± 8.8	1.5 (2.762, 0.238)	0.0199
Koo et al. 2012	Retrospective	At least one REM period of >/30 min duration in the treatment portion AND an increase in REM in the treatment portion of >/20%	95	56.7 ± 11.1	35.0 ± 7.0	6.7 ± 9.3	23.3 ± 15.1	16.5 (12.911, 20.089)	0.0001
Kushida et al. 2011	Prospective Randomized, controlled trial	-	57	48.8 ± 12	34.9 ± 8.0	13.1 ± 9.0	22.8 ± 8.4	9.7 (6.469, 12.931)	0.0001
Yaegashi et al. 2009	Retrospective	-	280	58.6 ± 14.7	25.7 ± 3.9	13.1 ± 6.2	18.1 ± 7.0	5.0 (3.902, 6.098)	0.0001
Osuna et al. 2008	Retrospective	6% or more increase in % REM sleep on titration night when compared to baseline PSG	179 (118 M + 61 F)	48.6 ± 4 (M) 51.6 ± 12.9 (F)[c]	33.7 ± 7.7 (M) 39.2 ± 8.2 (F)[c]	15.55	21.57	-	-
Drake et al. 2003	Prospective	-	71	50.7 ± 10.6	-	12.8 ± 5.6	19.1 ± 8.9	6.3 (3.833, 8.767)	0.0001
Verma et al. 2001	Retrospective	-	44	51.6	-	12.1 ± 8.3[a] 12.7 ± 9.0[b]	17.2 ± 8.1[a] 15.6 ± 8.6[b]	5.1 (1.624,8.576) 2.9 (−0.831, 6.631)	0.0045 0.1259
Randerath et al. 2001	Prospective	-	25	52.8 ± 9.0	31.4 ± 5.0	14.2 ± 6.7	17.1 ± 7.4	2.9 (−1.114, 6.914)	0.1529
Parrino et al. 2000	Retrospective	-	10	47.4 ± 5.3	>36	81 ± 30[d]	149 ± 32[d]	68 (38.86, 97.14)	0.0001
Collard et al. 1996	Prospective	-	80	52.1 ± 10.6	33.4 ± 6.6	17.8 ± 6.9	21.9 ± 9.5	4.1 (1.507, 6.693)	0.0021
Yamashiro and Kryger 1995	Prospective	-	107	52.3 ± 12.1	34.4 ± 8.2	11.2 ± 9.5	25.3 ± 14.4	14.1 (10.812, 17.388)	0.0001
Lamphere et al. 1989	Prospective	-	13	50.1 ± 11.6[e]	35.6 ± 9.5	9.2 ± 6.4	20.4 ± 8.7	11.2 (5.018, 17.382)	0.0010
Aldrich et al. 1989	Prospective	-	26	47	-	43.1 ± 5.4[d]	73.3 ± 6.9[d]	30.2 (26.749, 33.651)	0.0001
Issa and Sullivan 1986	Prospective	-	12	47.4	18.4 ± 2.0	18.4 ± 2.0	30.6 ± 2.0	12.2 (10.507, 13.893)	0.0001
Combined Means				53.65 ± 12.60	34.58 ± 11.20	13.82 ± 8.17	19.99 ± 10.06	6.17 (5.408, 6.931)	0.0001
			1252	1171	1119	1119			

Note: Osuna, Parrino & Aldrich studies were not included for combined means for REM sleep percentage given missing standard deviations for Osuna study and Parrino & Aldrich reported minutes rather than percentage. In Verma et al. study, only patients[a] who report improvement on CPAP were included for combined means

N sample size, MD mean difference, CI confidence interval

[a]Denotes: % REM sleep in patients who noted an improvement (CPAP PSG Likert scale score −diagnostic PSG Likert scale score > 0) and

[b]Denotes: % REM sleep in patients that did not note an improvement (CPAP PSG Likert scale score - diagnostic PSG Likert scale score less than or equal to 0)

[c]Denotes individual average for males and females respectively, i.e. 48.6 ± 4 for males (M), and 51.6 ± 12.9 for females (F)

[d]Denotes amount of REM sleep attained in minutes, not the Percentage of Total sleep time spent in REM

[e]Denotes average values for the entire cohort of 39 patient prior to randomization while other values listed herein depict the numbers obtained from 1st night CPAP titration cohort after randomization

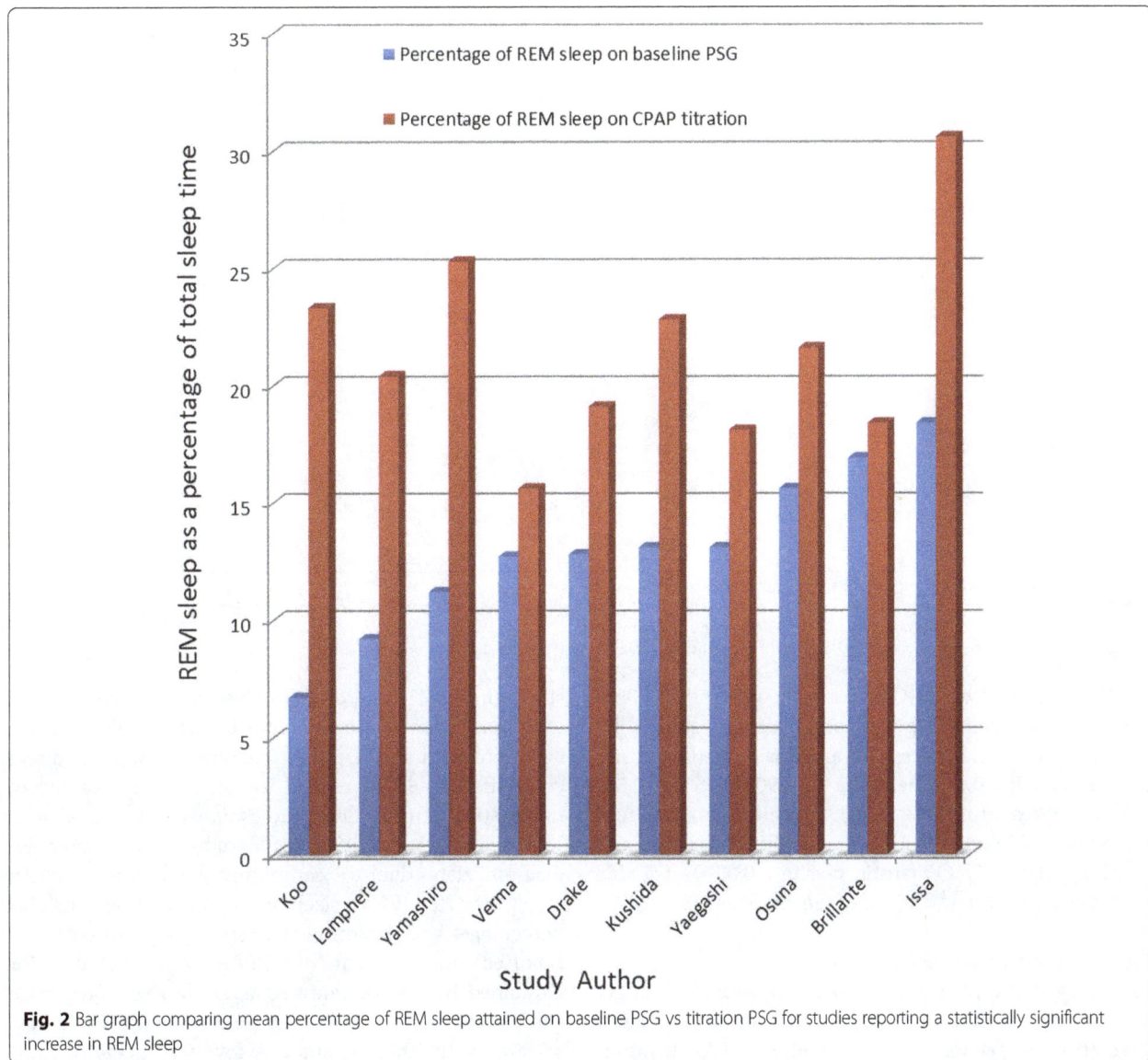

Fig. 2 Bar graph comparing mean percentage of REM sleep attained on baseline PSG vs titration PSG for studies reporting a statistically significant increase in REM sleep

more increase in duration of REM sleep on titration night compared to baseline PSG, Brillante et al. and Koo et al. found that 23% and 37% of patients respectively, met criteria for REM rebound. On the other hand, employing 6% or more increase in REM sleep duration on titration night compared to baseline PSG as the definition of REM rebound, Osuna et al. found that 46% patients met criteria for REM rebound. All except two studies (Yamashiro et al. and Koo et al.) used data derived from titration studies to calculate REM rebound (Table 2).

Mean differences and standardized mean differences

Based on polysomnography data, the CPAP REM percentage means ± standard deviations (M ± SD) in 1119 patients increased from 13.8 ± 8.2% to 20.0 ± 10.1% (a mean difference of 6.2%) which corresponds to a 44.6%

relative percentage increase of REM sleep during the CPAP treatment compared to baseline (Table 1). Analysis of studies using random effects modeling was performed for REM rebound percentage on titration with mean difference (MD) 7.86% [95% CI 5.01, 10.70], overall effect Z = 5.41, p-value <0.00001, Q statistic p-value <0.00001 (significant heterogeneity), $I^2 = 94\%$ (high inconsistency) (Fig. 3). The mean difference of 7.9% corresponds to a 57% relative percentage increase of REM sleep during the CPAP treatment compared to baseline. The risk of bias was high as the funnel plot for REM rebound percentage mean difference was significantly asymmetrically shaped. The sensitivity analysis demonstrated two sub-groups of studies that were non-heterogenous when combined, the first non-heterogenous sub-group comprised the studies by Yaegashi et al., Drake et al., Verma et al., Randerath

Table 2 REM rebound on CPAP titration: PSG parameters

Study, year	Baseline AHI	% of patients with REM rebound	Titration (T) or Split night (SN) study
Brillante et al. 2012	40.7 ± 26.1	23%	T
Koo et al. 2012	44.5 ± 28.8	37%	SN
Kushida et al. 2011	41.1 ± 31.6	-	T
Yaegashi et al. 2009	48.5 ± 20.2	-	T
Osuna et al. 2008	>10[a]	46%	T
Drake et al. 2003	62.0 ± 32.2	-	T
Verma et al. 2001	RDI >10[a]	-	T
Randerath et al. 2001	32.2 ± 18.1	-	T[c]
Parrino et al. 2000	67.9	-	T
Collard et al. 1996	24.2 ± 18.8	-	T
Yamashiro and Kryger 1995	23.6 ± 26.3	-	SN[b]
Lamphere et al. 1989	72.9 ± 21.5	-	T
Aldrich et al. 1989	69.6 ± 5.9	-	T
Issa and Sullivan 1986	57.6	-	T

[a]Denotes AHI cut off criteria for entry into the study, not the mean AHI
[b]Denotes that this study reported data from both Split night study as well as titration night study, but data tabulated represents Split night values as this was the study with first exposure to CPAP occurred and first REM rebound was witnessed
[c]Denotes PSG data collected from fixed CPAP setting, obtained using a manual CPAP titration 1–2 days prior

et al. and Collard et al. (Q-statistic $p = 0.62$ and $I^2 = 0\%$); while the second sub-group comprised the studies by Yamashiro et al., Lampere et al. and Issa et al. (Q-statistic $p = 0.54$ and $I^2 = 0\%$). The SMD is 0.90 [95% CI 0.59, 1.22], representing a large magnitude of effect (Cohen's guidelines) with an overall effect $Z = 5.60$, p-value <0.00001, Q statistic p-value <0.00001 (significant heterogeneity), $I^2 = 90\%$ (high inconsistency).

Predictive factors for REM rebound

Of the 14 studies, five studies (Brillante et al., Koo et al., Osuna et al., Verma et al. and Aldrich et al.) discussed predictive factors for REM rebound on CPAP titration (Table 3). High AHI on baseline PSG was found to be a predictive factor in all five studies, however a direct linear correlation could not be conclusively established between baseline AHI and "Delta REM" (denoting difference between percentage of REM sleep in post CPAP study and percentage of REM sleep in pre CPAP study), when data from all studies reporting REM sleep percentage were included (Fig. 4). Inability to establish direct correlation could be related to variability in rapidity of up-titration of individual studies as well as exclusion of Verma et al. and Aldrich et al. studies from scatter dot diagram data due to computing limitations; Aldrich et al. reported REM sleep in minutes rather than as percentages and in Verma et al. study, only patients who reported improvement on CPAP were included for combined means. Brillante et al. study also noted male gender and high arousal index on baseline PSG to be associated with REM rebound. A low percentage of REM sleep on baseline PSG was likely to result in greater "Delta REM" or REM rebound as found in three studies (Brillante et al., Koo et al. and Verma et al.). It was further corroborated when this inverse relationship was depicted on the scatter dot diagram when data from all

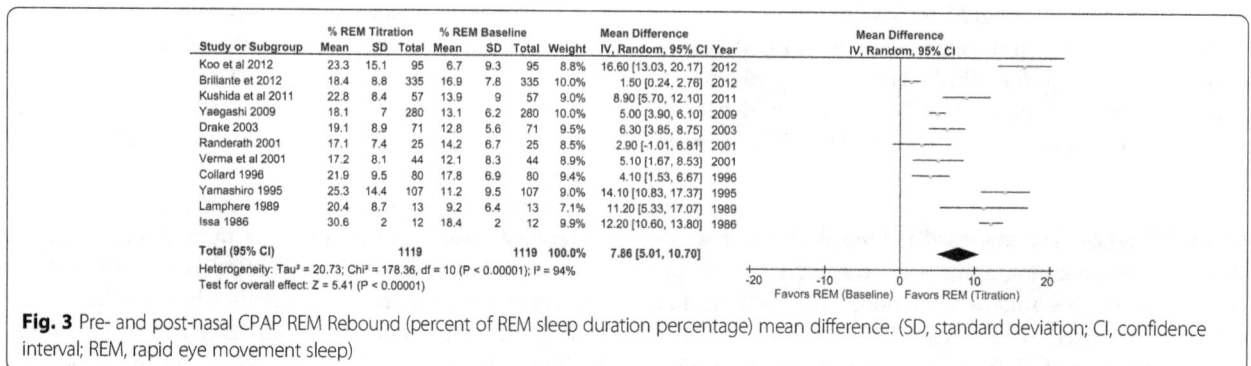

Fig. 3 Pre- and post-nasal CPAP REM Rebound (percent of REM sleep duration percentage) mean difference. (SD, standard deviation; CI, confidence interval; REM, rapid eye movement sleep)

Table 3 Predictive factors for REM rebound on CPAP titration

Study	High AHI on baseline PSG	Low % of REM sleep on baseline PSG	High arousal index on baseline PSG	Male gender	Low oxygen saturation on baseline PSG	High BMI
Brillante et al.	✓	✓	✓	✓	-	✗
Koo et al.	✓	-	-	-	-	-
Osuna et al.	✓	✓	-	-	-	✓
Verma et al.	✓	-	-	-	-	-
Aldrich et al.	✓	✓	-	-	✓	-

✓: Denotes that the parameter was studied and was found to be statistically significant factor for REM rebound
✗: Denotes that the parameter was studied but was not found to be statistically significant factor for REM rebound
- : Denotes that the parameter was not studied

studies reporting REM sleep percentage were included (Fig. 5). In the study by Osuna et al. (average BMI: 35.5 kg/m²), obesity was associated with REM rebound; however, the study by Brillante et al. (average BMI: 33.3 kg/m²) failed to find a statistically significant association between body weight and REM rebound. Low oxygen saturation on baseline PSG was associated with REM rebound as noted by Aldrich et al.

Study quality assessment
Overall, the studies included in this review met between four to eight out of a total of eight quality assessment

parameters, with most studies meeting five to six parameters. The quality of studies per "NICE guidelines" is outlined in Table 4.

Discussion
This systematic review and meta-analysis has five main findings. First, eleven of fourteen studies reported a statistically significant increase in REM sleep duration during titration night compared the baseline sleep study. While all studies report REM rebound, only a few studies define what REM rebound entails based on their statistical prediction models. Studies adopted cut-off

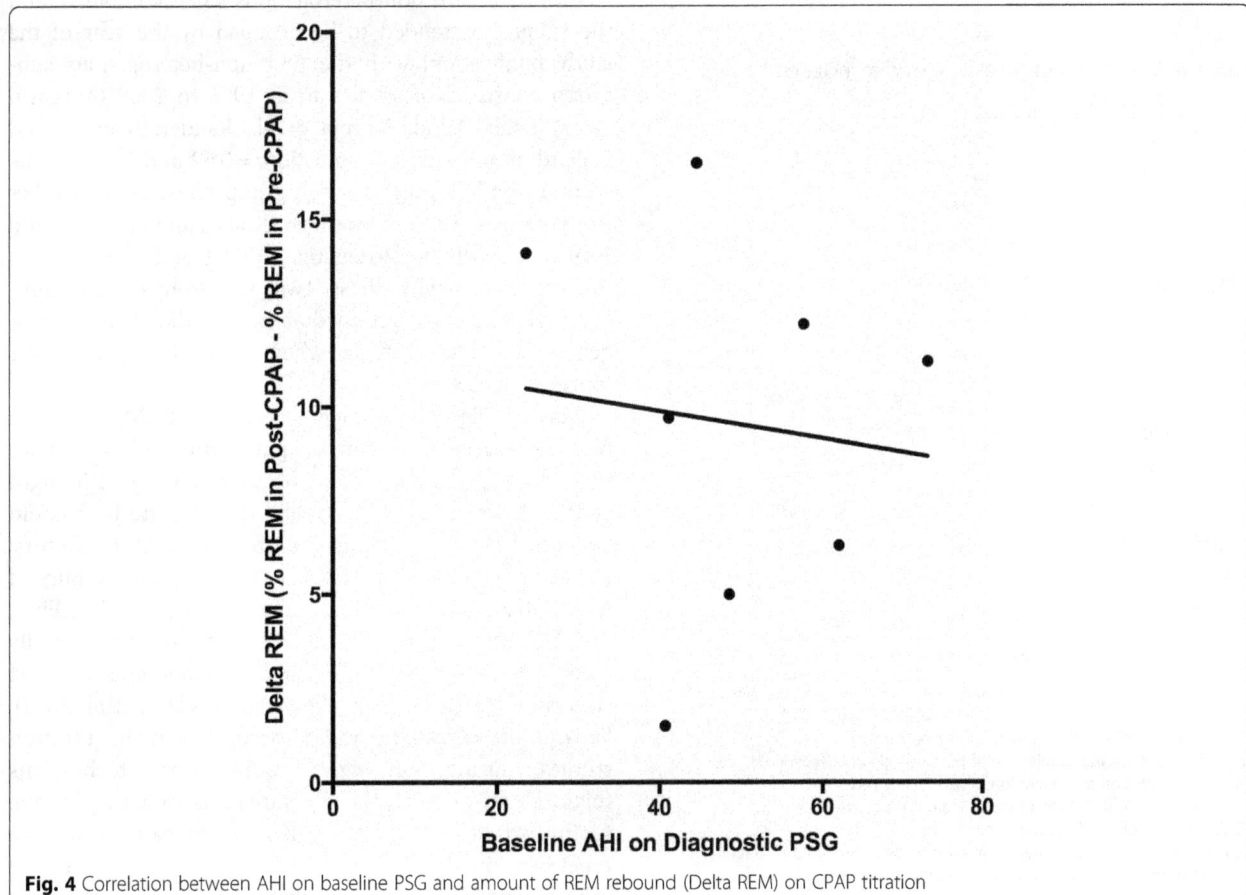

Fig. 4 Correlation between AHI on baseline PSG and amount of REM rebound (Delta REM) on CPAP titration

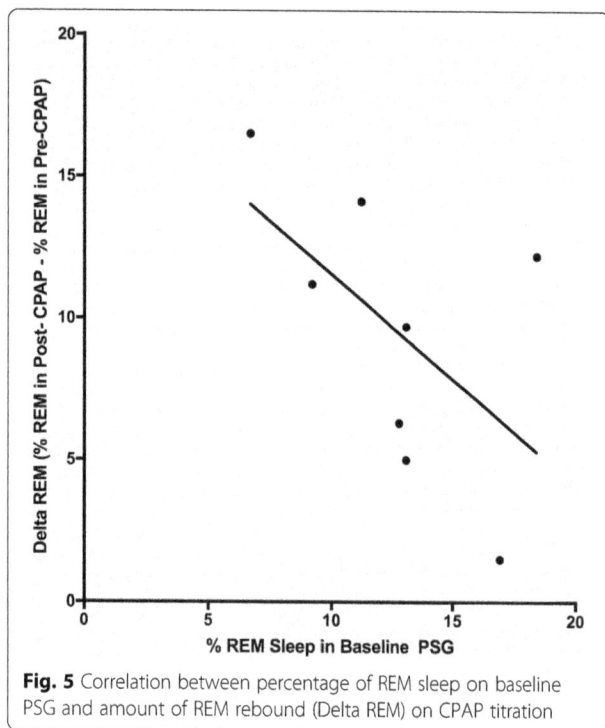

Fig. 5 Correlation between percentage of REM sleep on baseline PSG and amount of REM rebound (Delta REM) on CPAP titration

criteria of 6%-20% increase in percentage REM sleep on titration night when compared to baseline PSG to define REM rebound. Accepting a lower REM percentage increase as the cut -off criteria for REM rebound (when comparing REM percentage in titration study to REM percentage in baseline PSG study) leads to reporting a higher prevalence of REM rebound on CPAP titration. Accordingly, based on cut-off criteria used to define REM rebound, the prevalence of REM rebound varies between 23 and 46% in all patients undergoing CPAP titration study.

Second, when the specific cut-off criteria (in terms of duration of increase in REM sleep percentage) defining REM rebound are overlooked, the majority of patients undergoing a CPAP titration experience increased duration of REM sleep compared to their baseline sleep study. The percentage increase in REM sleep duration varies between 1.5 and 14% and may depend on certain polysomnographic and demographic factors. The mean difference of 7.86% corresponds to a 57% relative percentage increase of REM sleep during the CPAP treatment night compared to the baseline study. When evaluating the effect size based on Cohen's guidelines, the SMD is 0.90 [95% CI 0.59, 1.22], which is defined as a large effect. Interestingly, the sensitivity analysis demonstrated two sub-groups of studies that were non-heterogenous when combined, and the subgroups tended to be grouped by the year of the study publication; with the first non-heterogenous subgroup consisted of studies from 1996 to 2009 (Yaegashi et al., Drake et al., Verma et al., Randerath et al. and Collard et al.) with a Q-statistic $p = 0.62$ and $I^2 = 0\%$. The second non-heterogenous sub-group consisted of studies from 1986 to 1995 (Yamashiro et al., Lampere et al. and Issa et al.) with a Q-statistic $p = 0.54$ and $I^2 = 0\%$. It is unclear as to why these two sub-groups were non-heterogenous when grouped alone, but did cause heterogeneity and inconsistency when grouped as part of the fourteen studies.

Third, a high percentage increase in REM sleep was observed specifically during split night studies. A relatively high proportion of REM sleep during split night studies (compared to full night titration studies) could be multifactorial, associated with at least three factors: (A) the natural timing of REM sleep, (B) the rapidity of up-titrations and (C) the baseline severity of OSA. First, the PAP titration portion of split night study temporally coincides with timing for natural preponderance of REM sleep in the latter half of sleep period (Ciftci et al. 2008). Second, in contrast to dedicated, full night titration studies, during split-night studies, sleep technicians might be up-titrating the pressures relatively rapidly due to limited titration window leading to early, brief but repetitive bursts of saw tooth waves or low voltage mixed frequency REM spikes. Lastly, patients who

Table 4 Assessment of *quality of studies included in the systematic review

Study author	1	2	3	4	5	6	7	8
Brillante et al.	No	Yes	Yes	Yes	No	Yes	Yes	Yes
Koo et al.	No	Yes	Yes	Yes	No	No	Yes	Yes
Kushida et al.	Yes	Yes	Yes	Yes	Yes	Yes	Yes	Yes
Yaegashi et al.	No	Yes	Yes	Yes	No	Yes	Yes	Yes
Osuna et al.	No	Yes	No	Yes	No	Yes	Yes	Yes
Drake et al.	No	Yes	Yes	Yes	Yes	Yes	Yes	Yes
Verma et al.	No	Yes	Yes	Yes	No	Yes	Yes	Yes
Randerath et al.	No	Yes	Yes	Yes	Yes	Yes	Yes	Yes
Parrino et al.	No	Yes	No	Yes	No	No	Yes	Yes
Collard et al.	No	Yes	No	Yes	Yes	Yes	Yes	Yes
Yamashiro et al.	No	Yes	Yes	Yes	Yes	No	Yes	Yes
Lamphere et al.	No	Yes	No	Yes	Yes	No	Yes	Yes
Aldrich et al.	No	Yes	Yes	Yes	Yes	Yes	Yes	Yes
Issa et al.	No	No	No	Yes	Yes	No	Yes	Yes

*Quality assessment of the included studies checklist from questions from National Institute for Health and Clinical Excellence (NICE) 1–8:
1) Case series collected in more than one center?
2) Is the hypothesis/aim/objective of the study clearly described?
3) Are the inclusion and exclusion criteria clearly reported?
4) Is there a clear definition of the outcomes reported?
5) Were data collected prospectively?
6) Is there an explicit statement that patients were recruited consecutively?
7) Are the main findings of the study clearly described?
8) Are outcomes stratified?

undergo split night study typically have severe OSA. In such patients both high baseline AHI and high arousal index from sleep fragmentation, are being simultaneously resolved with PAP therapy, which may be promoting additional periods of restorative REM sleep. Immediate increased REM duration from CPAP use as early as after one night have been observed (Loredo et al. 2006; Issa and Sullivan 1986). So, it is plausible that the rebound REM increase occurs even within a few hours of initiation of CPAP, given that untreated OSA represents a state of several years of chronic partial sleep deprivation as well as sleep fragmentation.

We speculate that the quantity of REM rebound could depend upon rapidity of up- titrations as well how quickly the patient adapted to these up-titrations. In some studies, rapid CPAP up-titration may have led to early attainment of therapeutic pressure providing more time during sleep period to exhibit REM. In other studies, a more conservative and cautious approach may have lead to at least some REM sleep attained chronologically prior to attainment of therapeutic CPAP pressure leading to less REM rebound. Of note, about 5-20% patients may have experienced treatment emergent central sleep apnea or TECSA on first exposure to CPAP during these studies (Nigam et al. 2016). TECSA may have lead to increased arousal index and sleep fragmentation thereby limiting REM rebound which would be subsequently seen after several weeks of CPAP use in this cohort of CPAP users.

Fourth, certain polysomnographic and demographic factors could enhance REM rebound. Two such factors predicting enhanced Delta REM (and thereby predicting substantial REM rebound) as suggested in several studies include: 1) a lower amount of REM sleep on diagnostic PSG (strong association) and 2) a higher severity of OSA as noted by the AHI during diagnostic PSG (weak association, if any). Other possible associations include higher arousal index on baseline PSG, low oxygen saturation on baseline PSG, male gender, higher BMI and utilization of split-night PSG to study REM rebound. Additional research is needed to further evaluate the variables that predict which patients are more likely to experience REM rebound.

Fifth, almost half of the currently published studies were retrospective observational studies and prone to limitations of any retrospective study. There were differences amongst studies as to the definition of REM rebound. The sleep stage and respiratory events scoring rules have undergone considerable changes over the last few decades. Given the review includes studies conducted over last 30 years, the majority of the included studies were scored using Rechtschaffen and Kales manual for the scoring of sleep stages, while others were scored based on the American Academy of Sleep Medicine scoring manual introduced in 2007. The rules for scoring respiratory events have undergone considerable changes as well over the years, making it difficult to directly compare baseline AHIs reported by different authors; however, given that REM is defined based on the electroencephalogram, we believe that despite the differences in the AHI scoring criteria, the percentage of sleep scored for each of the sleep stages, including REM, should not change.

Limitations

We acknowledge that the expression "percentage" increase in REM sleep could arithmetically, sometimes get misconstrued as demonstrated by the following example: a doubling of REM sleep time from 5 to 10 min is not the same as a doubling of REM sleep time from 20 to 40 min. Therefore, we suggest that the percentage of relative increase in REM sleep should be interpreted cautiously in appropriate clinical and polysomnographic context. This "percentage" increase in REM sleep was chosen as they are conventional mathematical tools for data representation. Also, percentages are employed as a standard practice for reporting the proportion of the time spent in different sleep stages on a polysomnogram report. Unfortunately, as demonstrated by the above example, even a small amount of additional time spent in REM during the treatment night could translate to a significantly inflated percentage increase in REM sleep. Consistent with all systematic reviews, it is possible that we missed identifying studies that met our criteria; however, to decrease this possibility, we had two authors search independently. Additionally, our search was restricted to English-language manuscripts only, and there may have been additional studies in other languages. Lastly, as demonstrated by the funnel plot, there is a high risk of publication bias, therefore, it is possible that researchers with negative findings either never shared their findings, or those inferences may have been rejected after submission. Previous studies suggest that sleep stages (including REM stage) recovery after CPAP titration is not an instant "all-or-none phenomenon" but requires several days to weeks before complete return to normal control values (Parrino et al. 2005). This might have lead to underestimation of REM rebound as sleep reorganization is a dynamic adaptive process spanning several weeks, and our work only captured the initial phases of effective CPAP treatment. Our analysis was restricted to REM rebound in terms of duration and percentages; it did not include analysis of REM latency as this parameter was not recorded and shared by most constituent studies.

Conclusion

Significant increase in REM sleep duration can occur in the first CPAP titration night compared to REM sleep duration noted on the baseline sleep study. In studies reporting REM rebound, the REM sleep duration increased by 57% during the first CPAP titration night compared to the baseline sleep study. Although no consensus guidelines exist, various retrospective studies have outlined that 6-20% increase in percentage of REM sleep on titration night compared to baseline PSG could be indicative of REM rebound. The most crucial polysomnographic factor that predicts and promotes REM rebound is low amount of REM sleep attained on the diagnostic PSG. In order to increase the level of evidence, additional high quality, prospective studies will be required in the future.

Abbreviations
AHI: Apnea-hypopnea index; BMI: Body mass index; CI: Confidence interval; CPAP: Continuous positive airway pressure; EEG: Electrooculography; EMG: Electromyography; MD: Mean differences; MeSH: Medical Subject Headings; NREM: Non-rapid eye movement; OSA: Obstructive sleep apnea; PICOS: Patients, Intervention, Comparison, Outcomes, Study Design; PRISMA: Preferred Reporting Items for Systematic Reviews and Meta-Analyses; PSG: Polysomnogram; REM: Rapid eye movement; REVMAN: Review Manager; SD: Standard deviations; SDB: Sleep disorderd breathing; SMD: Standardized mean differences; SPSS: Statistical Package for Social Sciences

Acknowledgements
None.

Funding
None.

Authors' contributions
GN: Substantial contributions to the conception or design of the work; the acquisition, analysis, and interpretation of data for the work; AND Drafting and revising it critically for important intellectual content; AND Final approval of the version to be published; AND Agreement to be accountable for all aspects of the work in ensuring that questions related to the accuracy or integrity of any part of the work are appropriately investigated and resolved. MR: Substantial contributions to the conception of the work; the acquisition, analysis, and interpretation of data for the work; AND Drafting the work and revising it critically for important intellectual content; AND Final approval of the version to be published; AND Agreement to be accountable for all aspects of the work in ensuring that questions related to the accuracy or integrity of any part of the work are appropriately investigated and resolved. MC : Substantial contributions to the interpretation of data for the work; AND revising it critically for important intellectual content; AND Final approval of the version to be published; AND Agreement to be accountable for all aspects of the work in ensuring that questions related to the accuracy or integrity of any part of the work are appropriately investigated and resolved.

Authors' information
None.

Competing interests
The authors declare that they have no competing interests. Authors do not have anything to disclose, this study was not supported by industry. The views expressed in this manuscript are those of the authors and do not reflect the official policy or position of the Department of the Army, Department of Defense, or the US Government.

Author details
[1]Clay County Hospital, 911 Stacy Burk Drive, Flora, IL 62839, USA. [2]Division of Otolaryngology, Sleep Surgery, and Sleep Medicine, Tripler Army Medical Center, 1 Jarrett White Road, Tripler AMC, Honolulu, HI 96859, USA. [3]Sunnyside Community Hospital & Clinics, 208 N. Euclid, Grandview, WA 98930, USA.

References
Agnew Jr HW, Webb WB, Williams RL. Comparison of stage four and 1-rem sleep deprivation. Percept Mot Skills. 1967;24(3):851–8.

Aldrich M, Eiser A, Lee M, Shipley JE. Effects of continuous positive airway pressure on phasic events of REM sleep in patients with obstructive sleep apnea. Sleep. 1989;12(5):413–9.

Brillante R, Cossa G, Liu PY, Laks L. Rapid eye movement and slow-wave sleep rebound after one night of continuous positive airway pressure for obstructive sleep apnoea. Respirology. 2012;17(3):547–53.

Ciftci B, Ciftci TU, Guven SF. Split-night versus full-night polysomnography: comparison of the first and second parts of the night. Arch Bronconeumol. 2008;44(1):3–7.

Cohen J. Statistical power analysis for the behavioral sciences. Kawrence Erlbaum Associates: Hillsdale; 1988.

Collard P, Dury M, Delguste P, Aubert G, Rodenstein DO. Movement arousals and sleep-related disordered breathing in adults. Am J Respir Crit Care Med. 1996;154(2 Pt 1):454–9.

Drake CL, Day R, Hudgel D, Stefadu Y, Parks M, Syron ML, et al. Sleep during titration predicts continuous positive airway pressure compliance. Sleep. 2003;26(3):308–11.

Higgins JP, Thompson SG, Deeks JJ, Altman DG. Measuring inconsistency in meta-analyses. BMJ. 2003;327(7414):557–60.

Issa FG, Sullivan CE. The immediate effects of nasal continuous positive airway pressure treatment on sleep pattern in patients with obstructive sleep apnea syndrome. Electroencephalogr Clin Neurophysiol. 1986;63(1):10–7.

Koo BB, Wiggins R, Molina C. REM rebound and CPAP compliance. Sleep Med. 2012;13(7):864–8.

Kushida CA, Berry RB, Blau A, Crabtree T, Fietze I, Kryger MH, et al. Positive airway pressure initiation: a randomized controlled trial to assess the impact of therapy mode and titration process on efficacy, adherence, and outcomes. Sleep. 2011;34(8):1083–92.

Lamphere J, Roehrs T, Wittig R, Zorick F, Conway WA, Roth T. Recovery of alertness after CPAP in apnea. Chest. 1989;96(6):1364–7.

Lau J, Ioannidis JP, Schmid CH. Quantitative synthesis in systematic reviews. Ann Intern Med. 1997;127(9):820–6.

Loredo JS, Ancoli-Israel S, Kim EJ, Lim WJ, Dimsdale JE. Effect of continuous positive airway pressure versus supplemental oxygen on sleep quality in obstructive sleep apnea: a placebo-CPAP-controlled study. Sleep. 2006;29(4):564–71.

Nigam G, Pathak C, Riaz M. A systematic review on prevalence and risk factors associated with treatment- emergent central sleep apnea. Ann Thorac Med. 2016;11(3):202–10.

Osuna S, Siddiqui F, Vanegas MA, Walters AS, Chokroverty S. Prevalence and factors affecting REM and slow wave sleep rebound on CPAP titration study in patients with obstructive sleep apnea. Revista de la Facultad de Medicina. 2008;56(1):4–10.

Parrino L, Smerieri A, Boselli M, Spaggiari MC, Terzano MG. Sleep reactivity during acute nasal CPAP in obstructive sleep apnea syndrome. Neurology. 2000;54(8):1633–40.

Parrino L, Thomas RJ, Smerieri A, Spaggiari MC, Del Felice A, Terzano MG. Reorganization of sleep patterns in severe OSAS under prolonged CPAP treatment. Clin Neurophysiol. 2005;116(9):2228–39.

Randerath WJ, Galetke W, David M, Siebrecht H, Sanner B, Ruhle K. Prospective randomized comparison of impedance-controlled auto-continuous positive airway pressure (APAP(FOT)) with constant CPAP. Sleep Med. 2001;2(2):115–24.

Remmers JE, De Groot WJ, Sauerland EK, Anch AM. Pathogenesis of upper airway occlusion during sleep. J Appl Physiol Respir Environ Exerc Physiol. 1978;44(6):931–8.

Verma A, Radtke RA, VanLandingham KE, King JH, Husain AM. Slow wave sleep rebound and REM rebound following the first night of treatment with CPAP for sleep apnea: correlation with subjective improvement in sleep quality. Sleep Med. 2001;2(3):215–23.

16

Lung injury and inflammation response by chronic intermittent hypoxia in rats

Huan Lu[†], Xiaodan Wu[†], Cuiping Fu, Jing Zhou and Shanqun Li[*]

Abstract

Background: Chronic intermittent hypoxia is the primary pathophsiological feature of obstructive sleep apnea/hypopnea syndrome. The characteristics of CIH can be imitated by animal experiment models thus to study CIH related systemic organ injuries, including respiratory systems.

Methods: Sixteen male SD rats were randomly divided into two groups: CIH group ($n = 8$) and control group ($n = 8$). The CIH group was exposed to intermittent hypoxia circumstance for 5 weeks (8 h/day) and control group was placed in the same animal chamber exposed to normal air circumstance. Between the two groups, the inflammatory factors of IL-6 and TNF-α within serum and BALF were measured by ELISA; the structure and ultrastructure of lungs were evaluated by HE staining and electronmicroscopy. The nuclear factor-κB (NF-κB) in lung tissue was detected by Western blot.

Results: The concentration of IL-6 and TNF-α in serum in CIH group increased significantly (138.63 ± 43.82 vs. 41.82 ± 5.24 pg/ml and 126.62 ± 34.81 vs. 73.43 ± 5.72 pg/ml, both $P < 0.05$). The concentration of IL-6 and TNF-α in BALF in CIH group was higher than that in control group (67.1 ± 24.2 pg/ml vs 39.8 ± 21.5 pg/ml and 36.61 ± 19.17 pg/ml vs 20.31 ± 8.44 pg/ml, respectively, $P < 0.05$). In the HE staining of lung tissue, results showed that severe inflammatory cell infiltration in alveolar walls and alveolar spaces was found in CIH group and the histological score of CIH group is higher significantly (6.857 ± 0.553 vs. 2.286 ± 0.286 g, $P < 0.05$); In the electronmicroscopy of TypeIIalveolar cells, results showed that karyotheca and endoplasmic reticulum were damaged obviously in Type II alveolar cells. The NF-κB increased significantly in the CIH group compared with control group (0.43 ± 0.1 vs 0.22 ± 0.05, $P < 0.05$).

Conclusions: Animal experiment model can be used to imitate the pathophysiologic changes of CIH. There are systematic and local airway inflammation coexisting in CIH rats. CIH leads to inflammatory cell infiltration and organelle damages within lung tissues. We speculated that there was some correlation between inflammation and lung damages in CIH rats.

Keywords: Obstructive sleep apnea, Chronic intermittent hypoxia, Inflammation, NF-κB, Interleukin-6, Tumor necrosis factor-alpha, Rats

Background

Obstructive sleep apnea/hypopnea syndrome (OSAHS) is a common respiratory condition affecting approximately 3–7% of the middle-aged population (Lee et al. 2008; Tishler et al. 2003), characterized by apnea and hypopnea during sleep. Recurrent apnea and hyponea during sleep usually result in hypoxia/reoxygenation and

oxidative stress reaction, which can cause cell injury, inflammation and organ dysfunction (Spector 2000). Chronic intermittent hypoxia (CIH) is the primary feature of OSAHS. CIH represents a specific form of hypoxia, which differs from sustained hypoxia and resembles reperfusion injury. Oxidative stress and inflammation promoted by repeated cycles of hypoxia/reoxygenation have been proposed as possible underlying mechanisms, among others, predisposing to such as cardiovascular diseases, cerebrovascular diseases, metabolic diseases morbidity in OSAHS (Lavie 2003).

* Correspondence: li.shanqun@zs-hospital.sh.cn

[†]Equal contributors

Department of Pulmonary Medicine, Clinical Center for Sleep Breathing Disorder and Snoring, Zhongshan Hospital, Fudan University, 180 Fenlin Road, Shanghai 200032, China

Hypobaric hypoxia is a common animal model for hypoxic pulmonary hypertension. Pulmonary vasoconstriction and vascular remodeling mediated by hypoxia is the major pathophysiological characteristic of hypoxic pulmonary hypertension. Recent researches have found that chronic and intermittent hypoxia can both result in pulmonary hypertension through inducing pulmonary artery reconstruction (Fagan 2001). And clinical data also support the close connection between OSA and pulmonary hypertension (Ismail et al. 2015).

Moreover, systemic and local airway inflammation mediated by CIH/OSAHS could induce lung injury to some degrees which might aggravate existing respiratory diseases, such as asthma and COPD (Ioachimescu and Teodorescu 2013). However, elucidation of the basic mechanisms of inflammation damage is limited by the genetic heterogeneity of OSAHS patients and the presence of multiple confounding and comorbid conditions, including obesity. Animal models make it possible to study the causative mechanisms and the consequences of nocturnal respiratory events avoiding the confounding factors that occur in humans.

In this study, we used our patent rat CIH model (Patent number: ZL 2009 2 0067224.9) to study lung injury during exposure to CIH and its potential association with inflammation. We do these initial work to understand comprehensively and deeply the mechanism of OSAHS related lung injury.

Methods
Animals
Male Sprague-Dawley (SD) rats (130–150 g) were supplied by experimental animal centre of Zhongshan Hospital affiliated to Fudan University (Shanghai, China). The animals were housed individually at a constant temperature (23 ± 2 °C) at a relative humidity of 60% ± 2% on an automatically controlled 12 h light/dark cycle

(lights on at 07:00 AM). They had free access to food and water except during experiments that required otherwise. At the end of experiment, rats were anesthetized with pentobarbital sodium (40 mg/kg) intraperitoneally. All experiments were carried out in accordance with the National Institutes of Health Guide for the Care and Use of Laboratory Animals of China. Every effort was made to minimize the number of animals used and any pain and discomfort that they might experience.

Chronic intermittent hypoxia model
CIH model used in the present study were similar to our described previously (Fu et al. 2015; Liu et al. 2014). 16 rats were randomly divided into two groups, eight in each group. One group was exposed to intermittent air (IA) and the other served as control. CIH group was exposed to intermittent hypoxia (IH). Both groups underwent treatment from 09:00 to 17:00 daily for 5 weeks. IA and IH animals were placed in identical intermittent hypoxia chamber of our own design filled with nitrogen and oxygen or with air, using a gas delivery system which we described in detail previously. Briefly, the fracion of inspiration O_2 (FiO_2) in the IH chamber fluctuated between 6 and 21%, regulated by a gas control equipment through insufflation time and flow setting of nitrogen and oxygen. The oxygen concentration was measured automatically using an oxygen analyzer (Shanghai Medical Equipment, Shanghai, China). Every hypoxia/reoxygenation cycle took 1 min, the sequence is as follows: pure nitrogen for 30 s (FiO_2 decreased to about 6–7%)—rest for 10 s—pure oxygen for 20 s (FiO_2 increased to about 20–21%). For the control group, the chamber was filled with air and FiO_2 levels were kept stable at 20–21%. We took 10 points of two planes in the chamber: plane 1: point A_1, B_1, C_1, D_1, E_1, plane 2: point A_2, B_2, C_2, D_2, E_2 (Fig. 1a), the oxygen concentration changes of the 10 points were measured by the tester. After 10 cycles, we measured the oxygen

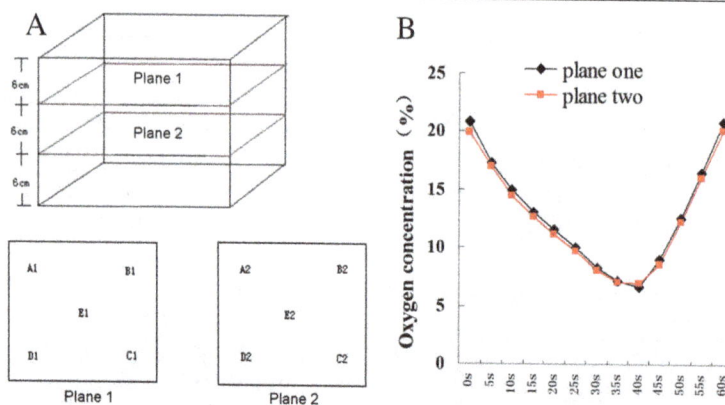

Fig. 1 Two planes and oxygen concentration change in the chamber. **a** Animal chamber is showed above. There are two planes and distribution of 10 points: the animals are placed in the plane 2; (**b**) The *black curve* represents plane one and the *red curve* represents plane two. Oxygen concentration in the chamber fluctuated between 6 and 7% to 20 and 21%

concentration of one point every 5 s for 5 cycles, then next point for 5 cycles. The average concentration of five points in each plane was taken for Y-axis, and the different time points of a cycle were taken for X-axis. The curve showed that oxygen concentration in the chamber first decreased and then increased to normal, it fluctuated between 6 and 7% to 20 and 21% (Fig. 1b). Intermittent hypoxia triggers a bewildering array of both detrimental and beneficial effects in multiple physiological systems. Our CIH protocol consists of severe hypoxia (2–8% inspired O2) and between 48 and 2,400 cycles/day (60 times/h*8 h = 480 cycles/day) which are prone to pathology (Navarrete-Opazo and Mitchell 2014).

Measurements

Wet/dry ratio measurement

Lung tissues were removed from rats after anesthesia. Right middle lobe was weighed and placed in a 60 °C drying oven. After drying for 72 h, it was weighed again, and then the wet/dry ratio was calculated.

Histology and electronmicroscopy

Right upper lobe was fixed in neutral formalin, embedded in paraffin wax, sliced and stained with hemagglutinin-esterase, then was observed in light microscope. The degree of lung injury was quantified based on the following (Su et al. 2003)@@: alveolar and interstitial edema, inflammatory infiltration, and hemorrhage. The severity of injury was graded for three variables: no injury = 0; injury to 25% of the field = 1; injury to 50% of the field = 2; injury to 75% of the field = 3; and diffuse injury = 4.

Right lower lobe was fixed in 4% glutaraldehyde and then 1% osmic anhydride, dehydrated by ethanol and acetone, embedded by 618 epoxy resin, sliced with thickness of 50 nm and dyed by uranyl acetate and lead citrate, then was observed in electronmicroscopy.

Western blot analysis

Lung tissues were lysed in a protein extraction buffer. The protease inhibitor of phenylmethylsulfonyl fluoride (PMSF) was added to the buffer with tissues. The samples were separated on 10% SDS-polyacrylamide gels, and then transferred to a nitrocellulose membrane. The primary antibodies were NF-κB (65KD) and β-actin (42KD) antibody (Abcam, USA). The stripe signals were detected by ECL kit (Beyotime, China).

Measurement of interleukin-6 (IL-6) and tumor necrosis factor-alpha (TNF-a) concentration in serum and bronchoalveolar lavage fluid (BALF)

After the experiment (the 36th day), 4–5 ml blood was collected from abdominal aorta of each rat in two groups, and then centrifuged at a rate of 3000 rpm for 15 min. The supernatant fluid was conserved in -70 °C refrigerator. Rats were exanguinated from abdominal arota, then a cannula was intubated into the left bronchus. The left lung of each rat was lavaged with a total of 9 ml neutral saline for three times with 3 ml each time. The lavaged fluid was collected and centrifuged (3000 r/min) for 15 min. The supernatant fluid was conserved in -70 °C refrigerator. The concentration of IL-6 and TNF-α in serum and BALF were measured by ELISA kit (DAKEWE, China).

Statistics

Measurement data are shown as $\bar{x} \pm S$. The comparisons of data among two groups were performed using independent sampler t-test. SPSS for windows Version 11.5 was used to do data processing. Significance was accepted when P values < 0.05.

Results

HE staining and electronmicroscopy of lung tissues (Fig. 2)

In the HE staining of lung tissue, lung tissue structure is normal in the control group rats (Fig. 2d, f); Results showed that there were significant lung tissue inflammatory injuries in the CIH group rats (Fig. 2e, g): alveolar septum widen, alveolar wall thicken, lymphocytes and mononuclear cells infiltrate, alveolar space lessen; little exudation within alveolar space, septal capillary open and congest mildly, focal nodular pneumonia lesions were found partly. The histological score of CIH group is much higher than that in the control group (6.857 ± 0.553 vs. 2.286 ± 0.286 g, $P < 0.05$).

In the electronmicroscopy of TypeIIalveolar cells, no abnormality was found in karyotheca and endoplasmic reticulum in the control group (Fig. 2a); Swelled nuclear membrane, outstretched endoplasmic reticulum, increased lamellar body and vacuolar degeneration were found in the CIH group (Fig. 2b and c).

Inflammation response of CIH rats (Fig. 3)

Weight changes (Fig. 3d)

There was no statistical difference of rats weight between two groups before the experiment. After the experiment (the 36[t]h day), body weight of rats in CIH group was lower than that in control group (359.11 ± 12.86 vs 469.61 ± 16.87 g, $P < 0.05$).

Wet/Dry ratio (Fig. 3c)

The wet/dry ratio of lung tissue in the CIH group is higher than that of in the control group (5.390 ± 0.460 vs 4.105 ± 0.481, $P < 0.05$). The lung wet-to-dry weight ratio reflects lung edema. Lung edema was found in the CIH group.

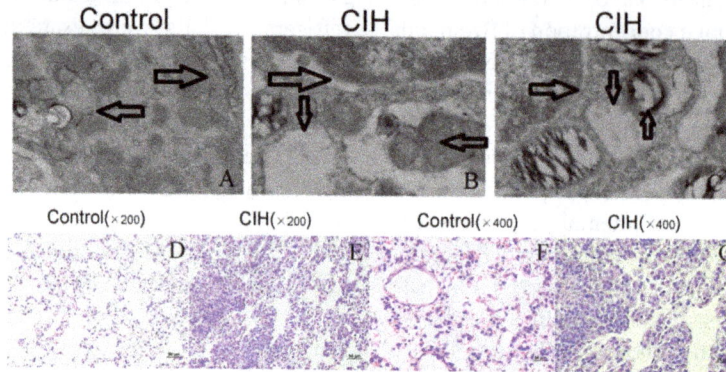

Fig. 2 Electronmicroscopy and Histopathology of lung tissue. **a-c** Ultrastructure of Type II alveolar cells under scanning electronmicroscope. **a** No change happened in karyotheca and endoplasmic reticulum in the control group; **b** Swelled nuclear membrane, outstretched endoplasmic reticulum and vacuolar degeneration appeared in the CIH group rats; **c** Swelled nuclear membrane, increased Lamellar body and vacuolar degeneration in the CIH group). → pointed to the karyotheca; ← pointed to endoplasmic reticulum; ↓ pointed to vacuolar degeneration; ↑ pointed to Lamellar body. **d-g** H&E staining of lung tissue (200× and 400×). **d, f** The structure of lung tissue is normal in the control group rats; (**e, g**) HE staining results showed that there were significant lung tissue inflammatory injuries in the CIH group rats: alveolar septum widen, alveolar wall thicken, lymphocytes and mononuclear cells infiltrate, alveolar space lessen; little exudation within alveolar space, septal capillary open and congest mildly, focal nodular pneumonia lesions were found partly

NF-κB (Fig. 3a, b)

NF-κB is a protein transcription factor that is required for maximal transcription of many proinflammatory molecules which are important in the generation of inflammation. In western blot analysis lung tissue, the NF-κB increased significantly in the CIH group compared with control group (0.43 ± 0.1 vs 0.22 ± 0.05, $P < 0.05$).

IL-6 and TNF-α (Fig. 3e)

IL-6 and TNF-α are pro-inflammatory factors secreted by mononuclear macrophage, vascular endothelial cell and T lymphocyte. The concentration of IL-6 and TNF-α in serum indicating systemic inflammation in CIH group were higher than that in control group (138.63 ± 43.82 vs 41.82 ± 5.24 pg/ml and 126.62 ± 34.81 vs 73.43

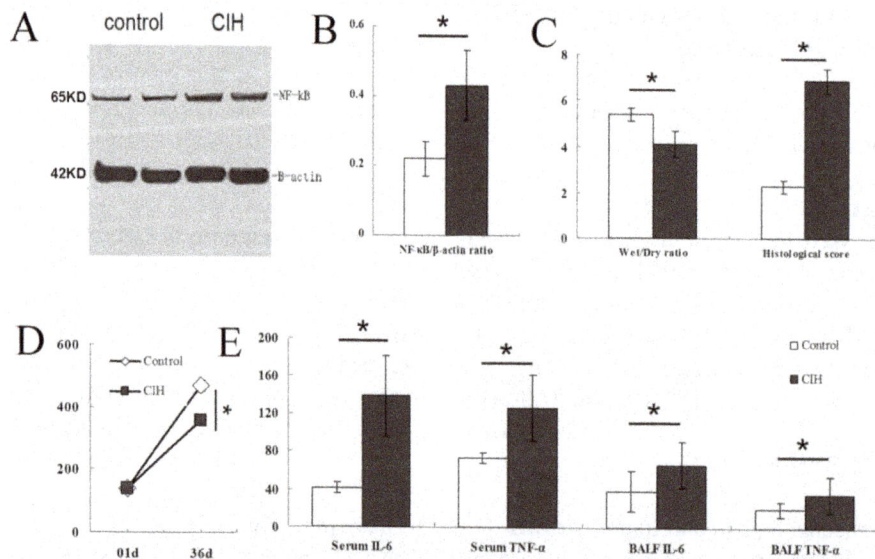

Fig. 3 Systematic and lung tissue local inflammation changes within CIH rats. **a** Western blotting results of NF-κB protein levels in the lung tissue; (**b**) Bar graph shows the statistic results of NF-κB protein levels; (**c**) Lung wet-to-dry ratio ($n = 8$) and histological scores ($n = 8$); (**d**) Body weight change of rats: 01d, the first day of experiment and 36d, the end of the experiment; (**e**) Concentration of IL-6 and TNF-α in serum and BALF. *, $P < 0.05$ compared with control group ($n = 8$). All results are means ± SEM

± 5.72 pg/ml, respectively, $P < 0.05$). The concentration of IL-6 and TNF-α in BALF indicating local airway inflammation in CIH group was higher than that in control group (67.1 ± 24.2 pg/ml vs 39.8 ± 21.5 pg/ml and 36.61 ± 19.17 pg/ml vs 20.31 ± 8.44 pg/ml, respectively, $P < 0.05$).

Discussion

Obstructive sleep apnea (OSA) is associated with repetitive nocturnal arterial oxygen desaturation and hypercapnia, large intrathoracic negative pressure swings, and acute increases in pulmonary artery pressure. CIH is the typical and primary pathophsiological feature of OSA. According to the hypoxia patterns, hypoxia model can be divided into hypobaric hypoxia, sustained hypoxia, intermittent continuous hypoxia and chronic intermittent hypoxia, among which CIH is the optimal model imitating the pathophsiological feature of OSA.

The core of pathophysiologic changes of CIH/OSA related multiple organs injury is inflammation response, including lung. Initial clinical study showed that OSAHS patients usually develop both systematic and local inflammation, and the former is characterized by elevation of inflammatory factors in plasma. Serum levels of different inflammatory markers were significantly increased in patients with the combination of sleep apnea, including hs-CRP, IL1-Ra, IL-8, IL-6, TNF-α, Rantes and sICAM. A meta-analysis addressed the profile of the inflammatory markers in OSAHS of multiple small size studies (Nadeem et al. 2013): Standardized pooled Mean differences were calculated to be 1.77 for CRP, 2.16 for IL-6, 1.03 for TNF-α, 4.22 for IL-8, 2.93 for ICAM, 1.45 for Selectins and 2.08 for VCAM. Continuous positive airway pressure (CPAP) is the primary treatment for OSAHS. Evidence shows that CPAP therapy reduces inflammation Severity. Another meta-analysis to study the effects of CPAP usage for patients with OSA significantly decreases serum inflammatory markers CRP, IL-6 and TNF-α (Baessler et al. 2013). IL-6 and TNF-α are pro-inflammatory factors secreted by mononuclear macrophage, vascular endothelial cell and T lymphocyte. In our study, systemic inflammation changes induced by CIH are apparent: IL-6 and TNF-α were significantly higher in CIH rats, which is an indirect index for successful CIH model. Animal models make it possible to study the causative mechanisms and the consequences of nocturnal respiratory events avoiding the confounding factors that occur in humans (such as obesity).

In addition to systemic inflammation, OSAHS patients also develop inflammation in local airway. Local inflammation is due to a structural and functional change of local airway, and congestion and edema of lung tissue resulted from recurrent obstruction and opening during sleep. Recurrent hypoxia/reoxygenation produces excessive oxygen free radicals, which injures local tissue and results in a high inflammatory factor status. Carpagnano et al. (Carpagnano et al. 2002) measured IL-6 in EBC of OSAHS patients and found a local inflammation in lower respiratory tract. Kensaku Aihara et al. found in OSAHS patients sputum IL-6, IL-8, TNF-α, and VEGF were significantly related to sputum neutrophil number, and sputum IL-8 and TNF-α were related to proximal airway resistance independently of BMI (Aihara et al. 2013). However, such study was mainly limited in clinical investigation. In our study, IL-6 and TNF-α in serum and BALF in CIH group was significantly higher than that in control group. Our results demonstrated both local inflammation and systemic inflammation were consistent with most of clinical study.

Transcription factor nuclear factor kB (NF-kB) is a master regulator of inflammatory gene expression and regulates cytokines such as TNF-a and IL-8 that contribute to atherosclerosis by inducing adhesion molecule expression (Hansson, 2005). Results on experiments animals and cell cultures have shown that IH activates a variety of transcription factors including the hypoxia-inducible factor-1 (HIF-1), NF-kB, c-fos (immediate early gene) and nuclear factor of activated T-cells (NFAT) (Nanduri et al. 2008), which regulate many genes that promote tissue perfusion and oxygenation (Garvey et al. 2009). In the lung tissue western blot results, the concentration of NF-kB in the CIH group increased significantly. The results suggested that chronic intermittent hypoxia activate inflammatory pathways in the lung tissue.

Inflammation in OSAHS can cause pathophysiologic change of several organs, and finally, the structure and function of organs are injured. The result showed the wet/dry ratio of CIH group was higher than that of control group, which hinted that CIH rats develop obvious edema of lung tissue. And pathological examination showed lung HE staining of CIH rats had all developed severe alveolar inflammation and some of them had developed diffuse lobular pneumonia. Our electronmicroscopy results showed that karyotheca and endoplasmic reticulum injuries of Type II alveolar cells were serious in the CIH group. Pulmonary edema as a resenting feature of sleep apnea syndrome has also been found in our animal model. Makarenko et al found that IH decreased transendothelial electrical resistance (TEER) suggesting attenuated endothelial barrier function which were induced by oxidative stress (Makarenko et al. 2014). Disruption of barrier function not only affects pulmonary gas exchange but also leads to pulmonary edema. Mild pulmonary edema, alteration of alveolarization process, and impairment of alveolar wall have been observed in the lung of subjects with OSA. CIH could produce a severe impact on pulmonary surfactant performance and may lead to collapse of the alveoli. Liang

Shao et al found that serum surfactant protein B (one of pulmonary surfactants) might be a potential biomarker to diagnose OSA (Shao et al. 2016).

Recent researches have found that chronic and intermittent hypoxia both can result in pulmonary hypertension through inducing pulmonary artery reconstruction. In our previous CIH rat experiments (Wu et al. 2011), echocardiogram results showed that compared to control group, the value of pulmonary arterial flow in CIH group increased significantly which could be due to vasoconstriction induced by repeated cycles of hypoxia/reoxygenation. Intermittent chronic hypoxia was used to mimic a severe hypoxic pulmonary hypertension (HPH) condition. Haifeng Jin et al found that chronic intermittent hypoxia-induced inflammation and excessive proliferation of pulmonary artery smooth muscle cells play important roles in the pathological process of hypoxic pulmonary hypertension (Jin et al. 2014). Chronic intermittent hypoxia elicits milder effects on pulmonary artery medial layer muscularization and subsequent right ventricular hypertrophy than chronic hypoxia (Ramirez et al. 2012). Clinical studies show that pulmonary hypertension associated with OSA appears to be mild and may be due to a combination of precapillary and postcapillary factors including pulmonary arteriolar remodeling and hyperreactivity to hypoxia and left ventricular diastolic dysfunction and left atrial enlargement (Sajkov and Mcevoy 2009). Inflammation participates in the initiation and progression of HPH by actively contributing to chronic vasoconstriction and remodeling of the pulmonary vessel wall. Hisashi Nagai et al (Nagai et al. 2015) demonstrated that pro-inflammatory pulmonary macrophages attenuate hypoxic pulmonary vasoconstriction via the activation of $\beta3AR/iNOS$ signaling in IH rats. It was a regret that we did not investigate the pressure change of pulmonary vessels.

In the clinical practice, OSA is more commonly seen in patients with obstructive lung diseases (OLD) such as asthma and COPD, perhaps as a result of shared risk factors and OSA is associated with worse clinical outcomes in patients with OLD, and continuous positive airway pressure therapy has potential beneficial effects on these vicious pathophysiological interaction. In OSA patients, local airway or systemic inflammatory state could exacerbate COPD or asthma which should be paid more attention by clinical physicians. Our animal results totally support the existing of systemic and local inflammation within lung of CIH.

Conclusions

In our CIH rats model, histopathology and electronmicroscopy results of lung tissue confirmed the damage effects. The changes of transcription factor NF-kB and pro-inflammatory factors IL-6 and TNF-α both indicated

the existing systemic and local inflammation which may induce the lung injuries. Further explorations of CIH related inflammation damage occurrence mechanism are needed. Our rat CIH model can be effectively used to imitate the pathophysiologic changes of CIH/OSA.

Acknowledgements
Thanks for ZiLong Liu PhD who provided professional and detailed writing services for this manuscript.

Funding
This work is supported by a research grant from Shanghai Committee of Science and Technology (No. 13430720500), Shanghai Leading Academic Discipline Project (No. B115) and National Natural Science Foundation of China (No. 81570081), and Shanghai family planning and health committee (No. 2016HP020).

Authors' contributions
SL and ZJ designed the study; HL, CF and WX all contributed to the completion of animal experiments; WX and ZJ assumed responsibility for the integrity of the data in the study; HL and WX analysed the data and HL wrote the paper; SL contributed to critical review and final approval of the manuscript. All of the authors read and approved the final manuscript.

Competing interests
The authors declare that they have no competing interests.

References
Aihara K, Oga T, Chihara Y, Harada Y, Tanizawa K, Handa T, Hitomi T, Uno K, Mishima M, Chin K. Analysis of systemic and airway inflammation in obstructive sleep apnea[J]. Sleep and Breathing. 2013;17(2):597–604.
Baessler A, Nadeem R, Harvey M, Madbouly E, Younus A, Sajid H, Naseem J, Asif A, Bawaadam H. Treatment for sleep apnea by continuous positive airway pressure improves levels of inflammatory markers - a meta-analysis[J]. J Inflamm (Lond). 2013;10:13.
Carpagnano GE, Kharitonov SA, Resta O, Foschino-Barbaro MP, Gramiccioni E, Barnes PJ. Increased 8-isoprostane and interleukin-6 in breath condensate of obstructive sleep apnea patients[J]. Chest. 2002;122(4):1162–7.
Fagan KA. Selected contribution: pulmonary hypertension in mice following intermittent hypoxia[J]. J Appl Physiol (1985). 2001;90(6):2502–7.
Fu C, Jiang L, Zhu F, Liu Z, Li W, Jiang H, Ye H, Kushida CA, Li S. Chronic intermittent hypoxia leads to insulin resistance and impaired glucose tolerance through dysregulation of adipokines in non-obese rats[J]. Sleep and Breathing. 2015;19(4):1467–73.
Garvey JF, Taylor CT, Mcnicholas WT. Cardiovascular disease in obstructive sleep apnoea syndrome: the role of intermittent hypoxia and inflammation[J]. Eur Respir J. 2009;33(5):1195–205.
Hansson GK. Mechanisms of disease-Inflammation, atherosclerosis, and coronary artery disease[J]. N Engl J Med. 2005;352(16):1685–95.
Ioachimescu OC, Teodorescu M. Integrating the overlap of obstructive lung disease and obstructive sleep apnoea: OLDOSA syndrome[J]. Respirology. 2013;18(3):421–31.
Ismail K, Roberts K, Manning P, Manley C, Hill NS. OSA and pulmonary hypertension: time for a new look[J]. Chest. 2015;147(3):847–61.
Jin H, Wang Y, Zhou L, Liu L, Zhang P, Deng W, Yuan Y. Melatonin attenuates hypoxic pulmonary hypertension by inhibiting the inflammation and the proliferation of pulmonary arterial smooth muscle cells[J]. J Pineal Res. 2014;57(4):442–50.
Lavie L. Obstructive sleep apnoea syndrome – an oxidative stress disorder[J]. Sleep Med Rev. 2003;7(1):35–51.

Lee W, Nagubadi S, Kryger MH, Mokhlesi B. Epidemiology of obstructive sleep apnea: a population-based perspective[J]. Expert Rev Respir Med. 2008;2(3):349–64.

Liu Z, Jiang L, Zhu F, Fu C, Lu S, Zhou J, Wu X, Bai C, Li S. Chronic intermittent hypoxia and the expression of orexin and its receptors in the brains of rats[J]. Sleep Biol Rhythms. 2014;12(1):22–9.

Makarenko VV, Usatyuk PV, Yuan G, Lee MM, Nanduri J, Natarajan V, Kumar GK, Prabhakar NR. Intermittent hypoxia-induced endothelial barrier dysfunction requires ROS-dependent MAP kinase activation[J]. AJP: Cell Physiology. 2014;306(8):C745–52.

Nadeem R, Molnar J, Madbouly EM, Nida M, Aggarwal S, Sajid H, Naseem J, Loomba R. Serum inflammatory markers in obstructive sleep apnea: a meta-analysis[J]. J Clin Sleep Med. 2013;9(10):1003–12.

Nagai H, Kuwahira I, Schwenke DO, Tsuchimochi H, Nara A, Ogura S, Sonobe T, Inagaki T, Fujii Y, Yamaguchi R, Wingenfeld L, Umetani K, Shimosawa T, Yoshida K, Uemura K, Pearson JT, Shirai M. Pulmonary macrophages attenuate hypoxic pulmonary vasoconstriction via β3AR/iNOS pathway in rats exposed to chronic intermittent hypoxia[J]. PLoS One. 2015;10(7): e131923.

Nanduri J, Yuan G, Kumar GK, Semenza GL, Prabhakar NR. Transcriptional responses to intermittent hypoxia[J]. Respir Physiol Neurobiol. 2008;164(1-2):277–81.

Navarrete-Opazo A, Mitchell GS. Therapeutic potential of intermittent hypoxia: a matter of dose[J]. Am J Physiol Regul Integr Comp Physiol. 2014;307(10):R1181–97.

Ramirez TA, Jourdan-Le SC, Joy A, Zhang J, Dai Q. Chronic and intermittent hypoxia differentially regulate left ventricular inflammatory and extracellular matrix responses.[J]. Hypertens Res. 2012;35(8):811–8.

Sajkov D, Mcevoy RD. Obstructive sleep apnea and pulmonary hypertension[J]. Prog Cardiovasc Dis. 2009;51(5):363–70.

Shao L, Li N, Yao X, Heizati M, Abdireim A, Wang Y, Abulikemu Z, Zhang D, Chang G, Zhou L, Hong J, Zhang Y, Kong J, Zhang X. Relationship between surfactant proteins B and C and obstructive sleep apnea: is serum SP-B concentration a potential biomarker of obstructive sleep apnea?[J]. Sleep and Breathing. 2016;20(1):25–31.

Spector A. Review: oxidative stress and disease[J]. J Ocul Pharmacol Ther. 2000;16(2):193–201.

Su X, Bai C, Hong Q, Zhu D, He L, Wu J, Ding F, Fang X, Matthay MA. Effect of continuous hemofiltration on hemodynamics, lung inflammation and pulmonary edema in a canine model of acute lung injury[J]. Intensive Care Med. 2003;29(11):2034–42.

Tishler PV, Larkin EK, Schluchter MD, Redline S. Incidence of sleep-disordered breathing in an urban adult population[J]. JAMA. 2003.

Wu X, Huang J, Kong D, Shao C, Zhou J, Lu S, Li S. Establishment of a rat chronic intermittent hypoxia model and evaluation by echocardiogram[J]. Fudan Univ J Med Sci. 2011;06:481–4.

17

A review of sleep disturbances following traumatic brain injury

José Rafael P. Zuzuárregui[1*], Kevin Bickart[2] and Scott J. Kutscher[3]

Abstract

Background: Sleep disorders are common following traumatic brain injury (TBI).

Methods: We review the literature regarding sleep disturbances in the acute and chronic phase following TBI in both the adult and pediatric population.

Results: Acute and chronic disruption of sleep commonly follows TBI and contributes to morbidity commonly seen post-injury in both adults and children. This includes the direct effect of TBI leading to sleep disruption, as well as sleep disorders resulting from TBI itself. Pre-TBI neurocognitive testing is important to determine a baseline prior to injury, while disrupted sleep can also prolong recovery after TBI. Early recognition of sleep disturbances post-injury can lead to earlier treatment and limit the sequelae of TBI, as well as assist in recovery.

Conclusion: We suggest that evaluation for sleep disturbances following TBI is a critical component of post-TBI assessment and management.

Keywords: Traumatic brain injury, Sleep disturbances, Insomnia, Hypersomnia, Obstructive sleep apnea, Circadian rhythm sleep disorder

Background

Subjective sleep disturbances and objective sleep disorders following traumatic brain injury (TBI) are common issues encountered in clinical practice. TBI is defined as an injury that includes transient amnesia, alteration or loss of consciousness that results from a force involving the head or body (Wickwire et al. 2016; Mathias and Alvaro 2012). TBI can be classified as mild, moderate or severe based on the presence and severity of the above symptoms, as well as neuroimaging characteristics. Reportedly, up to 1.7 million Americans suffers TBI yearly, with 70% of those deemed mild (Wickwire et al. 2016; Mathias and Alvaro 2012). Of those who sustain TBI, recent estimates suggest that 30–66% of patients experience some type of sleep disturbance (Wickwire et al. 2016; Mathias and Alvaro 2012; Nakase-Richardson et al. 2013; Chan and Feinstein 2015). Sleep disturbances in post-TBI patients can present acutely or can emerge as a chronic issue during the recovery phase, occasionally lasting years from the initial injury (Wickwire et al. 2016). Sleep disturbances and resultant sleep disorders can also impair the recovery process from TBI. Sleep disorders reported in post TBI patients include insomnia and hypersomnia syndromes, circadian rhythm disorders, and sleep related breathing disorders.

Recently, Mollayeva, et al. discussed the possible mechanisms of sleep disturbances following TBI (Mollayeva et al. 2016). These mechanisms are beyond the scope of this review, but may include disruption of neuronal networks involved in wakefulness and sleep directly related to acceleration-deceleration injuries to these axons, as well as direct injury to structures responsible for regulation of the circadian rhythm (Wickwire et al. 2016; Mollayeva et al. 2016). Genetic susceptibility to circadian rhythm disorders, changes in sleep duration, and changes in sleep architecture also appears to play a role in the individual risk of development of sleep disruption following TBI. Craniofacial anatomy prior to TBI also appears to predispose the individual to development of sleep-disordered breathing (Mollayeva et al. 2016).

* Correspondence: rafzuzu@bu.edu
[1]Division of Neurology, University of California, San Francisco, Fresno Center for Medical Education and Research, 155 N. Fresno St., Fresno 93701, CA, USA
Full list of author information is available at the end of the article

As a result, patients may experience a variety of sleep disturbances following TBI that emerge at different post-injury intervals (Table 1).

Previous studies have delineated TBI into the following time frames: acute phase occurring from 0 to 7 days, subacute phase occurring between 7 and 90 days, and chronic phase occurring greater than 90 days (Wickwire et al. 2016; Mollayeva et al. 2016). However, there is no current consensus on what constitutes these time frames as it relates to the emergence of sleep disturbances following TBI. The acute phase for sleep disruption has been described as occurring anywhere from 1 week up to one year post-injury, while the chronic phase has been felt to begin six months to a year following TBI (Wickwire et al. 2016; Nakase-Richardson et al. 2013; Chan and Feinstein 2015; Mollayeva et al. 2016; Pillar et al. 2003; Baumann et al. 2007; Sommerauer et al. 2013; Raikes and Schaefer 2016; Watson et al. 2007; Imbach et al. 2015). In this review, we designate the acute phase up to six months post-injury, with the chronic phase six months or greater.

Those who sustain TBI may suffer from hypersomnia and insomnia in the acute period post-injury (Wickwire et al. 2016; Baumann et al. 2007; Sommerauer et al. 2013; Raikes and Schaefer 2016; Watson et al. 2007; Imbach et al. 2015). Furthermore, central nervous system symptoms occurring as a result of TBI also may cause disruption of sleep (Pillar et al. 2003; Lavigne et al. 2015; Chaput et al. 2009; Minen et al. 2016; Hou et al. 2013; Jaramillo et al. 2016; Farrell-Carnahan et al. 2015; Bryan 2013; Holster et al. 2017). These include headache, tinnitus and/or vertigo. Mood disorders such as anxiety or depression that result from TBI are also common and may have a negative impact on sleep (Pillar et al. 2003; Chaput et al. 2009; Minen et al. 2016; Farrell-Carnahan et al. 2015; Bryan 2013; Holster et al. 2017). Sleep disturbances in the chronic phase are varied and include insomnia as well as circadian rhythm disruption (Wickwire et al. 2016; Mathias and Alvaro 2012; Nakase-Richardson

Table 1 Sleep Disturbances Following TBI in the Acute and Chronic Phase

Time period	Diagnosis
Acute	Hypersomnia
	Insomnia related to post-traumatic headache
	Insomnia related to post-traumatic mood disturbance
	Insomnia
Chronic	Insomnia
	Circadian rhythm disorders
	Obstructive sleep apnea
	Narcolepsy
	Chronic Traumatic Encephalopathy

et al. 2013; Chan and Feinstein 2015; Mollayeva et al. 2016; Pillar et al. 2003). In addition, the development of obstructive sleep apnea (OSA) and narcolepsy has also been described following TBI (Wickwire et al. 2016; Mathias and Alvaro 2012; Nakase-Richardson et al. 2013; Chan and Feinstein 2015; Mollayeva et al. 2016; Pillar et al. 2003). Here, we review commonly encountered sleep disturbances following TBI.

Methods

Two authors (JZ and KB) independently searched the international literature through February 2, 2017 for articles evaluating sleep disturbances following TBI, as well as the impact of sleep on cognition. Databases searched included PubMED/Medline and The Cochrane Library. The inclusion criteria: studies evaluating sleep disturbances in both adults and pediatric populations following TBI itself or direct sequelae resulting from TBI, as well as the impact of sleep on cognition. This includes the impact of sleep on neurocognitive testing in groups at high risk for TBI. An example of a search performed in PubMED/Medline is: ("sleep"[MeSH Terms] OR "sleep"[All Fields]) AND ("brain injuries, traumatic"[MeSH Terms] OR ("brain"[All Fields] AND "injuries"[All Fields] AND "traumatic"[All Fields]) OR "traumatic brain injuries"[All Fields] OR ("traumatic"[All Fields] AND "brain"[All Fields] AND "injury"[All Fields]) OR "traumatic brain injury"[All Fields]). There was no language restriction.

Sleep disturbances in the acute period following TBI
Hypersomnia

Increased sleep need is a significant issue in the acute period following TBI (Baumann et al. 2007; Sommerauer et al. 2013; Raikes and Schaefer 2016). A prospective study of 96 patients with TBI demonstrated that 22% experienced hypersomnia following TBI, defined as a sleep need of equal to or greater than 2 h when compared to pre-TBI sleep need (Baumann et al. 2007). Although no correlations were noted with regards to cerebrospinal fluid (CSF) hypocretin levels, polysomnography (PSG) or multiple sleep latency tests (MSLT), post-TBI patients reporting hypersomnia suffered more severe TBI than those without (Baumann et al. 2007). A retrospective case-control study ($n = 36$) showed that patients with hypersomnia based initially on actigraphy testing demonstrated increased stage 3 sleep on subsequent PSG testing when compared to controls (Sommerauer et al. 2013).

While it is clear that hypersomnia affects a significant number of patients following TBI, the length of time that this persists is variable. A recent prospective study ($n = 17$) used actigraphy to demonstrate that an increased sleep need might be seen in the acute period following

TBI, resolving one month post-injury (Raikes and Schaefer 2016). A larger prospective study ($n = 748$) showed that these changes persist up to one month, but may resolve by one year following TBI; however, increased sleep need was assessed via survey rather than actigraphy (Watson et al. 2007). Finally, a case-control study evaluating 42 patients with first-time TBI showed that sleep need was still significantly increased at 6 months when compared to controls (Imbach et al. 2015). The development of hypersomnia following TBI is a significant predictor of negative social outcomes, including subjective difficulties for patients at work, in relationships and various social settings (Chan and Feinstein 2015). This highlights the need for early assessment and treatment of hypersomnia.

Insomnia due to post-traumatic headache

Headache following TBI is a common symptom seen in 20–46.8% of patients with TBI ($n = 443$) (Lavigne et al. 2015; Chaput et al. 2009). This symptom can have a significant impact on quality of life both during wakefulness and sleep and can be seen irrespective of the severity of the injury. Multiple studies have been performed to evaluate the impact of post-traumatic headache (PTH) on sleep, with insomnia the most common symptom experienced (Minen et al. 2016; Hou et al. 2013). A retrospective cohort study ($n = 98$) showed that headache and insomnia are frequently comorbid conditions in the mild TBI population, with up to half of patients with PTH also suffering from insomnia (Hou et al. 2013). This study also showed that PTH portended a higher risk of development of insomnia when compared to severity of TBI, with estimates from 12.5 to 27% (Hou et al. 2013; Jaramillo et al. 2016). Finally, multiple studies have shown that insomnia appears to predict the persistence of PTH in TBI patients, leading to a vicious cycle where each symptom promotes the presence of the other. (Chaput et al. 2009; Hou et al. 2013).

Insomnia due to post-traumatic mood disturbances

Mood disturbances following TBI are also common, with estimates of prevalence of depression from 20 to 46% and anxiety from 24 to 61% ($n = 443$) (Chaput et al. 2009; Minen et al. 2016; Jaramillo et al. 2016). Depression and anxiety are often comorbid with PTH following TBI, with up to 33% of patients with TBI suffering from a mood disturbance and PTH (Minen et al. 2016). In addition, one study of 150 subjects and another of 168 subjects demonstrated that patients with TBI previously who suffered a repeat TBI were at higher risk for development of depression than those without previous TBI (Bryan 2013; Holster et al. 2017). Frequently, these patients often have poor sleep due to insomnia, with multiple studies demonstrating an increased association with depression and anxiety (Chaput et al. 2009; Minen

et al. 2016; Farrell-Carnahan et al. 2015; Bryan 2013; Holster et al. 2017). One review showed that the presence of insomnia in patients with TBI has a risk of depression six times higher than those who have suffered TBI without insomnia (Minen et al. 2016).

Insomnia

Insomnia has been demonstrated in the acute phase following TBI, with patients reporting difficulty in both initiation and maintenance of sleep (Chan and Feinstein 2015; Pillar et al. 2003; Lavigne et al. 2015; Chaput et al. 2009; Minen et al. 2016; Jaramillo et al. 2016). As noted above, this insomnia is typically seen comorbid with post-traumatic headache and mood disturbances (Lavigne et al. 2015; Chaput et al. 2009; Minen et al. 2016; Jaramillo et al. 2016). Some studies have suggested that insomnia is not independent of these issues following TBI, given the significant interaction between pain, depression and anxiety on sleep disturbance (Chan and Feinstein 2015; Lavigne et al. 2015; Chaput et al. 2009; Minen et al. 2016; Jaramillo et al. 2016). Further studies need to be performed to separate this interaction and define the true prevalence of acute insomnia development in the absence of post-traumatic symptoms.

Sleep disturbances in the chronic period following TBI

Insomnia

Insomnia is also a chronic issue following TBI. The prevalence of insomnia following TBI is varied, with anywhere from 10 to 84% of patients reporting insomnia symptoms up to three years following injury (Chan and Feinstein 2015; Mollayeva et al. 2016; Pillar et al. 2003; Hou et al. 2013; Ouellet et al. 2006; Viola-Saltzman and Musleh 2016; Zeitzer et al. 2009; Kempf et al. 2010). One small prospective study, however, found insomnia occurring in only three of 65 patients using actigraphy and PSG (Baumann et al. 2007).

The true prevalence of insomnia has been called into question as some studies have shown an overestimation of insomnia reported by patients with TBI when evaluated with subjective questionnaires and PSG (Ouellet and Morin 2006; Lu et al. 2015). While this may be an important consideration, other studies have used PSG to demonstrate increased sleep latency in patients with TBI, in addition to reduced sleep efficiency and increased sleep fragmentation (Ouellet and Morin 2006; Lu et al. 2015; Parcell et al. 2008; Williams et al. 2008).

Insomnia also appears to be an issue that may also worsen comorbid conditions related to TBI. As noted above, patient with insomnia following TBI are not only are at risk for development of PTH and post-traumatic mood disturbances, but the presence of these co-morbid problems can disrupt sleep and worsen insomnia symptoms

(Lavigne et al. 2015; Chaput et al. 2009; Minen et al. 2016; Hou et al. 2013; Jaramillo et al. 2016; Farrell-Carnahan et al. 2015).

Circadian rhythm disorders

Circadian rhythm disorders following TBI have not been well described in humans, with most early reports being case studies (Nagtegaal et al. 1997; Smits et al. 2000; Quinto et al. 2000). One study evaluated patients with insomnia following TBI with the use of actigraphy, saliva melatonin measurements, and body temperature measurement for the presence of a circadian rhythm sleep disorder (Ayalon et al. 2007). Of 42 patients in this study, 36% demonstrated evidence of either a delayed or advanced circadian rhythm. A recent study ($n = 18$) demonstrated that patients with TBI produced 42% less melatonin overnight when compared to controls, in addition to a delay in dim light melatonin onset by approximately 1.5 h (Grima et al. 2016). Another study ($n = 46$) showed that evening melatonin production is significantly lower in patients with TBI at least one year following injury when compared to controls (Shekleton et al. 2010). Although these studies clearly show a variability in the timing of melatonin production, it is unclear whether this finding is related to damage of intrinsic melatonin production or simply a change in circadian rhythm from TBI. In addition, these studies are unable to determine if circadian rhythm changes occurred after TBI as they did not evaluate patients prior to TBI.

Obstructive sleep apnea

The role of TBI in the development of obstructive sleep apnea (OSA) has been the subject of some debate. Some studies have shown that OSA appears to increase the risk of TBI, while other studies suggest that OSA is diagnosed more frequently post-injury. The etiology behind this finding is unclear, but may be related to craniofacial anatomy that places the patient at risk for subsequent development of OSA after TBI (Mollayeva et al. 2016). In one study ($n = 87$) that evaluated the prevalence of sleep disorders following TBI, PSG performed at three months post-injury demonstrated 23% of those with TBI had comorbid OSA (Castriotta et al. 2007). However, no baseline data was performed for comparison of OSA rates prior to TBI. A study by Guilleminault, et al. showed that 32% of patients ($n = 184$) with TBI were diagnosed with OSA post-injury (Guilleminault et al. 2000). However, the authors acknowledged that OSA may have been present in several patients prior to TBI. Several other studies evaluating the presence of OSA following TBI, found prevalence rates ranging from 11 to 61% (Wickwire et al. 2016; Mathias and Alvaro 2012; Baumann et al. 2007; Castriotta et al. 2007; Masel et al. 2001; Collen et al. 2012). In most cases, pre-TBI testing

with PSG was not available to confirm or rule out the presence of OSA prior to injury.

Nevertheless, recognition of OSA in patients with TBI is important due to the negative impact that it may have on cognition, which may be negatively impacted due to TBI itself.

Narcolepsy

Narcolepsy following TBI has been the subject of debate for many years, with the overall prevalence of narcolepsy following TBI estimated from 3 to 6% (Castriotta et al. 2007; Masel et al. 2001). While a CSF hypocretin deficiency has been noted in the acute post-injury period, normalization of these levels has also been found in a number of patients over time. One study demonstrated recovery of hypocretin levels to normal levels six months post-injury in 17 of 21 patients with EDS, while another study ($n = 27$) demonstrated that 19% of patients with narcolepsy without cataplexy developed symptoms within two years of suffering TBI (Baumann et al. 2007; Poryazova et al. 2011). Furthermore, pathologic examination of patients with severe TBI ($n = 44$) showed only mild damage to specific hypocretin neurons, while more widespread damage was seen in hypothalamic neurons involved in sleep-wake regulation (Baumann et al. 2005; 2009). Subsequently, the development of hypocretin deficient narcolepsy is questionable given the lack of specificity in damage to hypocretin neurons, as well as inconsistent presentation with regards to CSF hypocretin levels in hypersomnolence post TBI patients (Baumann et al. 2005). This is further reinforced by the demonstration of one such patient with narcolepsy following TBI in whom diffuse tensor imaging demonstrated injury to the ascending reticular activating system between the pons and hypothalamus, rather than the hypothalamus itself (Jang et al. 2016). The pathophysiology behind development of narcolepsy in post-TBI patients is likely of heterogeneous etiologies, and appears to differ from narcolepsy type I.

Despite the potential differences in pathophysiology, many post TBI patients appear to develop hypersomnolence consistent with that seen in type II narcolepsy. In contrast, very few patients appear to experience cataplexy as part of their symptomatology (Baumann et al. 2007). One study ($n = 37$) evaluated a group of patients with TBI who were HLA DQB1*0602 positive and found that seven patients (19%) developed narcolepsy with cataplexy after TBI (Poryazova et al. 2011). The authors suggested that these patients were genetically predisposed to the development of narcolepsy with cataplexy prior to TBI rather than cataplexy developing from TBI itself. Diagnostic testing with PSG and MSLT is often positive in patients with narcolepsy following TBI, with most studies using criteria of mean sleep latency < 5 min and ≥ 2 sleep onset rapid eye movement periods (Baumann et al. 2007; Castriotta et al. 2007; Poryazova et al. 2011; Jang et al. 2016). In light of these contrasting findings, it would seem that the use of PSG and MSLT for diagnosis for narcolepsy would be a more consistent diagnostic tool than use of CSF hypocretin levels.

Chronic traumatic encephalopathy

The recent discovery of chronic traumatic encephalopathy (CTE) has led to significant interest in research regarding this disease over the past fifteen years. CTE refers to a unique set of pathologic changes in the central nervous system that develop following traumatic brain injury, including a perivascular distribution of tau-positive neurofibrillary tangles in the neocortex (McKee et al. 2009). While CTE can have a significant impact on the neurocognitive profile of patients, as well as lead to neurodegeneration, literature regarding the impact of CTE on sleep is sparse (McKee et al. 2009). Although there has been some suggestion that OSA and insomnia may be risk factors for development of CTE, it is clear that poor sleep can negatively impact symptoms commonly seen in CTE, such as aggression, impulsivity and poor cognition (Quan 2014; Asken et al. 2016). At this time, research efforts have been sparse and have yet to elucidate the potential impact of sleep on the development of CTE.

Special considerations in the pediatric population

Even fewer investigations into sleep disturbances following TBI have been performed in the pediatric population, though interest has increased recently. Recent reviews of sleep disturbances in pediatric patients following TBI demonstrated that most studies focused on adolescents and used subjective measures to evaluate symptoms (Gagner et al. 2015; Hung et al. 2014; Beebe et al. 2007). However, sleep disturbances were common post-injury and included excessive daytime sleepiness, increased sleep latency and circadian rhythm disruption, though the latter was not as common (Gagner et al. 2015). One such prospective study of 15 patients demonstrated that sleep onset and maintenance difficulties were significantly increased in the TBI group when compared to their siblings (Sumpter et al. 2013). A similar recent prospective study evaluated 100 adolescent patients three to twelve months following TBI for sleep disturbances using questionnaires and actigraphy (Tham et al. 2015). Following TBI, patients not only reported poor sleep quality, but were also shown to have a shorter sleep duration and poorer sleep efficiency when compared to controls (Tham et al. 2015). This finding is in contrast to a previous study from the same authors ($n = 926$) that showed sleep disturbances were not significantly persistent three months post-injury (Tham et al. 2012). Despite recent interest, the dearth of information regarding sleep in pediatric TBI highlights the need for further research in this population.

Sleep and Neurocognition

Neurocognitive deficits are a well-known and disabling feature of TBI. As a result, neuropsychological testing has become a mainstay of post-injury evaluation. Various studies have revealed deficits in multiple neurocognitive domains following TBI, such as attention, visuospatial ability, memory and executive function (Carlsson et al. 1987; Konrad et al. 2011; Ponsford et al. 2008; De Beaumont et al. 2009; Himanen et al. 2006; Isoniemi et al. 2006; Monti et al. 2013). Others have demonstrated the utility of post-injury neuropsychological testing in predicting which patients develop chronic neurocognitive impairments (Carlsson et al. 1987; Konrad et al. 2011; Ponsford et al. 2008; De Beaumont et al. 2009; Himanen et al. 2006; Isoniemi et al. 2006; Monti et al. 2013). One such study ($n = 105$) showed that cognitive flexibility and reaction times testing in the emergency department predicted symptoms one month following TBI in the pediatric population (Brooks et al. 2016). Another study ($n = 61$) demonstrated that older age and male sex portended a higher risk of developing chronic deficits in visuospatial ability and visual memory (Himanen et al. 2006). Others have shown that repeated TBI, rather than age, was the major risk factor for permanent deficits (Carlsson et al. 1987).

While factors such as age, severity of trauma, number of prior traumatic brain injuries and timing of prior TBI have been shown to impact the outcome of neurocognitive testing, few studies have evaluated the impact of sleep on recovery (Albrecht et al. 2016; Gaudet and Weyandt 2017; Martindale et al. 2017; Lau et al. 2011; Sufrinko et al. 2015; Singh et al. 2016). Of these, one study ($n = 348$) demonstrated that patients with insomnia and reduced sleep times prior to TBI have a prolonged recovery post-injury as measured by the Immediate Post-concussion Assessment and Cognitive Test and Post-concussion Symptom Scale when compared to controls (Sufrinko et al. 2015). Another study demonstrated that poor sleep quality independently predicted cognitive dysfunction in post-TBI combat veterans when controlling for other variables such as PTSD, while others have corroborated that poor sleep prolonged cognitive recovery from TBI in non-combat patients (Martindale et al. 2017; Singh et al. 2016). Furthermore, sleep disturbances prior to TBI also increase the risk of post-concussive symptoms, which negatively impacts sleep and further contributes to prolonged recovery (Chan and Feinstein 2015; Lavigne et al. 2015; Chaput et al. 2009; Minen et al. 2016; Jaramillo et al. 2016; Singh et al. 2016).

Recently, a small group of studies have demonstrated the impact of various sleep metrics in the assessment of neurocognitive testing in TBI at baseline. One such study (n = 144) showed that athletes with low self-reported sleep quantity (68% of the subject's normal sleep quantity) performed worse on baseline neurocognitive testing than those with moderate (90%) or high sleep quantity (110%) (Mihalik et al. 2013). A subsequent study (n = 3686) showed that athletes without previous history of TBI with less than 7 h of sleep time prior to baseline neurocognitive testing had lower scores than those with more than 7 h of sleep (McClure et al. 2014).

Given the impact of poor sleep on baseline testing, sleep patterns prior to TBI should be considered by physicians when ordering or interpreting baseline neurocognitive testing. Postponement of neurocognitive testing should be considered if patients report a poor prior night of sleep. Finally, the development of sleep disturbances following TBI should be evaluated for and addressed in a timely fashion to improve recovery post-injury.

Treatment

Recovery from TBI can be negatively impacted by the aforementioned sleep disorders, highlighting the need for treatment of these conditions as they arise. Investigation into treatment of specific sleep disorders resulting from TBI, however, has been limited and largely based on current standard of care (Wickwire et al. 2016; Castriotta et al. 2009; Menn et al. 2014; Al-Adawi et al. 2006; Mignot 2012; Rao et al. 2015). For hypersomnia resulting from TBI, one randomized controlled trial (n = 117) showed that armodafinil 250 mg significantly reduced daytime sleepiness on Epworth Sleepiness scale and longer sleep latency on PSG (Menn et al. 2014). Methylphenidate did not show a significant impact on number of hours of sleep in TBI patients when compared to placebo (n = 30) (Al-Adawi et al. 2006). We recommend use of armodafinil and modafinil, but more potent stimulants may need to be used (Castriotta et al. 2009; Mignot 2012). Treatment of insomnia in TBI can be particularly challenging due to the comorbid conditions that arise from TBI itself and their respective impact sleep quality. Use of antidepressants for post-TBI mood disturbances is common, but the impact of these medications on cognitive recovery is not well studied (Rao et al. 2015). Agents with anticholinergic or heavy sedative qualities can worsen cognition and should be avoided if possible (Rao et al. 2015). Cognitive behavioral therapy is first line therapy for treatment of insomnia, but has not been well-evaluated in patients with insomnia resulting from TBI (Wickwire et al. 2016). Nevertheless, we recommend this therapy as first-line, which may also be a useful adjunct therapy for treatment of mood disorders resulting from TBI (Wickwire et al. 2016). Benzodiazepine-like agonists, such as zolpidem, are commonly used for the treatment of insomnia in the TBI population (Wickwire et al. 2016; Management

of Concussion/mTBI Working Group 2009). No randomized trials have evaluated the efficacy of these medications for insomnia following TBI. However, one study found that these medications may increase the risk of dementia in the TBI population, after controlling for the cognitive impact of insomnia (Chiu et al. 2015). If used at all, they should likely be limited to short term use. There are no trials that have explored melatonin in the treatment of circadian rhythm disorders due to TBI. One study showed that melatonin did not improve sleep latency, duration, or quality in this group (Kemp et al. 2004). In post-injury patients with OSA, we strongly recommend a trial of continuous positive airway pressure therapy to reduce the impact on sleep disordered breathing on cognition, which may already be impaired following TBI (Wickwire et al. 2016; Castriotta et al. 2009). Finally, treatment of narcolepsy resulting from TBI has not been well-studied and has focused on hypersomnia in this group. Similar to the recommendations above, modafinil and armodafinil should be tried first (Castriotta et al. 2009; Mignot 2012).

Conclusion

The impact of sleep disturbances on quality of life is well documented, with a particularly negative impact in patients with TBI in terms of cognitive and functional recovery from TBI (Wickwire et al. 2016; Mathias and Alvaro 2012; Chan and Feinstein 2015; Duclos et al. 2015; Mollayeva et al. 2016). This can occur directly from the sleep disturbances resulting from TBI or from a secondary exacerbation of common symptoms seen post-injury, such as headache, pain, mood disturbances or cognitive decline (Wickwire et al. 2016; Lavigne et al. 2015; Chaput et al. 2009; Minen et al. 2016; Hou et al. 2013; Jaramillo et al. 2016; Farrell-Carnahan et al. 2015; Duclos et al. 2015; Mollayeva et al. 2016; Ouellet et al. 2015; Theadom et al. 2016). A notable decrease of independence in performing activities of daily living in the recovery from TBI has been shown in patients with sleep disturbances post-injury, portending functional difficulties in the recovery period (Wickwire et al. 2016; Duclos et al. 2015). In addition to this, sleep disturbances also appear to prolong recovery from TBI (Mollayeva et al. 2016; Ouellet et al. 2015; Theadom et al. 2016). For these reasons, assessment and treatment for sleep disturbances following TBI is paramount to assist in improving quality of life and recovery from TBI itself.

Abbreviations

CSF: Cerebrospinal fluid; CTE: Chronic traumatic encephalopathy; MSLT: Multiple sleep latency tests; OSA: Obstructive sleep apnea; PSG: Polysomnography; PTH: Post-traumatic headache; TBI: Traumatic brain injury

Acknowledgements

The authors declare no acknowledgements.

Funding

The authors declare there was no funding for this study.

Authors' contributions

JZ conceived of the study, participated in its design and coordination, performed a literature search and helped to draft the manuscript. KB performed a literature search and helped to draft the manuscript. SK conceived of the study, participated in its design and coordination, and helped to draft the manuscript. All authors read and approved the final manuscript.

Competing interests

The authors declare that they have no competing interests.

Author details

[1]Division of Neurology, University of California, San Francisco, Fresno Center for Medical Education and Research, 155 N. Fresno St., Fresno 93701, CA, USA. [2]Department of Neurology, Stanford University School of Medicine, Stanford, USA. [3]Division of Sleep Medicine, Department of Psychiatry, Stanford University School of Medicine, Stanford, USA.

References

Al-Adawi S, Burke DT, Dorvlo AS. The effect of methylphenidate on the sleep-wake cycle of brain-injured patients undergoing rehabilitation. Sleep Med. 2006;7(3): 287–91.

Albrecht MA, Masters CL, Ames D, Foster JK, AIBL Research Group. Impact of mild head injury on neuropsychological performance in healthy older adults: longitudinal assessment in the AIBL cohort. Front Aging Neurosci. 2016;8:105.

Asken BM, Sullan MJ, Snyder AR, Houck ZM, Bryant VE, Hizel LP, McLaren ME, Dede DE, Jaffee MS, DeKosky ST, Bauer RM. Factors influencing clinical correlates of chronic traumatic encephalopathy (CTE): a review. Neuropsychol Rev. 2016;26(4):340–63.

Ayalon L, Borodkin K, Dishon L, Kanety H, Dagan Y. Circadian rhythm sleep disorders following mild traumatic brain injury. Neurology. 2007;68:1136–40.

Baumann CR, Bassetti CL, Valko PO, Haybaeck J, Keller M, Clark E, Stocker R, Tolnay M, Scammell TE. Loss of hypocretin (orexin) neurons with traumatic brain injury. Ann Neurol. 2009;66(4):555–9.

Baumann CR, Stocker R, Imhof HG, Trentz O, Hersberger M, Mignot E, Bassetti CL. Hypocretin-1 (orexin A) deficiency in acute traumatic brain injury. Neurology. 2005;65(1):147–9.

Baumann CR, Werth E, Stocker R, et al. Sleep-wake disturbances 6 months after traumatic brain injury: a prospective study. Brain. 2007;130:1873–83.

Beebe DW, Krivitzky L, Wells CT, Wade SL, Taylor HG, Yeates KO. Brief report: parental report of sleep behaviors following moderate or severe pediatric traumatic brain injury. J Pediatr Psychol. 2007;32(7):845–50.

Brooks BL, Daya H, Khan S, Carlson HL, Mikrogianakis A, Barlow KM. Cognition in the Emergency Department as a Predictor of Recovery after Pediatric Mild Traumatic Brain Injury. J Int Neuropsychol Soc. 2016;22(4):379–87.

Bryan CJ. Repetitive traumatic brain injury (or concussion) increases severity of sleep disturbance among deployed military personnel. Sleep. 2013;36(6):941–6.

Carlsson GS, Svärdsudd K, Welin L. Long-term effects of head injuries sustained during life in three male populations. J Neurosurg. 1987;67(2):197–205.

Castriotta RJ, Atanasov S, Wilde MC, Masel BE, Lai JM, Kuna ST. Treatment of sleep disorders after traumatic brain injury. J Clin Sleep Med. 2009;5(2):137–44.

Castriotta RJ, Wilde MC, Lai JM, Atanasov S, Masel BE, Kuna ST. Prevalence and consequences of sleep disorders in traumatic brain injury. J Clin Sleep Med. 2007;3(4):349–56.

Chan LG, Feinstein A. Persistent sleep disturbances independently predict poorer functional and social outcomes 1 year after mild traumatic brain injury. Head Trauma Rehabil. 2015;30(6):E67–75.

Chaput G, Giguère JF, Chauny JM, Denis R, Lavigne G. Relationship among subjective sleep complaints, headaches, and mood alterations following a mild traumatic brain injury. Sleep Med. 2009;10(7):713–6.

Chiu HY, Lin EY, Wei L, Lin JH, Lee HC, Fan YC, Tsai PS. Hypnotics use but not insomnia increased the risk of dementia in traumatic brain injury patients. Eur Neuropsychopharmacol. 2015;25(12):2271–7.

Collen J, Orr N, Lettieri CJ, Carter K, Holley AB. Sleep disturbances among soldiers with combat-related traumatic brain injury. Chest. 2012;142:622–30.

De Beaumont L, Théoret H, Mongeon D, Messier J, Leclerc S, Tremblay S, Ellemberg D, Lassonde M. Brain function decline in healthy retired athletes who sustained their last sports concussion in early adulthood. Brain. 2009; 132(Pt 3):695–708.

Duclos C, Beauregard MP, Bottari C, Ouellet MC, Gosselin N. The impact of poor sleep on cognition and activities of daily living after traumatic brain injury: a review. Aust Occup Ther J. 2015;62(1):2–12.

Farrell-Carnahan L, Barnett S, Lamberty G, Hammond FM, Kretzmer TS, Franke LM, Geiss M, Howe L, Nakase-Richardson R. Insomnia symptoms and behavioural health symptoms in veterans 1 year after traumatic brain injury. Brain Inj. 2015;29(12):1400–8.

Gagner C, Landry-Roy C, Lainé F, Beauchamp MH. Sleep-wake disturbances and fatigue after pediatric traumatic brain injury: a systematic review of the literature. J Neurotrauma. 2015;32(20):1539–52.

Gaudet CE, Weyandt LL. Immediate post-concussion and cognitive testing (ImPACT): a systematic review of the prevalence and assessment of invalid performance. Clin Neuropsychol. 2017;31(1):43–58.

Grima NA, Ponsford JL, St Hilaire MA, Mansfield D, Rajaratnam SM. Circadian melatonin rhythm following traumatic brain injury. Neurorehabil Neural Repair. 2016;30(10):972–7.

Guilleminault C, Yuen KM, Gulevich MG, Karadeniz D, Leger D, Philip P. Hypersomnia after head-neck trauma: a medicolegal dilemma. Neurology. 2000;54(3):653–9.

Himanen L, Portin R, Isoniemi H, Helenius H, Kurki T, Tenovuo O. Longitudinal cognitive changes in traumatic brain injury: a 30-year follow-up study. Neurology. 2006;66(2):187–92.

Holster JL, Bryan CJ, Heron EA, Seegmiller RA. Traumatic brain injury, sleep, and mental health: a longitudinal study of air force personnel pre- and post deployment to Iraq. J Head Trauma Rehabil. 2017;32(1):25–33.

Hou R, Han X, Sheng P, Tong W, Li Z, Xu D, et al. Risk factors associated with sleep disturbance following traumatic brain injury: clinical findings and questionnaire based study. PLoS One. 2013;8(10):e76087.

Hung R, Carroll LJ, Cancelliere C, Côté P, Rumney P, Keightley M, Donovan J, Stålnacke BM, Cassidy JD. Systematic review of the clinical course, natural history, and prognosis for pediatric mild traumatic brain injury: results of the international collaboration on mild traumatic brain injury prognosis. Arch Phys Med Rehabil. 2014;95(3 Suppl):S174–91.

Imbach LL, Valko PO, Li T, Maric A, Symeonidou ER, Stover JF, Bassetti CL, Mica L, Werth E, Baumann CR. Increased sleep need and daytime sleepiness 6 months after traumatic brain injury: a prospective controlled clinical trial. Brain. 2015;138:726–35.

Isoniemi H, Tenovuo O, Portin R, Himanen L, Kairisto V. Outcome of traumatic brain injury after three decades–relationship to ApoE genotype. J Neurotrauma. 2006;23(11):1600–8.

Jang SH, Seo WS, Kwon HG. Post-traumatic narcolepsy and injury of the ascending reticular activating system. Sleep Med. 2016;17:124–5.

Jaramillo CA, Eapen BC, McGeary CA, McGeary DD, Robinson J, Amuan M, et al. A cohort study examining headaches among veterans of Iraq and Afghanistan wars: associations with traumatic brain injury, PTSD, and depression. Headache. 2016;56(3):528–39.

Kemp S, Biswas R, Neumann V, Coughlan A. The value of melatonin for sleep disorders occurring post-head injury: a pilot RCT. Brain Inj. 2004;18:911–9.

Kempf J, Werth E, Kaiser PR, Bassetti CL, Baumann CR. Sleep-wake disturbances 3 years after traumatic brain injury. J Neurol Neurosurg Psychiatry. 2010;81(12):1402–5.

Konrad C, Geburek AJ, Rist F, Blumenroth H, Fischer B, Husstedt I, Arolt V, Schiffbauer H, Lohmann H. Long-term cognitive and emotional consequences of mild traumatic brain injury. Psychol Med. 2011;41(6):1197–211.

Lau BC, Collins MW, Lovell MR. Sensitivity and specificity of subacute computerized neurocognitive testing and symptom evaluation in predicting outcomes after sports-related concussion. Am J Sports Med. 2011;39(6):1209–16.

Lavigne G, Khoury S, Chauny JM, Desautels A. Pain and sleep in post-concussion/mild traumatic brain injury. Pain. 2015;156(Suppl 1):S75–85.

Lu W, Cantor JB, Aurora RN, Gordon WA, Krellman JW, Nguyen M, Ashman TA, Spielman L, Ambrose AF. The relationship between self-reported sleep disturbance and polysomnography in individuals with traumatic brain injury. Brain Inj. 2015;29(11):1342–50.

Management of Concussion/mTBI Working Group. VA/DoD clinical practice guideline for Management of Concussion/mild traumatic brain injury. J Rehabil Res Dev. 2009;46(6):CP1–68.

Martindale SL, Morissette SB, Rowland JA, Dolan SL. Sleep quality affects cognitive functioning in returning combat veterans beyond combat exposure, PTSD, and mild TBI history. Neuropsychology. 2017;31(1):93–104.

Masel BE, Scheibel RS, Kimbark T, Kuna ST. Excessive daytime sleepiness in adults with brain injuries. Arch Phys Med Rehabil. 2001;82:1526–32.

Mathias JL, Alvaro PK. Prevalence of sleep disturbances, disorders, and problems following traumatic brain injury: a meta-analysis. Sleep Med. 2012;13(7):898–905.

McClure DJ, Zuckerman SL, Kutscher SJ, Gregory AJ, Solomon GS. Baseline neurocognitive testing in sports-related concussions: the importance of a prior night's sleep. Am J Sports Med. 2014;42(2):472–8.

McKee AC, Cantu RC, Nowinski CJ, Hedley-Whyte ET, Gavett BE, Budson AE, Santini VE, Lee HS, Kubilus CA, Stern RA. Chronic traumatic encephalopathy in athletes: progressive tauopathy after repetitive head injury. J Neuropathol Exp Neurol. 2009;68(7):709–35.

Menn SJ, Yang R, Lankford A. Armodafinil for the treatment of excessive sleepiness associated with mild or moderate closed traumatic brain injury: a 12-week, randomized, double-blind study followed by a 12-month open-label extension. J Clin Sleep Med. 2014;10(11):1181–91.

Mignot EJ. A practical guide to the therapy of narcolepsy and hypersomnia syndromes. Neurotherapeutics. 2012;9(4):739–52.

Mihalik JP, Lengas E, Register-Mihalik JK, Oyama S, Begalle RL, Guskiewicz KM. The effects of sleep quality and sleep quantity on concussion baseline assessment. Clin J Sport Med. 2013;23(5):343–8.

Minen MT, Boubour A, Walia H, Barr W. Post-concussive syndrome: a focus on post-traumatic headache and related cognitive, psychiatric, and sleep issues. Curr Neurol Neurosci Rep. 2016;16(11):100.

Mollayeva T, Mollayeva S, Colantonio A. The risk of sleep disorder among persons with mild traumatic brain injury. Curr Neurol Neurosci Rep. 2016;16(6):55.

Mollayeva T, Mollayeva S, Shapiro CM, Cassidy JD, Colantonio A. Insomnia in workers with delayed recovery from mild traumatic brain injury. Sleep Med. 2016;19:153–61.

Monti JM, Voss MW, Pence A, McAuley E, Kramer AF, Cohen NJ. History of mild traumatic brain injury is associated with deficits in relational memory, reduced hippocampal volume, and less neural activity later in life. Front Aging Neurosci. 2013;5:41.

Nagtegaal JE, Kerkhof GA, Smits MG, Swart AC, van der Meer YG. Traumatic brain injury-associated delayed sleep phase syndrome. Funct Neurol. 1997;12(6):345–8.

Nakase-Richardson R, Sherer M, Barnett SD, et al. Prospective evaluation of the nature, course, and impact of acute sleep abnormality after traumatic brain injury. Arch Phys Med Rehabil. 2013;94(5):875–82.

Ouellet MC, Beaulieu-Bonneau S, Morin CM. Insomnia in patients with traumatic brain injury: frequency, characteristics, and risk factors. J Head Trauma Rehabil. 2006;21(3):199–212.

Ouellet MC, Beaulieu-Bonneau S, Morin CM. Sleep-wake disturbances after traumatic brain injury. Lancet Neurol. 2015;14(7):746–57.

Ouellet MC, Morin CM. Subjective and objective measures of insomnia in the context of traumatic brain injury: a preliminary study. Sleep Med. 2006;7(6):486–97.

Parcell DL, Ponsford JL, Redman JR, Rajaratnam SM. Poor sleep quality and changes in objectively recorded sleep after traumatic brain injury: a preliminary study. Arch Phys Med Rehabil. 2008;89(5):843–50.

Pillar G, Averbooch E, Katz N, Peled N, Kaufman Y, Shahar E. Prevalence and risk of sleep disturbances in adolescents after minor head injury. Pediatr Neurol. 2003;29:131–5.

Ponsford J, Draper K, Schönberger M. Functional outcome 10 years after traumatic brain injury: its relationship with demographic, injury severity, and cognitive and emotional status. J Int Neuropsychol Soc. 2008;14(2):233–42.

Poryazova R, Hug D, Baumann CR. Narcolepsy and traumatic brain injury: cause or consequence? Sleep Med. 2011;12(8):811.

Quan SF. Are sleep disturbances a risk for chronic traumatic encephalopathy? Only the shadow knows. J Clin Sleep Med. 2014;10(3):241–2.

Quinto C, Gellido C, Chokroverty S, Masdeu J. Posttraumatic delayed sleep phase syndrome. Neurology. 2000;54(1):250–2.

Raikes AC, Schaefer SY. Sleep quantity and quality during acute concussion: a pilot study. Sleep. 2016; [Epub ahead of print]

Rao V, Koliatsos V, Ahmed F, Lyketsos C, Kortte K. Neuropsychiatric disturbances associated with traumatic brain injury: a practical approach to evaluation and management. Semin Neurol. 2015;35(1):64–82.

Shekleton JA, Parcell DL, Redman JR, Phipps-Nelson J, Ponsford JL, Rajaratnam SM. Sleep disturbance and melatonin levels following traumatic brain injury. Neurology. 2010;74(21):1732–8.

Singh K, Morse AM, Tkachenko N, Kothare SV. Sleep disorders associated with traumatic brain injury-a review. Pediatr Neurol. 2016;60:30–6.

Smits MG, Nagtegaal JE. Post-traumatic delayed sleep phase syndrome. Neurology. 2000;55(6):902–3.

Sommerauer M, Valko PO, Werth E, Baumann CR. Excessive sleep need following traumatic brain injury. A case-control study of 36 patients. J Sleep Res. 2013; 22:634–9.

Sufrinko A, Pearce K, Elbin RJ, Covassin T, Johnson E, Collins M, Kontos AP. The effect of preinjury sleep difficulties on neurocognitive impairment and symptoms after sport-related concussion. Am J Sports Med. 2015;43(4):830–8.

Sumpter RE, Dorris L, Kelly T, McMillan TM. Pediatric sleep difficulties after moderate-severe traumatic brain injury. J Int Neuropsychol Soc. 2013;19(7):829–34.

Tham SW, Fales J, Palermo TM. Subjective and objective assessment of sleep in adolescents with mild traumatic brain injury. J Neurotrauma. 2015;32(11):847–52.

Tham SW, Palermo TM, Vavilala MS, Wang J, Jaffe KM, Koepsell TD, Dorsch A, Temkin N, Durbin D, Rivara FP. The longitudinal course, risk factors, and impact of sleep disturbances in children with traumatic brain injury. J Neurotrauma. 2012;29(1):154–61.

Theadom A, Starkey N, Jones K, Cropley M, Parmar P, Barker-Collo S, Feigin VL. Sleep difficulties and their impact on recovery following mild traumatic brain injury in children. Brain Inj. 2016;30(10):1243–8.

Viola-Saltzman M, Musleh C. Traumatic brain injury-induced sleep disorders. Neuropsychiatr Dis Treat. 2016;12:339–48.

Watson NF, Dikmen S, Machamer J, Doherty M, Temkin N. Hypersomnia following traumatic brain injury. J Clin Sleep Med. 2007;3:363–8.

Wickwire EM, Williams SG, Roth T, Capaldi VF, Jaffe M, Moline M, Motamedi GK, Morgan GW, Mysliwiec V, Germain A, Pazdan RM, Ferziger R, Balkin TJ, MacDonald ME, Macek TA, Yochelson MR, Scharf SM, Lettieri CJ. Sleep, sleep disorders, and mild traumatic brain injury. What we know and what we need to know: findings from a National Working Group. Neurotherapeutics. 2016;13(2):403–17.

Williams BR, Lazic SE, Ogilvie RD. Polysomnographic and quantitative EEG analysis of subjects with long-term insomnia complaints associated with mild traumatic brain injury. Clin Neurophysiol. 2008;119(2):429–38.

Zeitzer JM, Friedman L, O'Hara R. Insomnia in the context of traumatic brain injury. J Rehabil Res Dev. 2009;46(6):827–36.

18

Sleep problems in excessive technology use among adolescent: a systemic review and meta-analysis

Xi Mei[1,2*], Qi Zhou[1,2], Xingxing Li[1,2], Pan Jing[2], Xiaojia Wang[2] and Zhenyu Hu[1,2]

Abstract

Background: Inadequate sleep quantity and quality is a public health concern with an array of detrimental health outcomes. Portable technological devices have become a ubiquitous part of adolescents' lives and may affect their sleep duration and quality. The purpose of this study was to summarize published analyses of various technology uses and sleep outcomes and to examine whether there is an association between excessive technology use (ETU) and poor sleep outcomes in adolescents.

Method: We conduct a systematic review and meta-analysis. Pubmed, Embase, Science Direct, Google Scholar, Cochrane Library were used. Inclusion and exclusion criteria were performed. Only original research papers published from 1999 to 2018 and offcially reviewed by peers were included for analysis. We used the Review Manager 5.3 software for statistical analysis.

Results: Nineteen studies were included, and their quality was assessed. These studies involved 253,904 adolescents (mean [SD] age, 14.82 [0.83] years; 51.1% male). There was a strong and consistent association between ETU and sleep problems (odds ratio [OR], 1.33; 95% CI, 1.24–1.43) ($P < 0.00001$, $I^2 = 96\%$), reduced sleep duration (SMD, -0.25; 95% CI, -0.37-0.12) ($P < 0.00001$, $I^2 = 81\%$), and prolonged sleep onset latency (OR, 0.16; 95% CI, -0.02-0.34) ($P = 0.05$, $I^2 = 66\%$).

Conclusions: ETU has a significant effect on sleep duration in adolescents over 14 years of age, prolong the SOL of adolescents, and may lead to several sleep problems. Interventions must be developed to raise awareness of the potential health hazard to improve sleep hygiene through an integrated approach involving teachers, health care professionals, and parents.

Keywords: Excessive technology use, Sleep problems, Adolescents, Meta-analysis

Background

Sleep plays an important role in the growth of young people. The problem of sleep affects human cognition and social function, and is also a warning signal for a variety of diseases. Sleep disorders negatively affects several domains including school performance, mood regulation, cognitive process, and general health in adolescents (Dahl & Lewin, 2002; Gruber et al., 2012; Fredriksen et al., 2004; Wolfson & Carskadon, 1998). The USA National Sleep Foundation (NSF, 2006) recommends that adolescents sleep for no less than 9 hours a day (National Sleep Foundation, 2006), but in the USA, 75% of those 17 to 18 years old report insufficient sleep, and young people in other developed countries have the same phenomenon (National Sleep Foundation, 2014).

Teenagers now have multiple electronic devices such as smart phones and ipad. The daily watch on the screen has increased significantly. Excessive technology use (ETU) may contribute to the adolescent insufficient sleep. Previous study have found that sleep reduction appears to be aggravated by excessive use of technology devices such as TV viewing (Tynjala et al., 1993), internet use (Yen et al., 2008), video gaming (Weaver et al., 2010; Rehbein et al., 2010) and mobile telephone use

* Correspondence: meixi18401856@163.com
[1]Ningbo Key Laboratory of Sleep Medicine, Zhuangyu South Road No.1, Zhenhai District, Ningbo City 315201, Zhejiang Province, China
[2]Ningbo Kangning Hospital, Ningbo City 315201, Zhejiang Province, China

(Van den Bulck, 2007; Munezawa et al., 2011). ETU have been found to be associated with reduced sleep duration (Tynjala et al., 1993), delayed sleep onset latency (Tynjala et al., 1993; Weaver et al., 2010) and increased other sleep problems (Rehbein et al., 2010; Munezawa et al., 2011).

ETU in teenagers has been a hot spot of research for decades. A large number of academic literatures have reported related studies. However, the association between ETU and poor sleep outcomes has been underexplored, because the speed of technological devices developing has outpaced the research capabilities. In the current study, we present a systematic review to quantify the influence of ETU on sleep outcomes in a meta-analysis. Compared to previous study (Carter et al., 2016), we make a further exploration of sleep duration, sleep onset latency, as well as include several new related articles.

Method
Databases online
Pubmed, Embase, Science Direct, Google Scholar, Cochrane Library were used. We conducted extensive searches for studies published from 1999 using the terms "excessive Internet/technology use" or "problematic Internet/technology use" or "pathological Internet/technology use" or "Internet addiction" or "excessive computer/technology use" or "Internet gaming" or "computer gaming" or "Internet gaming addiction" combined with the terms "insomnia" or "sleep problems" or "sleep quality" or "sleep disorders" or "sleep disturbance" or "sleep deprivation". The year 1999 was chosen as the starting year for the search because that is when active empirical inquiry into the psychological factors affecting Internet addiction first began.

Study selection
This study was conducted following Preferred Reporting Items for Systematic Reviews and Meta-analyses (PRISMA) guidelines. After completing the search on the electronic databases, titles and abstracts of the identified articles were assessed for their suitability to be included in this research. Studies were included if they (1) were epidemiological studies of adolescents of school age between 11 and 20 years with appropriate study designs; (2) were cross-sectional, case-control and cohort studies that examined the relationship between ETU or problematic internet use and sleep problems including insomnia and poor sleep quality; (3) provided information of ETU and sleep outcomes in the shape of quantized data.

Exclusion criteria
Studies were excluded if they 1) did not provide sufficient information to calculate the aggregate prevalence and odds ratio (OR); 2) did not provide a specific definition or criteria for ETU or problematic internet use; 3) the authors did not respond to provide further information upon request including the psychiatric co-morbidity directly related to ETU (e.g. online gambling). Articles with abstracts that were written in the English language but had full texts written in non-English languages were excluded.

Quality assessment
The full texts of all relevant articles were retrieved, and their eligibility for inclusion was assessed. Two reviewers (Q.Z. and P. J.) independently assessed the methodological quality of all full-text articles, and discrepancies were resolved by a third reviewer (X.M.). We followed the guidelines in the Meta-analysis of Observational Studies in Epidemiology (MOOSE) statement for reporting (Stroup et al., 2000).

Definition of poor sleep quality
Since the Pittsburgh Sleep Quality Index (PSQI) (Buysse et al., 1989) was developed, based upon the International Statistical Classification of Disease and Related Health Problems, 10th edition (ICD-10) (World Health Organization, 1992) and the Diagnostic and Statistical Manual of Mental Disorders (DSM-V) (American Psychiatric Association, 2013) criteria for classification of insomnia, it was employed in plenty of original studies to assess insomnia and sleep disturbances. Furthermore, early awakenings, night awakenings, and long sleep onset latency were used to assess the sleep quality.

Technology and internet use
In this study, type of technology included PC, mobile phone, television, video games, and music. Internet was used for game, video, music, social communication, and study. A number of adolescents' time of usage was before sleep. In our study, we define the ETU as the problematic internet use (PIU) and excessive use of PC, cell phone, MP3 player, tablet, game console and TV as well as the technology use before sleep in bed and heavy use in daytime.

Measurement of association between technology use and sleep outcomes
Included studies measured the association between technology use and the influence on sleep using either regression slopes (β), correlation coefficients (r), or ORs. To ensure consistency in interpretation, studies that reported dichotomous data or logistic regression analyses of sleep quality and continues data of sleep duration were pooled in a meta-analysis.

Statistical analysis and heterogeneity

All statistical analyses were performed with Review Manager 5.3 using the random-effects models for aggregate prevalence and pooled OR. Statistical heterogeneity was assessed using the I^2 statistic. Dichotomous and continues data were respectively presented as OR and SMD with the associated 95% CIs, P values, and I^2 summary data. Heterogeneity exceeding 85% was explored using subgroup analyses. Subgroups to explore heterogeneity were classified by country.

Results

Study selection

A total of 297 studies were identified, and 67 full texts were reviewed, leading to 40 being excluded (Fig. 1). 23 studies involving 253,904 adolescent (mean [SD] age, 14.82 [0.83] years; 51.1% male) were included after

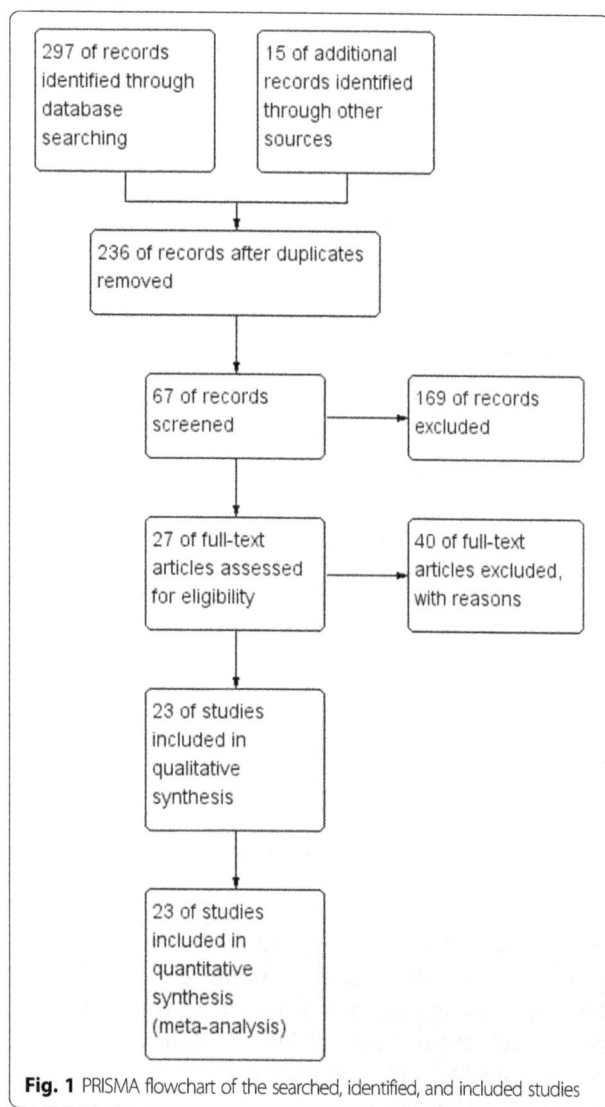

Fig. 1 PRISMA flowchart of the searched, identified, and included studies

assessed for methodological quality, with 4 excluded because of poor methods conduct or reporting.

Study characteristics

Table 1 showed characteristics of included studies. Author, publication year, country, study design and methods, participants (% male participants), case definition of technology exposure, exposure type of technology, age range (or average age) and sleep outcomes were listed.

Included studies were conducted in **Europe** ($n = 9$) (Arora et al., 2012; Arora et al., 2013; Arora et al., 2014; Bruni et al., 2015; Hysing et al., 2015; Van den Bulck, 2004; Lemola et al., 2014; Nuutinen et al., 2014; Punama-ki et al., 2006), **East Asia** ($n = 10$) (An et al., 2014; Cheung & Wong, 2011; Choi et al., 2009; Liu et al., 2017; Mak et al., 2014; Park, 2014; Park & Lee, 2017; Tan et al., 2016; Tamura et al., 2017; Kim et al., 2018), and **West Asia** ($n = 4$) (Fatih et al., 2013; Shochat et al., 2010; Sami et al., 2018; Hawi et al., 2018). Eight studies assessed the sleep duration of ETU and no excessive technology use (Arora et al., 2013; Arora et al., 2014; Fatih et al., 2013; Cheung & Wong, 2011; Choi et al., 2009; Lemola et al., 2014; Shochat et al., 2010; Hawi et al., 2018). Three studies assessed the sleep onset latency (Arora et al., 2014; Cheung & Wong, 2011; Shochat et al., 2010). Most of studies investigated association between the ETU and sleep problems.

Sleep outcomes

Sleep duration

Figure 2 shows the sleep duration of control and ETU groups. As can be seen, sleep duration of people in control condition is longer than that of ETU. The SMD is −0.25, and 95%CI is (−0.37, −0.12) ($P < .00001$, $I^2 = 81\%$). The large heterogeneity was due to the study by Choi2009, which recruited people of average age of 16.7 ± 1.0. People's average age or age range in other studies were 13.9 ± 2.0 of Arora2013, 11–13 of Arora2014, 16.04 ± 1.02 of Canan2013, 14.70 ± 2.02 of Cheung2010, 14.82 ± 1.26 of Lemola2014, 14.0 ± 0.8 of Shochat2010, 16.2 ± 1.0 of Hawi2018, respectively. After that study was excluded, the SMD was −0.30 (95% CI, −0.37, −0.23) ($P < .00001$, $I^2 = 21\%$). Considering the age range of subjects was large, we divided them into two groups: younger adolescents (average age ≤ 14 years) and older adolescents (average age > 14 years). The SMD of younger group is −0.30, and 95%CI is (−0.39, −0.20) ($P = 0.87$, $I^2 = 0\%$). The SMD of older group is −0.22, and 95% CI is (−0.41, −0.02) ($P < .00001$, $I^2 = 87\%$).

Sleep onset latency

Three studies reported sleep onset latency of frequent use group and control group (Fig. 3). Sleep onset latency

Table 1 Summary of studies included in the meta-analysis (n = 19)

Reference (author, year)	country	Study design & methods	Participants (% male participants)	Case definition of technology exposure and sleep outcomes	Exposure type of technology	Age range (or Average age)	Sleep Outcomevariable
An, 2014 (An et al., 2014)	China	cross-sectional school-based study	n = 13,723 (48%boys)	YIAT, PSQI, MSQA	Internet use	10.0–20.0 (15.26 ± 1.67)	Sleep quality
Arora, 2012 (Arora et al., 2012)	UK	cross-sectional school-based study	n = 624 (35.1%boys)	SSHS, TUQ	TV viewing; Video gaming; PC/laptop; Mobiles	11.0–18.0	Sleep quality
Arora, 2013 (Arora et al., 2013)	UK	cross-sectional school-based study	n = 632 (36.1%boys)	SSHS, TUQ	Computer use; Mobile telephone use; TV viewing; Video gaming	11.0–18.0 (13.9 ± 2.0)	Sleep duration
Arora, 2014 (Arora et al., 2014)	UK	cross-sectional study	n = 738 (54.5%boys)	SSHS, TUQ	Television; Video gaming; Mobile telephone; Music; Computer or laptop (study); Internet (social)	11.0–13.0	Sleep duration, sleep-onset latency, sleep problems including early awakening, difficulty falling to sleep, night awakenings
Bruni,2015 (Bruni et al., 2015)	Italy	cross-sectional study	n = 850 (42.8%boys)	SSHS, MPIQ, SPQ, Questionnaire on the use of technology	mobile phone-related activities; Internet-related activities	11.0–16.0 (13.53 ± 1.72)	Sleep quality
Canan, 2013 (Fatih et al., 2013)	Turkey	cross-sectional school-based study	n = 1956 (47.5%boys)	YIAT, Questionnaire of sleep quality	Chat rooms and Internet; messaging; Web surfing; playing online games; academic activities; Other Internet activities such as e-mail checking; reading online news; watching online videos; shopping.	14.0–18.0 (16.04 ± 1.02)	Sleep duration, sleep problems including early awakening, difficulty falling to sleep, night awakenings
Cheung, 2010 (Cheung & Wong, 2011)	Hong Kong	school-based cross-sectional study	n = 719 (60.4%boys)	PSQI, CIAS, GHQ-12	Internet use	10.0–20.0 (14.70 ± 2.02)	Sleep onset latency, Sleep duration, sleep quality
Choi, 2009 (Choi et al., 2009)	Korea	cross-sectional study	n = 2336 (57.5%boys)	YIAT, ESS	Internet use	16.7 ± 1.0	Sleep duration, sleep problems including early awakening, difficulty falling to sleep, night awakenings
Hysing, 2015 (Hysing et al., 2015)	Norway	A large cross-sectional population-based survey study	n = 9846 (46.5%boys)	HBSC	PC, cell phone, MP3 player, tablet, game console and TV.	16.0–19.0	Sleep problems
Jan, 2014 (Van den Bulck, 2004)	Belgium	cross-sectional study	n = 2546	Questionnaires of media use, sleep variables, activity level.	television-viewing; Computer-game playing; Internet use	14.76 ± 1.71	Sleep time
Lemola, 2014 (Lemola et al., 2014)	Switzerland	cross-sectional study	n = 362 (55.2%boys)	ISI, Media Use assess items.	TV or movies, play video games, talk on the phone or text, and spend time online on FaceBook or in chat rooms or surf the Internet	12.0–17.0 (14.82 ± 1.26)	Sleep duration, sleep difficulties
Liu, 2017 (Liu et al., 2017)	China	cross-sectional study	n = 1196 (53%boys)	MPAI, PSQI	mobile phone	14.0–20.0 (16.75 ± 0.94)	Sleep quality
Mak, 2014 (Mak et al., 2014)	Hong Kong	cross-sectional survey	n = 762 (57.6%boys)	PSQI, SQI, ESS, Questionnaires of	Screen viewing	12.0–20.0 (15.27 ± 1.70)	Sleep quality, daytime sleepiness

Table 1 Summary of studies included in the meta-analysis (n = 19) *(Continued)*

Reference (author, year)	country	Study design & methods	Participants (% male participants)	Case definition of technology exposure and sleep outcomes technology use	Exposure type of technology	Age range (or Average age)	Sleep Outcomevariable
Nuutinen, 2014 (Nuutinen et al., 2014)	Finland, France and Denmark.	a cross-sectional study	n = 5402 (47%boys)	HBSC	computer use	15.61 ± 0.37	Sleep habits
Park, 2014 (Park, 2014)	Korean	a cross-sectional study	n = 73,238 (52.4%boys)	YIAT, Questionnaires of sleep satisfaction	PIU	12.0–18.0 (15.06 ± 1.75)	Sleep satisfaction
Park, 2017 (Park & Lee, 2017)	Korean	a cross-sectional study	n = 70,696 (52.4%boys)	YIAT, Questionnaires of sleep satisfaction	PIU	12.0–18.0 (15.10 ± 1.75)	Sleep satisfaction
Punamaki, 2006 (Punamaki et al., 2006)	Finland	a cross-sectional study	n = 7292 (44.8%boys)	Questionnaires of ICT use and sleep habits	computer use; Mobile phone use	12.0–18.0	Sleeping habits
Shochat, 2010 (Shochat et al., 2010)	Israeli	a cross-sectional study	n = 449 (50.1%boys)	SSHS, EMFQ	electronic media	14.0 ± 0.8	Sleep duration, sleep onset latency, sleep habits
Tan, 2016 (Tan et al., 2016)	China	a cross-sectional study	n = 1661 (51.8%boys)	YIAT, PSQI	Internet use	12.0–18.0	Sleep disturbance
Sami, 2018 (Sami et al., 2018)	Israel	a cross-sectional study	n = 631 (45.5%boys)	YIAT, CASC	Internet use	12.0–18.0 (14.59 ± 1.53)	Sleep disturbance
Tamura, 2017 (Tamura et al., 2017)	Japan	a cross-sectional study	n = 295 (58.6%boys)	Questionnaires of mobile phone use, AIS	Mobile phone use	15.0–19.0 (16.2 ± 0.9)	Insomnia
Hawi, 2018 (Hawi et al., 2018)	Lebanon	a cross-sectional study	n = 524 (47.9%boys)	Questionnaires of sleep habit, IGD-20 Test	Internet game	15.0–19.0 (16.2 ± 1.0)	Sleep duration, sleep disturbance
Kim, 2018 (Kim et al., 2018)	Korea	a cross-sectional study	n = 57,426 (50.3%boys)	KYRBWS	Internet use	12.0–15.0 (13.5)	Sleep Satisfaction

YIAT Young Internet Addiction Test, *PSQI* Pittsburgh Sleep Quality Index, *MSQA* Multidimensional Sub-health Questionnaire of Adolescents, *SSHS* School Sleep Habits Survey, *TUQ* Technology Use Questionnaire, *MPIQ* Mobile Phone Involvement Questionnaire, *SPQ* Shorter Promis Questionnaire, *CIAS* Chinese Internet Addiction Scale, *GHQ-12* The 12-item version of General Health Questionnaire, *ESS* Epworth Sleepiness Scale, *HBSC* Health Behavior in School-aged Children, *ISI* Insomnia Severity Index, *MPAI* Mobile Phone Addiction Index, *SQI* Sleep Quality Index, *ICT* Information and Communication Technology, *EMFQ* Electronic Media and Fatigue questionnaire, *CASC* Child and Adolescent Sleep Checklist, *AIS* Athens Insomnia Scale, *IGD* Internet Gaming Disorder, *KYRBWS* Korea Youth Risk Behavior Web-based Survey

of people in control group is shorter than that of technology group ($P = 0.05$). The pooled SMD for sleep onset latency was 0.16 (95% CI, -0.02-0.34) (P = 0.05, $I^2 = 66\%$).

Sleep problems

There were data from 22 studies (An et al., 2014; Arora et al., 2012; Arora et al., 2014; Bruni et al., 2015; Fatih et al., 2013; Cheung & Wong, 2011; Choi et al., 2009; Hysing et al., 2015; Van den Bulck, 2004; Lemola et al., 2014; Liu et al., 2017; Mak et al., 2014; Nuutinen et al., 2014; Park, 2014; Park & Lee, 2017; Punama-ki et al., 2006; Shochat et al., 2010; Tan et al., 2016; Sami et al., 2018; Tamura et al., 2017; Hawi et al., 2018; Kim et al., 2018) that investigated association between the technology use and sleep problems (Fig. 4), including poor sleep quality (An et al., 2014; Arora et al., 2012; Bruni et al., 2015; Hysing et al., 2015; Lemola et al., 2014; Liu et al., 2017; Mak et al., 2014; Sami et al., 2018; Hawi et al., 2018), early awakenings (Arora et al., 2014; Fatih et al., 2013; Choi et al., 2009; Shochat et al., 2010), difficulty falling asleep (Arora et al., 2014; Fatih et al., 2013; Choi et al., 2009; Shochat et al., 2010), night awakenings (Arora et al., 2014; Fatih et al., 2013; Choi et al., 2009), less sleep quantity (Van den Bulck, 2004; Nuutinen et al., 2014; Park, 2014; Park & Lee, 2017; Punama-ki et al., 2006; Shochat et al., 2010; Kim et al., 2018) and insomnia (Cheung & Wong, 2011; Tan et al., 2016; Tamura et al., 2017). Three subgroups were classified by country. The OR of Asia subgroup was 1.55 (95% CI, 1.48–1.62) ($P = 0.24$, $I^2 = 23\%$). The large heterogeneity of Asia-China subgroup was due to the study of An2014. After that study was excluded, the pooled OR was 1.10 (95% CI, 1.05, 1.15) ($P = 0.002$, $I^2 = 79\%$). The large heterogeneity of Europe subgroup was due to the study of Jan2004, which recruited people of two average ages: first year: first year of secondary school (average age, 13 years); fourth year: fourth year of secondary school (average age, 16 years). After the study of Jan2004 was excluded, the OR was 1.24 (95% CI, 1.16, 1.33) ($P < .00001$, $I^2 = 80\%$).

In Asia subgroup, dichotomous data were available from study of Canan2013 that investigated sleep problem including difficulty falling asleep, night awakenings, and early morning awakenings, the prevalences of which in no frequent use population were 37.9, 36.0, 16.1% respectively, and the prevalences of frequent use population were 44.9, 44.1, 19.0% respectively. In the study of Choi2009, Tamura2017 and Park2017, dichotomous data were also available, and there was an increased odds of sleep problems in people who had frequently used a technology device. In the study of Park2014, the associations between sleep satisfaction and problematic internet use was

investigated [β coefficients (SE) were 0.47 (0.03)], and odd ratio adjusted for age, sex, residing region, perceived academic performance, family economic status, parents' level of education, and body mass index. In the recent study of Sami2018, Hawi2018, and Kim2018, the ORs were 1.70, 1.41, and 1.72 respectively.

In Asia-China subgroup, the associations between technology use and sleep quality was reported by An2014 [β coefficients (SE) were 0.894 (0.055)], Cheung2010 [β coefficients (SE) were 0.08 (0.01)], Liu2017 [β coefficients (SE) were 0.34 (0. 1033)]. In the study of Mak2014, the associations between technology use and sleep quality, and associations between technology use and excessive daytime sleepiness were accessed, and pooled OR was 1.14 (95% CI, 1.08, 1.20) ($P < 0.001$). In the study of Tan2016, the prevalence of problematic internet use was 17.2% among adolescents, with 40.0% of adolescents suffering from sleep disturbance, problematic internet use was found to be a significant predictor of sleep disturbance (β = 0.048, $P < 0.001$).

In Europe subgroup, study of Arora2012 developed a model adjusted for age, sex, ethnicity, activity, school, snacking, depression, bedroom sharing and morningness-eveningness. After conducting pathway analysis, the impact of frequent technology use to sleep quality was evaluated [β coefficients (SE) were 0.75 (0.27)]. In the study of Arora2014, the OR and 95% confidence intervals for the multinomial regression between technologies and sleep parameters were 1.41 [1.18, 1.68]. Correlation between internet/mobile phone use and sleep problems was reported in the study of Bruni2015 (β = 0.31, $P < 0.01$). In the study of Hysing2015, the long sleep onset latency and sleep deficit were contribute to sleep problems, the pooled OR was 1.26 (95% CI, 1.22, 1.30) ($P < 0.001$). The effect of weekday and weekend technology use on sleep problems was investigated by Jan2004, the pooled OR was 1.07 (95% CI, 1.05, 1.09) ($P = 0.16$, $I^2 = 36\%$). In the study of Lemola2014, regression models revealed that electronic media use in bed before sleep was related to sleep difficulties (β = 0.21, P < 0.001). In the study of Nuutinen2014, three countries' data were collected, the pooled OR was 1.22 (95% CI, 1.12, 1.33) ($P = 0.46$, $I^2 = 0\%$). Technology use including computer use and mobile phone use leaded to sleep problems in the study of Punamaki2006, the associations between technology use and sleep problems were reported in 12 and 14 years adolescents group and in 16 and 18 years adolescents group, the pooled OR was 1.24 (95% CI, 1.14, 1.35) ($P = 0.07$, $I^2 = 53\%$). In the study of Shochat2010, technology use included internet use and television use, the pooled OR for sleep problems was 1.11 (95% CI, 1.07, 1.15) ($P = 0.01$ $I^2 = 54\%$).

Discussion

The present study sought to quantify the relationships between technology uses and sleep outcomes in adolescent

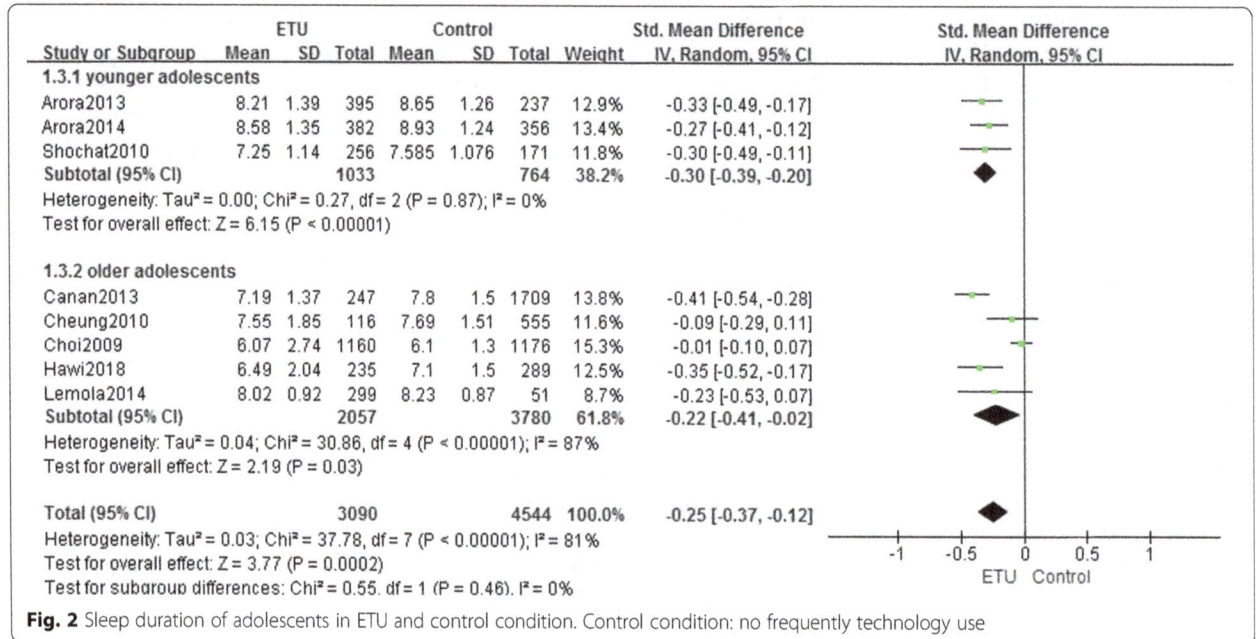

Fig. 2 Sleep duration of adolescents in ETU and control condition. Control condition: no frequently technology use

participants. The current meta-analysis ultimately contained results from 23 articles and involved combined sample sizes that ranged from 295 to 73,238 subjects, with 253,904 in total. This large sample could supply a considerable empirical basis for determining the contribution of technology overuses on poor sleep outcomes. In the first, ETU may disrupt the sleep by directly shortening or interrupting sleep time. In the second, the information on the Internet could be psychologically stimulating and affect the mood before sleep. Thirdly, the light emitted from the electronic screen may affect the circadian rhythm and physiological sleep (Cain & Gradisar, 2010; Hale & Guan, 2015; Chang et al., 2015). There may be other aspects of ETU that have not been found to damage sleep.

On the addictive aspect of technological devices or Internet use, young people may be more vulnerable than adults (Griffths & Hunt, 1998). They may be more likely to be affected by internal conditions because their brain and mental state are in development. An interesting result

of our meta-analysis was that studies in Asia, especially in Korea, reported larger effect sizes than Europe and Asia-China studies for outcome variables. This result was consistent with other findings (Winkler et al., 2013) indicating that culture-related differences in the study procedures as well as methodological differences may have caused this outcome. Meanwhile, sleep duration has significant differences among different age groups, while sleep onset latency does not (Ohayon et al., 2004). Our results indicated that ETU has a significant effect on sleep duration in adolescents over 14 years of age.

Although we have carried out a large number of sample analyses, our research still has some limitations. The limitations of research in this area include (1) the measurement error of self-reported data makes it difficult for us to determine the accuracy of the results, (2) in different articles the classification of the use of technology is different, and the definition of ETU is not the same (3) the speed of technology development is far beyond the

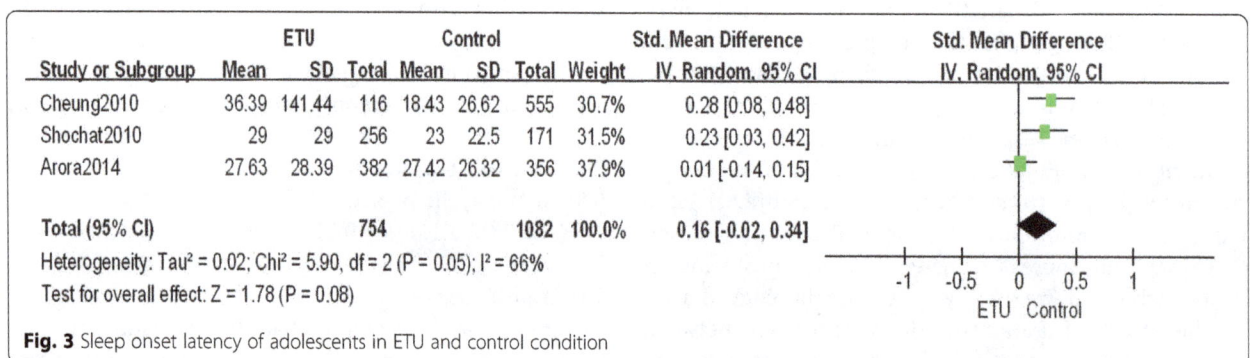

Fig. 3 Sleep onset latency of adolescents in ETU and control condition

Study or Subgroup	log[Odds Ratio]	SE	Weight	Odds Ratio IV, Random, 95% CI	Odds Ratio IV, Random, 95% CI
1.2.1 Asia					
Canan2013	0.2852	0.0831	4.9%	1.33 [1.13, 1.57]	
Choi2009	0.5008	0.0695	5.3%	1.65 [1.44, 1.89]	
Hawi2018	0.346	0.1052	4.3%	1.41 [1.15, 1.74]	
Kim2018	0.5423	0.0836	4.9%	1.72 [1.46, 2.03]	
Park2014	0.47	0.03	6.3%	1.60 [1.51, 1.70]	
Park2017	0.4187	0.0205	6.4%	1.52 [1.46, 1.58]	
Sami2018	0.53	0.1362	3.4%	1.70 [1.30, 2.22]	
Tamura2017	0.2624	0.4675	0.6%	1.30 [0.52, 3.25]	
Subtotal (95% CI)			36.1%	1.55 [1.48, 1.62]	
Heterogeneity: Tau² = 0.00; Chi² = 9.12, df = 7 (P = 0.24); I² = 23%					
Test for overall effect: Z = 19.25 (P < 0.00001)					
1.2.2 Asia-China					
An2014	0.8936	0.0551	0.0%	2.44 [2.19, 2.72]	
Cheung2010	0.08	0.01	6.5%	1.08 [1.06, 1.10]	
Liu2017	0.34	0.1033	4.3%	1.40 [1.15, 1.72]	
Mak2014	0.131	0.0276	6.3%	1.14 [1.08, 1.20]	
Tan2016	0.048	0.0146	6.5%	1.05 [1.02, 1.08]	
Subtotal (95% CI)			23.6%	1.10 [1.05, 1.15]	
Heterogeneity: Tau² = 0.00; Chi² = 14.34, df = 3 (P = 0.002); I² = 79%					
Test for overall effect: Z = 4.06 (P < 0.0001)					
1.2.3 Europe					
Arora2012	0.75	0.27	1.4%	2.12 [1.25, 3.59]	
Arora2014	0.3436	0.0909	4.7%	1.41 [1.18, 1.68]	
Bruni2015	0.31	0.1203	3.8%	1.36 [1.08, 1.73]	
Hysing2015	0.2311	0.0165	6.5%	1.26 [1.22, 1.30]	
Jan2004	0.0677	0.0096	0.0%	1.07 [1.05, 1.09]	
Lemola2014	0.21	0.0638	5.5%	1.23 [1.09, 1.40]	
Nuutinen2014	0.1989	0.0436	6.0%	1.22 [1.12, 1.33]	
Punamaki2006	0.2151	0.0429	6.0%	1.24 [1.14, 1.35]	
Shochat2010	0.1044	0.0187	6.4%	1.11 [1.07, 1.15]	
Subtotal (95% CI)			40.3%	1.24 [1.16, 1.33]	
Heterogeneity: Tau² = 0.01; Chi² = 35.63, df = 7 (P < 0.00001); I² = 80%					
Test for overall effect: Z = 6.39 (P < 0.00001)					
Total (95% CI)			100.0%	1.33 [1.24, 1.43]	
Heterogeneity: Tau² = 0.02; Chi² = 491.68, df = 19 (P < 0.00001); I² = 96%					
Test for overall effect: Z = 7.78 (P < 0.00001)					
Test for subgroup differences: Chi² = 116.00, df = 2 (P < 0.00001), I² = 98.3%					

0.7 0.85 1 1.2 1.5
ETU Control

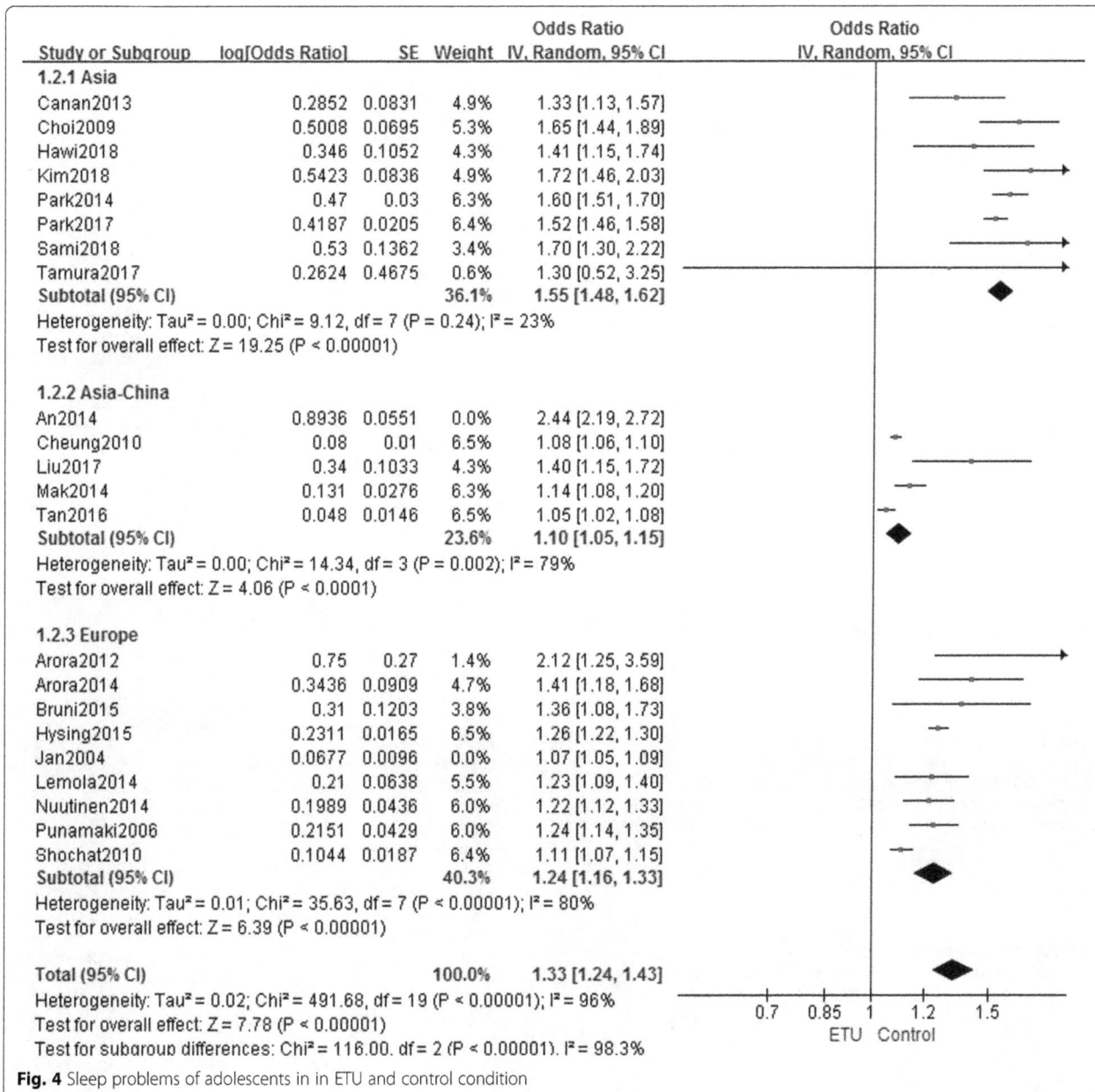

Fig. 4 Sleep problems of adolescents in in ETU and control condition

speed of research (4) the design of observational studies has its inherent weaknesses.

Despite these limitations, the results of our study have several suggestions and implications. A detailed investigation of sleep duration and sleep onset latency in the ETU subjects was carried out. The results suggesting that the deleterious association between screen-based technology overuse and sleep is a major public health problem in adolescents. We suggest that if a young people who own technological devices has a sleep problem it is possible to consider whether or not it is related to ETU. During the clinical visits by health visitors or school nurses, we also encourage screening of adolescents to identify whether their sleep is associated with ETU, meanwhile, formulating a treatment plan for a specific situation.

Conclusion

In this study, we summarized published articles of various technology uses and sleep outcomes. We suggested that there is a significant association between ETU and poor sleep outcomes in adolescents. ETU has a significant effect on sleep duration in adolescents over 14 years of age, prolong the SOL of adolescents, and may lead to several sleep problems. We recommend that interventions to minimize technology use need to be developed and evaluated. Parents should understand the effects of the ETU factor on adolescents' sleep and pay more attention to their sleep and make children go to bed earlier, so as to ensure sleep time and improve sleep quality. In addition, teachers and doctors must help parents to raise awareness of the potential health hazard and to improve sleep hygiene.

Abbreviations

CIAS: Chinese Internet Addiction Scale; EMFQ: Electronic Media and Fatigue questionnaire; ESS: Epworth Sleepiness Scale; ETU: Excessive Technology Use; GHQ-12: The 12-item version of General Health Questionnaire; HBSC: Health Behavior in School-aged Children; ICT: Information and Communication Technology; ISI: Insomnia Severity Index; MPAI: Mobile Phone Addiction Index; MPIQ: Mobile Phone Involvement Questionnaire; MSQA: Multidimensional Sub-health Questionnaire of Adolescents; PIU: Problematic Internet Use; PSQI: Pittsburgh Sleep Quality Index; SPQ: Shorter Promis Questionnaire; SQI: Sleep Quality Index; SSHS: School Sleep Habits Survey; TUQ: Technology Use Questionnaire; YIAT: Young Internet Addiction Test

Funding

This research was supported by Ningbo social development science and technology research project (grant No. 2014C50055).

Authors' contributions

Study concept and design: XM. Acquisition, analysis, or interpretation of data: All authors. Drafting of the manuscript: XM. Statistical analysis: QZ, XL. Obtained funding: XW. Administrative, technical, or material support: ZH. Study supervision: XW and ZH. All authors read and approved the final manuscript.

Competing interests

The authors declare that they have no competing interests.

References

American Psychiatric Association. Diagnostic and Statistical Manual of Mental Disorders 5th edn., 2013 , 51 (2) :4189–4189.

An J, Sun Y, Wan Y, Chen J, Wang X, Tao F. Associations between problematic internet use and adolescents' physical and psychological symptoms: possible role of sleep quality. J Addict Med. 2014;8:282–7.

Arora T, Hosseini-Araghi M, Bishop J, Yao GL, Thomas GN, Taheri S. The complexity of obesity in UK adolescents: relationships with quantity and type of technology, sleep duration and quality, academic performance and aspiration. Pediatric Obesity. 2012;8:358–66.

Arora T, Hussain S, Hubert Lam K-B, Lily Yao G, Neil Thomas G, Taheri S. Exploring the complex pathways among specific types of technology, self-reported sleep duration and body mass index in UK adolescents. Int J Obes. 2013; 37:1254–60.

Arora T, Emma B, Neil Thomas G, Taheri S. Associations between specific technologies and adolescent sleep quantity, sleep quality, and parasomnias. Sleep Med. 2014;15:240–7.

Bruni O, Sette S, Fontanesi L, Baiocco R, Laghi F, Baumgartner E. Technology use and sleep quality in preadolescence and adolescence. J Clin Sleep Med. 2015;11(12):1433–41.

Buysse DJ, Reynolds CF, Monk TH, Berman SR, Kupfer DJ. The Pittsburgh sleep quality index: a new instrument for psychiatric practice and research. Psychiatry Res. 1989;28:193–213.

Cain N, Gradisar M. Electronic media use and sleep in school-aged children and adolescents: a review. Sleep Med. 2010;11(8):735–42.

Carter B, Rees P, Hale L, et al. Association between portable screen-based media device access or use and sleep outcomes: a systematic review and Meta-analysis. JAMA Pediatr. 2016;170(12):1202–8.

Chang AM, Aeschbach D, Duffy JF, Czeisler CA. Evening use of light-emitting eReaders negatively affects sleep, circadian timing, and next-morning alertness. PNAS. 2015;112(4):1232–7.

Cheung LM, Wong WS. The effects of insomnia and internet addiction on depression in Hong Kong Chinese adolescents: an exploratory cross-sectional analysis. J. Sleep Res. 2011;20(2):311–7.

Choi K, Son H, Park M, Han J, Kim K, Lee B, Gwak H. Internet overuse and excessive daytime sleepiness in adolescents. Psychiatry Clin Neurosci. 2009; 63:455–62.

Dahl RE, Lewin DS. Pathways to adolescent health sleep regulation and behavior. J Adolesc Health. 2002;31:175–84.

Fatih CANAN, Osman YILDIRIM, Gjergji SINANI, Onder OZTURK, Tuba Yildirim USTUNEL, Ahmet ATAOGLU. Internet addiction and sleep disturbance symptoms among Turkish high school students. Sleep and Biological Rhythms. 2013;11:210–3.

Fredriksen K, Rhodes J, Reddy R, Way N. Sleepless in Chicago: tracking the effects of adolescent sleep loss during the middle school years. Child Dev. 2004;75:84–95.

Griffiths MD, Hunt N. Dependence on computer games by adolescents. Psychol Rep. 1998;82:475–80.

Gruber R, Michaelsen S, Bergmame L, et al. Short sleep duration is associated with teacher-reported inattention and cognitive problems in healthy schoolaged children. Nat Sci Sleep. 2012;4:33.

Hale L, Guan S. Screen time and sleep among school-aged children and adolescents: a systematic literature review. Sleep Med Rev. 2015;21:50–8.

Hawi NS, Samaha M, Griffiths MD. Internet gaming disorder in Lebanon: relationships with age, sleep habits, and academic achievement. J Behav Addictions. 2018;7(1):70–8.

Hysing M, Pallesen S, Stormark KM, Jakobsen R, Lundervold AJ, Sivertsen B. Sleep and use of electronic devices in adolescence: results from a large population-based study. BMJ Open. 2015;5:e006748.

Kim SY, Kim M-S, Park B, Kim J-H, Choi HG. Lack of sleep is associated with internet use for leisure. PLoS One. 2018;13(1):e0191713.

Lemola S, Perkinson-Gloor N, Brand S, Dewald-Kaufmann JF, Grob A. Adolescents' electronic media use at night, sleep disturbance, and depressive symptoms in the smartphone age. J Youth Adolescence. 2014; https://doi.org/10.1007/s10964-014-0176-x.

Liu Q-Q, Zhou Z-K, Yang X-J, Kong F-C, Niu G-F, Fan CY. Mobile phone addiction and sleep quality among Chinese adolescents: a moderated mediation model. Computers in Human Behavior. 2017; https://doi.org/10.1016/j.chb.2017.02.042.

Mak YW, Wu CST, Hui DWS, Lam SP, Tse HY, Yu WY, Wong HT. Association between screen viewing duration and sleep duration, sleep quality, and excessive daytime sleepiness among adolescents in Hong Kong. Int. J. Environ. Res. Public Health. 2014;11:11201–19. https://doi.org/10.3390/ijerph111111201.

Munezawa T, Kaneita Y, Osaki Y, Kanda H, Minowa M, Suzuki K, et al. The association between use of mobile phones after lights out and sleep disturbances among Japanese adolescents: a nationwide cross-sectional survey. Sleep. 2011;34:1013–20.

National Sleep Foundation. Sleep in America Poll 2006 19 June 2012. Available from: http://sleepfoundation.org/sites/default/files/2006_summary_of_findings.pdf.

National Sleep Foundation. Sleep in America Poll 2014: summary of findings. https://sleepfoundation.org/sites/default/files/2014-NSF-Sleep-in-Americapoll-summary-of-findings—FINAL-Updated-3-26-14-.pdf. Accessed 28 Sept 2016.

Nuutinen T, Roos E, Ray C, Villberg J, Valimaa R, Rasmussen M, Holstein B, Godeau E, Beck F, Leger D, Tynjala J. Computer use, sleep duration and health symptoms: a cross-sectional study of 15-year olds in three countries. Int J Public Health. 2014; https://doi.org/10.1007/s00038-014-0561-y.

Ohayon MM, Carskadon MA, Guilleminault C, Vitiello MV. Meta analysis of quantitative sleep parameters from childhood to old age in healthy individuals: developing normative sleep values across the human lifespan. SLEEP. 2004;27(7):1255–73.

Park S. Associations of physical activity with sleep satisfaction, perceived stress, and problematic internet use in Korean adolescents. Park BMC Public Health. 2014;14:1143.

Park S, Lee Y. Associations of body weight perception and weight control behaviors with problematic internet use among Korean adolescents. Psychiatry Res. 2017;251:275–80.

Punama-ki R-L, Wallenius M, Nyga rd C-H k, Saarni L, Rimpela A. Use of information and communication technology (ICT) and perceived health in adolescence: the role of sleeping habits and waking-time tiredness. J Adolesc. 2006; https://doi.org/10.1016/j.adolescence.2006.07.004.

Rehbein F, Kleimann M, Mossle T. Prevalence and risk factors of video game dependency in adolescence: results of a German nationwide survey. Cyberpsychol Behav Soc Netw. 2010;13:269–77.

Sami H, Dannielle L, Lihi D, Elena S. The effect of sleep disturbances and internet addiction on suicidal ideation among adolescents in the presence of depressive symptoms. Psychiatry Research. 2018; https://doi.org/10.1016/j.psychres.2018.03.067.

Shochat T, Flint-Bretler O, Tzischinsky O. Sleep patterns, electronic media exposure and daytime sleep-related behaviours among Israeli adolescents. Acta Paediatr. 2010; https://doi.org/10.1111/j.1651-2227.2010.01821.x.

Stroup DF, Berlin JA, Morton SC, Olkin I, Williamson GD, Rennie D, Moher D, Becker BJ, Sipe TA, Thacker SB. Meta-analysis of observational studies in epidemiology: a proposal for reporting. JAMA. 2000;283(15):2008–12.

Tamura H, Nishida T, Tsuji A, Sakakibara H. Association between excessive use of mobile phone and insomnia and depression among Japanese adolescents. Int J Environ Res Public Health. 2017; https://doi.org/10.3390/ijerph14070701.

Tan Y, Chen Y, Lu Y, Li L. Exploring associations between problematic internet use, depressive symptoms and sleep disturbance among southern Chinese adolescents. Int J Environ Res Public Health. 2016;13: 313. https://doi.org/10.3390/ijerph13030313.

Tynjala J, Kannas L, Valimaa R. How young Europeans sleep. Health Educ Res. 1993;8:69–80.

Van den Bulck J. Adolescent use of mobile phones for calling and for sending text messages after lights out: results from a prospective cohort study with a one-year follow-up. Sleep. 2007;30:1220–3.

Van den Bulck J. Television viewing, computer game playing, and internet use and self-reported time to bed and time out of bed in secondary-school children. SLEEP. 2004;27(1):101–4.

Weaver E, Gradisar M, Dohnt H, Lovato N, Douglas P. The effect of presleep videogame playing on adolescent sleep. J Clin Sleep Med. 2010;6:184–9.

Winkler A, Dörsing B, Rief W, Shen Y, Glombiewski JA. Treatment of internet addiction: a meta-analysis. Clin Psychol Rev. 2013;33:317–29.

Wolfson AR, Carskadon MA. Sleep schedules and daytime functioning in adolescents. Child Dev. 1998;69:875–87.

World Health Organization. The ICD-10 Classification of Mental and Behavioral Disorders: Clinical Description and Diagnostic Guidelines. The ICD-10. Geneva: World Health Organization; 1992.

Yen CF, Ko CH, Yen JY, Cheng CP. The multidimensional correlates associated with short nocturnal sleep duration and subjective insomnia among Taiwanese adolescents. Sleep. 2008;31:1515–25.

19

Hypopnea definitions, determinants and dilemmas: a focused review

Q. Afifa Shamim-Uzzaman[1]*, Sukhmani Singh[2] and Susmita Chowdhuri[3]

Abstract

Obstructive sleep apnea (OSA) is defined by the presence of repetitive obstructive apneas and hypopneas during sleep. While apneas are clearly defined as cessation of flow, controversy has plagued the many definitions of hypopneas, which have used variable criteria for reductions in flow, with or without the presence of electroencephalographic (EEG) arousal, and with varying degrees of oxygen desaturation. While the prevalence of OSA is estimated to vary using the different definitions of hypopneas, the impact of these variable definitions on clinical outcomes is not clear. This focused review examines the controversies and limitations surrounding the different definitions of hypopnea, evaluates the impact of hypopneas and different hypopnea definitions on clinical outcomes, identifies gaps in research surrounding hypopneas, and makes suggestions for future research.

Keywords: Obstructive sleep apnea, Hypopnea, Obstructive hypopnea, Central hypopnea

Introduction

Obstructive sleep apnea (OSA) is a common disorder, composed of apneas and hypopneas occurring at least five times per hour during sleep. Since polysomnographic identification in 1965, the notion of apneas (absence of airflow for > 10 s, Fig. 1) remains undisputed; however, the definition of hypopneas continues to evolve and their clinical impact debated over the years.

Bloch et al. first described 'hypopneas' as reductions in oxygen saturation that occurred in association with *reductions* in airflow instead of with *absence* of airflow, i.e., events suggestive of decreased ventilation that did not meet criteria for apneas. (Bloch et al., 1979) In this study "normal" asymptomatic volunteers had 40% more hypopneas than apneas (105 vs. 60, respectively) with frequent oxygen desaturation of $\geq 4\%$. (Bloch et al., 1979) Subsequently, in a small study comparing individuals with apneas alone vs. hypopneas alone ($n = 50$), Gould et al. noted no differences in age, weight, clinical symptoms, number of arousals (median 31/h vs. 20/h) or patterns of oxygen desaturation (median 45 vs. 40, 4% desaturation per hour) (Gould et al., 1988) between the two groups, and recommended changing the terminology

from "sleep apnea syndrome" to "sleep hypopnea syndrome," defined as 15 or more hypopneas per hour of sleep in conjunction with 2 or more major clinical features. Although the term "sleep hypopnea syndrome" did not gain much popularity, the terminology "sleep apnea-hypopnea syndrome" (SAHS) was used frequently, until the current term "obstructive sleep apnea" gained favor.

Objectives

In this focused review, our objective was to describe the variability in the definitions of hypopneas, limitations of technology that are used to detect hypopneas, and thereafter, make suggestions for future research to standardize hypopnea definition and detection. Our literature review also attempted to identify the potential clinical relevance of patients with hypopnea-predominant sleep apnea. These are outlined below.

Background
Defining moments for 'hypopnea'

Gould's definition of hypopnea was derived by comparing 75, 50% or 25% reductions in Respitrace thoraco-abdominal sum compared to thermocouple flow amplitude with arousal frequency and oxygen desaturations. (Gould et al., 1988) In this study, a 75% reduction in movement resulted in much fewer hypopneas than the number of desaturations or arousals and was excluded

* Correspondence: afifa@med.umich.edu
[1]VA Ann Arbor Heathcare Center and University of Michigan, 2215 Fuller Rd, Ann Arbor, MI 48105, USA
Full list of author information is available at the end of the article

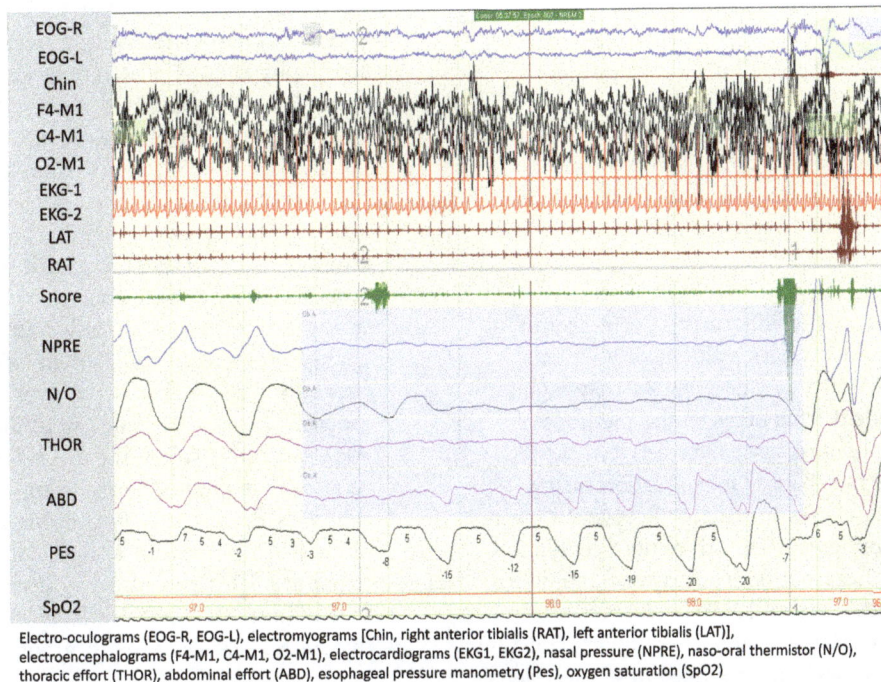

Electro-oculograms (EOG-R, EOG-L), electromyograms [Chin, right anterior tibialis (RAT), left anterior tibialis (LAT)], electroencephalograms (F4-M1, C4-M1, O2-M1), electrocardiograms (EKG1, EKG2), nasal pressure (NPRE), naso-oral thermistor (N/O), thoracic effort (THOR), abdominal effort (ABD), esophageal pressure manometry (Pes), oxygen saturation (SpO2)

Fig. 1 This figure shows an obstructive apnea. An apnea is a respiratory event lasting ≥10 s, characterized by a decrement in airflow of ≥90% from the baseline in the oronasal thermocouple signal. Clear crescendo effort in the abdominal belt suggests obstruction. Elevated and progressively increasing values in the Δ Pes during the event confirm the obstructive etiology

from consideration. While reductions in thoraco-abdominal movement of 25–50% were of similar accuracy and more accurate than the frequency of oxygen desaturation alone, the 50% reduction in effort was significantly closer to the arousal frequency than was the 25% reduction in thoraco-abdominal movement ($p < 0.05$). Hence, these authors defined 'hypopnea' as a "50% reduction in thoracoabdominal (Respitrace® sum) amplitude for 10 seconds or more when compared to the peak amplitude lasting for 10s or more that occurred within the previous 2 minutes in the presence of continued flow". (Gould et al., 1988)

In 1997, the AASM created a task force to delineate the criteria to identify and treat OSA. Their results, presented as a consensus statement commonly referred to as the "Chicago Criteria," defined hypopnea as a ≥ 50% decrement in airflow, or a < 50% reduction in airflow associated with either an oxygen desaturation or arousal. (Loube et al., 1999) Despite this, no uniform definition of 'hypopnea' was used amongst sleep laboratories within the United States for the next decade. (Moser et al., 1994; Redline & Sanders, 1997) A survey of 44 accredited sleep laboratories (labs) showed as many methods and definitions of hypopneas as number of labs. (Moser et al., 1994) Methods of detection included use of thermocouple, pneumotachograph, respiratory inductance plethysmography, intercostal electromyography, microphone or esophageal balloon. Additionally, the requirements for the degree of airflow reduction and oxygen desaturation also varied

widely. Moreover, 33 of the 44 labs used EEG arousal to fulfill the definition of hypopnea, even though there was no consistent definition of arousal at that time. This lack of precision precluded objective comparison of data from individual laboratories and raised doubts to the validity and reproducibility of hypopneas even within the same individual. In fact, Redline et al. (Redline et al., 2000) examined the effect of using 11 different criteria for scoring hypopneas on the prevalence of disease in a large community-based sample and reported that different approaches for measuring apnea-hypopnea index (AHI: number of apneas and hypopneas per hour of sleep) resulted in substantial variability in identifying and classifying sleep-disordered breathing.

Findings

A. Sources of variability in hypopnea detection

i)   Variability in flow measurements: Hypopnea detection implies determination of small changes in ventilation that accompany sleep disordered breathing; the amplitude of airflow is a measure of these changes. Sources of variability that contribute to poor reliability of these measurements of airflow include:

1)   positioning of thermo-elements, as slight displacements could produce major changes in signal amplitude,

2) alterations in proportion between nasal and oral breathing,

3) nasal cycle causing alterations in nasal airflow (which could change with changes in body position), (Cole & Haight, 1986)

4) variation in sensitivity and frequency response between different thermo-elements, (Berg et al., 1997)

5) displacement of the Respitrace® girdles that could alter signal amplitude.

ii) Type of device: Variability can also arise from the type of devices used during the recording. One study demonstrated that despite relatively high correlation coefficients between the methods of detecting hypopneas, agreement between the devices detecting changes in ventilation (using thermistor, nasal pressure and/or Respitrace®) were low, with poor agreement with minute ventilation measured by head-out body plethysmography in awake subjects. (Berg et al., 1997) The best agreement was noted with plethysmographic minute ventilations and the amplitudes of the summed Respitrace signals, and from the nasal-pressure signals. In fact, nasal-pressure measurements provided the greatest sensitivity and negative predictive values. Combination of nasal pressure and Respitrace® provided more consistent results – 86% sensitivity and 83% specificity – and better agreement between both methods (Cohen's K = 0.65).

iii) Observer reproducibility: Finally, Whyte et al. showed reproducibility in scoring of hypopneas by different observers. (Whyte et al., 1992) When two polysomnographers were asked to independently score both apneas and hypopneas on all-night polysomnograms of patients with OSA using the same methodology, there was close agreement between the polysomnographers for the number of hypopneas *(r* = 0.98; mean difference 11%) and for the number of apneas *(r* = 0.99; mean difference 8%). The agreement was similar for the durations of both hypopneas *(r* = 0.99; mean difference 13%) and apneas *(r* = 0.99; mean difference 11%). There was also close agreement between the total number of respiratory events scored with and without reference to the flow signal *(r* = 0.99; mean difference 1.4%) with a maximum under-recognition of 18 events per night in a subject with 237 apneas per night. (Whyte et al., 1992) Hence, it was possible for different observers to score hypopneas reliably.

iv) Variability in baseline: The lack of clear determination of "baseline" or normative values for each patient lends itself to inherent variability. If the baseline (SpO2, flow, EEG, muscle tone, etc) is not clear, variations from the baseline are subject to

interpretation. For example, subjective variations in detection of arousals can lead to variations in scoring hypopneas related to arousals. Since arousals can vary in their intensity and subsequent autonomic responses, (Azarbarzin et al. SLEEP 2014;37(4):645–653) they are not always detected by current scoring methods. The threshold visual intensity that causes different scorers to score arousals varies considerably, with some scoring arousals with minimal, equivocal changes in EEG whereas others score arousals only when the changes are unequivocal. When arousals are generally intense this is not a problem but when arousal changes are mild, large differences in AHI can arise. While the AASM scoring rules require that only arousal lasting 3 s be scored, the rules do not specify the minimum time difference between an arousal following a hypopnea. This can also can lead to variations in scoring arousals and ultimately to scoring hypopneas associated with arousals.

Attempts at reducing variability
Identification of factors affecting scoring:
A decade after the Chicago criteria, in an attempt to standardize definitions used by sleep laboratories and researchers, the American Academy of Sleep Medicine (AASM) published the *AASM Manual for the Scoring of Sleep and Associated Events* in 2007. This manual defined a hypopnea as a 30% reduction in airflow, as measured by the nasal pressure transducer flow signal, with a concomitant 4% drop in oxygen saturation; alternatively, a hypopnea was also defined as a 50% or greater decline in the flow signal associated with a 3% drop in oxygen saturation and/or an EEG arousal lasting at least 3 s in duration. (Iber et al., 2007) Controversy regarding the best definition led to the adoption of both definitions in the scoring manual; the first being referred to as rule "4A" (or "recommended") (Fig. 2) and the latter as rule "4B" (or "alternative") (Fig. 3).

However, the use of the recommended vs. alternative definitions of hypopnea led to highly variable apnea/hypopnea indices. Ruehland et al. scored the same 323 consecutive sleep studies using different hypopnea definitions and found considerable variability in the median apnea-hypopnea index (AHI, 8.3 vs. 14.9) as well as the hypopnea index (HI, 2.2 vs. 7.2) using the recommended and alternative definitions, respectively. (Ruehland et al., 2010) Greater than half of the inconsistencies in AHI was due to the inclusion of arousals in the alternative definition, and a quarter due to the reduction of the desaturation

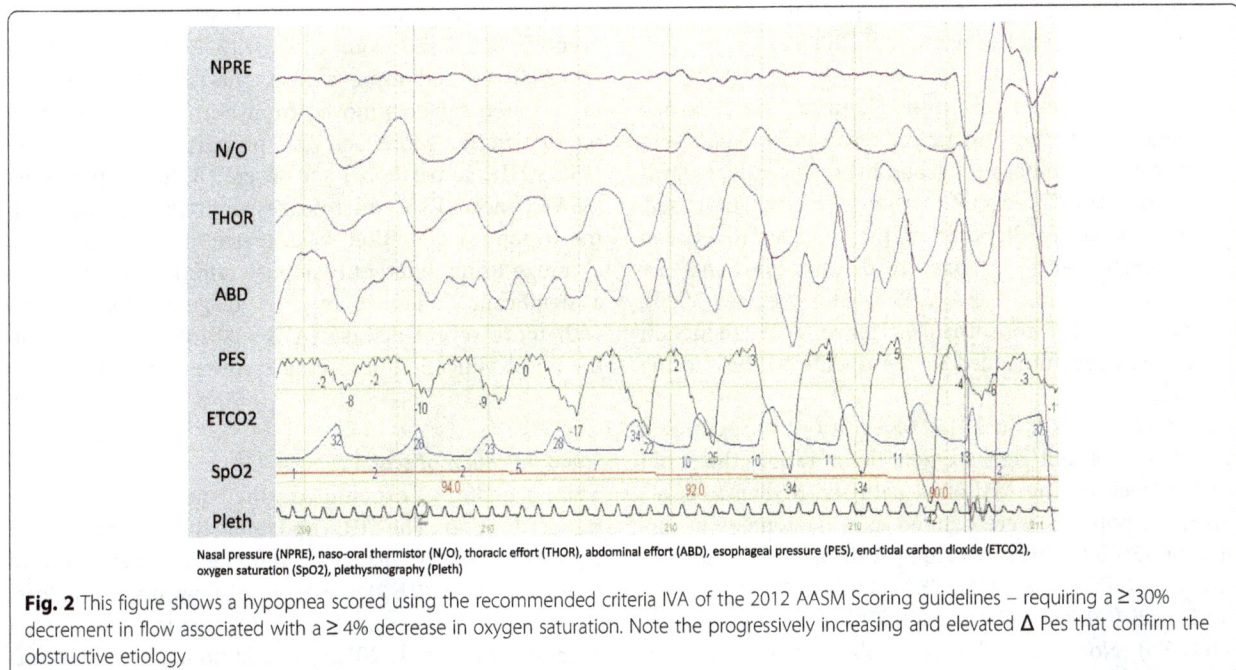

Nasal pressure (NPRE), naso-oral thermistor (N/O), thoracic effort (THOR), abdominal effort (ABD), esophageal pressure (PES), end-tidal carbon dioxide (ETCO2), oxygen saturation (SpO2), plethysmography (Pleth)

Fig. 2 This figure shows a hypopnea scored using the recommended criteria IVA of the 2012 AASM Scoring guidelines – requiring a ≥ 30% decrement in flow associated with a ≥ 4% decrease in oxygen saturation. Note the progressively increasing and elevated Δ Pes that confirm the obstructive etiology

requirement from 4 to 3%. (Ruehland et al., 2010) This translated to differences in the identification and classification of sleep apnea in the same patient. Hence, further clarification, with consideration of the clinical implications, was sought and is outlined below.

i) Effect of the arousal criterion on hypopnea scoring and classification of severity of sleep apnea The association between the arousal index and cardiovascular morbidities is not as robust as that of oxygen desaturation indices, below. However, correlations have been shown between the arousal index and hypertension (Sulit et al., 2006) as well as white matter disease in the

elderly. (Ding et al., 2004) In fact, the Cleveland Family Study showed a greater correlation of hypertension risk with the arousal index than with oxygen desaturation. This may, in part, be due to the activation of the sympathetic nervous system when arousals occur during sleep, (Loredo et al., 1999; Somers et al., 1993) and the resultant sleep fragmentation leads to clinically significant symptoms. (Bonnet, 1986; Thomas, 2006; Guilleminault et al., 2009) With respect to scoring, Guilleminault et al. showed that using criteria 4A to score hypopneas (i.e., a 30% flow reduction with 4% oxygen desaturation, without consideration of arousals) would have missed 40% of patients identified using the criteria incorporating arousals and who were responsive to positive airway

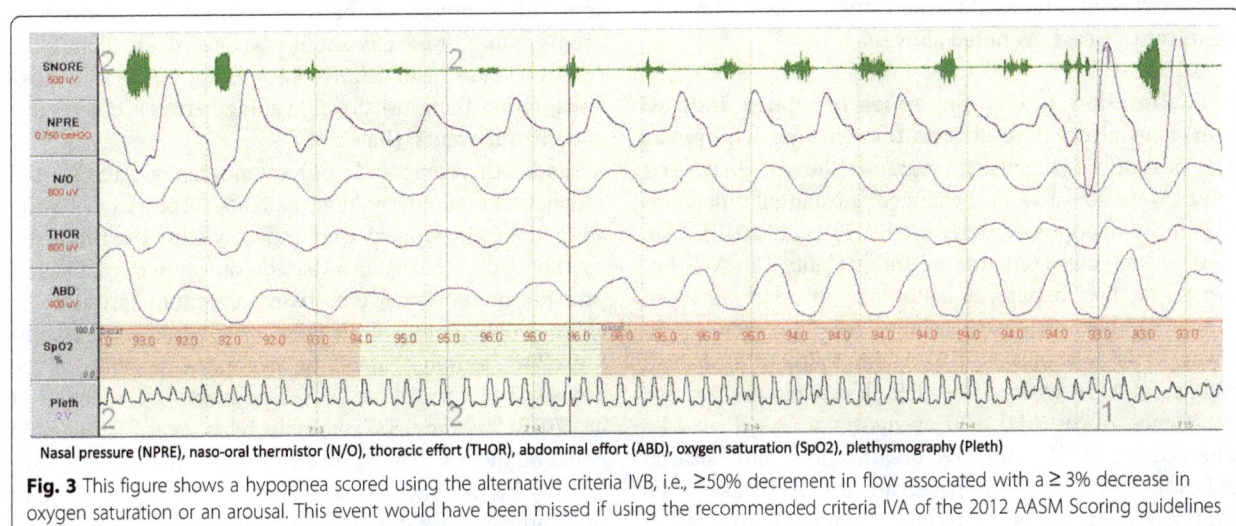

Nasal pressure (NPRE), naso-oral thermistor (N/O), thoracic effort (THOR), abdominal effort (ABD), oxygen saturation (SpO2), plethysmography (Pleth)

Fig. 3 This figure shows a hypopnea scored using the alternative criteria IVB, i.e., ≥50% decrement in flow associated with a ≥ 3% decrease in oxygen saturation or an arousal. This event would have been missed if using the recommended criteria IVA of the 2012 AASM Scoring guidelines

pressure (PAP) therapy (with both reductions in AHI and sleepiness). (Guilleminault et al., 2009)

ii) **Effect of oxygen criterion** There are clear, strong associations between obstructive respiratory events and cardiovascular events, stroke, and hyperglycemia, regardless of the SpO2 reduction criteria (3% vs. 4%) used. (Berry et al., 2012a) In addition, the correlation between AHIs scored with 3% oxygen desaturation and 4% oxygen desaturation was > 0.95 (Redline et al., 2000), showing excellent concordance. Hence, a 3% reduction criteria was recommended in the update to the scoring manual.

Of note, however, in 2015, Myllymaa et al. examined the effects of different oxygen desaturation threshold (ODT) levels on the AHI of 54 patients (Myllymaa et al., 2016). Hypopneas were defined as a decrement in airflow of ≥30% for over 10s along with one of the following: an ODT ≥ 2% (ODT2%), ODT ≥ 3% (ODT3%), ODT ≥ 4% (ODT4%), ODT ≥ 5% (ODT5%) or ODT ≥ 6% (ODT6%). Not only was there a significant increase in the median AHI with ODT3% vs. ODT4% (6.5 events/hr.; p = 0.003), different ODT's resulted in patients being classified under different categories of AHI severity. Using ODT3% instead of ODT4% resulted in a 44% increase (from 29.4 to 73.5%) in the number of patients with moderate or severe OSA (AHI ≥ 15). Thus, any changes in ODT, although slight, could result in significant differences in AHI, which could in turn, result in highly variable classifications of disease severity. (Myllymaa et al., 2016)

iii) **Effect of flow reduction criterion** Hypopneas defined with either 30% decrements in flow or 50% decrement in flow, if resulting in a desaturation or an arousal, carried clinical consequences, be it disrupted sleep, daytime sleepiness, or cardiovascular morbidity. However, a hypopnea based only on desaturation criteria alone (without arousals), would miss much clinically significant disease, as noted above.

iv) **Calibration model for apnea-hypopnea indices: Impact of alternative criteria for defining hypopneas** Analysis of 6441 polysomnograms showed that AHI values were sensitive and changed substantially depending on the hypopnea criteria used. (Ho et al., 2015) Also, there was greater concordance (or "stability") in AHI between the two hypopnea definitions as AHI increased above 30, but greater variability (or "divergence") at lower AHIs. (Ho et al., 2015) Additionally, in 2 Spanish cohorts of 1116 women and 939 elderly individuals, the prevalence of an AHI ≥30 events/h increased by 14% when using AHI with 3% desaturation plus arousal criterion (AHI3%a), compared to the AHI using 4% (AHI4%) desaturation criterion. (Campos-Rodriguez et al., 2016) The percentage of women with an AHI < 5 events/h decreased from 13.9% with AHI4 to 1.1% with the AHI3%a definition; almost one-third (31%) of the investigated subjects moved from normal to OSA labels or vice versa. Moreover, the proportion of moderate (15 ≤ AHI < 30 per hour) and severe (AHI ≥ 30 per hour) OSA changed 13.5 and 10%, respectively, depending on the hypopnea definition used. (Farre et al., 2015) Thus, although using different hypopnea criteria may not make a significant difference in OSA diagnosis for patients with more severe disease (AHI > 30), it could result in the misclassification of disease at lower AHI levels.

Standardization of scoring

These findings expounded the need for further standardization. The 2012 update to the scoring manual attempted to do just that, refining the definition of hypopnea to a 30% decrease in airflow lasting at least 10 s and associated a ≥3% SpO2 desaturation or an arousal. (Berry et al., 2012b) In addition, it included consensus definitions for obstructive and central hypopneas for the first time. From previous operational definitions used in heart failure with an obstructive event, obstructive hypopneas required any of the following indicators relative to baseline: paradoxical thoraco-abdominal movement, snoring, and inspiratory flattening of the flow signal whereas central hypopneas required the absence of all of these indicators (Fig. 4). Simply put, an *obstructive* hypopnea was a reduction in flow secondary to increased resistance of the upper airways (i.e., obstruction), whereas a *central* hypopnea was a result of decreased effort, not increased resistance (Fig. 5). However, the differences between central and obstructive hypopneas were not validated using esophageal catheter pressure changes, a gold standard measure of respiratory effort. Iber cautioned that given the substantial evidence supporting interaction between central and obstructive events, more emphasis should be placed on identifying causes such as heart failure, sleep disruption, and hypoxemia, rather than just distinguishing between obstructive and central events. (Iber, n.d.)

Randerath compared polysomnography (PSG) and esophageal manometry in 41 patients suspected of having sleep apnea; hypopneas were independently discriminated by blinded investigators based on either esophageal pressure or the visual PSG-based algorithm (presence or absence of flattening of the flow curve, paradoxical breathing effort, termination of the hypopnea, position of the arousal, and correlation with sleep stages). (Randerath et al., 2013) Of the 1837 scorable hypopneas, 1175 (64%) could be further defined by esophageal pressure and 1812 (98.6%) by the PSG-based algorithm; notably, evaluation of hypopneas using esophageal pressure was limited by

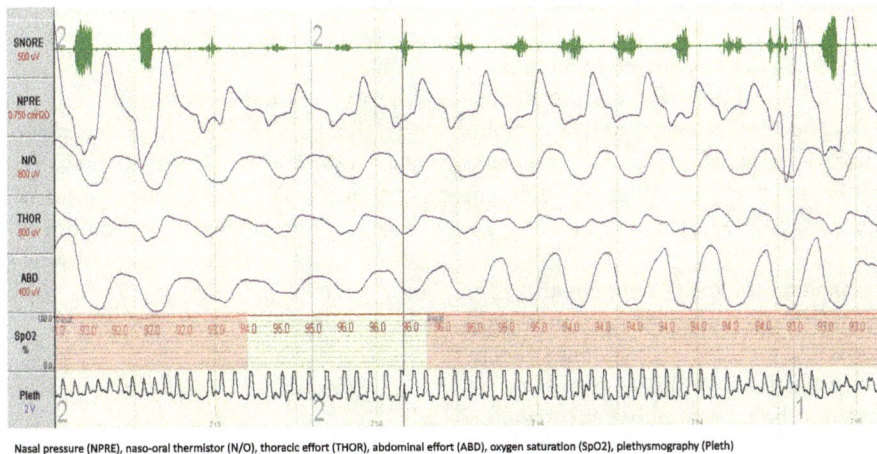

Nasal pressure (NPRE), naso-oral thermistor (N/O), thoracic effort (THOR), abdominal effort (ABD), oxygen saturation (SpO2), plethysmography (Pleth)

Fig. 4 An obstructive hypopnea. A hypopnea is classified as an obstructive hypopnea if the event meets all criteria for hypopnea and signs of obstruction (snoring, flow limitation, crescendo effort, or paradoxical breathing) are seen during the event

poor signal quality and artifact. Of those hypopneas that could be differentiated with both methods, using esophageal pressure as a reference, the PSG-based algorithm correctly defined 76.9% of central and 60.5% of obstructive hypopneas. However, because the esophageal manometry was not interpretable in 36% of their cases, the accuracy of a combined logic for hypopnea definition was only 68%. Thus, although 77% of central hypopneas were correctly identified, nearly 40% of obstructive events were misclassified. (Randerath et al., 2013) Thus, variability in the definitions of hypopneas has led to re-classification of the type and severity of OSA.

In a retrospective study, PSGs of 112 consecutive patients for suspected OSA were re-scored for respiratory events using either 2007 AASM recommended (AASM2007Rec), 2007 AASM alternate (AASM2007Alt), Chicago criteria (AASM1999), or 2012 AASMrecommended (AASM2012) respiratory event criteria (Duce et al., 2015). The median AHI using AASM2012 definitions, was approximately 90% greater than the AHI obtained using the AASM2007 recommended criteria, approximately 25% greater than the AASM2007Alt AHI, and approximately 15% lower than the AASM1999 AHI. These changes increased OSA diagnoses by approximately 20 and 5% for AASM2007Rec and AASM2007Alt, respectively. Minimal changes in OSA diagnoses were observed between AASM1999 and AASM2012 criteria. Differences between the AASM2007 using recommended criteria and AASM2012 hypopnea indices were

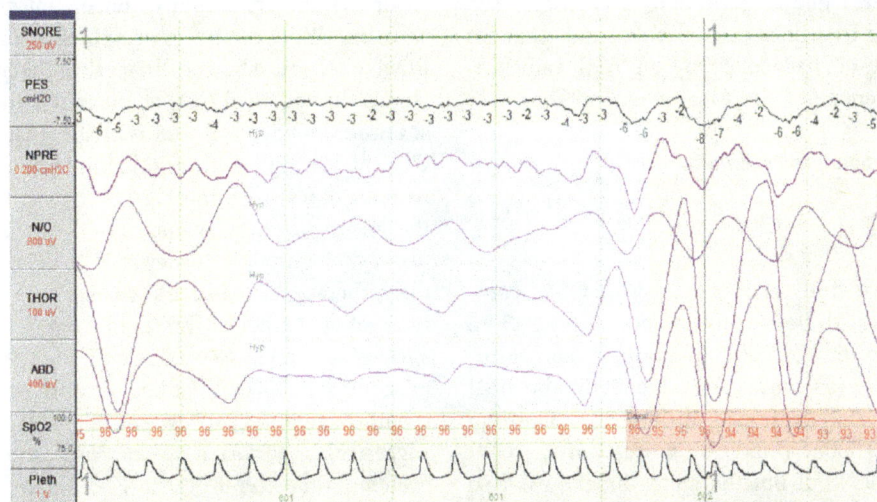

Nasal pressure (NPRE), naso-oral thermistor (N/O), thoracic effort (THOR), abdominal effort (ABD), oxygen saturation (SpO2), plethysmography (Pleth)

Fig. 5 A central hypopnea lacks the obstructive features seen in Fig. 4. The lack of elevated Pes values also confirms the central etiology of the hypopnea

predominantly due to the change in desaturation levels required.

Results from such studies point to the growing importance of finding consistent methods for scoring hypopneas. Approaches designed to "calibrate AHI thresholds to the event definitions employed" or create equations to measure AHI specific to the technology in different laboratories have been considered. (Ho et al., 2015)

Clinical factors determining the type of hypopnea

Although the diagnostic value of apnea-hypopnea indices (AHIs), as determined by different hypopnea definitions, has been evaluated by investigators, it is as yet unclear what determines the type of obstructive respiratory event an individual will have. Are there physiologic characteristics that predetermine whether an individual will have primarily apneas or primarily hypopneas? What underlying differences lead to some individuals having hypopneas associated with oxygen desaturations while others have hypopneas terminating in arousals? The literature detailing this, outlined below, is sparse.

Determinants of arousal-based vs. desaturation-based hypopneas

Tsai et al. reported that regardless of the hypopnea criteria used to define sleep apnea, there were no significant differences in patient *characteristics* [age, sex, body mass index (BMI), and neck circumference], or in consequent Epworth Sleepiness Scale, time spent at an SaO_2 below 90%, arousal index, or apnea index between patients with predominantly arousal-based hypopneas versus those with desaturation-based hypopneas. (Tsai et al., 1999) No patient characteristics predicted the type of hypopnea, regardless of which hypopnea scoring method was used; however, while the addition of arousal-based scoring criteria for hypopnea caused only small changes in the AHI, OSA defined solely by an AHI value increased the prevalence of OSA. (Tsai et al., 1999)

Determinants of hypopneas vs. apneas

i)   Effect of BMI

In a retrospective study of 90 adults with OSA, comparing two groups with body mass indices (BMI) ≥45 vs. BMI < 35, matched for age and gender, the hypopnea-to-apnea ratio (HAR) was significantly higher in the BMI ≥45 group (38.8 ± 50.7) compared to the BMI < 35 group (10.6 ± 16.5), $p = 0.0006$. (Mathew & Castriotta, 2014) The hypopnea index, but not the apnea index, was also higher in the BMI ≥45 vs. BMI < 35 group (28.7 ± 28.6 vs 12.6 ± 8.4, $p = 0.0005$), as was the AHI (35.5 ± 33.8 vs 22 ± 23, $p = 0.03$). In addition, the end-tidal CO2 was higher in the higher BMI group. However, the

hypopnea-to-apnea ratio did not appear to be influenced by the presence or absence of hypoventilation and was similar for those with or without obesity hypoventilation syndrome. (Mathew & Castriotta, 2014) In fact, BMI was the only significant predictor of HAR (adjusted r2 = 0.138; $p = 0.002$) when adjusting for age, gender, race, and ETCO2. Of note, a small sample size may have confounded the study findings. The authors suggested that different pathophysiologic mechanisms may have been involved in the generation of apneas and hypopneas.

ii)   Effect of Sex Hormones

A study of 118 patients with 'occlusive' sleep apnea syndrome, defined as daytime hypersomnolence and an AHI > 10/h, reported that, in women, only about 30% of respiratory events during sleep were occlusive apneas while 70% were hypopneas; conversely, in men, only 50% of events were hypopneas. The authors highlighted that both premenopausal and postmenopausal women had more hypopneas than apneas and "some of the most severely affected women were never observed to have complete cessation of airflow during sleep". (Leech et al., 1988) Notably, there were fewer sleep disordered breathing events associated with oxygen desaturation in women than men ($p < 0.003$); 19 women did not experience oxygen desaturation at all, and only three had a total of nine episodes of apnea, whereas 20 men accounted for 264 episodes of nocturnal oxygen desaturation or abnormal breathing. (Bloch et al., 1979)

Thus, gender differences exist in the prevalence of hypopneas, and these may be conferred by differences in upper airway anatomy or control of ventilation. The latter may be attributed to hormonal differences that in turn modify ventilatory responsiveness during sleep. Rowley et al. showed that the determinants of the change in end-tidal CO_2 at the apnea threshold included sex and menopausal status, with changes in end-tidal CO_2 at the apnea threshold highest in premenopausal women (4.6+/− 0.6 mmHg), with no difference between the postmenopausal women (3.1+/− 0.5 mmHg) and men (3.4+/− 0.7 mmHg) (Rowley et al., 2006). Hormone replacement therapy increased the change in end-tidal CO_2 (CO_2 reserve) at the apnea threshold from 2.9+/− 0.4 mmHg to 4.8+/− 0.4 mmHg ($P < .001$) indicating that estrogens and progestins stabilize breathing in women during non-rapid eye movement sleep. (Rowley et al., 2006) Moreover, studies suggest that testosterone increases the risk for central events during sleep in men. (Zhou et al., 2003; Chowdhuri et al., 2013)

Thus, although no patient characteristics can determine the predominant type of hypopnea (arousal- vs. desaturation-based) an individual may have, obesity and female sex may be associated with hypopnea-predominant OSA, rather than apnea-dominant.

Clinical consequences of hypopneas

Impact of differing definitions on clinical outcomes

The immediate consequences of hypopneas do not appear to differ from those of apneas. In 39 sleep apnea patients who underwent polysomnography, 80 events/subject were evaluated for clinical consequences — i.e., oxygen desaturation of ≥4% from the baseline, EEG arousal, and an increase in heart rate by 6 bpm. (Ayappa et al., 2005) Both apneas and hypopneas were not significantly different in frequency for oxygen desaturation (78% vs. 54%, respectively) arousals (63% vs.47%, respectively) and associated increase in heart rate (73% vs. 55%, respectively). In contrast, of the events with minimal (25–50%) amplitude reduction, only 25% caused desaturation, 42% arousal, and 42% heart rate increase. No specific consequence occurred after every event. Thus, the immediate consequences of individual respiratory events (oxygen desaturation, EEG arousal and heart rate) overlapped and were not specific to any particular event. The same may not hold true for excessive daytime sleepiness or for long term cardiovascular sequelae.

i) **Excessive daytime sleepiness** Hosselet et al. observed that the respiratory disturbance index (RDItotal), calculated from the sum of apneas, hypopneas and flow limitation events regardless of the level of desaturation or arousal (Hosselet et al., 2001), predicted daytime sleepiness. In this study, the highest sensitivity and specificity in separating patients with excessive daytime sleepiness (EDS) from patients without EDS (non-EDS) was provided by the RDItotal. For RDItotal, the optimal combination of sensitivity and specificity was obtained at a cutoff value of 18 events/h. However, the cutoff value of 5/h for the AHI per AASM results in sensitivity of 100% but specificity for EDS of only 15%.

Similarly, Ciftci et al. studied 90 patients who had an AHI > 5/h, scored according to the hypopnea definition of the AASM (Ciftci et al., 2004). The records of these patients were scored according to different hypopnea definitions (hypopnea-arousal, hypopnea-desaturation, hypopnea-effort). AHI (AASM), AHI (arousal), AHI (desaturation), and AHI (effort) were determined. Patients' daytime sleepiness was evaluated by the Epworth Sleepiness Scale (> 10). When all of three major symptoms (snoring, observed apnea, and daytime sleepiness) were found in a patient's history, the term "clinical OSAS" was applied. ESS was strongly correlated with each index. In addition, an AHI-AASM cutoff value > 5 had the highest sensitivity and specificity from the viewpoint of separation between EDS and non-EDS, and also between clinical OSAS and nonclinical OSAS. (Ciftci et al., 2004)

Chervin & Aldrich noted that the rate of apneas as opposed to the rate of hypopneas had a greater impact on the degree of excessive daytime sleepiness in patients with OSA (Chervin & Aldrich, 1998). In 1146 subjects (30% females), the mean number of apneas per hour of sleep (AI) was 14.3 ± 27.0 and the mean number of hypopneas per hour of sleep (HI) was 16.5 ± 16.1. A regression model showed that the AI explained 9.6% of the variance in mean sleep latency (MSL) ($p \leq 0.0001$) on Mean Sleep Latency Tests, after controlling for total sleep time, but the HI explained only 5.4% ($p \leq 0.0001$) of the variance. When AI, HI, and TST (total sleep time) were included in a single multiple-regression model, AI explained 8.3% of the variance in MSL and HI explained 4.0% ($p < 0.0001$ for each). The AHI during supine sleep (recorded in a subgroup of $n = 169$ subjects), the rate of apneas ($n = 1146$), and the rate of obstructive apneas were useful in explaining variation in measured levels of sleepiness; however, rates of hypopneas and central apneas were not as useful. The minimum recorded oxygen saturation ($n = 1097$) was as important as the AHI to the level of sleepiness. (Chervin & Aldrich, 1998)

ii) **Metabolism** In 2656 subjects from the Sleep Heart Health Study, hypopneas, even with mild degrees of oxygen desaturation of 2–3%, were associated with fasting hyperglycemia, independent of multiple covariates. Hypopneas were further stratified on the degree of associated oxyhemoglobin desaturation into: 0.0–1.9%, 2.0–2.9%, 3.0–3.9%, and ≥ 4.0% reductions in SaO2. Hypopneas based solely on the arousal criteria were not identified. The adjusted cumulative odds ratios for the hypopnea index (HI) and impaired fasting glucose were 1.15 (95% CI: 0.90–1.47), 1.44 (95% CI: 1.09–1.90), 2.25 (95% CI: 1.59–3.19) and 1.47 (95% CI: 1.13–1.92) respectively. (Stamatakis et al., 2008)

iii) **Stroke** Association between incident stroke and OSA using a hypopnea definition of ≥3% oxygen desaturation has been reported (Redline et al., 2010; Shahar et al., 2001) and may be somewhat stronger than the association with coronary heart disease or heart failure. This association of stroke and OSA may be mediated through ischemic pathways. *Potential mechanisms:* Andreas et al. simulated obstructed breaths using the Muller maneuver (generating high negative intrathoracic pressures against an obstruction) and showed a significant reduction in blood flow to the middle cerebral artery (MCA) during the period of obstruction, in conjunction with a drop in flow across the mitral and aortic valves. (Andreas et al., 1991) Using Doppler sonography, Netzer et al. showed that blood flow through the MCA was significantly reduced (i.e., > 50% reduction in velocity) more frequently with obstructive hypopneas (76%) and obstructive apneas (80%) than with central apneas (14%) ($p \leq 0.0001$); the level of reduced blood flow during obstructive apneas vs. obstructive hypopneas was not significantly different. However, there was a significant association between MCA blood flow reduction and the duration of obstructive hypopnea ($p < 0.05$), which was not seen with obstructive apneas or central apneas, although mean event durations were similar (18.1 ± 6.5 s for hypopnea, 17.2 ± 5.9 s for central apneas, and 14.8 ± 5.0 s for obstructive apneas; $p = 0.3$). Similarly, a statistically significant correlation ($p < 0.05$) was seen between the fall in oxygen saturation with obstructive hypopnea and reduction in MCA blood flow, not seen with central or obstructive apneas. (Netzer et al., 1998) Hence, the occurrence of MCA blood flow reduction increases as the duration of the obstructive hypopnea increases and its associated drop in oxygen saturation increases.

iv) Cardiovascular disease In a cohort of 6106 adults from the Sleep Heart Health Study hypopneas with $\geq 4\%$ oxygen desaturations were independently associated with cardiovascular disease, whereas hypopneas with less than a 4% desaturation or arousal only were not associated with prevalent cardiovascular disease, after controlling for apnea index, age, sex, race, body mass index, waist circumference, neck circumference, total cholesterol, smoking status, and hypertension. (Punjabi et al., 2008)

Mehra et al. found significant associations between SDB and the risk of atrial fibrillation and complex ventricular ectopy (CVE) amongst 2911 elderly men without heart failure where hypopneas were defined by a desaturation criterion of $\geq 3\%$. However, whether hypopneas predicted arrthymias was not investigated. The authors compared central vs. obstructive forms of sleep disordered breathing, and found that central sleep apnea was more strongly associated with atrial fibrillation (Odds Ratio 2.69, 95% CI: 1.61–4.47) than CVE (OR 1.27, 95% CI: 0.97–1.66) while OSA was associated with CVE, especially when associated with hypoxia; those in the highest hypoxia category had an increased odds of CVE (OR 1.62, 95% CI: 1.23–2.14) compared with those with the lowest associated hypoxia. (Mehra et al., 2009)

Proposed mechanisms for the arrhythmic potential of apneas and hypopneas include intermittent hypoxia leading to increased oxidative stress, systemic inflammation, and sympathetic activity; repetitive blood pressure elevations secondary to sympathetic activation; and excessive intrathoracic pressure changes leading to mechanical stress on the heart and blood vessel walls (including large caliber vessels such as the aorta). (Camen et al., 2013; Kohler & Stradling, 2010)

In patients with congestive heart failure (CHF), the criteria used to define hypopnea significantly influenced the AHI and the prevalence of sleep-disordered breathing (SDB). (Ward et al., 2013) The number of patients with CHF in whom SDB was diagnosed, using an AHI cutoff of $\geq 15/h$, increased by 16% using the AASM 'alternative' hypopnea rule ($\geq 50\%$ reduction in airflow with $\geq 3\%$ oxygen desaturation or arousal) compared with the 'recommended' hypopnea scoring rule ($\geq 50\%$ decrease in nasal airflow with a $\geq 4\%$ oxygen desaturation). Median AHI increased from 9.3/h to 13.8/h (median difference 4.6/h) and SDB prevalence increased from 29 to 46% with the AASM alternative scoring rule ($p < 0.001$). However, classification of SDB as OSA or central sleep apnea was not significantly altered by the hypopnea scoring rules.

Recent large scale studies in the non-sleep literature (McEvoy et al., 2016; Yu et al., 2017) boldly called into question the benefit of treating sleep apnea on cardiovascular outcomes and death. Although riddled with confounders such as non-adherence to PAP therapy, (McEvoy et al., 2016; Yu et al., 2017) different types of sleep apnea being treated (central vs. obstructive, (Yu et al., 2017) different modes of PAP therapy used, (Yu et al., 2017) and different diagnostic criteria for sleep apnea, (McEvoy et al., 2016) these studies raise important questions on the validity of comparing data using different recording and scoring methodologies.

Of the ten studies reviewed in Yu's meta-analysis (which included the McEvoy study), only 2 used any AASM criteria for scoring hypopneas, and though published in 2012 (Kushida et al., 2012) & 2015 (Huang et al., 2015), both of these used the 1999 Chicago Criteria. One study from Spain (Barbe et al., 2012) used a modification of the 2012 AASM criteria (scoring hypopneas with 50% decrement in flow associated with a 4% oxygen desaturation) while another (Bradley et al., 2005) scored hypopnea as a 50% decrement in flow only (without a consequence). The remaining six studies used cardiopulmonary or respiratory polygraphy, which could not measure arousals, so any arousal-based hypopneas would have been missed. Of these limited channel studies, three used a 4% oxygen desaturation index (ODI) of > 7.5 (Craig et al., 2012; McMillan et al., 2014) or > 12 (4%-drops from baseline/hour) (McEvoy et al., 2016) to diagnose sleep apnea; one (Parra et al., 2015) used a "discernible reduction in airflow or thoracic motion lasting >10 seconds and associated with a cyclical dip in SaO2 of > 3%" and calculated the AHI based on time in bed. In the remaining 2 studies (Cowie et al., 2015; Peker et al., 2016), scoring criteria were not clearly defined.

This raises many unanswered questions and reflects the current dilemmas. How did differences in diagnostic criteria affect the overall interpretation of the meta-analysis? Would the conclusions have been the same if there was a standardized definition of the disorder? Is it conceivable that treatment of apnea-predominant versus hypopnea predominant sleep apnea responded differently to PAP therapy? We currently do not have answers to these important questions.

v) Mortality In the clinical Spanish cohorts, AHI ≥30 events/h was associated with increased cardiovascular mortality risk in women after adjusting for multiple covariates, regardless of the AHI4%, AHI3% or AHI3%-arousal hypopnea definition, whereas in elderly individuals the mortality risk was higher in those diagnosed using the AHI4% and AHI3% definitions but not using the AHI3%a definition. (Campos-Rodriguez et al., 2016)

Summary & recommendations
A. Technical specifications
While a number of studies have investigated the physiology and clinical significance of hypopneas, the data are sparse and inconclusive, mainly because the definitions and diagnostic methods have varied across studies. Thus, there remains a crucial gap in knowledge regarding the clinical presentation and prognosis of hypopneas. A clear, standard, and consistent definition of hypopnea is vital to this understanding. How can we claim that sleep apnea has consequences if the disorder itself is not clearly defined?

To this end, we recommend that the following specific, concrete recommendations be incorporated into the scoring guidelines:

i) Clear definition of, or guidance on, determination of baseline values for flow or SpO_2. With today's technological advancements, digital methods to determine these, especially when the pre-event signals are unstable, could be helpful to avoid subjectivity.

ii) Criteria for identification of poor or unreliable signals (e.g., EEG, flow or SpO2 signals) and guidance on when to exclude these from the calculation of respiratory events or sleep time.

iii) Clear guidelines on arousal criteria that minimize subjectivity and bias.

iv) Specifications on the use of sensors that meet specific performance calibration criteria.

Clinical impact
Few studies have reported on the impact of the different definitions of hypopneas on chronic medical conditions. Also, studies evaluating the clinical impact of these variable definitions of respiratory events on cardiovascular or neurocognitive sequelae are lacking. Specifically, whether combinations of respiratory events, hypoxia and EEG arousals have variable physiological effects on daytime sleepiness, cardiovascular morbidity and mortality cannot be ascertained from these studies.

There are no data available regarding effects of sleep hypopneas in patients with asthma, COPD or other lung and/or neuromuscular diseases. Whether treatment of 'hypopnea-predominant' OSA leads to reduced cardiovascular morbidity or mortality or metabolic and neurocognitive dysfunction is also not known. And, although studies suggest that sleep apnea may be related to adverse clinical consequences such as cardiovascular disease, stroke, abnormal glucose metabolism, excessive daytime sleepiness, and increased mortality; further research is still needed to determine the *effect* that treating sleep apnea has on these condition.

Conclusion
Notwithstanding the numerous attempts at standardizing the scoring rules, the qualitative nature of scoring flow via visual inspection causes inter-observer variability, and the semi-quantitative sensors (thermistors, nasal prongs, or thoraco-abdominal bands) used to obtain uncalibrated signals for flow or effort, all lead to a level of uncertainty when scoring hypopneas. And several unanswered questions still remain regarding the final impact of using these variable hypopnea definitions for the diagnosis of OSA. Therefore, we emphasize the importance of standardizing the scoring of hypopneas across all sleep labs, regardless of their status of accreditation by the AASM.

Future research needs to focus on carefully delineating the pathophysiological significance and long-term clinical implications of the various hypopnea definitions and hypopneas per se on neurocognitive, cardiovascular and metabolic outcomes.

Abbreviations
AASM: American Academy of Sleep Medicine; AHI: Apnea-Hypopnea Index; AI: Apnea Index; CI: Confidence Interval; COPD: Chronic Obstructive Pulmonary Disease; CVE: Complex Ventricular Ectopy; EDS: Excessive daytime sleepiness; EEG: Electroencephalogram; EMG: Electromyogram; ETCO2: End-tidal Carbon Dioxide; HAR: Hypopnea-to-apnea Ratio; HI: Hypopnea Index; IL-6: Interleukin-6; MCA: Middle Cerebral Artery; MSL: Mean Sleep Latency; ODT: Oxygen Desaturation Index; OSA: Obstructive Sleep Apnea; OSAS: Obstructive Sleep Apnea Syndrome; PSG: Polysomnography; RDI: Respiratory Disturbance Index; SAHS: Sleep Apnea-Hypopnea Syndrome; SaO2/SpO2: Oxygen saturation; SDB: Sleep disordered breathing; SE: Standard Error; TST: Total Sleep Time

Funding
No funding was provided for the development of this manuscript.

Author's contributions
All authors participated in the review of the literature and in the writing of this manuscript. All authors read and approved the final manuscript.

Competing interests

The authors declare that they have no competing interests.

Author details

[1]VA Ann Arbor Heathcare Center and University of Michigan, 2215 Fuller Rd, Ann Arbor, MI 48105, USA. [2]Oakland University, Rochester, MI, USA. [3]John D. Dingell VA Medical Center and Wayne State University, Detroit, MI, USA.

References

Andreas S, et al. Doppler echocardiographic analysis of cardiac flow during the Mueller manoeuver. Eur J Clin Investig. 1991;21(1):72–6.

Ayappa I, et al. Immediate consequences of respiratory events in sleep disordered breathing. Sleep medicine. 2005;6(2):123–30.

Barbe F, et al. Effect of continuous positive airway pressure on the incidence of hypertension and cardiovascular events in nonsleepy patients with obstructive sleep apnea: a randomized controlled trial. JAMA. 2012;307(20):2161–8.

Berg S, et al. Comparison of direct and indirect measurements of respiratory airflow: implications for hypopneas. Sleep. 1997;20(1):60.

Berry RB, et al. Rules for scoring respiratory events in sleep: update of the 2007 AASM manual for the scoring of sleep and associated events. J Clin Sleep Med. 2012a;8(5):597–619.

Berry RB, et al. The AASM manual for the scoring of sleep and associated events. Rules, Terminology and Technical Specifications. Darien, Illinois: American Academy of Sleep Medicine; 2012b.

Bloch A, et al. Sleep apnea, hypopnea and oxygen desaturation in normal subjects. N Engl J Med. 1979;300:513–7.

Bonnet MH. Performance and sleepiness as a function of frequency and placement of sleep disruption. Psychophysiology. 1986;23(3):263–71.

Bradley TD, et al. Continuous positive airway pressure for central sleep apnea and heart failure. N Engl J Med. 2005;353(19):2025–33.

Iber C, Ancoli-Israel S, Chesson AL Jr. Quan SF for the American Academy of Sleep Medicine. The AASM manual for the scoring of sleep and associated events: rules, terminology and technical specifications. 1st ed. Westchester, IL: American Academy of Sleep Medicine; 2007.

Campos-Rodriguez F, et al. Impact of different hypopnea definitions on obstructive sleep apnea severity and cardiovascular mortality risk in women and elderly individuals. Sleep Med. 2016;27-28:54–8.

Chervin RD, Aldrich MS. Characteristics of apneas and hypopneas during sleep and relation to excessive daytime sleepiness. Sleep. 1998;21(8):799–806.

Chowdhuri S, et al. Testosterone conversion blockade increases breathing stability in healthy men during NREM sleep. Sleep. 2013;36(12):1793–8.

Ciftci TU, Kokturk O, Ozkan S. Apnea-hypopnea indexes calculated using different hypopnea definitions and their relation to major symptoms. Sleep and Breathing. 2004;8(03):141–6.

Cole P, Haight JS. Posture and the nasal cycle. Annals of Otology, Rhinology & Laryngology. 1986;95(3):233–7.

Cowie MR, et al. Adaptive servo-ventilation for central sleep apnea in systolic heart failure. N Engl J Med. 2015;373(12):1095–105.

Craig SE, et al. Continuous positive airway pressure improves sleepiness but not calculated vascular risk in patients with minimally symptomatic obstructive sleep apnoea: the MOSAIC randomised controlled trial. Thorax. 2012;67(12):1090–6.

Ding J, Nieto F, Beauchamp N Jr. Sleep-disordered breathing and white matter disease in the brainstem in older adults. Sleep. 2004;27(3):474–9.

Duce B, Milosavljevic J, Hukins C. The 2012 AASM respiratory event criteria increase the incidence of hypopneas in an adult sleep center population. J Clin Sleep Med. 2015;11(12):1425–31.

Farre R, et al. A step forward for better interpreting the apnea-hypopnea index. Sleep. 2015;38(12):1839–40.

Gould G, et al. The sleep hypopnea syndrome. Am Rev Respir Dis. 1988;137(4):895–8.

Guilleminault C, Hagen C, Huynh N. Comparison of hypopnea definitions in lean patients with known obstructive sleep apnea hypopnea syndrome (OSAHS). Sleep and Breathing. 2009;13(4):341–7.

Ho V, et al. Calibration model for apnea-hypopnea indices: impact of alternative criteria for hypopneas. Sleep. 2015;38(12):1887–92.

Hosselet J-J, et al. Classification of sleep-disordered breathing. Am J Respir Crit Care Med. 2001;163(2):398–405.

Iber C. Are We Ready to Define Central Hypopneas? Sleep. 2013;36(3):305-306. https://doi.org/10.5665/sleep.2434.

Iber C. Are we ready to define central hypopneas? Sleep. 36(3):363–8.

Iber C, et al. The AASM manual for the scoring of sleep and associated events: rules, terminology and technical specifications: American Academy of Sleep Medicine; 2007.

Kohler M, Stradling JR. Mechanisms of vascular damage in obstructive sleep apnea. Nat Rev Cardiol. 2010;7(12):677–85.

Kushida CA, et al. Effects of continuous positive airway pressure on neurocognitive function in obstructive sleep apnea patients: the apnea positive pressure long-term efficacy study (APPLES). Sleep. 2012;35(12):1593–602.

Leech JA, et al. A comparison of men and women with occlusive sleep apnea syndrome. Chest. 1988;94(5):983–8.

Loredo JS, et al. Relationship of arousals from sleep to sympathetic nervous system activity and BP in obstructive sleep apnea. CHEST Journal. 1999;116(3):655–9.

Loube DI, et al. Indications for positive airway pressure treatment of adult obstructive sleep apnea patients: a consensus statement. Chest. 1999;115(3):863–6.

Mathew R, Castriotta RJ. High hypopnea/apnea ratio (HAR) in extreme obesity. J Clin Sleep Med. 2014;10(4):391–6.

McEvoy RD, et al. CPAP for prevention of cardiovascular events in obstructive sleep apnea. N Engl J Med. 2016;375(10):919–31.

McMillan A, et al. Continuous positive airway pressure in older people with obstructive sleep apnoea syndrome (PREDICT): a 12-month, multicentre, randomised trial. Lancet Respir Med. 2014;2(10):804–12.

Mehra R, et al. Nocturnal arrhythmias across a spectrum of obstructive and central sleep-disordered breathing in older men: outcomes of sleep disorders in older men (MrOS sleep) study. Arch Intern Med. 2009;169(12):1147–55.

Moser NJ, et al. What is hypopnea, anyway? Chest. 1994;105(2):426–8.

Myllymaa K, et al. Effect of oxygen desaturation threshold on determination of OSA severity during weight loss. Sleep and Breathing. 2016;20(1):33–42.

Netzer N. Blood flow of the middle cerebral artery with sleep-disordered breathing correlation with obstructive hypopneas. Stroke. 1998;29(1):87–93.

Parra O, et al. Efficacy of continuous positive airway pressure treatment on 5-year survival in patients with ischaemic stroke and obstructive sleep apnea: a randomized controlled trial. J Sleep Res. 2015;24(1):47–53.

Peker Y, et al. Effect of positive airway pressure on cardiovascular outcomes in coronary artery disease patients with nonsleepy obstructive sleep apnea. The RICCADSA randomized controlled trial. Am J Respir Crit Care Med. 2016;194(5):613–20.

Punjabi NM, et al. Sleep-disordered breathing and cardiovascular disease: an outcome-based definition of hypopneas. Am J Respir Crit Care Med. 2008;177(10):1150–5.

Randerath WJ, et al. Evaluation of a noninvasive algorithm for differentiation of obstructive and central hypopneas. Sleep. 2013;36(3):363–8.

Redline S, Sanders M. Hypopnea, a floating metric: implications for prevalence, morbidity estimates, and case finding. Sleep. 1997;20(12):1209–17.

Redline S, et al. Effects of varying approaches for identifying respiratory disturbances on sleep apnea assessment. Am J Respir Crit Care Med. 2000;161(2):369–74.

Redline S, et al. Obstructive sleep apnea–hypopnea and incident stroke: the sleep heart health study. Am J Respir Crit Care Med. 2010;182(2):269–77.

Rowley J, et al. The determinants of the apnea threshold during NREM sleep in normal subjects. Sleep. 2006;29(1):95–103.

Ruehland W, et al. The New AASM Criteria for Scoring Hypopneas: Impact on the Apnea Hypopnea Index. Sleep 32: 150–157, 2009. Year Book of Pulmonary Disease. 2010;2010:244–5.

Shahar E, et al. Sleep-disordered breathing and cardiovascular disease: cross-sectional results of the sleep heart health study. Am J Respir Crit Care Med. 2001;163(1):19–25.

Somers VK, et al. Sympathetic-nerve activity during sleep in normal subjects. N Engl J Med. 1993;328(5):303–7.

Stamatakis K, et al. Fasting glycemia in sleep disordered breathing: lowering the threshold on oxyhemoglobin desaturation. Sleep. 2008;31(7):1018–24.

Sulit L, Storfer-Isser A, Kirchner H. Differences in poly-somnography predictors for hypertension and impaired glucose tolerance. Sleep. 2006;29(6):777–83.

Thomas RJ. Sleep fragmentation and arousals from sleep—time scales, associations, and implications. Clin Neurophysiol. 2006;117(4):707–11.

Tsai WH, et al. A comparison of apnea–hypopnea indices derived from different definitions of hypopnea. Am J Respir Crit Care Med. 1999;159(1):43–8.

20

Treating insomnia with medications

J. F. Pagel[1,4*] (iD), Seithikurippu R. Pandi-Perumal[2] and Jaime M. Monti[3]

Abstract

Insomnia is a conspicuous problem in modern 24 h society. In this brief overview, medications used to treat insomnia such as hypnotics, sedatives, medications inducing sedation as a side effect, medications directed at the sleep-associated circadian neuroendocrine system, and agents utilized in treating insomnia-inducing sleep diagnoses such as restless leg syndrome are discussed. The newer GABA-effective hypnotics are the only medications with demonstrated effectiveness in treating chronic insomnia with the majority of evidence supporting treatment efficacy for cognitive-behavioral therapy and short acting GABA-receptor agonists. In patients with comorbid insomnia the use of hypnotics can improve outcomes and potentially reduce morbidity and mortality associated with the use of more toxic medications. Except in individuals whose insomnia is secondary to circadian disturbance, mood disorder/depression and/or restless leg syndrome , there is minimal evidence supporting the efficacy of other medications used to treat insomnia despite their widespread use. Sedatives and other medications used off-label for sedative side-effects are a contributing factor to drug induced hypersomnolence, a factor in more than 30% of motor accident deaths. Hypnotic medications with low toxicity, addictive potential, minimal next day sleepiness, and an otherwise benign side-effect profile can be utilized safely and effectively to treat and improve function and quality of life for patients suffering from insomnia. These are the agents that should be exclusively classified as hypnotics and utilized to induce sleep when medications are required to treat the complaint of insomnia. Other pharmacological agents producing sedation (sedatives and agents used off-label for sedative side-effects) should be used cautiously for the treatment of insomnia due to the increased risk of next day sleepiness as well as for known toxicities and adverse side effects.

Keywords: Insomnia, Medications, Hypnotics, Sedatives, Benzodiazepine

Introduction

Insomnia, defined as the subjective perception of difficulty with sleep initiation, duration, consolidation, or quality that occurs despite adequate opportunity for sleep, is a conspicuous problem in modern 24-h society (Sateia et al. 2017). Episodes of acute or transient insomnia each year affect > 80% of adults. Chronic insomnia (> 3 months in duration) includes difficulty falling asleep, insufficient sleep, or perceived nonrestorative sleep producing daytime complaints of somnolence, fatigue, irritability, or difficulty concentrating and performing everyday tasks, and has a population prevalence of approximately 14 % (Hauri 2005; *NIH State of the Science Conference Statement on Manifestations and Management of Chronic Insomnia in Adults Statement, Journal of Clinical Sleep Medicine* 2005). Chronic insomnia is significantly associated with a decrease in quality of life measures, the exacerbation of co-morbid diagnoses, and an increased likely-hood for developing mood disorders / de[ression (Sateia et al. 2017). While there are dozens of insomnia-associated sleep diagnoses, any medical or psychiatric disorder or environmental stress that produces nighttime discomfort is likely to induce insomnia. Medications for treating insomnia are classified as hypnotics, sedatives, medications inducing sedation as a side effect, medications directed at the sleep-associated circadian neuroendocrine system, and agents utilized in treating insomnia-inducing sleep diagnoses such as restless leg syndrome (RLS) (Curry et al. 2006; Bhat et al. 2008).

Sleep hygiene and cognitive behavioral therapies

Sleep behaviors must be addressed for any patient presenting with insomnia. Insomnia can be treated without medications, using sleep hygiene combined with

* Correspondence: pueo34@gmail.com
[1]University of Colorado School of Medicine, Couthern Colorado Residency Program, Pueblo, CO, USA
[4]Rocky Mountain Sleep, 1306 Fortino Blvd, Pueblo, CO 81008, USA
Full list of author information is available at the end of the article

cognitive and behavioral therapies (CBT). This approach avoids potential drug side effects and toxicities and has shown long-term persistence in treating chronic insomnia that can be superior to results obtained using drug therapies (Morin 2005). Sleep hygiene refers to environmental factors, dietary approaches, drugs, and a lack of required sleep facilitating approaches that can induce insomnia. Insomnia inducing drugs include caffeine, nicotine, weight loss preparations, and activating agents of both prescription and abuse. CBT extends sleep hygiene into the use of sleep facilitating cognitive and behavioral approaches for treating insomnia (Finley and Perlis 2014). CBT has proven its usefulness in treating chronic insomnia, working best when administered by a trained provider over several extended visits (Riemann and Perlis 2009). Insomnia treatment can be limited to the use of hygiene and CBT, but such an approach has clear limitations. Behavioral approaches are rarely effective in treating acute and transient episodes of insomnia and have limited usefulness in treating comorbid insomnia. CBT requires patient interest and effort and as a clinical approach is unavailable to many affected individuals due to both cost and limitations in provider access (Lichstein et al. 2005). Even when appropriately utilized, CBT does not work for every patient (Trauer et al. 2015).

Sleep neurophysiology

From a behavioral stand-point, sleep is a complex, reversible behavioral state of perceptual disengagement from, and unresponsiveness to, the environment (Carskadon and Dement, 2011). To this point, no specific anatomical site or required neurochemical trigger has been identified. Neuroanatomical structures in the CNS are affected globally by sleep associated changes in neurochemical, electrophysiological and neuroendocrine systems.

The neurochemistry of sleep

Sleep is a global state involving multiple factors and systems, with no single neurochemical identified as necessary for modulating sleep (Brown et al. 2012). In most cases, the CNS effects of drugs can be ascribed to primary effects on specific neurotransmitters and neuromodulators. Most hypnotics affect GABA, the primary negative neurotransmitter in the CNS, or affect specific neuromodulators of GABA that include serotonin, acetylcholine, and dopamine (Pagel 2017). Other drugs, particularly those classified as sedatives, induce sedation by antagonizing one or more of the central activating neuromodulators. These activating neuromodulators include serotonin, norepinephrine, histamine, acetylcholine, dopamine, and orexin. Other substances known to affect sleep include adenosine, substance P, corticotrophin releasing factor (CRF), thyrotrophin releasing factor (TRF), vasoactive intestinal peptide (VIP),

neurotensin, muramyl peptides, endotoxins, cytokines [interleukin-1B, tumor necrosis factor-α], interleukin 1B, tumor necrosis factor-α (TNFα), prostaglandin D2 (PGD2) and melanin concentrating hormone (MCH) (García-García et al. 2009; Urade and Hayaishi 2011; Pabst et al. 1999). Sedation is among the most common effects and/or side effects of prescription medications. The list of agents inducing sedation as an effect and/or side effect is extensive and includes most medication classifications (Table 1) (Pagel 2017). Sedation is commonly induced by over the counter (OTC) preparations (particularly anti-histamines), and commonly used drugs of abuse such as cannibis and ethanol. When the use of

Table 1 Medications Not Classified As Sedative/Hypnotics Inducing Daytime Sleepiness As A Side Effect

Medication Class	Neurochemical Basis For Sleepiness
Antiparkinsonian Agents	Dopamine Receptor Agonists
Antimuscarinic/ Antispasmodic	Varied effects
Skeletal Muscle Relaxants	Varied Effects
Alpha- Adrenergic Blocking Agents	Alpha-1 Adrenergic Antagonists
Beta-Adrenergic Blocking Agents	Beta Adrenergic Antagonists
Gamma-Hydroxy-Butyrate	GABA Agonist
Opiate Agonists	Opioid Receptor Agonists (General Cns Depression)
Opiate Partial Agonists	Opioid Receptor Agonists (General Cns Depression)
Anticonvulsants	
Barbiturates	GABA Agonist
–Benzodiazepines	GABA Agonist
- Hydantoins	Neurotransmitter effect poorly defined - electrophysiolic?
- Succinimides	Neurotransmitter effect poorly defined - electrophysiolic?
Other Antidepressants	
- Maoi	Norepinephrine, 5ht & Dopamine
- Ssri	Serotonin Uptake Inhibition
-Agents With Mixed Effects	Serotonin, Dopamine, & Norepinephrine
Other Antipsychotics	Dopamine Receptor Blockage, Varied Effects On Histaminic, Cholinergic And Alpha Adrenergic Receptors
Other Benzodiazepines Not Used For Sedation	GABA Agonist
Anxiolytics, misc. Sedative & hypnotics	GABA Agonist, Varied Effects
Antitussives	Neurotransmitter Effect Poorly Defined
Antidiarrhea agents	Neurotransmitter Effect Poorly Defined - Opioid In Some Cases
Antiemetics	Antihistamine & Varied Effects
Genitourinary Smooth Muscle Relaxants	Neurotransmitter Effect Poorly Defined

these agents is coupled with the use of sedating prescriptions, additive sedation, toxicity, and side-effects increase the danger of life-threatening over-dose (National Institue on Drug Abuse: National Institutes of Health 2015).

The electrophysiology of sleep

In the clinical laboratory, sleep is defined by its electroencephalography (EEG) in concert with electromyography (EMG), electrooculography (EOG) and other telemetry. Using polysomnographic recordings, sleep can be classified into rapid eye movement (REM) sleep and non-rapid eye movement (NREM) sleep. The NREM sleep is further classified into 3 sleep stages namely Stage N1 sleep, Stage N2 sleep, and stage N3 sleep (also known as slow wave sleep, delta sleep or deep sleep), based primarily on the occurrence of synchronous physiologic EEG potentials. Drowsy awake with eyes closed is defined by the presence of alpha - the frequency with the most power on spectral analysis. Sleep onset (Stage N1) is generally defined as occurring at the point in which there is a decline of alpha rhythm (9–11 Hz) to less than 50% of the recorded epoch. Stage N2 sleep is denoted by bursts of sleep spindles at sigma frequency (11–16 Hz) and K-complex events - electrophysiological down states known to negatively affect the general tendency of neurons to develop spike potential activity (Cash et al. 2009). Deep sleep (stage N3 sleep) occurs in association with delta frequency oscillations (0.5–1.5 Hz). REM sleep is characterized by bursts of intracranial theta (5–8 Hz), with alpha and gamma oscillations noted in scalp recordings, associated with conjugate eye movements and diminished skeletal EMG activity. Medications producing CNS-related behavioral effects generally affect background EEG frequencies (Mamdema and Danhof 1992). In most cases, a consistent pattern of EEG change produced by a drug is associated with a consistent pattern of behavioral change (Hermann and Schaerer 1986). Psychoactive drugs produce alterations in physiologic EEG rhythms consistent across therapeutic classifications and utilized to predict the behavioral activity of new preparations, drug interactions and toxicities (Blume 2006) (Table 2).

The neuroendocrinology of sleep

Sleep regulation is a complex interaction between the homeostatic and the endogenous circadian processes (Borbély et al. 2016). The circadian processes of sleep are largely controlled by the suprachiasmatic nucleus (SCN) in the hypothalamus (Dai et al. 1998; Hofman et al. 1996; Swaab et al. 1985; Vimal et al. 2009). This internal human clock responds to external factors with the greatest influence being exposure to light/dark (LD) cycle (Lewy et al. 1980; Morin 2015). The other important element to the timing of the sleep/wake cycle is the endogenously produced neural hormone melatonin, produced by the pineal gland in response to signals from the SCN. Melatonin can induce sedation, an effect sometimes utilized to assist children in tolerating medical procedures (Johnson et al. 2002). In addition to regulation of the sleep/wake cycle, body temperature and numerous other processes vary with circadian rhythm (Sack et al. 2007). Externally introduced

Table 2 Consistent quantitative alteration in physiologic EEG frequencies induced by psychoactive medications

Class of drugs	Eeg frequencies					Treatment indications
	Delta (0.5–1.5 Hz)	Theta (5.5–8.5 Hz)	Alpha (8.5–11 Hz)	Sigma (12–16 Hz)	Beta/Gamma (21–32 Hz)	
Benzodiazepines (BZDs)			Decrease	Increase	Increase	Anxiety Sedation
Barbiturates				Increase	Increase	Anxiety Sedation Epilepsy
Tricyclic Antidepressants (TCAs)	decrease	Decrease			Increase	Depression
SSRI Antidepressants	decrease		Increase			Depression Anxiety OCD
Amphetamines	decrease	Decrease			increase	Somnolence Narcolepsy AD/HD
Opiates	increase		decrease			Pain
Anticonvulsants Phenytoin, valproate, carbamazepine		increase				Epilepsy
Gamma hydroxy butyrate (GHB)	increase					Cataplexy Narcolepsy
Classic Neuroleptics		increase	decrease	decrease		Schizophrenia Psychosis

melatonin can be utilized to reset circadian rhythms of sleep and body core temperature through its actions on the SCN (Abbott et al. 2014).

The optimal hypnotic

Sleep-inducing drugs (hypnotics) are medications specifically designed to induce sleepiness directly after intake. Optimal agents affect cognitive performance during this period while inducing minimal sleepiness in the waking day after use. An optimal hypnotic would have low toxicity and addictive potential, as well a minimal side effect profile (Oswald 1970). Among the first hypnotics, and an agent still in use is chloral hydrate - the original "Mickey Finn" - slipped into the drinks of unsuspecting marks for the purposes of criminal activity. Unfortunately, this medication is difficult to use since the LD-50 (potentially fatal dose) is quite close to the therapeutic dose. In the years leading up to the 1970's, rapidly acting barbiturates were commonly utilized for their hypnotic effects. Unfortunately, these medications, also drugs of abuse, had a significant danger of overdose and contributed to an era that was characterized in part by deaths due to overdoses of sleeping pills. These medications and similar barbiturate-like medications [Methaqualone (Quaalude, Sopor) Glutethimide (Doriden), Ethchlorvynol (Placidyl), Methyprylon (Nodudar)] have limited availability and are rarely used due to limited efficacy, cognitive effects, the potential for abuse and lethal toxicity associated with overdose (Oswald 1970). Today their primary therapeutic uses include executions and facilitated euthanasia (Lossignol 2008).

Most currently utilized hypnotics affect the widely dispersed negative neurotransmitter GABA. In the 1970's benzodiazepines (GABA agonists) were first marketed as hypnotics. Some of these agents had an extremely short duration of action [Triazolam (Halcion)]. While this agent-induced minimal next day somnolence, use was associated with daytime memory impairment, particularly at higher dosages (Roehrs et al. 2000; Adam and Oswald

1989). In the 1990's newer agents were developed and marketed that had selective effects on GABA receptors including Zolpidem (Ambien), Zaleplon (Sonata), Eszopiclone (Estorra) and Indiplon. While all hypnotics have abuse potential for individuals with addictive histories and personalities, these agents have been noted to have minimal additive potential (Hajak et al. 2003). These agents are less likely to have deleterious side effects than most OTC treatments for insomnia, however, with increased use, more side effects including next effects on driving have been reported. This effect as well as next day rebound insomnia has particularly been reported for higher doses of zolpidem (Verster et al. 2002). In many cases, MVA's occurred in the period of somnolence and cognitive impairment during the first few hours after ingestion. Comparatively normal results on psychomotor tests can be obtained 3.25 h. after zaleplon ingestion and 6.25 h. after zopiclone ingestion (Paul et al. 2003). While these agents have excellent efficacy with minimal side effects, at higher doses these agents can exhibit benzodiazepine-like effects. Idiosyncratic reactions of persistent daytime somnolence and/or memory loss have been reported. Some patients will report next day sedation after the nighttime use of these agents, as well as demonstrate an increased error rate in driving tests (Verster et al. 2007). Such information was forthcoming only after these drugs became generic and widely utilized in clinical practice. Most sedating drugs if adopted into such widespread use would also be at least as likely to demonstrate epidemiological effects on MVA's and MVA associated deaths. In the elderly, chronic use of sedating drugs (particularly those with anti-cholinergic side effects) can be associated with an increased risk for falls, and confusion (American Geriatrics Society 2015). Reported next day sleepiness and other side effects associated with hypnotic use are summarized in Table 3.

The newer GABA-effective hypnotics are the only medications with demonstrated effectiveness in treating chronic insomnia (*NIH State of the Science Conference*

Table 3 Hypnotics - Agents Utilized To Induce Sleep With Minimal Next Day Sleepiness After Used Based On Pharmacodynamics, Clinical Trials, And/Or Performance Testing

Drug & Class	1/2 Life	Next Day Sleepiness [Clinical Trials]	Toxicity And/Or Significant Side Effects
Short acting gaba agonist - triazolem	1–2 HR.	Anecdotal and per survey [placebo Equivalent]	Antegrade Amnesia, Confusion At Higher Dose
GABA selective agents - zaleplon	1 HR.	[Placebo Equivalent]	No consistent reports [not in widespread use]
Zolpidem	1.5 HR.	Anecdotal [placebo Equivalent] Per survey when dosed outside pharmacodynamic profile and in the elderly	Symptomatic Parasomnias, Next night rebound insomnia
Eszopiclone	6 HR.	Anecdotal [placebo Equivalent]	Possible Parasomnia Associations [Agent Not In Widespread Generic Use]

Statement on Manifestations and Management of Chronic Insomnia in Adults Statement, Journal of Clinical Sleep Medicine 2005). According to the NIH, the majority of evidence supports the efficacy of cognitive-behavioral therapy and short acting benzodiazepine receptor agonists in the treatment of chronic insomnia, at least in the short term. Chronic insomnia is often, however, a lifelong illness, and the longest clinical trials for these agents have been one year in duration. These agents can be safely utilized chronically or in an "as needed" (prn) basis in individuals with both short and long term insomnia (Morin and Espie 2003; Schutte-Rodin et al. 2008). Except in individuals whose insomnia is secondary to circadian disturbance, mood disorder/depression and/or restless leg syndrome, there is minimal evidence supporting the efficacy of other medications used to treat insomnia despite their widespread use (*NIH State of the Science Conference Statement on Manifestations and Management of Chronic Insomnia in Adults Statement, Journal of Clinical Sleep Medicine* 2005; Morin, Medalie and Cifu 2017).

Sedatives

Sedatives induce calming and reduce arousal during waking. At the extreme end of the spectrum of use, sedative agents are utilized in anesthesia. The sedative category included the opiates, a drug class developed from the domesticated poppy with evidenced utilization from neolithic archeologic sites (5000–7000 B. C.) (Heinrich 2013). At the dawn of medicine as a specialty, among the few agents useful as a medication was laudanum - a tincture of opium that mixed with water or wine was used as a soporific even for crying infants. Most sedative drugs selectively affect specific neurotransmitters and neuromodulators in the CNS (Schwartz 2000). Multiple factors and systems are involved. Sedative drugs can exert primary effects either at the inhibitory neurotransmitter gamma-Aminobutyric acid (GABA), or on sedating neuromodulators. Others potentiate sedation by antagonizing one of the widely dispersed central activating neuromodulators: serotonin, norepinephrine, dopamine, histamine, and orexin.

Many patients suffering from chronic insomnia are hyperaroused, unable to fall asleep even after minimal sleep the night before. Treatment of this hyperarousal presenting clinically as agitation and sometimes anxiety can produce improved sleep. Unfortunately, sedation and reduced arousal are variants of the same cognitive calming effect. Because of this, sedatives induce daytime sleepiness in many users. The idea sedative agent, like the ideal hypnotic, should have low toxicity, low addiction potential, and a benign side effect profile.

Fifty years ago, longer acting benzodiazepines, particularly Diazepam (Valium) preempted the role of opiates in sedation. Some of these agents had active breakdown products that produced an extraordinarily long active half-life (11 days) (Oswald 1970). The prolonged effect is one of waking calming and sedation, associated with increased auto accidents and falls with hip fractures. Medium 1/2 life agents including alprazolam, temazepam, and lorazepam affect next day performance tests (Ray et al. 1989). The use of these agents may be associated with an increased level of next day MVA's (Ceutel 1995; Buysse 1991).

Other sedating agents affect the GABA neuromoduators - acetylcholine, dopamine, and serotonin. Most of these agents are classified as sedating antidepressants. Sedating antidepressants include the tricyclics (amitryptiline, imipramine, nortriptyline, etc.), and atypical antidepressants: Trazodone (Deseryl), and Mirtazapine (Remeron). Trazondone is among the most widely prescibed agents for inducing sleep. There are few studies addressing the efficacy this off-label approach to treating insomia, but there are more describing trazadone's significant side-effects including next day sleepiness and psychomotor impairment in the elderly (Mendelson 2005). Among the SSRI's, Paroxetine (Paxil) can induce mild sedation. Use of sedating antidepressants has been associated with declines in daytime performance, driving test performance, and an increased potential for involvement in motor vehicular accidents (Volz and Sturm 1995). Both tricyclic and atypical antidepressants are widely used as a hypnotics despite significant next day sedation (Settle 1998).

Many of the sedating medications treat hyperarousal by antagonizing the wake-producing neuromodulating systems: serotonin, norepinephrine, dopamine, histamine, and orexin. Both prescription and over the counter (OTC) agents are marketed for sedative effects produced pharmacologically by antagonizing orexin, histamine, and norepinephrine.

Antihistamines and antipsychotics induce sedation based on their antihistaminic effects (Monti et al. 2016). Over the counter sleeping pills contain sedatingH-1 antihistamines, usually diphenhydramine, hydroxyzine or triprolidine (Monti and Monti 2000). These agents induce sedation with acute use, and often induce increased daytime sleepiness and cognitive impairment persisting into the day following nighttime use (O'Hanlon and Ramaekers 1995). In comparative studies, driving performance at 2.5 h. after administration of 50 mg. of diphenhydramine is worse than in individuals with a blood alcohol concentration (BAC) of 0.1% - the level of legal intoxication in most states (Wiler et al. 2000). Nighttime drug use can produce drowsiness severe enough to affect next day performance and driving tests (Gango et al. 1989). Sedation is infrequent with H2 antagonists (e.g. cimetidine, ranitidine, famotidine, and nizatidine), but somnolence as a side effect is reproducible in susceptible individuals (White and Rumbold 1988). Sedation is a common side effect of the traditional antipsychotics, with chlorpromazine and thioridazine somewhat more sedating than haloperidol. Clinical studies have shown a high incidence of persistent sedation with clozapine (46%) with less frequent reports of sedation with risperidone, olanzapine, sertindole and quetiapine (Monti et al. 2016). The sedation associated with these agents is most likely associated with their known effects on histaminic receptors.

Doxepin, a sedating psychotropic agent with pronounced histamine (H-1) receptor antagonism exerts at least part of its effects by antagonizing orexin (Krystal et al. 2013). Suvorexant, is an orexin antagonist designed to lower waking arousal (Norman and Anderson 2016). Currently, it is being heavily marketed as a hypnotic (Rhyne and Anderson 2015). As based on performance and driving tests, this agent is known to produce a dose-related next day increase in somnolence for all age groupings tested (Farkus 2013). Sedative drug effects on daytime sleepiness are summarized in Table 4.

Other agents inducing sedation

Many other agents induce significant sedation as part of their clinical effect or as an untoward side-effect.

Clinically these agents are sometimes used off-label for their sedative effects. Among antihypertensives in wide use, the complaints of tiredness, fatigue and daytime sleepiness are commonly associated with drugs having antagonistic effects at the norepinephrine neuroreceptor (Dimsdale 1992). The complaints of tiredness, fatigue and daytime sleepiness (2–4.3%) associated with beta-blocker use may occur secondary to disturbed sleep or direct action of the drug. Beta-blocking drugs with vasodilating properties (e.g. carvedilol, labetalol) are also associated with reported fatigue and somnolence (3–11%). Sedation is among the most common side effects reported for the alpha-2 agonists clonidine and methyldopa (30–75%) (AHFS 2003). Alpha-1 antagonists (e.g. terazosin, prazosin) are sometimes associated with transient sedation. Prazosin, a norepinephine antagonist, has demonstrated value in treating insomnia associated with PTSD nightmares (Raskind et al. 2003). Clonidine is sometimes utilized to treat the agitation and insomnia that result from using amphetamines to treat AD/HD in pediatric patients (Ming et al. 2011).

Sedation is a common side effect induced by anti-epileptic drugs, reported at levels of 70% with phenobarbitol, 42% with carbamazepine and valproate, and in 33% of patients using phenytoin and primidone

Table 4 Sedatives - Agents Used To Induce Sleep And Sedation With Significant Next Day Sleepiness After Used Based On Pharmacodynamics, Clinical Trials, And/Or Performance Testing

CLASS (DRUG) [Neuromodulator Effected]	1/2 LIFE	Next Day Sleepiness [Clinical Trials]	Next Day Effects On Performance & Driving Tests	Toxicity And/Or Significant Side Effects
Antidepressants - tricyclics (amitriptyline etc.) [serotonin]	10–20 HR.	Significant	Significant With Minimal Study	Anticholinergic, Respiratory suppression in overdose
- Atypicals (trazadone, mirtazapine) [serotonin]	traza- done (8 h) mirtaza-pin 20–40 HR.	Significant	Significant With Minimal Study	Respiratory Suppression In Overdose
H1 antihistamine Diphinhydramine, hydroxyzine, triprolidine) [histamine]	2–12 HR.	Significant	Significant - Multiple studies	Confusion [Black Boxed For The Elderly]
Antipsychotic - Olanzapine [histamine]	6–8 HR.	Significant	Significant with minimal study	Potentially persistent extra-pyramidal Side effects
- Doxepin [histamine, orexin]	1/2–15 h. (dose based) active metabolite	Significant	Significant With Minimal Study	Potentially persistent extrapyramidal Side effects
Gaba agonists - medium 1/2 life benzodiazepi-nes (estalolam, clonazepam, temezepam, etc.) [GABA]	7–10 HR.	Significant	Significant Multiple studies	Disinhibition
- Long 1/2 life benzodiazepi- nes (flurezepam, diazepam, etc.) [GABA]	Up To 11 Days	Significant	Significant Multiple studies	Disinhibition Falls in the elderly
Orexin antagonists (suvorexant) [orexin]	10–22 HR.	Significant	Significant	Unknown New agent

Key: the term "Significant" indicates comparison to placebo or hypnotics

(Schweitzer et al. 2003). In clinical trials sedation is reported as a side effect to treatment with topiramate (15–27%) at at levels of 5–10% for gabapentin, lamotrigine, vigabatrin, and zonisamide (AHFS 2003). The neurochemical basis for the sedation induced by many of these agents remains poorly defined except for those agents know to have GABA agonist effects (e.g. gabapentin, phenobarbitol) (Westbrook 2000). Some drugs may act by glutamate antagonism and others by having direct effects on CNS electrophysiology (Pagel 1996). In individuals being treated with such medications for seizure disorders, the clinical differential between medication effects and sedation secondary to recurrent seizures can be difficult to determine (Manni and Tartara 2000).

Almost all drugs with CNS activity induce sleepiness as a side effect in some patients (Bittencourt et al. 2005; Guilleminault and Brooks 2001). The sedative side effects of some of these agents are clinically utilized in specific situations. However, sleepiness is a common and often-unwanted side effect for many types of prescription medications including commonly used antitussives, skeletal muscle relaxants, antiemetics, antidiarrheal agents, genitourinary smooth muscle relaxants, and others (Table 1). These sedative side effects can limit the use of these agents in patients in which the level of persistent daytime sleepiness affects waking. All sedating agents can contribute to an increased risk for motor vehicular accidents.

Drug induced Hypersomnolence

Drug induced hypersomnolence is a significant problem in today's society. Approximately 30% of traffic deaths in the United States can be attributed at least in part to the use of ethanol - the most commonly abused sedating medication (Department of Transportation (US), National Highway Traffic Safety Administration (NHTSA) 2015). Sedating drugs other than ethanol are contributing factors in 16% of motor vehicular accidents (Berning et al. 2015).While not nearly as great a risk factor for driving as alcohol, marijuana may nearly double the risk of having a vehicle collision (Sewell et al. 2009). In the United States, marijuana users are about 25% more likely to be involved in an MVA than drivers with no evidence of marijuana use (Compton and Berning 2015).

The prescription and OTC medications known to increase the risk of sleepiness-related crashes include longer acting benzodiazepine anxiolytics, sedating antihistamines (H1 class), and tricyclic antidepressants (TCAs). The risks are higher with higher drug doses and for people taking more than one sedating drug simultaneously (Ceutel 1995; Gengo and Manning 1990; Van Laar et al. 1995). Since a high percentage of the population uses drugs of abuse as well as medications for underlying illness, the use of multiple sedating drugs use

has increasingly become a problem. In 1993, about one in eight drivers were using more than one drug, but by 2010, it was closer to one in five. The number of drivers dying in MVA's with three or more sedating drugs in their system increased from 11.5 to 21.5% during this period. Among drivers who tested positive for any drug, 48% also tested positive for alcohol (Disney et al. 2011).

Comorbid insomnia

The term secondary insomnia has historically been applied to patients with insomnia associated with either a medical or psychiatric condition or a primary sleep disorder. Until 2005 the NIH guidelines regarded such insomnia as being a consequence of the primary diagnosis. This led to recommendations that indicated the key was treating the primary or underlying condition with the assumption that this would, in turn, lead to resolution of insomnia. In 2005 the NIH convened another "State of the Science" conference to review the manifestations and management of chronic insomnia (*NIH State of the Science Conference Statement on Manifestations and Management of Chronic Insomnia in Adults Statement, Journal of Clinical Sleep Medicine* 2005). The committee concluded that most cases of insomnia are comorbid with other conditions. The concern over continuing to use the term "secondary" insomnia is that in many cases we do not have clear proof of cause and effect and, of greater concern; the use of the term may lead to under-treatment of insomnia. This recommendation to view insomnia as comorbid has to lead to a shift in treatment paradigms. While identification and treatment of the "primary" condition remain a priority, concurrent treatment of insomnia is now viewed as desirable. In general treatment of comorbid insomnia is now essentially the same as treating primary insomnia with a growing number of studies confirming that this approach is effective (Morin and Benca 2012; Sateia and Nowell 2004; Winkelman 2015). Treatment of insomnia can often improve the symptoms of the "primary" or a comorbid condition.

Circadian system disturbances

Sleep disorders related to circadian rhythm are caused by a misalignment of the approximately 24-h endogenous circadian rhythm and the "normal" 24 h day/night cycle (Melatonin can act as a hypnotic and is a useful adjunct to treatment in individuals with circadian disturbance (Pandi-Perumal et al. 2008). Prescription synthetic analogs of melatonin such as rameleton are available. Sleep tendency and reduced sleep latency are affected from 1 3/4–4 3/4 h post ingestion (Stone et al. 2000). Melatonin has been used as a hypnotic with inconsistent results (Monti et al. 2013). The impact of this agent on next day performance is generally considered to be minimal. Next day psychomotor test results may not be affected, although one study has demonstrated significant effects on next day deviation of lateral position in driving tests (Mets et al. 2011).

Melatonin and light exposure have proven especially effective when used to treat Delayed Sleep Phase Syndrome most prevalent in adolescents and young adults (Pandi-Perumal et al. 2008). Patients with this syndrome have difficulty falling asleep at the desired bedtime, often falling asleep between 2 and 6 AM and then, if their lifestyle permits, sleeping approximately a normal 8 h, awakening at between 10 AM and 2 PM. Individuals with this common disorder often suffer from chronic insufficient sleep time with all its daytime consequences. Treatment involves exposure to bright light at the proper time in the circadian phase response curve. In the case of delayed phase syndrome, this is after the nadir of body temperature. Treatment with 10,000 lx for 30 min on awakening and timed melatonin administration in the early evening 3–6 h before sleep time (before the Dim Light Melatonin Onset (DLMO) or 12+ hours before the temper nadir are effective. Since melatonin can be soporific so caution needs to be exercised if used when the patient has wakeful activities to perform. Advanced Sleep Phase Syndrome (ASPS) is the mirror image of DSPS with patients sleep onset and awakening both several hours earlier than desired with the total sleep period remaining fairly normal. This is less common than DSPS and tends to occur more in middle-aged to elderly adults. Treatment options are similar to those for delayed phase syndrome with the timing of treatment designed to delay rather than advance the circadian rhythm. In shift workers, melatonin can be used to help shift the worker's circadian rhythm as required. When taken before bedtime in the early morning it can improve sleep quality. For individuals suffering from Jet Lag Disorder melatonin can be used to speed the adjustment to the new time zone (Brown et al. 2009; Srinivasan et al. 2010). Visually blind and incarcerated individuals can have non-24 h. and free-running circadian patterns that can be responsive to melatonin agonists such as tasimelteon (Neubauer et al. 2015).

Restless legs syndrome and periodic leg movement disorder
Restless Legs Syndrome (RLS) is a common neurologic condition marked by the urge to move, particularly the legs, which occurs primarily at rest in the evening or bedtime. The essential criteria for making the diagnosis include: 1) The urge to move the legs, usually accompanied or caused by uncomfortable and unpleasant sensations in the legs; 2) The urge to move or unpleasant sensations begin or worsen with rest or inactivity; 3) The urge to move or unpleasant sensations are partially or totally relieved by movement; 4) The urge to move or

unpleasant sensations are worse in the evening (Verma and Kushida 2014). Sleep disruptionand complaints of decreased quality of life is present in 3/4 of the patients with the syndrome (Allen and Earley 2001). A majority of RLS patients will have repetitive periodic limb movements (PLMS) on polysomnogram. The RLS/PLMD has a genetic basis and increases with age so that in the geriatric population (> 80 years) over 30% of individuals may meet criteria for the diagnosis. RLS/PLMD is also more common in children with AD/HD, patients in renal failure, individuals with low serum ferritin levels (< 50), and in patients taking some medications such including antidepressants, antiemetics and antihistamines (Phillips et al. 2006).

The treatment of the sleep disruption, primarily sleep onset, relies predominately on the treatment of the RLS rather than the treatment of resultant insomnia. Dopaminergic agonists have become the primary initial treatment for RLS. Pramipexole and ropinirole have both received FDA approval for this indication and are used in doses low relative to their use for Parkinson's Disease. Pramipexole is used in a range of 0.125 to 2 mg and ropinirole at 0.25 to 4 mg. Dopaminergic agents, especially pramipexole, can induce significant somnolence as well as sleep attacks in some individuals (Micalief et al. 2009). Benzodiazepines have been used, historically clonazepam but also temazepam. There are no recent studies of the efficacy of these but historically they have been useful and still have a role when side effects limit the use of the dopaminergic agents or in combination in refractory cases. When lack of response or side effects are still present opioids with significant addictive potential in this situation such as codeine or oxycodone are sometimes utilized (Comella 2014). Gabapentin, and pregablin used off-label to treat RLS/PLMD induce significant hypersomnolence, interact with opiates, and have been described as drugs of abuse (Schifarno 2014). A varient of these agents, the alpha-2-delta ligand gabapentin enacarbil recently approved as a treatment for RLS is known to induce significant sedation and dizziness (Lee et al. 2011).

Insomnia associated with sleep apnea and its treatment
Obstructive sleep apnea (OSA) induces daytime sleepiness in a significant percentage of affected individuals. Both apnea severity and the level of daytime sleepiness affecting waking function can be negatively affected by the concomitant use of sedatives - particularly opiates and ethanol (Pagel 2017). In a subset of individuals with OSA, breathing disruption contributes to disordered sleep and insomnia. The treatment of OSA with positive airway pressure (PAP) can improve sleep quality for such individuals (Nigram et al. 2017). However for others, PAP therapy can exacerbate insomnia (particularly in those patients with co-morbid PTSD) (Nigram et al. 2016). At altitude and in patients with concomitant

heart failure, PAP therapy can induce the development of complex / central apnea - a diagnosis associated with significant complaints of insomnia (Pagel et al. 2011).

Comorbid psychiatric disorders

Psychiatric disorders commonly comorbid with insomnia include major depression, bipolar mood disorder, anxiety disorders, psychotic disorders, and amnestic disorders such as Alzheimer's disease. Estimates of the incidence of insomnia with these diagnoses are in the 50–75% range (Grandner and Perlis 2015). The most common psychiatric association is with the diagnosis of depression in which insomnia and depression have a circular or bidirectional relationship (Sateia and Nowell 2004). There are several studies that show that insomnia patients are at risk to develop depression. In a large study of young adults over a period of 20 years, 2 weeks of insomnia or longer predicted major depressive episodes and major depressive disorders (Buysse et al. 2008). Recurrent insomnia can also be the earliest sign that a patient in remission from their depression is at risk of a relapse (Breslau et al. 1996). Chronic insomnia problems may contribute to the persistence of depression. This issue is of particular importance in light of the significant rate of residual sleep disturbance in persons who have been otherwise successfully treated for depression (Ohayon and Roth 2003). Insomnia persisting after treatment of depression can be the most refractory symptom of depression. Drawing on data from a large interventional study of enhanced care for depressed elderly persons, the investigators found that persistent insomnia was associated with a 1.8 to 3.5 times greater likelihood of remaining depressed, compared with the population without continued sleep disturbance (Perlis et al. 1997). The relationship between insomnia and depression is further complicated by the fact that many common anti-depressants, especially the selective serotonin reuptake inhibitors (SSRI's), can induce disturbed sleep (McCrae and Lichstein 2001). In patients with insomnia and a psychiatric diagnosis treatment options include those also used for primary insomnia, either pharmacologic treatment, cognitive behavior treatment (psychological and behavioral) or a combination of both. Eszopiclone has been studied in patients with major depression along with the simultaneous use of fluoxetine (Fava et al. 2006). The combination was well tolerated and resulted in a rapid improvement in sleep. Of note, there was also a more rapid and larger antidepressant response. This does not suggest an antidepressant effect of eszopiclone but rather suggests that improved sleep has a beneficial effect on depression. This makes a strong case for the comorbid approach to treatment, simultaneous treatment of the two entities rather than the traditional approach of waiting for insomnia to improve as a result of treating depression. Combining treatment with antidepressants with cognitive-behavioral therapy for insomnia also demonstrated that the combined treatment was superior to the antidepressants alone both in terms of depression outcome (61.5% vs 33.3% remission, respectively) and insomnia outcome (50% vs 7.7% remission, respectively) (Manber et al. 2008). A similar result occurred with the use of eszopiclone with escitalopram for generalized anxiety disorder compared to the escitalopram alone (Pollack et al. 2008).

Comorbid pain

Chronic pain leads to poor sleep in a majority of patients (Cheatle et al. 2016). Pain can be an acute or chronic part of a broad range of medical ailments but most commonly cancer, rheumatologic disorders and headache. Chronic pain and sleep disruption produce a cycle of pain causing poor sleep and poor sleep leading to greater pain (Abad et al. 2008). Management is suggested as follows: diagnosis of the sleep problem, emphasis on sleep hygiene and then CBT techniques followed by pharmacologic interventions including medications for both pain and insomnia (Riemann and Perlis 2009) In rheumatologic disorders treatment of sleep with hypnotics or sedating antidepressants improves sleep but also improves pain tolerance. It should be noted that the United States is currently in the midst of an epidemic of opiate use that is resulting in a large number of deaths. Hypnotics have reduced side-effects, less addiction potential, and much lower toxicity than the opiates often used to treat chronic pain.

Other comorbid medical conditions

Patients with respiratory problems often have disruption of their sleep. COPD patients frequently have fragmented sleep (Crinion and McNicholas 2014). This can improve with oxygen if hypoxia is part of the problem. While Obstructive Sleep Apnea commonly induces daytime sleepiness, it can induce disturbed sleep as well (Talih et al. 2017). About a 1/3 of asthma patients who are poorly controlled have nocturnal asthma attacks that interfere with their sleep and may lead to daytime symptoms. Patients with gastroesophageal reflux often have sleep disruption for the reflux. In addition, reflux can trigger asthma attacks in vulnerable patients. Patients with end-stage renal disease suffer from a variety of sleep disorders with a very high prevalence (Parish 2009). These can include insomnia, sleep apnea and a high incidence of secondary RLS. Menopause is associated with insomnia which can respond to treatment with hormones but also with treatment using a hypnotic (Soares et al. 2006). Chronic neurological conditions including Parkinsons disease are associated with significant insomnia, as are gastrointestinal disorders inducing pain and/or reflux, nocturia and enuresis, and other sleep associated disorders such as narcolepsy (Sateia et al. 2017).

The appropriate use of hypnotic and sedative medications

Sedative/hypnotic agents were among the first known phamaceudical therapies. Many have had significant toxicities and side effects. Some with addictive potential have developed into major drugs of abuse that continue to negatively effect our modern society. For the physician addressing the patient complaint of insomnia, these agents can be difficult to appropriately utilize. This brief overview argues that today there are medications with very low toxicity, addictive potential, minimal next day sleepiness, and an otherwise benign side-effect profile that can be utilized safely and effectively to treat and improve function and quality of life for patients suffering from insomnia. These are the agents that should be exclusively classified as hypnotics and utilized as the first line of agents to induce sleep when medications are required to treat the complaint of insomnia (Table 3). The other pharmacological agents producing sedation (sedatives and others used off-label for sedative side-effects) should be used cautiously for the treatment of insomnia due to the increased risk of next day sleepiness as well as for known toxicities and adverse side effects (Tables 1 & 4).

Abbreviations

24h: twenty-four hour; AD/HD: attention deficit hyperactivity disorder; ASPS: Advanced sleep phase syndrome; BAC: Blood alcohol concentration; CBT: cognitive and behavioral therapies; CNS: Central nervous system; COPD: chronic obstructive pulmonary disease; CRF: corticotrophin releasing factor; DLMO: Dim light melatonin onset; DSPS: Delayed sleep phase syndrome; EEG: electroencephalography; EMG: electromyography; EOG: electrooculography; FDA: Federal drug administration; GABA: gamma amino-butyric acid; Hz: hertz; LD: Light dark; LD-50: lethal dose 50%; MCH: melanin concentrating hormone; MVA's: Motor vehicular accidents; NIH: National Institute of Health; NREM: non-rapid eye movement; OSA: Obstructive sleep apnea; OTC: over the counter; PAP: positive airway pressure; PGD2: prostaglandin D2; PLMD: Periodic limb movement disorder; PLMS: periodic limb movements; PTSD: Post traumatic Stress Disorder; REM: Rapid eye movement; RLS: Restless Leg Syndrome; SCN: suprachiasmatic nucleus; SSRI's: Selective serotonin reuptake inhibitors; TCAs: Tricyclic antidepressants; TNF a: tumor necrosis factor-α; TRF: thyrotrophin releasing factor; VIP: vasoactive intestinal peptide

Acknowledgements

JF Pagel wishes to acknowledge the influence and training of Vernon Pegram PhD.

Authors' contributions

All authors contributed to this text. All authors read and approved the final manuscript.

Competing interests

The authors declare that they have no competing interests.

Author details

[1]University of Colorado School of Medicine, Couthern Colorado Residency Program, Pueblo, CO, USA. [2]Somnogen Canada Inc, College Street, Toronto, ON, Canada. [3]School of Medicine Clinics Hospital, University of the Republic, Montevideo, Uruguay. [4]Rocky Mountain Sleep, 1306 Fortino Blvd, Pueblo, CO 81008, USA.

References

Abad VC, Sarinas PSA, Guilleminault C (2008) Sleep and rheumatologic disorders. Sleep medicine reviews 12(3) .

Abbott S, Soca R, Zee P. Circadian Rhythm Sleep Disorders. In: Pagel J, Pandi-Perumal S, editors. Primary Care Sleep Medicine. 2nd ed. NY: Springer; 2014. p. 297–310.

Adam K, Oswald I. Can a rapidly-eliminated hypnotic cause daytime anxiety. Pharmacopsychiatry. 1989;22:115–9.

AHFS. Drug Information. Bethesda: American society of health-system pharmacists; 2003.

Allen R, Earley C. Restless leg syndrome: a review of clinical and neurophysiological features. J Clin Neurophysiol. 2001;18:128–47.

American Geriatrics Society. Updated beers criteria for potentially inappropriate medication use in older adults. J Am Geriatr Soc. 2015;63:1–20.

Berning A, Compton R, Wochinger K. Results of the 2013–2014 National Roadside Survey of alcohol and drug use by drivers. Washington, DC: NHTSA; 2015. (DOT HS 812 118). https://www.nhtsa.dot.gov/sites/nhtsa.dot.gov/files/812118-roadside_survey_2014.pdf. Accessed 2 June 2017.

Bhat A, Shafi F, Sohl A. Pharmacotherapy of insomnia. Expert Opin Pharmacother. 2008;9:351–62.

Bittencourt LR, Silva RS, Santos RF, Pires ML, Mello MT. Excessive daytime sleepiness. Rev Bras Psiquiatr. 2005;27(Suppl 1):16–21. http://www.scielo.br/pdf/rbp/v27s1/en_24471.pdf

Blume WT. Drug effects on EEG. J Clin Neurophysiol. 2006;23(4):306–11. Review. PMID: 16885705

Borbély AA, Daan S, Wirz-Justice A, Deboer T. The two-process model of sleep regulation: a reappraisal. J Sleep Res 2016;25(2):131–143. doi: 10.1111/jsr.12371. http://onlinelibrary.wiley.com/doi/10.1111/jsr.12371/epdf.

Breslau N, Roth T, Rosenthal L, et al. Sleep disturbance and psychiatric disorder: a longitudinal epidemiological study of young adults. Biol Psychiatry. 1996;39:411–8.

Brown GM, Pandi-Perumal SR, Trakht I, Cardinali DP. Melatonin and its relevance to jet lag. Travel Med Infect Dis 2009;7(2):69–81. doi: 10.1016/j.tmaid.2008.09.004.

Brown RE, Basheer R, McKenna JT, Strecker RE, RW MC. Control of Sleep and Wakefulness. Physiol Rev. 2012;92(3):1087–187. https://doi.org/10.1152/physrev.00032.2011. http://physrev.physiology.org/content/92/3/1087.full.pdf

Buysse D, Angst J, Gamma A, Ajdacic V, Eich D, Rossler W. Prevalence, course, and comorbidity of insomnia and depression in young adults. Sleep. 2008;31:473–80.

Buysse DJ. In: Monk TM, editor. Drugs Affecting Sleep Sleepiness and Performance in Sleep sleepiness and Performance. West Sussex, England: John Wiley & Sons; 1991. p. 4–31.

Carskadon M. Dement WC. Monitoring and Staging Human Sleep. In: Kryger MH, Roth T & Dement WC, editors. Principles and Practice of Sleep Medicine. 5th ed. St. Louis: Elsevier Saunders; 2011. 16–26.

Cash SS, Halgren E, Dehghani N, Rossetti AO, Thesen T, Wang C, Devinsky O, Kuzniecky R, Doyle W, Madsen JR, Bromfield E, Eross L, Halász P, Karmos G, Csercsa R, Wittner L, Ulbert I. The human K-complex represents an isolated cortical down-state. Science. 2009;324(5930):1084–7. https://doi.org/10.1126/science.1169626.

Ceutel C. Risk of traffic accident injury after a prescription for a benzodiazepine. Ann Epidemiol. 1995;5(3):239–44.

Cheatle MD, Foster S, Pinkett A, Lesneski M, Qu D, Dhingra L. Assessing and managing sleep disturbance in patients with chronic pain. Sleep Med Clin. 2016;11(4):531–41. https://doi.org/10.1016/j.jsmc.2016.08.004.

Comella C. Treatment of restless leg syndrome. Neurotherapeutics. 2014;11:177–87.

Compton RP, Berning A. Traffic Safety Facts Research Note: drugs and alcohol crash risk. Washington: NHTSA; 2015. Available at URL: http://www.nhtsa.gov/staticfiles/nti/pdf/812117-Drug_and_Alcohol_Crash_Risk.pdf. Accessed 2 June 2017

Crinion SJ, McNicholas WT. Sleep-related disorders in chronic obstructive pulmonary disease. Expert Rev Respir Med. 2014;8(1):79–88. https://doi.org/10.1586/17476348.2014.860357. 24378218

Curry DT, Eisenstein RD, Walsh JK (2006) Pharmacologic Management of Insomnia: past, present and future. Psychiatric clinics of North America vol 29 #4 .

Dai J, Swaab DF, Van der Vliet J, Buijs RM. Postmortem tracing reveals the organization of hypothalamic projections of the suprachiasmatic nucleus in the human brain. J Comp Neurol. 1998;400(1):87–102.

Department of Transportation (US), National Highway Traffic Safety Administration (NHTSA). Traffic Safety Facts 2014 data: alcohol-impaired driving. Washington: NHTSA; 2015. available at URL: http://www-nrd.nhtsa.dot.gov/Pubs/812231.pdf. (Last accessed June 02, 2017)

Dimsdale JE. Reflections on the impact of antihypertensive medications on mood, sedation, and Neuropsychologic functioning. Arch Intern Med. 1992; 152(1):35–9. https://doi.org/10.1001/archinte.1992.00400130061005.

Disney L, Pelkey S, Wipperman M, Yi H. from CSR; Caces F, Rank K, Zobeck T. from ONDCP (2011) Drug Testing and Drug-Involved Driving of Fatally Injured Drivers in the United States: 2005–2009. http://www.whitehouse.gov/ondcp/drugged-driving.

Farkus R. Suvorexant safety and efficacy - FDA. 2013. www.fda.gov/downloads/.../UCM354215.pdf. Accessed 2 June 2017.

Fava M, McCall WV, Krystal A, Wessel T, Ruben R, Caron J, Amato D, Roth T. Eszopiclone co-administered with fluoxetine in patients with insomnia coexisting with major depressive disorder. Biological Psycyiatry. 2006;59:1052–60.

Finley J, Perlis V. Cognitive Behavioral Therapy of Chronic Insomnia. In: Pagel J, Pandi-Perumal S, editors. Primary Care Sleep Medicine. 2nd ed. NY: Springer; 2014. p. 67–82.

Gango F, Gabos C, Miller J. The pharmacodynamics of diphenhydramine-induced drowsiness and changes in mental performance. Clin Pharm & Therapeutics. 1989;45(1):15–21.

García-García F, Acosta-Peña E, Venebra-Muñoz A, Murillo-Rodríguez E. Sleep-inducing factors. CNS Neurol Disord Drug Targets. 2009;8(4):235–44. 19689305

Gengo F, Manning C. A review of the effects of antihistamines on mental processes related to automobile driving. J Allergy Clin Immunol. 1990;86:1034–9.

Grandner MA, Perlis ML. Treating insomnia disorder in the context of medical and psychiatric comorbidities. JAMA Intern Med. 2015;175(9):1472–3. https://doi.org/10.1001/jamainternmed.2015.3015. 26147221

Guilleminault C, Brooks SN. Excessive daytime sleepiness: a challenge for the practising neurologist. Brain. 2001;124(Pt 8):1482–91. 11459741

Hajak G, Muller WE, Wittchen HU, Pittrow D, Kirch W. Abuse and dependence potential for the non-benzodiazepine hypnotics zolpidem and zopiclone: a review of case reports and epidemiological data. Addiction. 2003;98(10):1371–8.

Hauri P. (Task Force Chair) The international classification of sleep disorders – diagnostic and coding manual (ICD-11), American Academy of sleep medicine (2005) .

Heinrich M. Ethnopharmacology and Drug Discovery. In: Reference module in chemistry, molecular sciences and chemical engineering. New York: Elsevier; 2013.

Hermann WM, Schaerer E. Pharmaco-EEG: computer EEG analysis to describe the projection of drug effects on a functional cerebral level in humans. In: Lopes da Silva FH, Strom Van Leevwen W, Redmond A, editors. Handbook of electroencephalography and clinical neurophysiology. Vol. 2. Clinical applications of computer analysis of EEG and other neurophysiological signals. Amsterdam: Elsevier; 1986. p. 385–445.

Hofman MA, Zhou JN, Swaab DF. Suprachiasmatic nucleus of the human brain: an immunocytochemical and morphometric analysis. Anat Rec. 1996;244(4):552–62. 8694290

Johnson K, Page A, Williams H, Wassemer E, Whitehouse W. The use of melatonin as an alternative to sedation in uncooperative children undergoing an MRI examination. Clin Radiology. 2002;57:502–6.

Krystal AD, Durrnace HH, Scharf M, Jochelson P, Rogowski R, Ludington E, Roth T. Efficacy and safety of doxepin 1 mg and 3 mg in a 12 week sleep laboratory and outpatient trial of elderly subjects with chronic primary insomnia. Sleep. 2013;33:1553–61.

Lee D, Ziman R, Perkins T, Poceta J, Walters A. A randomized, double-blind, placebo-controlled study to assess the efficacy and tolerability of gabapentin enacarbil in subjects with restless leg syndrome. J Clin Sleep Med. 2011;14:282.

Lewy AJ, Wehr TA, Goodwin FK, Newsome DA, Markey SP. Light suppresses melatonin secretion in humans. Science. 1980;210(4475):1267–9. 7434030

Lichstein K, Nau S, McCrae C, Stone K. Psychological and Behavioral Treatments for Secondary Insomnias. In: Kryger M, Roth T, Dement W, editors. Principles and Practice of Sleep Medicine; 2005.

Lossignol D. Euthanasia: medications and medical procedures. Rev Med Brux. 2008;29:435–40.

Mamdema JW, Danhof M. Electroencepalogram effect measures and relationships between pharmacokinetics and pharmachodynamics of centrally acting drugs. Clin Pharmacokinet. 1992;23:191–215.

Manber R, Edinger JD, Gress JL, San Pedro-Salcedo MG, Kuo TF, Kalista T. Cognitive behavioral therapy for insomnia enhances depression outcome in patients with comorbid major depressive disorder and insomnia. Sleep. 2008; 31(4):489–95.

Manni R, Tartara A. Evaluation of sleepiness in epilepsy. Clin Neurophysiol. 2000; 111(suppl. 2):S111–4.

McCrae CS, Lichstein KL. Secondary insomnia: diagnostic challenges and intervention opportunities. Sleep Med Rev. 2001;5(1)

Medalie L, Cifu AS. Management of Chronic Insomnia Disorder in adults. JAMA. 2017;317(7):762–3. https://doi.org/10.1001/jama.2016.19004. 2824134

Mendelson WB. A review of the evidence for the efficacy and safety of trazadone in insomnia. J clin Psychiatry. 2005;66:469–76.

Mets MA, de Vries JM, de Senerpont Domis LM, Volkerts ER, Olivier B, Verster JC. Next-day effects of ramelteon (8 mg), zopiclone (7.5 mg), and placebo on highway driving performance, memory functioning, psychomotor performance, and mood in healthy adult subjects. Sleep. 2011;34(10):1327–34. https://doi.org/10.5665/SLEEP.1272.

Micalief J, Rey M, Eusebio A, Audebert C, Rouby F, Jouve E, Tardieu S, Blin O. Antiparkinsonism drug-induced sleepiness: a double-blind placebo-controlled study of L-dopa, bromocriptine and pramipexole in healthy subjects. British J Clin Pharm. 2009;87(3):333–40.

Ming X, Mulvey M, Moherty S, Patel V. Safety and efficacy of clonidine and clonidine extended-release in the treatment of children and adolescents with attention deficit and hyperactivity disorders. Adolesc Health Med Ther. 2011;2:105–12.

Monti JM, Monti D. Histamine H_1 receptor antagonists in the treatment of insomnia. Is there a rational basis for use? CNS Drugs13; 2000. p. 87–96.

Monti JM, Torterolo P, Lagos P. Melanin-concentrating hormone control of sleep waking behavior. Sleep Med Rev. 2013;17:293–8.

Monti JM, Torterolo P, Pandi Perumal SR. The effects of second generation antipsychotic drugs on sleep variables in healthy subjects and patients with schizophrenia. Sleep Med Rev. 2016;33:51–7.

Morin CM. Psychological and Behavioral Treatments for Primary Insomnia. In: Kryger M, Roth T, Dement W, editors. Principles and Practice of Sleep Medicine; 2005.

Morin CM, Benca R. Chronic insomnia. Lancet. 2012;379(9821):1129–41. https://doi.org/10.1016/S0140-6736(11)60750-2.

Morin CM, Espie C. Insomnia: a clinical guide to Assesment and treatment. New York: Kluwer Academic / Plenum Publishers; 2003. p. 101–19.

Morin LP. A Path to Sleep Is through the Eye (1,2,3). eNeuro. 2015;2(2) https://doi.org/10.1523/ENEURO.0069-14.2015. eCollection 2015 Mar-Apr

National Institue on Drug Abuse: National Institutes of Health. "Overdose Death Rates". Bethesda; 2015. https://www.ncbi.nlm.nih.gov/pmc/articles/PMC4553644. Accessesd 4 Feb 2018.

Neubauer DN, BaHammam AS, Pandi-Perumal SR. Tasimelteon. Milestones in Drug Therapy. 2015;49:261–9. https://doi.org/10.1007/978-3-319-11514-6_13. https://link.springer.com/chapter/10.1007%2F978-3-319-11514-6_13

Nigram G, Camacho M, Riaz M. Rapid eye movement sleep (REM) rebound on initial exposure to CPAP therapy: a systemic review and meta-analysis. Sleep Science and Practice. 2017;1:13.

Nigram G, Pathak C, Riaz M. A systemic review on prevalence and risk factors associated with treatment-emergent sleep apnea. Annals of Thoracic Medicine. 2016;11:202.

NIH State of the Science Conference Statement on Manifestations and Management of Chronic Insomnia in Adults Statement, Journal of Clinical Sleep Medicine (2005) 1, #4, 412–421. https://consensus.nih.gov/2005/insomniastatement.htm.

Norman JL, Anderson SL. Novel class of medications, orexin receptor antagonists, in the treatment of insomnia - critical appraisal of suvorexant. Nat Sci Sleep. 2016;8:239–47. https://doi.org/10.2147/NSS.S76910. eCollection 2016.

O'Hanlon JF, Ramaekers JG. Antihistamine effects on actual driving performance in a standard driving test: a summary of Dutch experience. 1989-94. Allergy. 1995;50:234–42.

Ohayon MM, Roth T. Place of chronic insomnia in the course of depressive and anxiety disorders. J Pscyhiatr Res. 2003;56:497–502.

Oswald I. Sleep, New York, Penguin Books Ltd. ISBN. In: 9780140207439, vol. 13; 1970. p. 157.

Pabst MJ, Beranova-Giorgianni S, Krueger JM. Effects of muramyl peptides on macrophages, monokines, and sleep. Neuroimmunomodulation. 1999;6(4): 261–83.

Pagel JF. Pharmachologic alterations of sleep and dream: a clinical framework for utilizing the electrophysiological and sleep stage effects of psychoactive medications. Human Psychopharmachology. 1996;11:217–23.

Pagel JF (2017) Drug induced Hypersomnolence, in Hyperpersomnolence, A. S. BaHammam (Ed.) Sleep Med Clin. ;12(3):383–393.

Pagel JF, Kawiatkowski C, Parnes B. The effects of altitude associated central apnea on the diagnosis and treatment of OSA: comparative data from three different sites in the mountain west. J Clin Sleep Med. 2011;7(6):610–5.

Pandi-Perumal SR, Trakht I, Spence DW, Srinivasan V, Dagan Y, Cardinali DP. The roles of melatonin and light in the pathophysiology and treatment of circadian rhythm sleep disorders. Nat Clin Pract Neurol. 2008;4(8):436–47. https://doi.org/10.1038/ncpneuro0847. Epub 2008 Jul 15. PMID: 18628753.

Parish J. Sleep-related problems in common medical conditions. Chest. 2009; 136(2):563–72.

Paul MA, Gray G, Kenny G, Pigeau RA. Impact of melatonin, zaleplon, zopiclone, and temazepam on psychomotor performance. Aviat Space Environ Med. 2003;74:1263–70.

Perlis ML, Giles DE, Buysse DJ. Self-reported sleep disturbance as a prodromal symptom in recurrent depression. J Affect Disord. 1997;42:209–12.

Phillips B, Hening W, Britz P, Manning D. Prevalence and correlates of restless leg syndrome: results from the 2005 National Sleep Foundation poll. Chest. 2006; 129:76–80.

Pollack M, Kinrys G, Krystal A, McCall WV, Roth T, Schaefer K, Rubens R, Roach J, Huang H, Krishnan R. Eszopiclone Coadministered with escitalopram in patients with insomnia and comorbid generalized anxiety disorder. Arch Gen Psychiatry. 2008;65(5):551–62.

Raskind MA, Peskind ER, Kanter ED, et al. Reduction of nightmares and other PTSD symptoms in combat veterans by prazosin: a placebo-controlled study. Am J Psychiatry. 2003;160(2):371–3.

Ray WA, Griffen MR, Downey W. Benzodiazepines of long and short elimination half life and the risk of hip fracture. JAMA. 1989;262:3303–7.

Rhyne DN, Anderson SL. Suvorexant in insomnia: efficacy, safety and place in therapy. Ther Adv Drug Saf. 2015;6(5):189–95. https://doi.org/10.1177/ 2042098615595359. https://www.ncbi.nlm.nih.gov/pmc/articles/PMC4591519/ pdf/10.1177_2042098615595359.pdf

Riemann D, Perlis ML (2009) The treatment of chronic insomnia: a review of benzodiazepine receptor agonists and psychological and behavioral therapies. Sleep medicine reviews. Vol 13(3).

Roehrs T, Carskadon MA, Dement WC, Roth T. Daytime Sleepiness and Alertness. In: Kryger M, Roth T, Dement W, editors. Principles and practice of sleep medicine. 3rd ed. Philadelphia: Saunders company; 2000. p. 43–53.

Sack RL, Auckley D, Auger RR, Carskadon MA, Wright KP, Vitiello M, Zhdanova IV. Circadian rhythm sleep disorders: part I, basic principles, shift work and jet lag disorders. Sleep. 2007;30(11):14841501.

Sateia MJ, Buysse DJ, Krystal AD, Neubauer DN, Heald JL. Clinical practice guideline for the pharmacologic treatment of chronic insomnia in adults: an American Academy of sleep medicine clinical practice guideline. J Clin Sleep Med. 2017;13(2):307–49.

Sateia MJ, Nowell PD. Insomnia. Lancet. 2004;364(9449):1959–73.

Schifarno F. Misuse and abuse of pregabalin and gabapentin, cause for concern? CNS Drugs. 2014;28:491–6.

Schutte-Rodin S, Broch L, BuysseD, Dorsey C, Sateia M. Clinical guideline for the evaluation and Management of Chronic Insomnia in adults. J Clin Sleep Med. 2008;4:487–504.

Schwartz JH. Neurotransmitters. In: Kandel ER, Schwartz JH, Jessell TM, editors. Principles of Neural Science. 4th ed. New York: McGraw Hill; 2000. p. 280–97.

Schweitzer PK, Muehlbach MJ, Walsh JK. MedicalDrugs affecting sleep, sleepiness and performance. Am J Geriatr Psychiatry. 2003;11:205–13.

Settle EC. Antidepressant drugs: disturbing and potentially dangerous adverse effects. J Clin Psychiatry. 1998;59(S16):25–9.

Sewell R, Poling J, Sofuoglu M. The effect of cannabis compared with alcohol on driving. Am J Addict. 2009;18(3):185–93. https://doi.org/10.1080/ 10550490902786934.

Soares CN,Joffe H, Rubens R, Caron J, Roth T, Cohen L (2006) Eszopiclone in patients with insomnia during perimenopause and early Postmenoause. Obstetrics and Gynecolgoy 108(6) .

Srinivasan V, Singh J, Pandi-Perumal SR, Brown GM, Spence DW, Cardinali DP. Jet lag, circadian rhythm sleep disturbances, and depression: the role of melatonin and its analogs. Adv Ther. 2010;27(11):796–813. https://doi.org/10. 1007/s12325-010-0065-y. 20827520

Stone BM, Turner C, Mills SL, Nicholson AN. Hypnotic activity of melatonin. Sleep. 2000;23(5):663–70.

Swaab DF, Fliers E, Partiman TS. The suprachiasmatic nucleus of the human brain in relation to sex, age and senile dementia. Brain Res. 1985;342(1):37–44. 4041816

Talih FR, Ajaltouni JJ, Tamim HM, Kobeissy FH. Risk of obstructive sleep apnea and excessive daytime sleepiness in hospitalized psychiatric patients. Neuropsychiatr Dis Treat. 2017;13:1193–200. https://doi.org/10.2147/NDT. S131311. eCollection 2017.

Trauer M, Doyle J, Shantha M, Rajaratham D. Cognitive behavioral therapy for chronic insomnia: a systemic review and meta-analysis. Ann Intern Med. 2015;163:191–204.

Urade Y, Hayaishi O. Prostaglandin D2 and sleep/wake regulation. Sleep Med Rev. 2011;15(6):411–8.

Van Laar M, et al. Acute and subchronic effects of nefazodone and imipramine on highway driving, cognitive functions, and daytime sleepiness in healthy adult and elderly subjects. J Clin Psychopharmacol. 1995;15(1):30–40.

Verma N, Kushida C. Restless Legs and PLMD. In: Pagel J, Pandi-Perumal S, editors. Primary Care Sleep Medicine. 2nd ed. NY: Springer; 2014. p. 339–44.

Verster J, Volkerts E, Olivier B, Johnson W, Liddicoat L. Zolpidem and traffic safety - the importance of treatment compliance. Curr Drug Saf. 2007;2(3):220–6.

Verster JC, Volkerts ER, Schreuder AHCML, et al. Residual effects of middle-of-the-night administration of zaleplon and zolpidem on driving ability, memory functions, and psychomotor performance. J Clin Psychopharmacol. 2002;22: 576–83.

Vimal RL, Pandey-Vimal MU, Vimal LS, Frederick BB, Stopa EG, Renshaw PF, Vimal SP, Harper DG. Activation of suprachiasmatic nuclei and primary visual cortex depends upon time of day. Eur J Neurosci. 2009;29(2):399–410. https://doi. org/10.1111/j.1460-9568.2008.06582.x.

Volz HP, Sturm Y. Antidepressant drugs and psychomotor performance. Neuropsychobiology. 1995;31:146–55.

Westbrook G. Seizures and Epilepsy. In: Kandel ER, Schwartz JH, Jessell TM, editors. Principles of Neural Science. 4th ed. New York: McGraw Hill; 2000. p. 199–935.

White JM, Rumbold GR. Behavioural effects of histamine and its antagonists: a review. Psychopharmacology. 1988;95(1):1–14.

Wiler J, Bloomfield J, Woodworth G, Grant A, Layton T, Brown T, McKenzie D, Baker T, Watson G. Effects of fexofenadine, diphenhydramine, and alcohol on driving performance: a randomized, placebo-controlled trial in the Iowa driving simulator. Ann Intern Med. 2000;132:354–63.

Winkelman JW. Insomnia Disorder. N Engl J Med. 2015;373(15):1437–44. https:// doi.org/10.1056/NEJMcp1412740. http://familymed.uthscsa.edu/residency08/ mmc/Insomnia_Disorder.pdf

21

Prevalence, predictors and effects of shift work sleep disorder among nurses in a Nigerian teaching hospital

Benson A. Fadeyi[1,2]* (iD), Abiodun O. Ayoka[1], Michael B. Fawale[3], Quadri K. Alabi[1,4], Adeniyi M. Oluwadaisi[1,2] and Joseph G. Omole[1]

Abstract

Background: This study evaluated the prevalence, predictors and effects of Shift Work Sleep Disorder (SWSD) among nurses in a Nigerian teaching hospital.

Methods: Eighty-eight nurses (44 each from the pool of shift and non-shift nurses), who emerged by simple random sampling, participated in the study. Socio-demographic data and health complaints were obtained with questionnaires. Each participant was assessed with Epworth sleepiness scale (ESS), insomnia severity index (ISI) and sleep log, while SWSD cases were ascertained by applying the International Classification of Sleep Disorders (ICSD-2) criteria. Body mass index, blood pressure, body temperature and salivary cortisol levels were also determined.

Results: Generally, results showed that the shift group; comprising of shift nurses, recorded higher values of biophysical profiles and more health complaints than the non-shift group (control); comprising of non-shift nurses. Also, 19 (43.2%) of the shift nurses fulfilled the criteria for SWSD, on this basis, the shift group was divided into two: SWSD ($n = 19$) and No SWSD ($n = 25$). And within the shift group, the SWSD group had higher systolic ($p = 0.014$), diastolic ($p = 0.012$), and mean arterial ($p = 0.009$) blood pressures; they also recorded higher temperature ($p = 0.001$), higher salivary cortisol levels ($p = 0.027$) and more health complaints.

Conclusion: The results of this study indicate that rotating shift work among nurses is associated with increased level of health complaints and physiologic indices of stress as well as sleep impairment.

Keywords: Nurses, Shift work sleep disorder, Circadian rhythm, Cortisol, Nigerian-Africans

Background

Shift work is an employment practice designed to make use of, or provide service across, all 24 h of the clock each day of the week (often abbreviated as 24/7). The practice typically sees the day divided into shifts and sets periods of time during which different groups of workers perform their duties. The term "shift work" includes both long-term night shifts and work schedules in which employees change or rotate shifts (U.S. Congress Office of Technology Assessment 1991; Institute for Work and Health; 2014; Grosswald 2004). In Nigeria, shiftwork is

prevalent among factory workers and nurses (Omoarukhe 2012). Nurses engage in shift work schedule as a means of providing uninterrupted and round-the-clock care to patients in the hospital (Isah et al. 2008). In the Nigerian hospital under study i.e. Federal teaching hospital, Ido-Ekiti (FETHI) the shift arrangement in the work schedule of nurses involves the morning shift (8 am–4 pm), afternoon shift (1 pm–8 pm) and night shift (8 pm–8 am). While some nurses work on non-shift basis (permanent morning), some work on rotating shift basis; thereby alternating between morning, afternoon and night shifts.

Shift work sleep disorder (SWSD) is a sleep disorder that is typified by sleepiness and insomnia, which can be attributed to an individual's work schedule (Flo et al., 2012). And according to the International Classification

* Correspondence: fadbenus@yahoo.com
[1]Department of Physiological Sciences, Faculty of Basic Medical Sciences, College of Health Sciences, Obafemi Awolowo University, Ile-Ife, Nigeria
[2]Department of Dental and Oral Surgery, Federal Teaching Hospital, Ido-Ekiti, Ekiti State, Nigeria
Full list of author information is available at the end of the article

of Sleep Disorders (ICSD-3), SWSD is characterized by insomnia or sleepiness that occurs in association with shift work (American Academy of Sleep Medicine 2014). The diagnostic criteria for SWSD, as defined by the American Academy of Sleep Medicine (AASM)'s International Classification of Sleep Disorders-3 (ICSD-3) (American Academy of Sleep Medicine 2014) include: (a) There is a report of insomnia and/or excessive sleepiness, accompanied by a reduction of total sleep time, which is associated with a recurring work schedule that overlaps the usual time for sleep; (b) the symptoms have been present and associated with the shift work schedule for at least 3 months; (c) sleep log and actigraphy monitoring (where possible and preferably with concurrent light exposure measurement) for at least 14 days (work and free days) demonstrate a disturbed sleep and wake pattern; (d) the sleep and/or wake disturbance are not better explained by another current sleep disorder, mental disorder, medication use, poor sleep hygiene, or substance use disorder. While the criteria in the American Academy of Sleep Medicine (AASM)'s International Classification of Sleep Disorders-2 (ICSD-2) (American Academy of Sleep Medicine 2005) include: (i) complaints of insomnia or excessive sleepiness temporally associated with a recurring work schedule in which work hours overlap with the usual time for sleep, (ii) symptoms must be associated with the shift work schedule over the course of at least 1 month, (iii) sleep log or actigraphic monitoring for ≥7 days demonstrates circadian and sleep-time misalignment; (iv) sleep disturbance is not better explained by another sleep disorder, mental disorder, a medical or neurological disorder, medication use or substance use disorder (American Academy of Sleep Medicine 2005). The total daily sleep time is usually shortened and sleep quality is less in those who work night shifts compared to those who work day shifts (Liira et al. 2015). Many of the people suffering from SWSD remain undiagnosed and untreated, the consequences of which include: reduced productivity, lowered cognitive performance, increased likelihood of accidents, high risk of morbidity and mortality and decreased quality of life (Knutson 2003). There is need therefore, to study SWSD in relation to its prevalence, predictors and possible effects, with a view to providing useful recommendations to shift-workers and their employers on the effective coping strategies with shift work schedules. Also, emerging evidence raises serious concern about the potential impact of SWSD on health outcomes. The data generated from this study has the potential of driving new guidelines and directing policies regarding shiftwork practices in Nigeria.

Methods

Participant

Ethical clearance was obtained from Ethics and Research Committee of FETHI, while written informed consent was obtained from all the participants. The participants were members of FETHI nursing staff between the ages of 22–45 years. Eighty-eight (88) of them drawn into two groups of forty-four (44) each; shift group and non-shift group (control) participated in this study. The shift group comprised of nurses who worked on shift basis (rotating shift), while the non-shift group comprised of nurses who worked between 8 am and 4 pm on working weekdays (Monday to Friday). The participants emerged as follows: out of a total nursing staff population of one hundred and fifty-nine (159), the total number of nurses who work on non-shift basis is sixty-eight (68), while the remaining nurses (91) work on shift basis. Using FETHI nursing staff register, numbers were assigned to the nurses; the non-shift nurses were assigned numbers ranging from 1 to 68, while the shift nurses were assigned numbers ranging from 1 to 91. Forty-four (44) random numbers within the range of 1 to 68 were then electronically generated, the corresponding numbers (on FETHI non-shift nursing staff register) to the numbers so generated were the non-shift nurses recruited into this study and this represented the non-shift group. Again, forty-four (44) random numbers, this time within the range of 1 to 91 were electronically generated and the corresponding numbers (on FETHI non-shift nursing staff register) to the numbers so generated were the shift nurses recruited into this study, this represented the shift group. Nursing mothers and individuals with history of chronic medical illnesses, such as: Diabetes Mellitus; Chronic Kidney Disease (CKD); Chronic Obstructive Pulmonary Disease; Obstructive Sleep Apnea Syndrome (OSAS); Central Sleep Apnea Syndrome (CSAS); Hypertensive Heart Disease; Cancers, and psychiatric diseases, which can cause sleep disruption were excluded. Also excluded were individuals who were on drugs that alter sleep pattern such as the benzodiazepines, barbiturates, antihistamines, quinazolinones, antidepressants, antipsychotics and melatonin.

Measurements

Anthropometric measurements

The height and weight of each participant were measured by the investigators and trained research assistants in accordance with the World Health Organization (WHO) multinational monitoring of trends and determinants in cardiovascular disease criteria (Böthig 1989). To measure height, the participant was asked to take off his/her hats or head ties and shoes, stand with his/her back to a vertical rigid measure calibrated to the nearest 0.1 centimeter (cm). They were asked to hold their heads and look straight in front of them. A flat rule was placed on the highest point on the participant's head (scalp) at right angles to the vertical rule. The point at which the hand-held rule touched the vertical rule was the participant's height. To measure weight, the weighing scale was placed on a hard, straight surface, and the participants were asked to take off their shoes and empty their pockets and stand on the weighing scale while they looked straight ahead of them. Height and weight were measured to the nearest 0.1 cm and 0.1 kilogram (kg), respectively. Body mass index (BMI), a measure of body adiposity, was calculated using the formula weight (kg) divided by the square of height (meter squared; m^2) (Keys et al. 1972).

Blood pressure measurement

Blood pressure measurements were done with digital sphygmomanometer of appropriate cuff size per participant. The participants were asked to sit and take a rest of at least 5 min. The cuff of the sphygmomanometer was then tied round the left arm (without any intervening clothing) and with the lower edge of the cuff an inch above the cubital fossa of flexed arm of the subject, the cuff is inflated and measurement taken. Measurements were taken between 8 am and 9 am.

Measurement of body temperature

The body temperature of each participant was measured at the axilla, by placing the digital thermometer in a central position (in the armpit), the arm is then adducted close to the chest wall and the thermometer is left in this position until it beeps. The displayed value is then recorded. Measurements were taken between 8 am and 9 am.

Assessment of sleepiness

Epworth Sleepiness Scale (ESS) is an effective instrument used to measure average daytime sleepiness. The ESS differentiates between average sleepiness and excessive daytime sleepiness that requires intervention. The individual self-rates his/her likelihood of dozing in eight different situations. Scoring of the answers is 0–3, with 0 being "would never doze" and 3 being "high chance of dozing". A sum of 11 or more from the eight individual scores reflects above normal daytime sleepiness and need for further evaluation (Johns 1991). The validity and reliability of ESS has been tested in different groups of individuals across the healthcare continuum. It has also been used previously among populations in Nigeria (Drager et al. 2010; Ozoh et al. 2013; Obaseki et al. 2014).

Assessment of insomnia

This was done by using the Insomnia Severity Index (ISI). ISI is a standardized and validated tool for assessing insomnia (Bastien et al. 2001). The ISI has seven questions with scores for each question ranging from 0 to 4. The scores for the seven answers were added up to get a total score. Total score categories of ISI are: 0–7 = No clinically significant insomnia, 8–14 = Sub threshold insomnia, 15–21 = Clinical insomnia (moderate severity), 22–28 = Clinical insomnia (severe). A score of 10 or more was used as the cut off for insomnia in this study.

Sleep pattern monitoring

Participants' sleep pattern was monitored using a 30-day sleep log. The sleep log was filled by participant having been instructed on how to use it. Important components of the sleep log included time of retiring to bed, estimated time taken to fall asleep, time of final awakening, as well as the time/length of in-between awakening(s) before the final awakening. Total sleep duration (nocturnal and daytime) as well as sleep efficiency were calculated from the sleep log as follows;

Total time in bed (TB) in minutes. = time between bedtime and rise time.
Total time awake (TA) in minutes = total time of in-between awakening(s) before the final awakening.
Total sleep time (TS) in minutes = (TB) − (TA)
Sleep efficiency (E) = (TS) / (TB) × 100%.

Salivary cortisol analysis

Samples of participants' saliva were collected between 8 am and 9 am using a salivette. Participants were asked not to eat before salivary collection and they were asked to do gentle rinsing of their mouths with water, after which 4 ml of saliva was collected into a labelled salivette. The analysis of the saliva samples was done at the chemical pathology laboratory of FETHI, using enzyme immunoassay testing; the principle of which followed the competitive binding scenario.

Statistical analysis

All data collected were entered into and analyzed with the Statistical Package for Social Sciences (SPSS) for windows, version 21.0 (IBM Corporation, Armonk, NY). Means, standard deviations, proportions and percentages were determined as appropriate. Tests of significance for differences and associations were done using Pearson's Chi-Square and Yate's continuity corrections were carried out where applicable. Student's independent t-test was used for mean comparisons. P-values of less than 0.05 were taken to be statistically significant. A binary logistic regression was run to estimate the adjusted odd ratios for all the identified predictors of SWSD.

Results

Comparison of socio-demographic characteristics between the SWSD, no SWSD and non-shift groups

The shift group was divided into two groups; SWSD and No SWSD groups, based on the assessment of SWSD or not among the participants. Comparing the groups; SWSD versus No SWSD, SWSD versus controls, and No SWSD versus control were comparable across all socio-demographic characteristics as seen in Table 1. However, there was no significant difference in all the compared parameters (Table 1).

Comparison of health complaints and occupational accident between the SWSD, no SWSD and non-shift groups

Participants in the SWSD group were more likely to complain of frequent headaches ($p = 0.045$), generalized muscle ache ($p = 0.005$) and lack of concentration ($p = 0.003$) compared with the No SWSD group. The SWSD group, compared with the control group, was more likely to report frequent headaches ($p = 0.003$), generalized muscle ache ($p = 0.003$), lack of concentration ($p < 0.001$), fatigue ($p = 0.029$), menstrual irregularities ($p = 0.043$), and needle stick injury ($p = 0.012$). The No SWSD group, compared with the control group, were more likely to report menstrual irregularities ($p = 0.039$) (Table 2).

Comparison of anthropometric and biophysical profiles between SWSD, no SWSD and non-shift groups

The groups show no significant difference in their BMI scores and pulse pressure. However, the SWSD group compared with the No SWSD group had higher systolic blood pressure ($p = 0.014$), diastolic blood pressure ($p = 0.012$) and mean arterial blood pressure ($p = 0.009$). The SWSD group had higher temperature (°C) than the No SWSD group ($p < 0.001$) and the control group ($p < 0.001$). The No SWSD group had higher temperature than the control group ($p = 0.001$). The SWSD group had higher cortisol level (ng/ml) than the No SWSD group ($p = 0.027$) and the control group ($p < 0.004$) (Table 3).

Comparison of sleep parameters between SWSD, no SWSD and non-shift groups

The SWSD group had lower nocturnal sleep duration than the control group ($p < 0.001$), higher daytime sleep duration than the control group ($p < 0.001$), lower sleep efficiency than the No SWSD group ($p = 0.002$), higher ESS scores than both the No SWSD group and the control group ($p < 0.001$), higher proportion of participants reporting excessive daytime sleepiness than the No SWSD and control groups ($p < 0.001$), higher ISI score than the control group ($p = 0.028$), and higher proportion of participants reporting insomnia than the control

Table 1 Comparison of socio-demographic characteristics between SWSD, No SWSD and non-shift group

Variables	Shift group		Non-shift group	p1	p2	p3
	SWSD n = 19	No SWSD n = 25	n = 44			
Age (yrs) (Mean ± SD)	34.7 ± 4.1	35.7 ± 5.1	36.7 ± 4.8	0.980	0.425	0.399
Age group (yrs) n (%)						
26–30	3 (15.8)	4 (16.0)	3 (6.8)	0.797	0.417	0.682
31–35	6 (31.6)	11 (44.0)	22 (50.0)			
36–40	6 (31.6)	5 (20.0)	9 (20.5)			
41–45	4 (21.1)	5 (20.0)	10 (2.7)			
Gender n (%)						
Male	6 (31.6)	6 (24.0)	17 (38.6)	0.576	0.593	0.215
Female	13 (68.4)	19 (76.0)	27 (61.4)			
Ethnicity n (%)						
Yoruba	17 (89.4)	23 (8.0)	41 (93.2)	0.405	0.815	0.638
Igbo	1 (5.3)	2 (8.0)	2 (4.5)			
Hausa	1 (5.3)	0 (0.0)	1 (2.3)			
Others						
Smoking n (%)	1 (5.3)	0 (0.0)	0 (0.0)	0.432	0.302	Constant
Alcohol n (%)	3 (15.8)	0 (0.0)	1 (2.3)	0.073	0.078	1.000
Coffee n (%)	3 (15.8)	0 (0.0)	1 (15.8)	0.073	0.145	1.000
Kola nut n (%)	2 (10.5)	0 (0.0)	1 (2.3)	0.181	0.443	1.000

p1 SWSD vs No SWSD groups; p2 SWSD vs non-shift Groups; p3 No SWSD vs non-shift Groups
BMI Body mass index, *SBP* Systolic blood pressure

Table 2 Comparison of health complaints and occupational accident between the SWSD, No SWSD and non-shift Groups

Variables	Shift group		Non-shift group	p1	p2	p3
	SWSD $n = 19$	No SWSD $n = 25$	$n = 44$			
Frequent headache n (%)	6 (31.6)	2 (8.0)	2 (4.5)	**0.045**	**0.003**	0.957
Generalized Muscle Ache n (%)	7 (36.8)	1 (4.0)	2 (4.5)	**0.005**	**0.003**	1.000
Lack of Concentration n (%)	8 (42.1)	2 (8.0)	1 (2.3)	**0.021**	**< 0.001**	0.612
Fatigue n (%)	6 (31.6)	6 (24.0)	3 (6.8)	0.576	**0.029**	0.096
Backache n (%)	4 (21.1)	5 (20.0)	3 (6.8)	0.932	0.225	0.210
Aches in the Feet n (%)	3 (15.8)	3 (12.0)	1 (2.3)	1.000	0.145	0.260
Indigestion n (%)	3 (15.8)	4 (16.0)	2 (4.5)	0.985	0.314	0.239
Menstrual Irregularities n (%)	4 (21.1)	5 (20.0)	1 (2.3)	1.000	**0.043**	**0.039**
Number of complaints (mean ± SD)	2.2 ± 2.0	1.1 ± 1.7	0.3 ± 1.2	0.226	**0.004**	0.130
Needle Stick Injury n (%)	5 (26.3)	3 (12.0)	1 (2.3)	0.223	**0.012**	0.260

p1 SWSD vs No SWSD groups; p2 SWSD vs non-shift Groups; p3 No SWSD vs non-shift Groups
Bold enteries are statistically significant

group ($p = 0.088$). The No SWSD group, compared with the control group, had lower nocturnal sleep duration ($p < 0.001$), higher daytime sleep duration ($p < 0.001$) and had no report of excessive daytime sleepiness ($p = 0.043$) (Table 4).

Logistic regression of the predictors of shift work sleep disorder among the shift subjects

Table 5 shows the predictors of SWSD among the shift subjects on bivariate analysis. However, none of these factors independently predicted SWSD upon regression analysis (Table 5).

Discussion

In this study, all the participants essentially were in the same age range, with the shift group having a mean age of 35.7 ± 4.6 while the controls had a mean age of 36.7 ± 4.8. No significant difference existed between the groups on account of age and sex. However, majority of the participants in both groups were female. The female gender dominance in the study population is consistent with the finding of Ulrich (2010). Although this study found no association between gender and SWSD, this is contrary to the findings of lower risk for the female gender reported by Flo et al., 2012. The dominant ethnicity of the

Table 3 Comparison of anthropometric and biophysical profiles between SWSD, No SWSD and non-shift Groups

Variables	Shift group		Non-shift group	p1	p2	p3
	SWSD $n = 19$	No SWSD $N = 25$	$n = 44$			
BMI(kg/m^2) (Mean ± SD)	24.8 ± 2.6	24.3 ± 3.9	23.8 ± 2.6	0.630	0.191	0.571
• Normal weightn (%)	13 (68.4)	15 (60.0)	34 (77.3)	0.565	0.459	0.128
• Overweightn (%)	6 (31.6)	10 (40.0)	10 (22.7)			
SBP (mmHg)(Mean ± SD)	122.1 ± 13.2	113.2 ± 9.9	118.9 ± 12.8	**0.014**	0.364	0.060
• Normal n (%)	17 (89.5)	25 (100.0)	41 (93.2)	0.181^F	0.633^F	0.549^F
• High n (%)	2 (10.5)	0 (0.0)	3 (6.8)			
DBP (mmHg) (Mean ± SD)	74.0 ± 7.9	68.4 ± 6.2	71.1 ± 7.6	**0.012**	0.165	0.143
• Normal n (%)	18 (94.7)	25 (100.0)	43 (97.7)	0.432*	0.516*	1.000*
• High n (%)	1 (5.3)	0 (0.0)	1 (2.3)			
PP(mmHg) (Mean ± SD)	48.1 ± 10.1	44.8 ± 7.1	47.8 ± 10.1	0.210	0.913	0.073
MABP (mmHg) (Mean ± SD)	90.0 ± 8.7	83.3 ± 6.9	87.0 ± 8.6	**0.009**	0.178	0.078
Temperature (°C) (Mean ± SD)	38.0 ± 0.5	37.2 ± 0.7	36.8 ± 0.2	**< 0.001**	**< 0.001**	**0.001**
Cortisol (ng/ml) (Mean ± SD)	15.1 ± 3.2	12.8 ± 2.1	12.3 ± 2.0	**0.027**	**< 0.004**	0.735

p1 SWSD vs No SWSD groups; p2 SWSD vs non-shift Groups; p3 No SWSD vs non-shift Groups
SWSD Shift Work Sleep Disorder, BMI Body mass index, SBP Systolic blood pressure
FFisher's exact
*Stands for liklihood ratio
Bold enteries are statistically significant

Table 4 Comparison of sleep parameters between SWSD, No SWSD and non-shift Groups

Variables	Shift group		Non-shift group	p1	p2	p3
	SWSD $n = 19$	No SWSD $n = 25$	$n = 44$			
Nocturnal sleep duration[a] (Mean ± SD)	5.8 ± 1.4	5.9 ± 1.1	7.2 ± 1.3	0.922	**< 0.001**	**< 0.001**
• < 7 h n (%)	11 (57.9)	15 (60.0)	16 (36.4)	0.888	0.113	0.058
• 7–9 h n (%)	8 (42.1)	10 (40.0)	28 (63.6)			
Daytime sleep duration[a] (Mean ± SD)	2.7 ± 0.8	2.4 ± 0.6	1.0 ± 0.6	0.672	**< 0.001**	**< 0.001**
Sleep efficiency[a] (Mean ± SD)	75.9 ± 11.7	85.9 ± 9.2	86.3 ± 10.6	**0.002**	**0.001**	0.893
ESS score (Mean ± SD)	12.6 ± 2.8	5.3 ± 2.7	6.1 ± 3.8	**< 0.001**	**< 0.001**	0.356
• EDS n (%)	17 (89.5)	0 (0)	7 (15.9)	**< 0.001**[F]	**< 0.001**[F]	**< 0.001**[Y]
• No EDS (%)	2 (10.5)	25 (100.0)	37 (84.1)			
ISI score (Mean ± SD)	8.4 ± 3.6	6.6 ± 2.3	5.8 ± 2.5	0.207	**0.028**	0.453
• Insomnia n (%)	2 (10.5)	0 (0)	0 (0)	0.181[F]	0.088[F]	–
• No insomnian (%)	17 (89.5)	25 (100.0)	44 (100.0)			

P1 SWSD vs No SWSD groups; p2 SWSD vs non-shift Groups; p3 No SWSD vs non-shift Groups
SWSD Shift Work Sleep Disorder, *ESS* Epworth Sleepiness Scale, *EDS* Excessive daytime sleepiness, *ISI* Insomnia Severity Index
[a]Average of nocturnal sleep duration over 30 days
FFisher's exact
YYates corrected
Bold enteries are statistically significant

participants in this study was Yoruba, understandably so, since the study was carried out at a location in Nigeria that is dominated by the Yoruba ethnic nationality (Falola and Heaton 2008), even though no statistically significant difference was observed in the representation of ethnicity in the study groups. The prevalence of substance use was low across the groups and it was in the form of smoking, alcohol, coffee and kola nut consumption. The shift group reported a higher proportion of participants with substance use. This is consistent with the findings of Lasebikan and Oyetunde 2012, who reported that shift nurses are more involved in substance use than non-shift nurses. This may be borne out of repeated need to stay awake and be alert on duty during the natural sleep period.

Health complaints in the form of frequent headaches, generalized muscle aches, lack of concentration, fatigue, backache, aches in the feet, indigestion and menstrual irregularities cut across the shift and non-shift groups. On a general note, the shift group, compared to the control group had higher proportion of participants reporting symptoms on each of the afore-listed health complaints, however there was significant differences only in the reports of lack of concentration, fatigue, and menstrual irregularities. Within the shift group, reports of health complaints were most likely to be present in the SWSD group. Previous studies have reported similar pattern in the report of health problems among shift workers (Costa 1994; Knutson 2003). The reason for these health complaints may be due to the various circadian dysrhythmias associated with shift duty; for example circadian disruption was reported to be associated with fatigue (Cole et al. 1990), digestive disorders (Lennernäs et al. 1994) and cardiovascular diseases (Knutsson and Bøggild 2000). We also found out that a higher proportion of the shift nurses reported occupational accident in the form of needle stick injury compared with the non-shift nurses, also more shift nurses in the SWSD group reported needle stick injury than the shift nurses without SWSD; this points to the vulnerability of the shift nurses with SWSD. The occurrence of needle stick injury is of note, especially as human immunodeficiency virus and other blood-borne infections may be transmitted through such means (Steven 2007). Although this study did not consider the risk of motor vehicle accidents between participants in the two groups of study, there has been documentation of incidents of motor vehicle accidents among night shift workers. A recent study in Iran made an alarming discovery of increased motor vehicle accidents among night shift workers (Saadat et al. 2018).

In the present study, both the shift and control groups showed no significant difference on account of their

Table 5 Logistic regression of the predictors of shift work sleep disorder among the shift subjects

Variable	Odds ratio	95% CI	p value
Headache	0.170	0.006–5.227	0.311
Muscle ache	3.371	0.130–87.726	0.465
Lack of concentration	5.021	0.597–42.227	0.138
Salivary cortisol	1.210	0.817–1.794	0.341
Systolic BP	1.064	0.968–1.169	0.199
Diastolic BP	0.945	0.791–1.129	0.530
Sleep efficiency	0.933	0.841–1.035	0.189

CI confidence interval, *BP* blood pressure

mean BMI scores. Also, the three groups of SWSD, No SWSD and non-shift showed no significant difference when assessed on the basis of their BMI score. However, a downward trend in the BMI scores was observed from SWSD to No SWSD to the non-shift groups (Table 3). Studies by Scheer et al. (2009); Delezie and Challet (2011), had reported higher BMI scores among shift workers. The exact mechanisms linking shift work to higher BMI scores are still developing, but proposed pathways include reduced leisure time for physical activity, difficulty in maintaining a healthy diet or increased consumption of energy-dense foods to combat fatigue, and reduced quality and quantity of sleep (Antunes et al. 2010).

In the present study, there were no significant differences in the blood pressure indices (systolic blood pressure, diastolic blood pressure, mean arterial blood pressure and pulse pressure) between the shift nurses and the nurses who work non shift. This is in tandem with the study of Sfreddo et al. (2010), which found no association between shift work and the incidence of hypertension. However, McCubbin et al. (2010), reported a direct relationship between working night shift and blood pressure dysregulation, especially in individuals with positive family history of hypertension. The study by McCubbin et al. (2010), further revealed that stress caused by shift work may have adverse effects on the cardiovascular system both through direct mechanisms as well as by indirect influences. The observation, in this study, of insignificant difference between the shift and non-shift groups on account of blood pressure parameters, may be due to the fact that the participants in this study fall under the age group which have lower tendency for hypertension in addition to the fact that the participants are medically-inclined and as such may have taken necessary precautionary measures to prevent high blood pressure.

We observed a statistically significantly higher mean body temperature among the shift nurses as compared to the nurses who work non-shift (controls). Comparison between the three groups of SWSD, No SWSD and non-shift group also show significant differences in mean body temperature (°C), with the SWSD group recording the highest mean body temperature and the non-shift recording the least (Table 3). Study by Colquhoun and colleague also found a higher body temperature among shift workers (Colquhoun and Edwards 1970).

The secretion of cortisol (a major glucocorticoid secreted by the adrenal cortex) follows a diurnal rhythm, with the highest in the morning and the lowest in the night. In addition, the secretion of cortisol increases in stressful situations (Smith et al. 2009). In this study, we found a direct relationship between cortisol level and working on shift basis; higher cortisol levels were recorded among nurses who work on shift basis than those who work non-shift. It is also note-worthy that even among the shift group, the SWSD group recorded a significantly higher cortisol level. This higher cortisol level among the shift group may partly explain some of the symptoms/complaints reported by the nurses who work rotating shift.

The mean nocturnal sleep duration (over a 30-day period) for shift nurses was significantly lower than that of the nurses in the control group. Within the shift group, the SWSD group had lower mean nocturnal sleep duration than the No SWSD group (Table 4). Also, the mean daytime sleep duration (over a 30-day period) for shift nurses was significantly higher than that of the controls group, and within the shift group, the SWSD group recorded a higher mean daytime sleep duration (Table 4). It can be inferred from this that the shift nurses had inadequate nighttime sleep duration (worse among the SWSD group) which they try to make up for in the day; this is a sleep time misalignment of some sort. The mean ESS and ISI scores were significantly higher among the shift group than the controls. Also a significantly higher proportion of the shift nurses had excessive daytime sleepiness; these, coupled with a better sleep efficiency among the non-shift nurses point to the existence of SWSD among the shift nurses. Although individuals with symptoms and history suggestive of CKD, OSAS and CSAS were exempted from this study, it is important to note that both OSAS and CSAS are implicated in excessive daytime sleepiness and nighttime insomnia (American Academy of Sleep Medicine 2014). In addition, association has been established between CKD and OSAS (Nigam et al. 2017), and also between CKD and CSAS (Nigam et al. 2016). Previous studies had reported a prevalence level of 10% in a community-based sample (Drake et al. 2004), while Waage et al. (2009), reported a prevalence of 23.3% among oil rig workers. These figures are lower than what was reported by Flo et al. (2012a, 2012b); 43.3% (among nurses) and what we found out in this current study; 43.2%. It is instructive to know that these high prevalence levels were both reported among nurses.

Bivariate analysis showed the predictors of SWSD among the shift nurses and the identified predictors were: headache, muscle ache, lack of concentration, high salivary cortisol level, high diastolic blood pressure and low sleep efficiency. On logistic regression analyses however, these factors did not independently predict SWSD.

Limitations

The fact that none of the identified predictors of SWSD independently predicted the condition may be a limitation of some sort of this study. Also, by conducting this study in a region of Nigeria that is dominated by a particular tribe, the study was rubbed of variability. Therefore, a larger and more varied study population and variable testing may be necessary in future studies. Another shortcoming of this study is that the study lasted a month, hence sleep monitoring was done for 30 days and ICSD-2 diagnostic criteria was applied, thereby limiting the application of ICSD-3 (American Academy of Sleep Medicine 2014). In addition, actigraph monitoring was not done, but a 30-day sleep log was employed. However, by using standardized and validated instruments and by recruiting heterogenous subjects in a profession that is almost entirely homogenous, we sought to bring strength to this study.

Conclusion

Evidence from this study suggest that rotating shift work among nurses is associated with increased level of health complaints and physiologic indices of stress as well as sleep impairment. The prevalence of SWSD among shift nurses in this study was 43.2%. The factors that predicted SWSD in the study sample were headache, muscle ache, lack of concentration, high salivary cortisol level, high diastolic blood pressure and low sleep efficiency.

Abbreviations

CKD: Chronic Kidney Disease; COPD: Chronic Obstructive Pulmonary Disease; CSAS: Central Sleep Apnea Syndrome; ESS: Epworth Sleepiness Scale; FETHI: Federal Teaching Hospital, Ido-Ekiti; ICSD-2: International Classification of Sleep Disorders-2nd edition; ICSD-3: International Classification of Sleep Disorders-3rd edition; ISI: Insomnia Severity Index; OSAS: Obstructive Sleep Apnea Syndrome; SWSD: Shift Work Sleep Disorder; WHO: World Health Organization

Authors' contributions

BAF, AOA and MBF made significant contributions to conception, design, experimentation, acquisition and interpretation of data and writing of manuscript. QKA, AMO and JGO made substantial contribution in interpretation of data and revising the manuscript for intellectual content. All authors read and approved the final manuscript.

Competing interests

The authors of this manuscript declare no competing interests.

Author details

[1]Department of Physiological Sciences, Faculty of Basic Medical Sciences, College of Health Sciences, Obafemi Awolowo University, Ile-Ife, Nigeria. [2]Department of Dental and Oral Surgery, Federal Teaching Hospital, Ido-Ekiti, Ekiti State, Nigeria. [3]Department of Medicine (Neurology Unit), Faculty of Clinical Sciences, College of Health Sciences, Obafemi Awolowo University, Ile-Ife, Nigeria. [4]Department of Haematology and Blood Transfusion, Faculty of Basic Medical Sciences, College of Medicine, Afe-Babalola University, Ado-Ekiti, Ekiti State, Nigeria.

References

American Academy of Sleep Medicine (AASM). International classification of sleep disorders, revised: Diagnostic and coding manual. 2nd edn. (ICSD-2). Westchester: AASM; 2005.

American Academy of Sleep Medicine (AASM). In: Darien IL, editor. International classification of sleep disorders. 3rd ed. United States: American Academy of Sleep Medicine; 2014.

Antunes LC, Levandovski R, Dantas G, Caumo W, Hidalgo MP. Obesity and shift work: Chronobiological aspects. Nutr Res Rev. 2010;23(1):155–68.

Bastien CH, Vallieres A, Morin CM. Validation of the insomnia severity index as an outcome measure for insomnia research. Sleep Med. 2001;2:297–307.

Böthig S. WHO MONICA Project: objectives and design. Int J Epidemiol. 1989; 18(3):S29–37.

Cole RJ, Loving RT, Kripke DF. Psychiatric aspects of shiftwork. Occup Med. 1990; 5:301–14.

Colquhoun WP, Edwards RS. Circadian rhythms of body temperature in shift Workers at a Coalface. Br J Ind Med. 1970;27(3):266–72.

Costa G. The impact of shift and night work on health. Appl Ergon. 1994;27(1):922.

Delezie J, Challet E. Interactions between metabolism and circadian clocks: reciprocal disturbances. Ann N Y Acad Sci. 2011;1243:30–46.

Drager LF, Genta PR, Pedrosa RP, Nerbass FB, Gonzaga CC, Krieger EM, et al. Characteristics and predictors of obstructive sleep apnea in patients with systemic hypertension. Am J Cardiol. 2010;105(8):1135–9.

Drake CL, Roehrs T, Richardson G, Walsh JK, Roth T. Shift work sleep disorder: prevalence and consequences beyond that of symptomatic day workers. Sleep. 2004;27:1453–62.

Falola T, Heaton MM. A history of Nigeria. Cambridge: Cambridge University Press; 2008. p. 23. ISBN 0-521-68157-X

Flo E, Pallesen S, Magerøy N, Moen BE, Grønli J. Shift work disorder in nurses assessment, prevalence and related health problems. PLoSONE. 2012b;7(4):e33981.

Flo E, Pallesen S, Magerøy N, Moen BE, Grønli J, Nordhus IH, Bjorvatn B. Shift Work Disorder in Nurses – Assessment, Prevalence and Related Health Problems. PLoS One. 2012a;7(4):e33981.

Grosswald B. The effects of shift work on family satisfaction. Families in Society. 2004;85(3):413–24.

Institute for Work & Health, Ontario, Canada. Fact Sheet, Shiftwork (PDF). Retrieved. 2014: 09-25.

Isah EC, Iyamu OA, Imoudu GO. Health effects of night shift duty on nurses in a university teaching hospital in Benin. Nigeria: Niger J Clin Pract. 2008;11(2):144–8.

Johns M. A new method for measuring daytime sleepiness: the Epworth sleepiness scale. Sleep. 1991;14:540–5.

Keys A, Fidanza F, Karvonen MJ, Kimura N, Taylor HL. Indices of relative weight and obesity. J Chronic Dis. 1972;25:329–43.

Knutson A. Health disorders of shift workers. Occup Med (Lond). 2003;53:103–8.

Knutsson A, Bøggild H. Shiftwork and cardiovascular disease: review of disease mechanisms. Rev Environ Health. 2000;15:359–72.

Lasebikan VO, Oyetunde MO. Burnoutamong nurses in a Nigerian general hospital: prevalence and associated factors. ISRN Nurs. 2012; https://doi.org/10.5402/2012/402157.

Lennernäs M, Hambraeus L, Åkerstedt T. Nutrient intake in day and shift workers. Work Stress. 1994;8:332–42.

Liira J, Verbeek JH, Costa G, Driscoll TR, Sallinen M, Isotalo LK, Ruotsalainen JH. "Pharmacological interventions for sleepiness and sleep disturbances caused by shift work" The Cochrane database of systematic reviews. 8. JAMA. 2015; 313(9):961–2.

McCubbin JA, Pilcher JJ, Moore DD. Blood pressure increases during a simulated night shift in persons at risk for hypertension. Int J Behav Med. 2010;17(4): 314–20.

Nigam G, Camacho M, Chang ET, Riaz M. Exploring sleep disorders in patients with chronic kidney diseases. Nat Sci Sleep. 2018;10:35–43.

Nigam G, Pathak C, Riaz M. A systematic review of central sleep apnea in adult patients with chronic kidney disease. Sleep Breath. 2016;20(3):957–64.

Obaseki D, Kolawole B, Gomerep S, Obaseki J, Abidoye I, Ikem R, et al. Pre- valence and predictors of obstructive sleep apnea syndrome ina sample of patients with type2 Diabetes Mellitus in Nigeria. Niger Med J. 2014;55(1):24–8.

Omoarukhe, Omowumi. Management of Swift Work in Nigeria and its implications for labour – management relations, Green Thesis. 2012.

Ozoh O, Okubadejo N, Akanbi M, Dania M. High-risk of obstructive sleep apnea and excessive daytime sleepiness among commercial intra-city drivers in Lagos metropolis. Niger Med J. 2013;54(4):224–9.

Saadat S, Karbakhsh M, Saremi M, Alimohammadi I, Ashayeri H, Fayaz M, Sadeghian F, Rostami R. A prospective study of psychomotor performance of driving among two kinds of shift work in Iran. Electron Physician. 2018;10: 6417–25. https://doi.org/10.19082/6417.

Scheer FA, Hilton MF, Mantzoros CS, Shea SA. Adverse metabolic and cardiovascular consequences of circadian misalignment. Proc Natl Acad Sci. 2009;106(11):4453–8.

Sfreddo C, Fuchs SC, Merlo ÁR, Fuchs FD. Shift work is not associated with high blood pressure or prevalence of hypertension. PLoS One. 2010;5(12):e15250.

Smith JL, Gropper SA, Groff J. Advanced nutrition and human metabolism. Belmont: Wadsworth Cengage Learning; 2009. p. 247. ISBN 0-495-11657-2

Steven B. Environmental and occupational medicine. 4th ed. Philadelphia: Wolters Kluwer/Lippincott Williams & Wilkins; 2007. p. 745. ISBN 978-0-7817-6299-1

U.S. Congress Office of Technology Assessment. Biological Rhythms: Implications for the Worker. 1991.

Ulrich B. Gender diversity and nurse-physician relationships. Virtual Mentor. 2010; 12:41–5.

Waage S, Moen BE, Pallesen S, Eriksen HR, Ursin H, Akerstedt T, et al. Shift work disorder among oil rig workers in the North Sea. Sleep. 2009;32:558–65.

22

Impact of blue-depleted white light on pupil dynamics, melatonin suppression and subjective alertness following real-world light exposure

Jamie M. Zeitzer[1,2]* (iD), Raymond P. Najjar[1,3], Cheng-Ann Wang[1] and Mirelle Kass[1,4]

Abstract

Background: The non-image forming system, which conveys light information to circadian and sleep centers in the brain, is optimized to respond to short wavelengths of light (blue). Exposure to white light with reduced blue content can cause lower than expected circadian and sleep responses. These findings, however, come from controlled laboratory conditions that may not be entirely accurate when attempting to apply them to most real-world settings. It was our intention to examine whether, under ecologically-valid circumstances, a blue-depleted white light had a diminished impact on sleep and circadian functions as compared to an equiluminant white light.

Methods: In Study 1, seven healthy, young individuals were exposed to a series of one-minute light pulses (32, 100 or 140 lx) produced either by a standard white light emitting diode (LED) or an LED light with reduced blue content. Pupil responses were measured with an infrared pupillometer. In Study 2, ten healthy, young individuals participated in two overnight evaluations. On one of the nights, participants received three hours of 150 lx of a standard white LED starting at habitual bedtime. The protocol on the alternate night was identical except an LED with reduced blue content was used (both lights were identical to those used in Study 1). Saliva samples were collected every 20–30 min for determination of melatonin concentrations and subjective sleepiness was assessed hourly with the Stanford Sleepiness Scale. In both studies, pre-light exposure baseline was real-world ambulatory light exposure.

Results: Study 1. The post-illumination pupil response (PIPR) to 32 lx was increased in response to the standard as compared to blue-depleted LED ($p < 0.05$, paired t-test). PIPR did not differ between lighting conditions at higher illuminances. Study 2. Neither salivary melatonin concentrations nor subjective sleepiness scores were different between lighting conditions.

Conclusions: While the absence or reduction of blue light has the physiologic capacity to reduce the impact of light on non-image forming photoreceptive functions, under a pre-exposure lighting environment closer to that which is found in the real world, no such differences are observed except for pupil responses to moderately dim light.

Keywords: Light, Blue light, Short wavelength light, Melatonin, Alertness, Pupil

* Correspondence: jzeitzer@stanford.edu
[1]Department of Psychiatry and Behavioral Rhythms, Stanford University, Stanford, CA 94305, USA
[2]Mental Illness Research Education and Clinical Center, VA Palo Alto Health Care System, Palo Alto, CA 94304, USA
Full list of author information is available at the end of the article

Background

While retinal photoreception is mostly thought of as the basis of "image formation", the retina underlies a number of non-image forming functions as well. Notable among these are synchronizing the timing of the circadian clock (Czeisler et al., 1989), suppressing pineal melatonin production (Zeitzer et al., 2000), increasing alertness (Cajochen et al., 2000), and changing pupil size (Alpern & Campbell, 1962). In mammals, while rods and cones are the main contributors to conscious visual perception, a combination of rods, cones, and melanopsin contribute to non-image forming photoreception. Melanopsin is a light-absorbing pigment expressed in the intrinsically photosensitive retinal ganglion cells (ipRGCs) and conveys the eponymous intrinsic photosensitivity (Berson et al., 2002). ipRGCs project widely to the brain (notably the hypothalamus) to convey information about the overall intensity of light (Nelson & Takahashi, 1991).

Melanopsin has a peak sensitivity in the blue range of the light spectrum (Newman et al., 2003) and the spectral sensitivity of sustained melatonin suppression also peaks in the blue light range (~ 460 nm) (Brainard et al., 2001). The peak photopic sensitivity for conscious image formation is, however, in the green portion of the spectrum (555 nm). As such, it has been theorized that exposure to broad spectrum white light that has been depleted of or has minimal short wavelengths (blue light) would not alter conscious visual perception but would minimally activate non-image forming photoreceptive functions (McBean et al., 2016). This would be notable for extended (hours) light stimuli as the response to shorter light stimuli is likely more driven by cones (Gooley et al., 2010). In one study of spectrally-altered polychromatic light, blue-depleted white light (~ 239 lx, normal room lighting) was not different from normal white light in terms of its impact on sleep latency, melatonin suppression, and sleepiness (Santhi et al., 2011). In a separate study, authors found that 50 lx of blue-depleted white light (~ 50 lx, low room lighting) was less effective at melatonin suppression and caused less enhancement of electroencephalographic measures of alertness than 50 lx of normal white light (Rahman et al., 2017). In this latter study, however, participants spent 8 h in moderate room lighting (~ 88 lx) prior to receiving the experimental light which likely sensitized the responses to the low intensity light (Smith et al., 2004; Chang et al., 2011).

The purpose of this experiment was to test under real-world conditions whether a commercially-available LED-based lamp that emitted a broad spectrum white light had greater impacts on pupil function, subjective alertness and melatonin suppression than a commercially-available LED-based bulb that emitted a broad spectrum, blue-depleted white light.

Methods

Study 1

We examined seven participants (four male, 3 female) during a single 3-h session. Five were Caucasian, one was Asian, and one identified as multiple races. They were aged 21–29 (26 ± 3.4 years, mean ± SD). Participants came to the laboratory between 4 and 7 h after their typical wake time, following a night during which they had at least 7 h in bed allotted towards sleep (self-reported). All participants were in good self-reported physical and mental health, not depressed (< 28 on the Center for Epidemiologic Studies Depression Scale (Radloff, 1977)), without sleep disorders (< 6 on the Pittsburgh Sleep Quality Index (Buysse et al., 1989)), of intermediate chronotype (Horne & Östberg, 1976), were not regular smokers, and did not have an alcohol use disorder (< 20 on the Alcohol Use Disorders Identification Test; lack of proximal alcohol use was confirmed upon entry to the laboratory with salivary alcohol test). All participants had normal color vision (Ishihara plate test (Ishihara, 2007)), lacked self-reported ocular pathologies, and did not use medications that impacted ocular function or pupil size. Female participants were not pregnant, as confirmed upon entry to the laboratory with a urinary pregnancy test. All procedures were approved by the Stanford University Institutional Review Board and conformed to the principals outlined in the Declaration of Helsinki.

Following completion of screening questionnaires and determination of eligibility, participants took part in an approximately three-hour examination of their pupil responses to light. During this examination, participants were seated and placed their chin on a chin rest and rested their forehead on a temple bar, all of which fixed the distance between the eyes and an experimental light source both within and between participants. A head-mounted infrared eye tracker (ViewPoint USB-60 × 3 Binocular Pupillometry system, Arrington Research, Scottsdale AZ) was placed on the participant's head and was used to record pupil size (recorded at 60 Hz) throughout the study. Once the eye tracker was in place, participants were exposed to 30 min of darkness. Following this dark adaptation, participants were exposed to a series of 1-min light pulses, each of which were separated by 10 min of darkness (to allow for partial dark adaptation of rhodopsin), that were produced by one of two lamps – (1) a standard broad spectrum (white) LED (EcoSmart BR30, 2700 K, color rendering index = 95, Home Depot, Atlanta GA) the spectrum of which is generated by blue LED exciting phosphors, or (2) a blue-depleted white LED (BlueFree in a 9.525 cm diameter bulged reflector casing, 2700 K, color rendering index = 78, Soraa, Fremont CA) that has a significantly reduced short wavelength light (blue) component (Fig. 1) as its

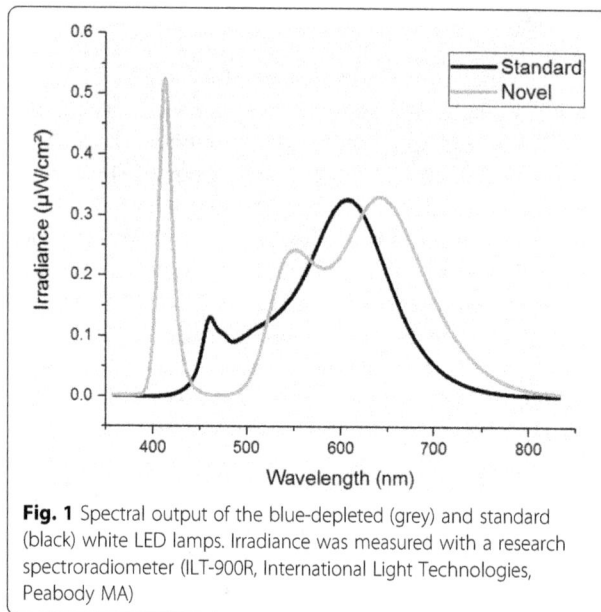

Fig. 1 Spectral output of the blue-depleted (grey) and standard (black) white LED lamps. Irradiance was measured with a research spectroradiometer (ILT-900R, International Light Technologies, Peabody MA)

spectrum is generated by violet LED exciting phosphors. Lamps were placed behind an ultraviolet-filtering, clear plastic panel fitted with neutral density filters (Roscolux neutral gray, #398; Rosco, Stamford CT) and a diffuser (Roscolux tough white diffusion #116; Rosco, Stamford CT). The two lamps were each calibrated to produce three different illuminances: 32 lx (log photon flux: 13.6 $\log_{10}(1/cm^2/s)$), 100 lx (log photon flux: 14.1 $\log_{10}(1/cm^2/s)$), and 140 lx (log photon flux: 14.2 $\log_{10}(1/cm^2/s)$) (corneal illuminances confirmed in situ with an ILT1700 Research Photometer, International Light Technologies, Peabody MA; photon flux determined with ILT-900R, International Light Technologies, Peabody MA and converted using the Lucas toolbox (Lucas et al., 2014)). Light was presented in a diffuse circle at a 21° visual angle. All illuminances used were in the photopic range (i.e., the different illuminances would have differential impact on cones but a similar, saturating impact on rods). During the experiment, each of the two lamps produced each of the three illuminances once (six different light exposures), with the order of the exposures being randomized separately for each participant (randomization from Random.org), with an additional 1-min light exposure from the standard LED lamp being the first in all cases (calibration). Pupil dynamics were analyzed offline with ViewPoint EyeTracker (Arrington Research, Scottsdale AZ) and macros developed in Excel (v.16.0.4549.1000, Microsoft, Redmond WA). Following the final 10-min dark exposure to assess pupil redilation, the experiment was concluded, and the participant was discharged from the study.

For each participant, the eye with the best pupillometric signal-to-noise ratio was selected. Artifacts (notably, eye blinks) were manually removed and pupil data were smoothed (Loess with fourth-degree polynomial) before analyses. Pupil size was calculated as the width of an elliptical contour fitted by the Arrington software. Baseline pupil size was calculated as the median pupil size during the 25 s of darkness preceding each light exposure. Pupil constriction was baseline-adjusted such that: % *pupil constriction from baseline* $= \left(\frac{baseline\ pupil\ size - pupil\ size}{baseline\ pupil\ size}\right) \times 100$ (Joyce et al., 2016). Multiple pupillometric parameters were calculated, including: peak phasic constriction (largest acute reduction in pupil size), sustained pupil constriction (median of constricted pupil size 10 post light-onset to 5 s pre light-offset), and the post-illuminance pupil response (PIPR), which has been shown to be representative of ipRGC activity (Adhikari et al., 2015) (Fig. 2) and calculated as the percent pupil constriction from baseline 6 s after light-offset. The time from light onset to peak constriction (constriction speed) and from light offset to 90% of baseline (re-dilation speed) were also calculated. All pupil analyses were conducted blind to the specific illuminance and lamp being tested.

Study 2

We examined a separate 10 participants (five male, five female) in a randomized, double-blind cross-over trial. Six were Caucasian and four were Asian. They were aged 25–35 years (29 ± 3.0 years, mean ± SD). All participants were in good health and passed the same screening as reported in Study 1.

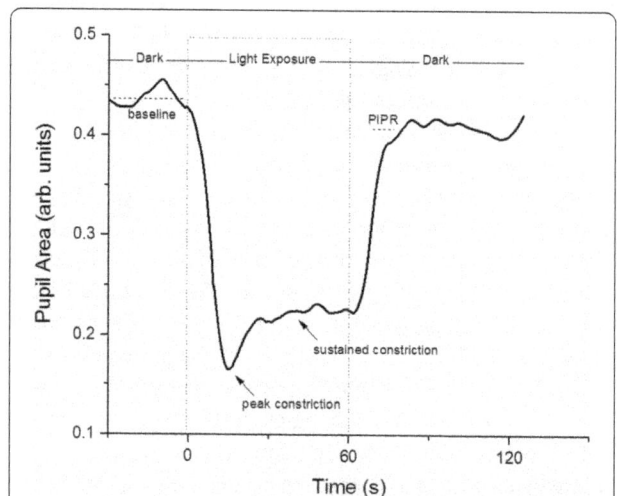

Fig. 2 A representative tracing of pupil area as it changes in response to a sixty-second light exposure that is preceded and followed by darkness. In each exposure, we quantitate the baseline in darkness, the peak constriction, the sustained constriction, and the PIPR starting 6 s after the cessation of the light

Following consent and screening, participants were scheduled for two overnight stays at the Zeitzer laboratory at the VA Palo Alto Health Care System. Each stay was at least one week apart. During the week prior to entry into the laboratory, participants kept a regular sleep/wake schedule such that all bed and wake times were within ±30 min of a participant-set target time and 7–9 h apart. Compliance with this schedule was confirmed through examination of self-reported sleep logs and continuous wrist actigraphy (Motionlogger, Ambulatory Monitoring, Ardsley NY), a useful proxy for determining sleep/wake patterns (Ancoli-Israel et al., 2003). One divergence from the schedule was permitted – otherwise participants were rescheduled. Habitual bedtime was calculated as the mid-point of the at-home sleep schedule minus four hours. The timing of all laboratory procedures were based off this calculation. For young individuals with a regular sleep/wake schedule and an intermediate chronotype, determination of habitual sleep timing is a useful approximation of the position of the endogenous circadian clock (Duffy et al., 1998).

Participants arrived at the laboratory for the overnight study approximately four hours prior to their target bedtime. Once an accurate sleep schedule was verified, participants were brought to the room in which they would spend the next 14 h. The room is specially designed for the conduct of circadian studies. There are no windows and all lighting is controlled by a panel outside of the room. The walls are painted with a highly reflect-ive titanium-dioxide-based white paint and all of the surfaces are white or covered in white sheets. Upon entry into the room, the lights were dimmed (< 10 lx in any angle of gaze, ILT1700 Research Photometer, International Light Technologies, Peabody MA). Room lighting was produced with evenly spaced fluorescent lamps (Philips F32 T8, 3500 K) controlled by an electronic ballast. For the next 14 h, participants lay in bed and rested in either a semirecumbent (during periods of wake) or flat (during periods of sleep) position. Saliva samples were collected every 30 min (Salivette, Sarstedt, Newton NC), with 90 mL of water being provided after each saliva sample and removed 10 min prior to the subsequent saliva collection. Collection of saliva under conditions of constant dim light and constant posture is both sufficient and necessary for the accurate collection of unattenuated concentrations of melatonin (Duffy & Dijk, 2002). A Stanford Sleepiness Scale (SSS) (Hoddes et al., 1973) was obtained hourly following a saliva sample collection. The SSS is a Likert-like scale from 1 to 7, with higher numbers indicating greater sleepiness.

At habitual bedtime, the overhead dim light was turned off and the experimental light was turned on for three hours. The experimental light was fixed to the foot of the bed in an aluminum reflector such that the front of the light was facing the participant. During the experimental light exposure, saliva sample collection frequency was increased to every 20 min. The experimental light was one of two conditions: a standard white light LED or a blue-depleted white LED, both identical to those used in Study 1 (Fig. 1). Both lights were calibrated to a target of 150 lx at corneal level in a typical angle of gaze. By matching the lux units, the lights should have had a similar impact on image forming perception. The visit number (1 or 2) during which participants received the standard or blue-depleted white light was determined a priori through a random number generator (Random.org). The allocation was double-blind as neither the participant nor the laboratory technician administering the light knew which bulb was the standard and which was the blue-depleted. There was no obvious difference in the perceptual quality or color of the light emitted from the two lamps in the laboratory environment and the lamps were designated as "A" and "B" by the primary investigator (JMZ) – the laboratory technician was unaware of the matching of the A/B designation and the type of lamp being used. During the three hours of experimental light exposure, participants were kept awake by a laboratory technician and asked to look at the LED lamp, alternating every ten minutes between a gaze fixed at the lamp and free gaze around the room. During both the free and fixed gaze components, participants were not permitted to avoid light exposure by hiding their eyes or directing their gaze downward (e.g., no reading was allowed). Illuminance during the fixed and free periods was recorded with the ILT1700 Research Photometer at the end of each of these periods, estimating the average angle of gaze. Three hours after habitual bedtime, all lighting was turned off and the participant was allowed to sleep ad libitum. Upon arising, the participant was given a standard hospital breakfast, and could leave the unit.

Saliva samples were immediately frozen (– 20 °C) and placed in storage at – 80 °C within one week of collection. Saliva samples were assayed as a single batch in duplicate using a salivary melatonin enzyme-linked immunosorbent assay (ALPCO, Salem NH) per the manufacturer's instructions. Published intra-and inter-assay coefficients of variation are 6.1–13.0% with an assay sensitivity of 0.3 pg/mL. The assay microplate was read using a Multiskan FC Microplate Photometer (Thermo Scientific, Waltham MA). One of the 10 participants had a failed melatonin assay and insufficient saliva to conduct a repeat assay; the melatonin data from this participant were excluded. The three hours prior to habitual sleep onset, during which participants were in dim light, was denoted as the "baseline". Melatonin levels were expected to be rising to their elevated nocturnal levels during the baseline. The three hours after habitual bedtime, during which participants were exposed to the experimental light, was denoted as the "light exposure". Melatonin data during the baseline and light exposure were integrated over time using the trapezoidal method. Integrated melatonin concentrations during each hour of the light exposure was separately calculated.

Statistical analyses, as specified below, were performed using either OriginPro 2017 (v.b9.4.0220, OriginLab Corporation, Northampton MA) or Excel (v.16.0.4549.1000, Microsoft, Redmond WA). Z-score transformation was done for visualization purposes only (see Fig. 3). The mean and standard deviation of each participant's melatonin data were determined and the individual values were z-score transformed as $z = (X-\mu)/\sigma$, such that X = sample value, μ = population mean, and σ = population standard deviation.

Results

Lamp characteristics

The standard white LED has broad coverage of the visible wavelengths, with a major peak at 607 nm (orange) and a minor peak at 461 nm (blue) (Fig. 1). The blue-depleted white LED has similar coverage, but lacks blue wavelengths and has a major peak at 413 nm (violet) and secondary peaks at 641 nm (red) and 551 nm (green) (Fig. 1). Due to the difference in the lamp output in the blue region of visible light (450–495 nm), at the target of 150 lx, the corresponding α-opic melanopic lux is 77.0 for the standard white LED and 46.0 for the blue-depleted white LED (Lucas et al., 2014), a 40% reduction in the drive on melanopsin.

Study 1

Following the stable pupil size observed under conditions of darkness, the pupil rapidly constricted to a minimum size in response to both lights (Fig. 2). There was a slight but stable relaxation of the constriction over the next 55 s,

remaining throughout the remainder of the light stimulus. At the cessation of the light stimulus, the pupil size re-dilated to approximately 90% of baseline size within approximately 9 s. The pupil remained constricted greater than baseline in darkness for several seconds before returning to full dilation. Baseline (darkness) pupil size was not different within participants ($p = 0.15$, repeated measure one-way ANOVA). Visual and statistical inspection of the plots revealed no differences in pupillometric parameters between the higher (100, 140 lx) lighting conditions of the two lamps (Table 1). Responses to 32 lx, however, appeared to be lamp-specific. There was no difference between the lamps in terms of phasic ($p = 0.51$, paired t-test) or sustained ($p = 0.42$, paired t-test) constriction, nor was there a difference in the constriction speed ($p = 0.36$, paired t-test). The re-dilation speed in response to the blue-depleted white light at 32 lx was, however, 58% faster ($p < 0.05$, paired t-test) and the PIPR was also reduced by 45% with the blue-depleted white light ($p < 0.05$, paired t-test) as compared to the standard white LED (Table 1).

Study 2

The same lamps were used in Study 2 as were used in Study 1 (Fig. 1), but were calibrated prior to the experiment to produce 150 lx at corneal level. During the study, exposure to the standard white LED was 150 ± 3.24 lx during the fixed gaze and 151 ± 2.70 during the free gaze. Exposure to the blue-depleted white LED was 153 ± 4.60 lx during the fixed gaze and 152 ± 5.05 during the free gaze. There was no difference in the photopic illuminance received during the fixed and free ($p = 0.11$, repeated measure two-way ANOVA) or between the blue-depleted and standard white LED lamps ($p = 0.15$, repeated measure two-way ANOVA).

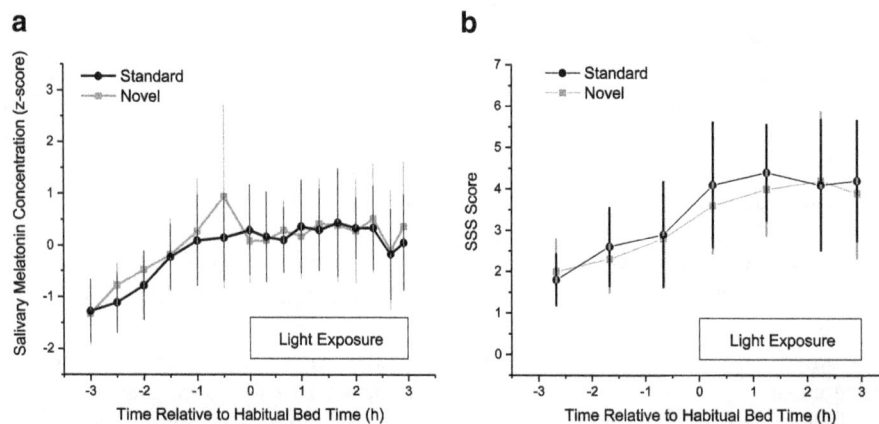

Fig. 3 Changes in salivary melatonin concentration (**a**) and SSS values (**b**) during the baseline (< 10 lx, − 3 → 0 h) and experimental light exposure (150 lx, 0 → 3 h) for both the blue-depleted (grey) and standard (black) white LED lamps. Melatonin data were z-score transformed and averaged prior to plotting. Mean ± SD are shown

Table 1 Pupil responses to light

Blue-Depleted White LED

Illuminance	Baseline (arb. unit)	Phasic max constriction (%)	Sustained constriction (%)	Constriction Slope (%/s)	Dilation Slope (%/s)	PIPR 6 s (%)
32 lx	0.46 ± 0.072	−64 ± 5.8	−56 ± 4.2	− 8.2 ± 2.3	7.7 ± 1.0*	− 11 ± 6.7*
100 lx	0.43 ± 0.095	−63 ± 8.3	−54 ± 6.8	− 8.5 ± 3.5	7.1 ± 4.1	− 10 ± 13
140 lx	0.48 ± 0.056	− 67 ± 5.8	− 60 ± 4.7	−8.5 ± 2.1	6.4 ± 3.2	−19 ± 18

Standard White LED

Illuminance	Baseline (arb. unit)	Phasic max constriction (%)	Sustained constriction (%)	Constriction Slope (%/s)	Dilation Slope (%/s)	PIPR 6 s (%)
32 lx	0.45 ± 0.087	−62 ± 10	− 53 ± 11	− 7.2 ± 2.5	4.9 ± 1.8	−20 ± 3.5
100 lx	0.45 ± 0.097	− 65 ± 4.3	−57 ± 3.3	−9.2 ± 2.1	7.8 ± 2.8	−10 ± 11
140 lx	0.45 ± 0.094	−66 ± 4.5	−57 ± 6.5	−7.8 ± 2.3	5.1 ± 2.7	−23 ± 16

Comparison of pupil responses to two different lamps – a blue-depleted white LED (top) and a standard white LED (bottom) – to three different illuminances of light. Light-induced changes in pupil size were normalized to percent of baseline pupil size. *$p < 0.05$ using a paired Student t-test. Data are presented as mean ± SD

Melatonin concentrations during the baseline portion prior to exposure to the blue-depleted or standard white LED lighting were similar ($p = 0.33$, paired t-test) as the expected rise of melatonin occurred in the hours prior to habitual bed time (Fig. 3a). There was no obvious impact of either light source on salivary melatonin concentrations (Fig. 3a). Melatonin concentrations during the full exposure ($p = 0.40$, paired t-test) or during any single hour of exposure (p's > 0.37, paired t-tests) to the blue-depleted white light was indistinguishable from that observed during the same time of exposure to the standard white light.

SSS scores during the baseline portion prior to exposure to the blue-depleted or standard white LED lighting were similar ($p = 0.78$, paired t-test). The expected rise in subjective sleepiness occurred around the time of habitual bedtime and this level of sleepiness was maintained throughout the three hours of light exposure (Fig. 3b). There was no obvious difference in the impact of the two light sources on SSS scores ($p = 0.21$, paired t-test).

Discussion

At a low illuminance of 32 lx, the blue-depleted white LED light (40% lower melanopsin stimulation) had significantly less of an impact on the post-illumination pupil response (PIPR) than a broad spectrum white LED light, and did so without impacting melatonin or subjective sleepiness. At higher illuminances (≥100 lx), there were no differences in light-induced PIPR, melatonin suppression, or relief of subjective sleepiness between the two light sources.

Our pupil findings are consistent with the theory that the PIPR is driven by melanopsin. At the lower illuminance tested, PIPR was reduced in response to the light that had 40% less drive on melanopsin. We did not, however, observe an impact of the lights on phasic constriction, which is also thought to be influenced by melanopsin. The partial (40%) reduction in melanopic drive

and the relatively small number of participants may have contributed to our inability to detect such a difference. We also used an extended (60 s) light stimulation; shorter light stimulations (e.g., 1 s) may have revealed more differences in PIPR at the higher intensities. The pupil responses to light that are dependent upon cones were not differentially impacted by the two lights tested.

None of the other non-image forming functions that we tested, however, were impacted by the reduction of melanopsin drive in the blue-depleted white light. Previous studies have indicated that 150 lx of white light is sufficient to suppress melatonin and decrease subjective sleepiness (Zeitzer et al., 2000; Cajochen et al., 2000). It must be noted, however, that these measures of light-induced changes were conducted after extended (> 40 h) exposure to no greater than dim light. In the current study, participants arrived to the lab after exposure to real-world environments and were in dim light (< 10 lx) for only three hours prior to the experimental light exposure. Previous studies (Smith et al., 2004; Chang et al., 2011; Rufiange et al., 2007; Zeitzer et al., 2011) have demonstrated that the impact of light on non-image forming functions, such as those presented in this report, is sensitized by previous exposure to dim light. It is, therefore, possible that at increased intensities we may have observed the expected changes in melatonin and alertness. Under the ecologically relevant conditions to which most individuals are exposed, however, we do not observe meaningful changes in melatonin or alertness after exposure to normal room light intensities. Individuals who lack exposure to bright indoor or outdoor light, however, might benefit from exposure to blue-depleted white light (Rahman et al., 2017).

Given the previous literature, had we sensitized the non-image forming system with many hours of dim or room light prior to exposure or increased the intensity of the experimental light exposure, we might have observed a difference in the impact of the two lamps on melatonin suppression and subjective alertness. We did not design the experiment as such since previous studies had already established the biological capacity of the non-image forming photoreceptive system to have a peak response to long duration blue light. We, rather, were concerned with the potential real-world use of white light lamps that had diminished impact on melanopsin and, at least for subjective sleepiness and melatonin suppression, we did not observe an advantage of the blue-depleted white LED lamp. We did not explicitly examine objective alertness or circadian phase shifting here, but these two processes operate in a similar intensity range as subjective alertness and melatonin suppression (Zeitzer et al., 2000; Cajochen et al., 2000) and might have similar outcomes. Future research could examine the utility of such lamps as sleep-permissive light sources in environments in which individuals have consistent exposure to lower levels of daytime lighting (e.g., submarines, winter time in extreme northern latitudes, all day low intensity office lighting).

Conclusions

After exposure to a real-world daytime lighting environment, except for pupil responses to moderately dim light, there are no difference in non-imaging forming responses to broad spectrum white light and a broad spectrum white light with reduced blue content.

Abbreviations

ANOVA: Analysis of variance; ipRGC: Intrinsically photosensitive retinal ganglion cells; LED: Light emitting diode; PIPR: Post-illumination pupillary response; SSS: Stanford Sleepiness Scale

Acknowledgements
We wish to thank Ms. Chun-Ping Liao for conduct of the melatonin assays and Dr. Aurélien David of Soraa for helpful discussions of lighting and facilitating the implementation of this study.

Funding
This research was conducted using a grant from Soraa Inc. The company provided both material and financial support. The company was not involved in the design, conduct, or analysis of the research, nor were they involved in the writing of this manuscript.

Authors' contributions
JMZ designed and analyzed the study. RPN analyzed the pupil data. C-A Wang conducted the study. MK assisted in data analyses. All authors read and approved the final manuscript.

Competing interests
The authors declare no competing interests directly relevant to this manuscript. None of the authors have any financial holdings or relationships with the funder, Soraa (see below).

Author details
[1]Department of Psychiatry and Behavioral Rhythms, Stanford University, Stanford, CA 94305, USA. [2]Mental Illness Research Education and Clinical Center, VA Palo Alto Health Care System, Palo Alto, CA 94304, USA. [3]Department of Visual Neurosciences, Singapore Eye Research Institute, Singapore 169856, Singapore. [4]Present address: Connecticut College, New London, CT, USA.

References
Adhikari P, Zele AJ, Feigl B. The post-illumination pupil response (PIPR). Invest Ophthalmol Vis Sci. 2015;56:3838–49.

Alpern M, Campbell FW. The spectral sensitivity of the consensual light reflex. J Physiol. 1962;164:478–507.

Ancoli-Israel S, Cole R, Alessi C, Chambers M, Moorcroft W, Pollack CP. The role of actigraphy in the study of sleep and circadian rhythms. Sleep. 2003;26:342–92.

Berson DM, Dunn FA, Takao M. Phototransduction by retinal ganglion cells that set the circadian clock. Science. 2002;295:1070–3.

Brainard GC, Hanifin JP, Greeson JM, Byrne B, Glickman G, Gerner E, Rollag MD. Action spectrum for melatonin regulation in humans: evidence for a novel circadian photoreceptor. J Neurosci. 2001;21:6405–12.

Buysse DJ, Reynolds CF III, Monk TH, Berman SR, Kupfer DJ. The Pittsburgh sleep quality index: a new instrument for psychiatric practice and research. Psychiatry Res. 1989;28:193–213.

Cajochen C, Zeitzer JM, Czeisler CA, Dijk D-J. Dose-response relationship for light intensity and ocular and electroencephalographic correlates of alertness in humans. Beh Brain Res. 2000;115:75–83.

Chang AM, Scheer FA, Czeisler CA. The human circadian system adapts to prior photic history. J Physiol. 2011;589:1095–102.

Czeisler CA, Kronauer RE, Allan JS, Duffy JF, Jewett ME, Brown EN, Ronda JM. Bright light induction of strong (type 0) resetting of the human circadian pacemaker. Science. 1989;244:1328–33.

Duffy JF, Dijk D-J. Getting through to circadian oscillators: why use constant routines? J Biol Rhythm. 2002;17:4–13.

Duffy JF, Dijk D-J, Klerman EB, Czeisler CA. Later endogenous circadian temperature nadir relative to an earlier wake time in older people. Am J Phys. 1998;275:R1478–87.

Gooley JJ, Rajaratnam SM, Brainard GC, Kronauer RE, Czeisler CA, Lockley SW. Spectral responses of the human circadian system depend on the irradiance and duration of exposure to light. Sci Transl Med. 2010;2:31ra33.

Hoddes E, Zarcone V, Smythe H, Phillips R, Dement WC. Quantification of sleepiness: a new approach. Psychophysiology. 1973;10:431–6.

Horne JA, Östberg O. A self-assessment questionnaire to determine morningness-eveningness in human circadian rhythms. Intl J Chronobiol. 1976;4:97–110.

Ishihara S. Ishihara's tests for colour deficiency. Tokyo: Kanehara Trading Inc.; 2007.

Joyce DS, Feigl B, Zele AJ. The effects of short-term light adaptation on the human post-illumination pupil response. Invest Ophthalmol Vis Sci. 2016;57: 5672–80.

Lucas RJ, Peirson SN, Berson DM, Brown TM, Cooper HM, Czeisler CA, Figueiro MG, Gamlin PD, Lockley SW, O'Hagan JB, et al. Measuring and using light in the melanopsin age. Trends Neurosci. 2014;37:1–9.

McBean AL, Najjar RP, Schuchard RA, Hall CD, Wang C-A, Ku B, Zeitzer JM. Standing balance and spatiotemporal aspects of gait are impaired upon nocturnal awakening in healthy late middle-aged and older adults. J Clin Sleep Med. 2016;12:1477–86.

Nelson DE, Takahashi JS. Sensitivity and integration in a visual pathway for circadian entrainment in the hamster (Mesocricetus auratus). J Physiol. 1991; 439:115–45.

Newman LA, Walker MT, Brown RL, Cronin TW, Robinson PR. Melanopsin forms a functional short-wavelength photopigment. Biochemist. 2003;42:12734–8.

Radloff LS. The CES-D scale: a self-report depression scale for research in the general population. Appl Psychol Meas. 1977;1:385–401.

Rahman SA, St Hilaire MA, Lockley SW. The effects of spectral tuning of evening ambient light on melatonin suppression, alertness and sleep. Physiol Behav. 2017;177:221–9.

Rufiange M, Beaulieu C, Lachapelle P, Dumont M. Circadian light sensitivity and rate of retinal dark adaptation in indoor and outdoor workers. J Biol Rhythm. 2007;22:454–7.

23

Validation of minute-to-minute scoring for sleep and wake periods in a consumer wearable device compared to an actigraphy device

Joseph Cheung[1,2*] ⓘ, Jamie M. Zeitzer[1,2,3], Haoyang Lu[2] and Emmanuel Mignot[1,2*]

Abstract

Background: Actigraphs are widely used portable wrist-worn devices that record tri-axial accelerometry data. These data can be used to approximate amount and timing of sleep and wake. Their clinical utility is limited, however, by their expense. Tri-axial accelerometer-based consumer wearable devices (so-called fitness monitors) have gained popularity and could represent cost-effective research alternatives to more expensive devices. Lack of independent validation of minute-to-minute accelerometer data for consumer devices has hindered their utility and acceptance.

Methods: We studied a consumer-grade wearable device, Arc (Huami Inc., Mountain View CA), for which minute-to-minute accelerometer data (vector magnitude) could be obtained. Twelve healthy participants and 19 sleep clinic patients wore on their non-dominant wrist, both an Arc and a research-grade actigraph (Actiwatch Spectrum, Philips, Bend OR) continuously over a period of 48 h in free-living conditions. Time-stamped data from each participant were aligned and the Cole-Kripke algorithm was used to assign a state of "sleep" or "wake" for each minute-long epoch recorded by the Arc. The auto and low scoring settings on the Actiwatch software (Actiware) were used to determine sleep and wake from the Actiwatch data and were used as the comparators. Receiver operating characteristic curves were used to optimize the relationship between the devices.

Results: Minute-by-minute Arc and Actiwatch data were highly correlated ($r = 0.94$, Spearman correlation) over the 48-h study period. Treating the Actiwatch auto scoring as the gold standard for determination of sleep and wake, Arc has an overall accuracy of $99.0\% \pm 0.17\%$ (SEM), a sensitivity of $99.4\% \pm 0.19\%$, and a specificity of $84.5\% \pm 1.9\%$ for the determination of sleep. As compared to the Actiwatch low scoring, Arc has an overall accuracy of $95.2\% \pm 0.36\%$, a sensitivity of $95.7\% \pm 0.47\%$, and a specificity of $91.7\% \pm 0.60\%$ for the determination of sleep.

Conclusions: The Arc, a consumer wearable device in which minute-by-minute activity data could be collected and compared, yielded fundamentally similar sleep scoring metrics as compared to a commonly used clinical-grade actigraph (Actiwatch). We found high degrees of agreement in minute-to-minute data scoring for sleep and wake periods between the two devices.

Keywords: Consumer wearable, Validation, Sleep monitoring, Actigraphy

* Correspondence: cheungj@stanford.edu; mignot@stanford.edu
[1]Stanford University Center for Sleep Sciences and Medicine, Palo Alto, CA, USA
Full list of author information is available at the end of the article

Background

Actigraphs are portable wrist-worn devices that record tri-axial accelerometry data (i.e., gross movement in three directions). By imputing sleep patterns from accelerometry data, actigraphs have been used for nearly 30 years to objectively quantify longitudinal sleep patterns in research studies (Ancoli-Israel et al. 2003). The premise of the algorithms that have been developed for such imputation is to assume that the wearer is asleep when not moving and to determine when gross body movements are large and/or long enough to suggest that the wearer is awake (Cole et al. 1992; Sadeh et al. 1991). More recently, actigraphs have been used in clinical practice, especially in the monitoring and treatment of insomnia-related disorders (Ancoli-Israel et al. 2003; Kushida et al. 2001; Morgenthaler et al. 2007). Wide-spread use has however been limited by the high cost of these devices.

There has been a massive increase in the use of accelerometers in recent years as they are found in most cell phones and wrist-worn fitness trackers. Many of these devices use the accelerometer to track movement for use in both sleep and exercise tracking. As these are consumer devices, the algorithms that translate 'raw movement' data into 'sleep/wake' activity are proprietary. Despite the raw data that is used to impute sleep and wake not being made available to researchers, the whole-night sleep measures of a few of these devices have been validated to varying degrees (de Zambotti et al. 2016; Bianchi 2017; Roomkham et al. 2018). In order to perform proper validation studies, however, an important criterion is to have access to minute-by-minute raw data, as is available in research/clinical-grade actigraphs.

The objective of this study was to examine the feasibility of using a low-cost consumer grade wearable device as an actigraph device for sleep monitoring (see Table 1 for device specifications). We identified a low-cost wearable device, the Amazfit Arc (Huami, Inc), in which minute-by-minute activity data could be obtained. To our knowledge, this is the first study comparing the raw minute-by-minute accelerometry data obtained from a low-cost consumer wearable device to that obtained

from a clinical-grade actigraph in estimating sleep parameters in free-living conditions.

Methods

Twelve community-dwelling participants without significant self-reported health issues or sleep disorders and twenty-two sleep clinic patients at the Stanford University sleep clinic were recruited to participate in this study. Three of the sleep clinic participants did not complete the study due to missing data: two had missing Actiwatch data and one did not return the devices. In all, 31 participants completed the study, 20 of whom were female and 11 male, with a mean (±SD) age of 40.1 ± 7.9 years (range, 19–72). Of the 19 participants recruited from the sleep clinic (mean BMI of 25.2 ± 0.9), 16 were later diagnosed with obstructive sleep apnea (OSA, mild to severe), three were diagnosed with hypersomnia (one patient was diagnosed with hypersomnia and OSA), one was diagnosed with delayed sleep -wake phase disorder, two have hypertension. All participants wore on their non-dominant wrist both an Arc and Actiwatch Spectrum continuously over a period of 48 h in free-living conditions outside of the sleep clinic (i.e., two nights of data). Participants completed a custom sleep diary concomitant with wearing the actigraphs. Arc devices (six devices) were purchased from Huami Inc. (Mountain View, CA). Actiwatch Spectrum devices (three devices) were purchased from Philips Respironics (Bend, OR). Both Arc and Actiwatch devices were configured to store data as the integral of activity occurring in 60 s segments. Time synchronization was performed across the Arc and Actiwatch devices at the beginning of each participant's study period. A Samsung Android (version 7.1.1) smartphone installed with the Amazfit app (version 1.0.2) was used to communicate with Arc devices. The app was used to synchronize the Arc devices before and after the study period. Minute-by-minute accelerometer data were obtained from the Huami Inc's cloud (https://github.com/huamitech/rest-api/wiki; last accessed May 7, 2018). Actiwatch data were retrieved using Philips Actiware (version 6.0.9).

Time stamps were used to align minute-by-minute data from both devices. Sleep diary data were used to set the time in bed window. Spearman's correlations were used to compare the raw values of the Arc and Actiwatch devices on a minute-by-minute basis in each participant. Actiwatch data in Actiware were also converted into "sleep" and "wake" using the built-in algorithms on both "auto" and "low" settings. For the Arc device, data were cleaned by removing a series of default output values of "20" while device was inactive. To determine the occurrence of wake, we first determined a *Wake Threshold Value* = (Σall *activity during mobile time/mobile time*) $* k$; such that k is a constant and

Table 1 Comparison of consumer- and research-grade actigraphs

	Amazfit Arc	Philips Actiwatch Spectrum
Cost[a]	$70	$900–1000
Accelerometers	MEMS tri-axial	Piezo-electric tri-axial
Accelerometer sampling rate	25 Hz	32 Hz
Weight	20 g	31 g
Recording time	30 days	60 days
Battery life (one charge)	20 days	60 days
Light sensor	None	Yes

[a]Manufacturer suggested retail price at the time of this study. g gram

mobile time is the total time of minute epochs where activity is ≥ 2. We then used the Cole-Kripke algorithm (Cole et al. 1992) to derive a window adjusted activity value for each 1-min epoch: $Total\ Activity = E_0 + E_1 * 0.2 + E_{-1} * 0.2 + E_2 * 0.04 + E_{-2} * 0.04$; such that E_0 is the activity level in the one-minute epoch of interest, E_1 is one minute later and E_{-1} is one minute earlier, and so on. If the *Total Activity* in a given one-minute epoch is less than or equal to the *Wake Threshold Value*, the epoch is scored as sleep. If the *Total Activity* in a given one-minute epoch is greater than the *Wake Threshold Value*, the epoch is scored as wake. The Actiwatch uses $k = 0.88888$ in its auto scoring method. In Actiwatch's low scoring method, a *Wake Threshold Value* of 20 is used. A secondary algorithm (Kripke et al. 2010; Webster et al. 1982; Jean-Louis et al. 2001) was used to automatically determine sleep onset time and sleep offset time. The algorithm scans the initial minute-by-minute scoring of each time in bed window. Within each window, the beginning of the first five or more consecutive sleep minutes was defined as sleep onset time. Epochs that were initially scored as sleep, before such an onset time, were rescored as wake. Similarly, the end of the last five or more consecutive sleep minutes was defined as sleep offset time. Any epochs that were initially scored as sleep, after such an offset time, were rescored as wake.

Using a receiver operating characteristic (ROC) analysis, we explored a range of constants to select an optimal value for *Wake Threshold Value* determination in the Arc, using the results from the Actiwatch as the "gold standard". To determine the relative accuracy of the Arc device, we compared minute-by-minute sleep and wake assignments in both devices and calculated the overall accuracy [(True Positive (TP) + True Negative (TN))/total], sleep sensitivity [TP / (TP+ False Negative (FN))] (same as wake specificity), sleep specificity [TN/(TN + False Positive (FP))] (same as wake sensitivity), and wake precision [TN/(TN + FN)]. Summary results on total sleep time (TST) and wake after sleep onset (WASO) were calculated. Data are presented as mean ± SEM except where noted.

Results

We compared minute-by-minute data obtained from both the Arc and Actiwatch devices over the 48-h study period from all 31 participants. The overall patterns observed between the Arc and Actiwatch appear to be quite similar (Fig. 1).

Within participants, absolute activity for the Actiwatch and Arc devices were highly correlated ($r = 0.94 \pm 0.005$, range: 0.87–0.98, $n = 31$; Spearman correlation). Movement data from in-bed periods were also well correlated ($r = 0.89 \pm 0.01$, range: 0.73–0.96, n = 31; Spearman correlation). The absolute difference in values obtained from the Actiwatch and Arc were approximately 9-fold different in magnitude (linear regression of all data, slope ± SD = 0.11 ± 0.02) (Fig. 2).

To determine a *Wake Threshold Value* that would yield optimal correspondence between the minute-by-minute score of the Arc and Actiwatch, we compared sensitivity and specificity of a series of *Wake Threshold Values* using ROC analysis (Fig. 3). For the Actiwatch analysis in which the *Wake Threshold Value* was determined on auto setting, a k constant of 1.1 used for the Arc data was determined to produce an optimal alignment. For the Actiwatch analysis in which the *Wake Threshold Value* was determined on low setting (a high sensitivity with a threshold value of 20), a threshold value of 5 used for the Arc data produced an optimal alignment.

Using the *Wake Threshold Values* determined in the ROC analysis, we then examined the accuracy,

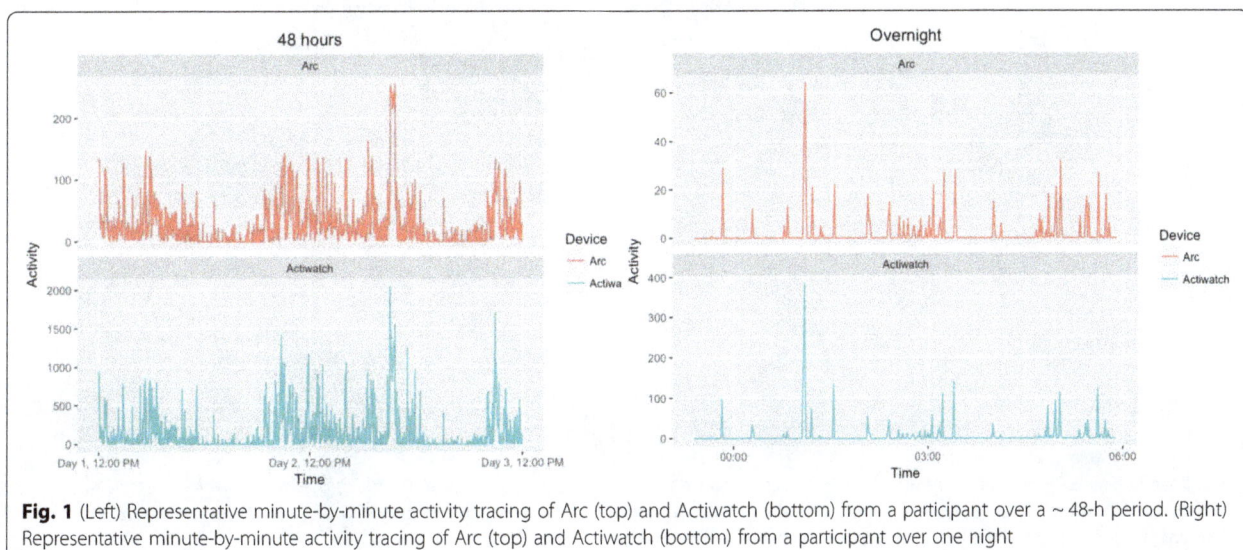

Fig. 1 (Left) Representative minute-by-minute activity tracing of Arc (top) and Actiwatch (bottom) from a participant over a ~ 48-h period. (Right) Representative minute-by-minute activity tracing of Arc (top) and Actiwatch (bottom) from a participant over one night

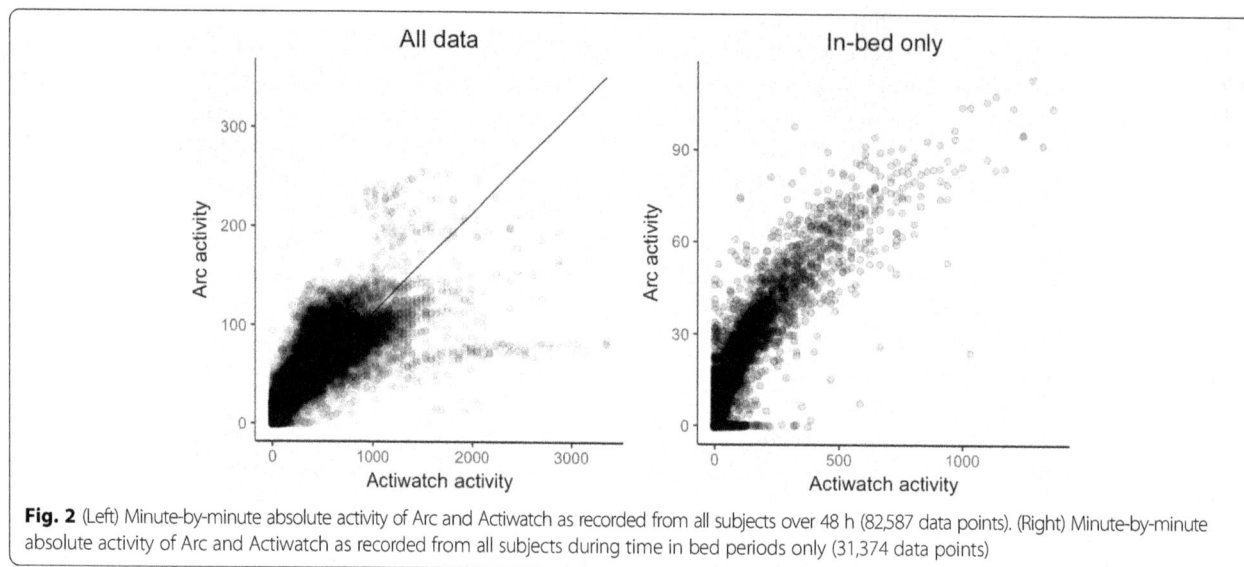

Fig. 2 (Left) Minute-by-minute absolute activity of Arc and Actiwatch as recorded from all subjects over 48 h (82,587 data points). (Right) Minute-by-minute absolute activity of Arc and Actiwatch as recorded from all subjects during time in bed periods only (31,374 data points)

sensitivity, specificity, and precision of the imputed sleep/wake as determined by the Arc (Table 2). For the most part, there was good correspondence in the determination of sleep and wake by the Arc and Actigraph. Using the auto setting for scoring of the Actigraph data (corresponding to 1.1 on the Arc), there was a slight underscoring of wake with near perfect determination of sleep. Using the low setting for scoring of the Actigraph data (corresponding to 5 on the Arc), there was greater sensitivity for wake at the cost of a slight underscoring of sleep. We also split our data into those from healthy participants only ($n = 12$) and those from sleep patients ($n = 19$). The observed concordance between Arc and Actiwatch (auto setting) was similar, with an overall accuracy of 99.6% in the healthy group and 98.7% in the sleep patient group.

To examine the possibility of systematic bias in overall sleep parameter scoring, we generated Bland-Altman plots to visually inspect the level of agreement between Arc and Actiwatch derived results (Fig. 4). Comparing Arc (using k constant of 1.1) and Actiwatch auto setting, overall bias (discrepancy) in estimating TST was − 0.44 min over one sleep period. The spread of the differences is observed to be even, with no bias in overestimation or underestimation of TST. For WASO, overall bias in estimating WASO over one sleep period was 0.35 min. In comparison to Actiwatch low setting (shown in Fig. 4), the overall bias in estimating TST was − 4.5 min over one sleep period. In this case, it appears that using a threshold of 5 in Arc (compared to a threshold of 20 used in Actiwatch)

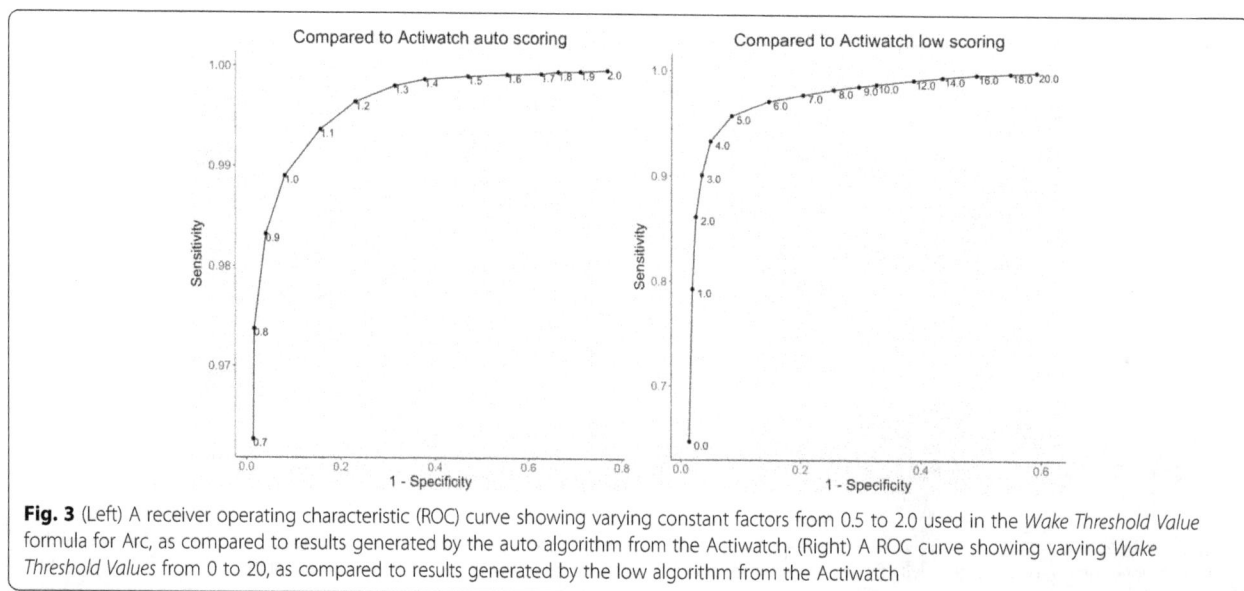

Fig. 3 (Left) A receiver operating characteristic (ROC) curve showing varying constant factors from 0.5 to 2.0 used in the *Wake Threshold Value* formula for Arc, as compared to results generated by the auto algorithm from the Actiwatch. (Right) A ROC curve showing varying *Wake Threshold Values* from 0 to 20, as compared to results generated by the low algorithm from the Actiwatch

Table 2 Overall accuracy and comparative performance of Arc in detecting sleep/wake during the main sleep periods, in comparison to gold-standard determination of "sleep" and "wake" Actiwatch using the preset auto and low settings of the Actiwatch software

	Overall Accuracy	Sleep Sensitivity (wake specificity)	Sleep Specificity (wake sensitivity)	Wake Precision
"Auto" setting	99.0% ± 0.17%	99.4% ± 0.19%	84.5% ± 1.9%	81.2% ± 2.3%
"Low" setting	95.2% ± 0.36%	95.7% ± 0.47%	91.7% ± 0.60%	83.6% ± 1.2%

results in a slight underestimation of TST for the Arc device. In terms of WASO, overall bias in estimating WASO over one sleep period was 3.9 min, with a slight overestimation using the Arc device.

Discussion

In comparing the accuracy of Arc, a consumer wearable device, against a clinical/research-grade actigraphy device, Philips Actiwatch (Spectrum), we find that the consumer device performs similarly in the estimation of sleep parameters. Despite lower absolute (approximately 9-fold) value of activity recorded by the Arc, sufficient signal-to-noise ratio was present to impute sleep and wake states. This is likely because the Cole-Kripke algorithm (Cole et al. 1992) is robust and utilizes *relative* movement data for the determination of sleep and wake. Using ROC analyses to objectively determine thresholds for the Arc device, we were also able to faithfully recapitulate the commonly used auto and low scoring settings on the Actiwatch device. The device performed similarly well in both a patient population (OSA, disrupted sleep) and a control population.

To our knowledge, this is the first validation study where minute by minute accelerometer data (vector

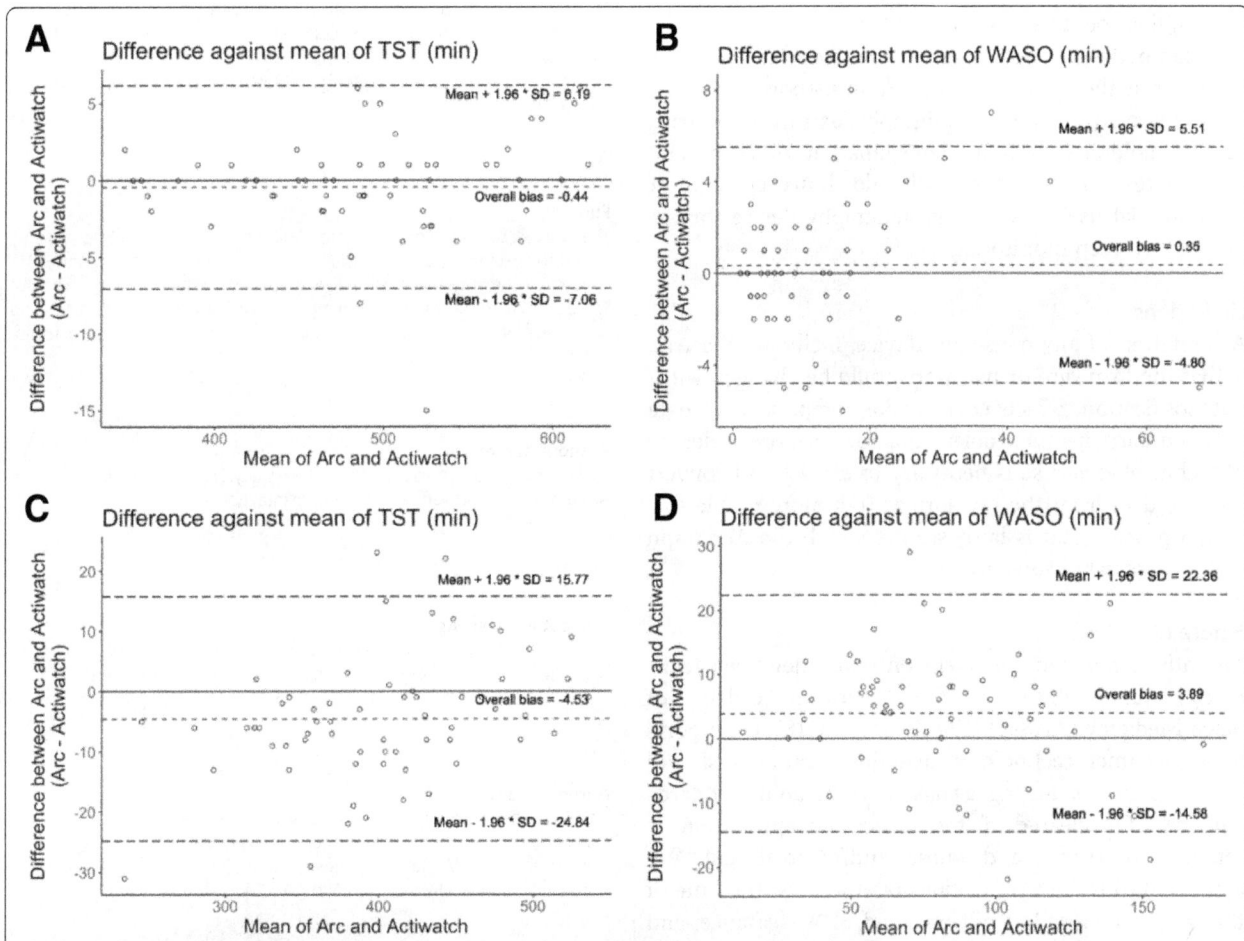

Fig. 4 a Bland-Altman plot of TST estimated by Arc as compared to Actiwatch. **b** Bland-Altman plot of WASO estimated by Arc as compared to Actiwatch. Data shown represent comparison of Arc using a constant factor of 1.1 in the wake threshold formula comparing to results generated by the auto algorithm from the Actiwatch. **c** Bland-Altman plot of TST estimated by Arc as compared to Actiwatch. **d** Bland-Altman plot of WASO estimated by Arc as compared to Actiwatch. Data shown represent comparison of Arc using a wake threshold of 5 comparing to results generated by the low algorithm from the Actiwatch

magnitude) from a consumer wearable device was compared to an actigraph in sleep monitoring. Previous studies have compared whole night summary data from wearables, including a recent study (Lee et al. 2017) comparing another consumer wearable (Fitbit Charge HR) with an actigraph (Actiwatch 2). These report good accuracy for sleep evaluation between the two devices, however, only sleep summary data were examined.

Besides the price difference, there are other differences between the Arc and the Actiwatch. While present on the Actiwatch, the Arc lacks a light sensor, a feature often useful in identifying bed and wake times. The Actiwatch is also capable of storing data at a higher average resolution (e.g., 15 s and 30s epochs) in comparison to the Arc. On the other hand, the Arc device is capable of recording raw accelerometer data at 25 Hz resolution. The Arc device also remotely uploads its data to a secure portal, eliminating the need for participants to come to the laboratory to have data from the actigraph downloaded, which is necessary with the Actiwatch. For longer duration longitudinal studies, this could be of significant benefit.

In comparing the Arc device to the Actiwatch, we use the latter as the "gold standard". Future studies will need to compare Arc to polysomnography, as this is the true, current gold standard in determination of sleep and wake states. The current results do, however, support the potential use of Arc as an actigraphy device for the purpose of sleep monitoring.

Limitations
A limitation of any consumer device, including the Arc, is that the firmware or hardware could be changed without notification, which could make comparison of data between participants problematic. Furthermore, a degree of technical expertise is necessary to extract and convert the Arc data from the raw format to a more usable format, a process that is fairly seamless with the Actigraph and its associated software.

Future directions
Recently, a position statement on consumer sleep technology was published by the American Academy of Sleep Medicine (AASM) (Khosla et al., 2018). It supports that consumer technology including wearables should require rigorous testing against current gold standards and be FDA-cleared if the device or application is intended to render a diagnosis and/or treatment. We agree with this AASM position statement. At the time of this work, the Arc has not obtained FDA clearance, and therefore, should not replace existing clinical diagnostic procedure in the diagnosis of sleep conditions. However, we think that this work is a step forward in examining and validating a consumer wearable and provides supporting evidence for the Arc as an inexpensive

actigraphy tool for sleep research. Concomitant validation of the Actiwatch and of the Arc consumer-grade device against overnight polysomnography will be an important next step to determine full equivalence.

Conclusions
The Arc, a consumer wearable device, can be used as an actigraph for sleep monitoring and is able to produce sleep parameters that are comparable to a research-grade actigraph.

Abbreviations
OSA: Obstructive sleep apnea; PSG: Polysomnography; ROC: Receiver operating characteristic; TST: Total sleep time; WASO: Wake after sleep onset

Acknowledgements
We thank Ms. Eileen Leary for assistance in writing the IRB protocol. We thank Ms. Kary Newman and Ms. Polina Davidenko for assisting in patient recruitment and data collection. This work was supported by the Stanford Clinical and Translational Science Award to Spectrum (UL1 TR001085) and Stanford University Department of Psychiatry Small Grant Program. JC is supported by NIH K23NS101094.

Funding
This work was supported by Stanford Clinical and Translational Science Award to Spectrum (UL1 TR001085), and a Stanford University Department of Psychiatry Small Grant Program. JC is supported by NIH NINDS K23NS101094. The device maker Huami, Inc. was not involved in the design, conduct, funding, or analysis of the research, nor were they involved in the writing of this manuscript.

Authors' contributions
JC, JMZ and EM designed and analyzed the study. HL assisted in data analyses. All authors read and approved the final manuscript.

Competing interests
The authors declare that they have no competing interests. None of the authors have any financial holdings or relationships with the device maker Huami, Inc.

Author details
[1]Stanford University Center for Sleep Sciences and Medicine, Palo Alto, CA, USA. [2]Department of Psychiatry and Behavioral Sciences, Stanford University, Stanford, CA, USA. [3]Mental Illness Research Education and Clinical Center, VA Palo Alto Health Care System, Palo Alto, CA, USA.

References
Ancoli-Israel S, Cole R, Alessi C, Chambers M, Moorcroft W, Pollak CP. The role of Actigraphy in the study of sleep and circadian rhythms. Sleep. 2003;26(3): 342–92.

Validation of minute-to-minute scoring for sleep and wake periods in a consumer wearable device...

213

Bianchi MT. Sleep devices: wearables and nearables, informational and interventional, consumer and clinical. Metabolism Elsevier Inc. 2017:1–10. https://doi.org/10.1016/j.metabol.2017.10.008.

Cole RJ, Kripke DF, Gruen W, Mullaney DJ, Gillin JC. Automatic sleep/wake identification from wrist activity. Sleep. 1992;15(5):461–9.

de Zambotti M, Godino JG, Baker FC, Cheung J, Patrick K, Colrain IM. The boom in wearable technology: cause for alarm or just what is needed to better understand sleep? Sleep. 2016;39(9):1761–2. https://doi.org/10.5665/sleep.6108.

Jean-Louis G, Kripke DF, Cole RJ, Assmus JD, Langer RD. Sleep detection with an accelerometer Actigraph: comparisons with polysomnography. Physiol Behav. 2001;72(1–2):21–8. https://doi.org/10.1016/S0031-9384(00)00355-3.

Khosla S, Deak MC, Gault D, Goldstein CA, Hwang D, Kwon Y, et al. Consumer sleep technology: an American Academy of sleep medicine position statement. J Clin Sleep Med. 2018;14(5):877–80. https://doi.org/10.5664/jcsm.7128

Kripke DF, Hahn EK, Grizas AP, Wadiak KH, Loving RT, Steven Poceta J, Shadan FF, Cronin JW, Kline LE. Wrist Actigraphic scoring for sleep laboratory patients: algorithm development. J Sleep Res. 2010;19(4):612–9. https://doi.org/10.1111/j.1365-2869.2010.00835.x.

Kushida CA, Chang A, Gadkary C, Guilleminault C, Carrillo O, Dement WC. Comparison of Actigraphic, polysomnographic, and subjective assessment of sleep parameters in sleep-disordered patients. Sleep Med. 2001;2(5):389–96. https://doi.org/10.1016/S1389-9457(00)00098-8.

Lee H-A, Lee H-J, Moon J-H, Lee T, Kim M-G, In H, Cho C-H, Kim L. Comparison of wearable activity tracker with Actigraphy for sleep evaluation and circadian rest-activity rhythm measurement in healthy young adults. Psychiatry Investigation. 2017;14(2):179. https://doi.org/10.4306/pi.2017.14.2.179.

Morgenthaler T, Alessi C, Friedman L, Owens J, Kapur V, Boehlecke B, Brown T, et al. Practice parameters for the use of Actigraphy in the assessment of sleep and sleep disorders: an update for 2007. Sleep. 2007;30:519–29.

Roomkham S, Lovell D, Cheung J, Perrin D. Promises and Challenges in the Use of Consumer-Grade Devices for Sleep Monitoring. IEEE Reviews in Biomedical Engineering. 2018;XX(X):1–1. https://doi.org/10.1109/RBME.2018.2811735.

Sadeh A, Lavie P, Scher A, Tirosh E, Epstein R. Actigraphic home-monitoring sleep-disturbed and control infants and young children: a new method for pediatric assessment of sleep-wake patterns. Pediatrics. 1991;87(4):494–9.

Webster JB, Kripke DF, Messin S, Mullaney DJ, Wyborney G. An activity-based sleep monitor system for ambulatory use. Sleep. 1982;5(4):389–99. https://doi.org/10.1093/sleep/5.4.389.

24

Obstructive sleep apnea syndrome and sleep disorders in individuals with occupational injuries

Stig Solbach[1], Katrin Uehli[1], Werner Strobel[2], Stefanie Brighenti-Zogg[1], Selina Dürr[1], Sabrina Maier[1], Michel Hug[1], Roland Bingisser[3,4], Jörg Daniel Leuppi[1,4] and David Miedinger[1,4]*

Abstract

Background: Some sleep disorders are known risk factors for occupational injuries (OIs). This study aimed to compare the prevalence of obstructive sleep apnea syndrome (OSAS) in a population of patients with OIs admitted to the emergency room (ER) with hospital outpatients as controls.

Methods: Seventy-nine patients with OIs and 56 controls were recruited at the University Hospital of Basel, Switzerland between 2009 and 2011. All patients completed a questionnaire and underwent a full-night attended polysomnography (PSG). We considered an apnea–hypopnea index (AHI) > 5 as an abnormal finding suggestive of a diagnosis of OSAS.

Results: Patients with OIs did not differ from controls regarding sex, age, body mass index, and job risk of OI. Patients with OIs tended to have an abnormal AHI ($n = 38$ [48%] vs. $n = 16$ [29%], odds ratio [OR] = 2.32 [95% confidence interval (CI):1.05–5.13]), and a higher AHI (8.0 vs. 5.6 events/h; Cohen's d 0.28, $p = 0.028$) compared with controls. Patients with OIs also had abnormal limb movement index, arousal index, and signs of sleep bruxism compared with controls. Compared with 36 controls (66%), 70 patients with OIs (89%) had either excessive daytime sleepiness (EDS), and/or an abnormal finding during PSG (OR = 4.32, 95% CI:1.65–11.52). However, patients with OIs did not differ from controls regarding EDS or oxygen desaturation index.

Conclusions: Patients treated in the ER for OI had more abnormal findings suggestive of OSAS or other sleep disorders compared with a control group of hospital outpatients. Screening for these conditions should be part of the postaccident medical investigation.

Keywords: Obstructive sleep apnea syndrome, Occupational accidents, Sleep fragmentation, Polysomnography, Excessive daytime sleepiness

Background

Obstructive sleep apnea syndrome (OSAS) is a respiratory sleep disorder with recurrent episodes of hypopnea, apnea, and associated arousals leading to fragmented sleep and, therefore, excessive daytime sleepiness (EDS) (Gharibeh and Mehra 2010). Studies in the general population of Switzerland reported a prevalence of 23.4% in women and 49.7% in men (Heinzer et al. 2015). OSAS is a potential risk factor for hypertension and cardiovascular disease and is associated with type 2 diabetes (Fava et al. 2011; Reichmuth et al. 2005). Studies have shown that salespersons, drivers, seamen, engine and motor operators, and cooks and stewards are at increased risk of being diagnosed with OSAS (Li et al. 2008).

The European Agency Eurostat defined an accident at work according to the European Statistics on Accidents at Work as "a discrete occurrence in the course of work which leads to physical or mental harm" (European Statistics on Accidents at Work (ESAW) 2013). In 2013, there were around 3.1 million nonfatal accidents in the European Union (EU-28), which led to an absence of at

* Correspondence: david.miedinger@unibas.ch
This study was performed at the University Hospital in Basel, Switzerland
[1]Cantonal Hospital Baselland, University Clinic of Medicine, CH-4410 Liestal, Switzerland
[4]Medical Faculty, University of Basel, Basel, Switzerland
Full list of author information is available at the end of the article

least 4 days from work and predominately affected male workers (Key figures on Europe 2016). We previously reviewed the published literature and estimated that 13% of occupational injuries (OIs) could be attributed to sleep problems (Uehli et al. 2014; Uehli et al. 2013). Impaired self-reported sleep quality, sleep duration, and daytime sleepiness were significant risk factors for work injuries such as musculoskeletal injuries (Uehli et al. 2014; Uehli et al. 2013). OSAS and EDS can be considered as established risk factors for road traffic accidents and have been suggested to be important causes for injuries at the workplace (Garbarino et al. 2011; Arita et al. 2015; Akkoyunlu et al. 2013; Lindberg et al. 2001; Suzuki et al. 2005). However, the latter investigations were based on questionnaires about symptoms of OSAS, such as snoring and EDS, as well as self-reported or registered data on injuries occurring at work. It has been shown that OSAS screening questionnaires have a limited sensitivity and specificity of around 77 and 53%, respectively, to diagnose OSAS in patients without history of sleep disorders (Abrishami et al. 2010). Retrospective assignment of injury status by questionnaire or consulting registries is prone to recall bias or underreporting.

In contrast, objective assessment using full-night attended polysomnography (PSG)—the gold standard for diagnosis of OSAS—might provide more reliable results at the time of injury. This would allow immediate counseling of the affected worker and quick initiation of evidence-based interventions to treat OSAS and EDS to decrease the risk for future and maybe more severe or even fatal OIs.

n this study, we investigated the prevalence of OSAS and other sleep disorders and symptoms of EDS in a sample of individuals who attended the emergency room (ER) of a tertiary hospital due to OI and compared them with a sample of hospital outpatients without recent history of injury at the workplace. Our hypothesis was that individuals with OI would have a higher prevalence of OSAS related sleep abnormalities in PSG than outpatients without OI.

Methods

We included patients aged between 17 and 65 years who attended the ER of the University Hospital of Basel, Switzerland, for treatment of a work-related injury (occupational injury patients [OIPs]). We enrolled males and females who fulfilled the following inclusion criteria: (1) aged between 16 and 65 years, (2) admission to hospital ER for a work-related injury on the day or subsequent day of injury, (3) moderate-to-serious injury severity (Grossmann et al. 2011), (4) sufficient German language skills, and (5) able to complete the questionnaire. During the same period, patients who were treated for acute conditions in the surgical outpatient

department and who did not report workplace-related injuries in the last 3 months were recruited as controls (CONs). All participants were required to have a theoretical work capacity of 100% and to be employed at least 50% of the full-time equivalent.

All participants completed the Epworth Sleepiness Scale (ESS), a questionnaire to evaluate EDS (Johns 1991). We considered an ESS score of > 10 points as indicative of EDS. Furthermore, we collected data related to the injury and the type of work they performed when injured and measured the patient's body weight and height. Work injury types were defined on the basis of groups of work injury variables that had been identified by factor analysis as published previously (Uehli et al. 2013). Patients' job risk was classified as "high risk" or "low risk" by a trained study nurse reading the relative work injury risk from the Swiss national accident statistics based on the respondent's primary job, age, and gender (Swiss National Accident Insurance Fund (Suva) 2009). The patient's job risk was classified as "high risk" if his relative work injury risk was greater than the 3-year Swiss average.

Within 2 weeks after the OI, patients were investigated in the sleep laboratory. All subjects underwent a full-night attended PSG. A trained medical assistant monitored the patients and their recordings during the night to ensure continuous recording of data. We recorded chest and abdomen movements, nasal flow, pulse oximetry, electrocardiogram, submental and tibial electromyogram, electroencephalogram, and electrooculogram, accompanied by a microphone and infrared camera for monitoring purposes. Sleep data were analyzed by a trained physician qualified and experienced in the analysis of sleep studies, who was blinded with respect to group allocation of the patient (OIP or CON group). The PSG data were collected using RemLogic (Embla, Broomfield CO, USA). The AHI was calculated based on 2007 AASM Manual for Scoring Sleep and Associated Events. Hypopnea was defined as a reduction of airflow by at least 30% and followed by a drop in oxygen saturation of at least 4% from baseline for at least 10 s. Apnea was defined as an airflow limitation of more than 90% of baseline. Sleep bruxism was assessed based on electromyogram activity. A cutoff of > 5 was chosen to define an abnormal PSG result for the apnea–hypopnea index (AHI), oxygen desaturation index (ODI), limb movement index (LMI), and arousal index.

We used IBM SPSS Statistics version 24 for statistical analysis. Descriptive statistics were computed as mean and standard deviation. We used the Mann–Whitney U test for continuous variables and Fisher's exact test for proportions. For continuous variables effect size expressed as Cohen's d was calculated. The Shapiro–Wilk test was used to examine whether data were normally distributed and histograms were assessed visually. The significance level was set at $p < 0.05$.

Results

A total of 144 participants were enrolled (79 OIP, 66 CON) and underwent a full-night attended PSG. However, we lost PSG data for 10 controls due to hard disk failure on the sleep laboratory computer. These individuals were excluded from further analysis. One individual in the OIP group was previously diagnosed with OSAS but refused treatment and was therefore included in the analysis.

Figure 1 shows the distribution of patients in the OIP and CON groups according to occupational categories of the International Standard Classification of Occupations, 1988. There was no difference between the OIP and CON groups regarding job risk for work-related injuries according to the Swiss National Accident Statistics 2007 edition (OIP $n = 38$ [48%] classified as "high risk" vs. CON $n = 23$ [41%] classified as "high risk," $p = 0.484$). The proportion of females between groups did not differ significantly (OIP $n = 32$ [41%] vs. CON $n = 29$ [53%], $p = 0.217$), and there was no difference in age (OIP 36 ± 13 years vs.

CON 39 ± 13 years; Cohen's d – 0.23, $p = 0.110$) or body mass index (BMI) (OIP 25.8 ± 5.0 kg/m^2 vs. CON 24.7 ± 4.12 kg/m^2; Cohen's d 0.24, $p = 0.145$).

The results obtained by full-night attended PSG are presented in Table 1. The proportion of patients with an abnormal AHI as well as the mean AHI was higher in the OIP than the CON group. In contrast, there was no significant difference in the proportion of patients with an abnormal ODI or the mean ODI between the OIP and CON groups. Furthermore, patients in the OIP group comprised a higher proportion of individuals with signs of sleep bruxism and abnormal LMI and arousal index than the CON group.

Nine individuals each in the OIP and CON groups had an abnormal ESS score (equivalent to 11 and 16% in the OIP and CON groups, respectively; OR 0.67 [95% CI: 0.22–2.01]). There was also no difference in mean ESS score between the OIP and CON groups (OIP 7.2 ± 3.5 vs. CON 6.3 ± 4.1; Cohen's d 0.24, $p = 0.190$).

We stratified patients in the OIP group according to AHI severity and saw that an increased AHI was associated with increasing age, BMI, and ESS and was present in higher proportion of males (Table 2).

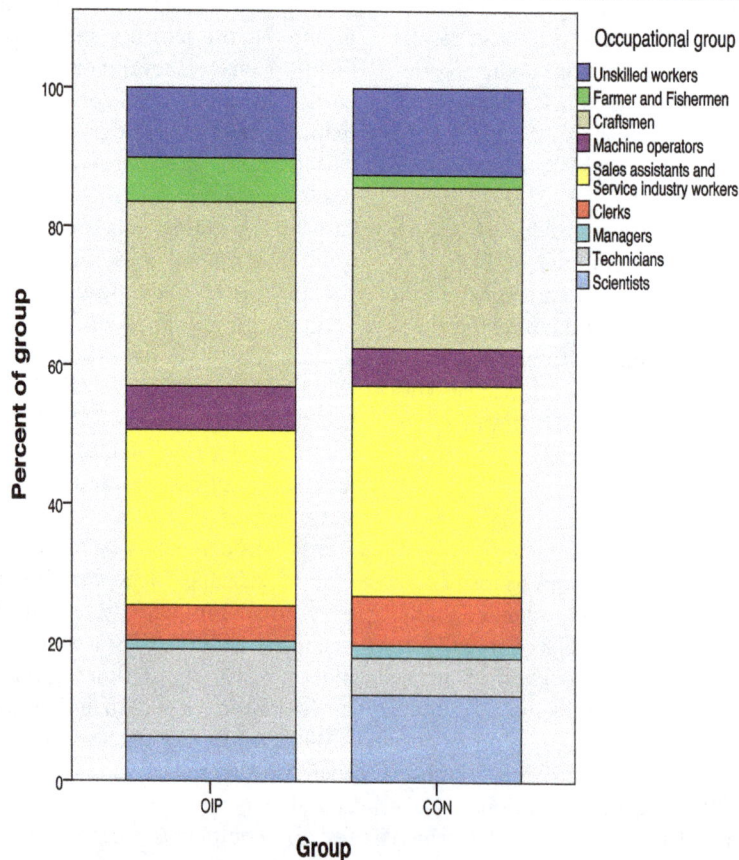

Fig. 1 Distribution of patients in the OIP and CON groups according to occupational categories of the International Standard Classification of Occupations (ISCO-88) (Bundesamt für Statistik 2017). Legend: OIP = occupational injuries patients, CON = controls

Table 1 Individuals with excessive daytime sleepiness or abnormal findings during the sleep study with full-night attended polysomnography

	OIP group	CON group	
Total sleep time (min)	5.7 (±1.1)	5.5 (±1.1)	Cohen's d 0.18, $p = 0.210$
AHI > 5 (n)	38 (48%)	16 (29%)	OR 2.32 (1.05–5.13)
AHI (events/h)	8.0 (±9.5)	5.6 (±7.2)	Cohen's d 0.28, $p = 0.028$
ODI > 5 (n)	13 (17%)	9 (16%)	OR 1.03 (0.37–2.87)
ODI (events/h)	3.7 (±6.8)	3.0 (±6.5)	Cohen's d 0.11, $p = 0.698$
LMI > 5 (n)	52 (66%)	22 (40%)	OR 2.98 (1.38–6.46)
LMI (events/h)	11.87 (±12.4)	7.59 (±8.1)	Cohen's d 0.41, $p = 0.030$
Sleep bruxism (n)	8 (10%)	1 (2%)	OR 6.20 (0.75–138.08)
Arousal index > 5 (n)	57 (72%)	28 (51%)	OR 2.59 (1.19–5.67)
Arousal index (events/h)	9.5 (±8.8)	6.9 (±5.8)	Cohen's d 0.35, $p = 0.011$
Breathing-related arousals (events/h)	6.0 (±6.6)	4.4 (±5.7)	Cohen's d 0.26, $p = 0.036$
Unspecified arousals (events/h)	2.7 (±1.6)	2.6 (±1.6)	Cohen's d 0.06, $p = 0.584$
Abnormal PSG finding (n)	67 (85%)	35 (64%)	OR 3.35 (1.38–8.25)

Data are presented as mean (SD) or frequency (%) and odds ratio OR (95% confidence interval (CI)) or effect size (Cohen's d) and p-value. Abnormal PSG finding was defined as at least one abnormal finding in the following categories: AHI > 5, ODI > 5, LMI > 5, sleep bruxism, arousal index > 5

When considering the results of the ESS and the full-night attended PSG, 70 patients in the OIP group (89%) and 36 controls (66%) had either EDS and/or an abnormal finding (OR 4.32 95% CI: 1.65–11.52). However, there was no difference in age, gender, BMI, and gender for individuals with or without EDS, respectively (age 39.9 ± 14.9 years vs. 37.3 ± 12.1 years; Cohen's d 0.19 $p = 0.964$; BMI 24.6 ± 4.0 kg/m^2 vs. 25.4 ± 4.7 kg/m^2; Cohen's d – 0.18 $p = 0.595$; 7 females (39%) vs. 54 females (47%), $p = 0.617$).

Injury mechanism, type, location, and tasks during which work-related injuries occurred in the OIP group are shown in Table 3. Most of the patients were admitted for musculoskeletal injuries and wounds located at the extremities, and most injuries occurred while handling tools, machines, or loading and while moving at the workplace. The two most common injury mechanisms were stepping, caught/hit/crushed/struck by an object, or overloading.

Discussion

Individuals treated for OIs in the ER of a tertiary hospital in Switzerland and investigated with full-night attended PSG were found to have abnormal findings more frequently, such as elevated AHI and arousal index compatible with a diagnosis of OSAS compared with a control group of patients treated for other conditions in the same hospital. Furthermore, individuals with OIs were found to have a higher LMI and signs of sleep bruxism compared with controls. Our findings confirm previous studies suggesting that untreated OSAS and other sleep disorders need to be considered as important risk factors for injuries that occur at the workplace. Information about workers regarding symptoms and complications of OSAS together with PSG screening and subsequent treatment may offer an opportunity to decrease their risk of future injuries.

Our results support our primary hypothesis that an abnormal AHI is more frequent in patients with OI than in outpatients without OI. However, the differences in terms of prevalence of abnormal and mean AHI were relatively small and may be considered clinically insignificant. In post hoc analysis we compared several objective parameters obtained during the full-night attended PSG and found differences between patients with OI and without OI that were statistically significant

Table 2 Stratification of OIP group according to the apnea–hypopnea index (AHI)

	AHI < 5 (n = 39)	AHI 5–9.9 (n = 21)	AHI 10–14.9 (n = 9)	AHI > 15 (n = 10)
Age (years)	30.05 (9.7)	38.38 (12.3)	45.11 (14.0)	44.1 (12.7)
BMI (kg/m^2)	24.89 (3.7)	25.88 (4.8)	24.88 (2.6)	29.92 (8.4)
ESS	6.26 (4.2)	4.57 (3.3)	9.22 (3.7)	7.40 (3.9)
Gender (males)	21 (53.8%)	12 (57.1%)	6 (66.7%)	8 (80%)

Data are presented as mean (SD) or frequency (%)

Table 3 Distribution of different work injury types according to apnea–hypopnea index (AHI) in the OIP group ($n = 79$)

	AHI > 5 ($n = 38$)	AHI ≤5 ($n = 41$)	All OIP
Caught, hit	12	11	23
Handling, carrying	5	4	9
Side task	15	12	27
Tool, machine	13	13	26
Object	20	22	42
Cut, open wound	18	23	31
Musculoskeletal injury, fall	22	18	40
Extremities	37	37	74

Data are presented as the number of individuals with a certain work injury type. "Caught, hit": Being caught, hit, crushed, or struck; "Handling, carrying": Handling or carrying loads by hand or using a handling device; "Side task": Carrying out a side task such as walking around, cleaning, tidying, changing clothes or taking a break; "Tool, machine": Involving a tool or machine, that is, for cutting, assembling, forming, lifting, or digging; "Object": Involving an object, that is, obstacles, inventory, ladders, or building parts; "Cut, open wound": Being cut or open wound; "Musculoskeletal injury, fall": Musculoskeletal injury or slip, trip, or fall; "Extremities": Extremity, that is, hands, arms, legs, or feet

and would suggest that other sleep disorders may also be related with OI but the statistical significance did not pass Bonferroni correction for multiple testing. Therefore, these findings need to be confirmed in appropriately designed future studies.

OIs are caused by acute exposure to physical agents at the workplace, such as mechanical energy, electricity, chemicals and ionizing radiation, or by a sudden lack of essential agents, such as oxygen or heat. Injury events are caused by a complex interaction between factors associated with materials and equipment, the work environment, and the worker (Castillo et al. 2011). OIs represent a serious public health concern. It is estimated that every day approximately 1020 workers die as a result of OIs, and more than 960,000 workers are hurt because of accidents in the workplace (Hamalainen et al. 2009). Personal and occupational factors were found to be associated with an increased risk of OI and, as we have previously reported, approximately 13% of OIs can be attributed to sleep problems of any kind reflected by impaired sleep quality or quantity, breathing-related sleep problems, or the use of sleep medication (Uehli et al. 2014). Researchers analyzing data from the Canadian Community Health Survey (CCHS) found the strongest associations between work injury and sleep problems in men in trades and transportation jobs, women in processing and manufacturing jobs, and women who work rotating shifts (Kling et al. 2010).

Our sample of patients with OIs mainly consisted of individuals classified as craftsmen or sales assistants and service industry workers. According to the Swiss occupational health statistics male craftsmen of all ages and female craftsmen up to the age of 24 years have a high risk for OI.

The same is true for young male sales assistants and service industry workers (Swiss National Accident Insurance Fund (Suva) 2009). Our analysis did not reveal a systematic difference between OIP and CON regarding job risk for work-related injuries, proportion of males in the sample, age or BMI. We considered patients undergoing outpatient surgery as appropriate controls as they were 1) also engaged in regular employment and 2) were living and working in the hospitals catchment area and would therefore most likely have sought care for work-related injury in the same hospital.

In this study, individuals admitted with OIs were more frequently found to have findings compatible with a diagnosis of OSAS during sleep compared with the control group without OIs. These findings confirm previous research suggesting that OSAS might be a potential risk factor for injuries in the workplace. Ulfberg et al. investigated OI claims reported to the Occupational Injury Statistics register in Sweden in patients suffering from sleep-disordered breathing and in employed age-matched controls. They found that the risk of OI was increased in heavy snorers and patients with OSAS (Ulfberg et al. 2000). Similarly, Lindberg et al. reported an increased risk of OI in male snorers using questionnaires on snoring and EDS, as well as occupational accident reports to a national register (Lindberg et al. 2001). Acciantoli et al. studied workers with and without OSAS after full-night attended PSG and a questionnaire on self-judged work performance. Workers with OSAS reported to be affected by OI in the past more than those with normal sleep patterns (Accattoli et al. 2008). Furthermore, the authors stated that those with OSAS reported more difficulties with memory, impaired vigilance, concentration, ability to perform monotonous tasks, responsiveness, learning new tasks, and manual ability, and that the findings were associated with OSAS severity (Accattoli et al. 2008). Hassani et al. studied hospital workers in Iran using the Berlin questionnaire and data on self-reported OI. The workers classified as high risk for OSAS in the screening questionnaire were found to have a higher risk for self-reported accidents than those with a low-risk classification (Hassani et al. 2015). Finally, Hirsch and co-workers investigated patients with symptoms of OSAS referred to the sleep laboratory and reviewed occupational injury claims in the 5 years preceding the sleep study. They reported a twofold increase in the odds for OI in individuals with OSAS. Similar to our study, no consistent relationship between OI and OSA severity was found and EDS was not associated with OI (Hirsch Allen et al. 2016). Their study approach was different: The OI status was determined by using data obtained from the workers compensation board and only included OI cases that resulted in at least 1 day of absence from work and it is therefore possible that the actual number of OI is much higher when considering the fact that not all OI are reported and do not necessarily lead to lost workdays. Moreover, the interval between OI and the diagnosis of OSAS was much longer and the authors did not consider other abnormal sleep study findings that could be risk factors for OI.

In our study, we could not detect significant differences in the mean ODI and proportion of individuals with abnormal ODI. Our findings suggest that the cause of increased risk of OI is more attributable to fragmentation of sleep, rather than to recurrent severe desaturations. Factors affecting workers' arousal and attentiveness are known to be associated with an increased injury risk (Ulfberg et al. 2000). Fortunately, studies investigating drivers on a road safety platform, using a driving simulator and neuropsychological tests, have shown that impairments in vigilance, attention, and alertness seem to be partially reversible if individuals with OSAS undergo treatment with continuous positive airway pressure (CPAP). Mazza et al. showed that patients with OSAS with untreated OSAS had slower reaction times leading to a lengthening of vehicle stopping distance and an increased number of collisions compared with individuals without OSAS. These differences were no longer present after a 3-month period of CPAP treatment (Mazza et al. 2006). Orth et al. reported improvements in attention and alertness and a decrease in accident frequency and concentration faults in driving simulation and neuropsychological testing after initiation of CPAP treatment (Orth et al. 2005). As well as showing signs of immediate treatment success, there is evidence for an effect of CPAP treatment on road traffic accident rate (Yamamoto et al. 2000; Barbe et al. 2007). The use of oral appliances or hypoglossal stimulation therapy has not yet been shown to improve work performance or to reduce OI rate (Rabelo Guimaraes Mde and Hermont 2014). This emphasizes the importance of early detection and initiation of CPAP treatment to decrease the risk of OI (besides its well-known effect on cardiovascular risk reduction). Our findings confirm previously reported associations of age, BMI, and male gender with elevated AHI but not with ESS. This suggests that individuals with risk factors should be specifically targeted and counseled about OSAS and its associated adverse outcomes, even if they have not yet suffered an OI and do not report EDS.

We found a higher leg movement index in individuals with OI compared with controls. This finding either could reflect a reaction to breathing-related arousal or could be a result of underlying restless legs syndrome. Restless legs syndrome has been shown to disrupt sleep length, sleep quality, and daytime alertness and to impair quality of life and work productivity (Stevens 2015). A recent systematic review reported an association of sleep bruxism with sleep-related arousal, but a clear causative link with OSAS is still questionable (Jokubauskas and Baltrusaityte 2017). Until now, there has been no published evidence showing that individuals with restless

legs syndrome or sleep bruxism are at higher risk of injuries. However, a recent study investigating firefighters with sleep questionnaires found that in individuals positively screened for restless legs syndrome, insomnia and shift work disorder had an increased risk of self-reported motor vehicle crashes, near crashes, nodding off or falling asleep while driving, and injuries in and out of work (Barger et al. 2015). Based on this, we suggest that patients with OIs should be screened for symptoms of restless legs syndrome and sleep bruxism, and that further studies are required to investigate the impact of these conditions on work safety outcomes.

Previous research has shown that workers with EDS have a more than twofold higher risk of sustaining an OI than workers without EDS (Melamed and Oksenberg 2002). The ESS questionnaire was designed to measure EDS but is frequently used in clinical practice—despite its limited diagnostic performance—to screen for OSAS (Osman et al. 1999). Our findings confirm that most individuals with only slightly abnormal AHI would probably not report EDS and that the ESS would therefore not be useful to identify these individuals. As our study results suggest, most would not be identified by nocturnal pulse oximetry either. Using only questionnaires to screen for OSAS has some limitations. Even specific screening questionnaires have only moderate diagnostic performance mainly due to their relatively low specificity (Abrishami et al. 2010; Ramachandran and Josephs 2009). Moreover, questionnaires, such as the ESS, have been shown to be prone to underreporting when used in the workplace setting (Parks et al. 2009). Therefore, authors have advocated screening for OSAS in commercial drivers using combined methods, such as data from questionnaires, physician-obtained history, BMI measurements, and functional tests and to complete the investigation with specific tests, such as portable monitors or full-night attended PSG (Kales and Straubel 2014).

We have previously reported an association between poor sleep quality, measured as low sleep efficiency, as well as a short sleep duration with injury during side tasks (Uehli et al. 2013). In the present analysis, the OIP group showed the most frequent work injury types involved an object (obstacles, inventory, ladders, or building parts), a musculoskeletal injury or slip, trip, or fall, or extremities (hands, arms, legs, or feet). However, the distribution of work injury type was similar in patients with abnormal and normal AHI measurements.

Our findings need to be interpreted with caution. We conducted our study in a hospital in the city center of Basel with nearby large production and service industries. The location of the hospital therefore probably attracted a high proportion of workers in industrial and service companies situated in the catchment area. Patients working in the primary sector (farming, fishing, foresting) were underrepresented in our study sample. Full-night attended PSG is an expensive diagnostic procedure and its availability is limited in many countries. However, studies have shown that portable monitors for home sleep testing in addition to clinical data (e.g., BMI) can be used to identify patients with OSAS without incurring greater costs (Gurubhagavatula et al. 2013). Eijsvogel et al. showed that a two-step screening with a questionnaire and a nasal flow recording was a promising way to screen for OSAS in a healthy working population (Eijsvogel et al. 2016). Administration of the questionnaire and the sleep investigation were carried out in the 2 weeks following the OI. We could not determine the impact of an OI on the outcome of the sleep investigation. Based on the available evidence from several studies, we believe that sleep-disordered breathing is the main cause of OI and that any reverse effect can probably be neglected. Although the use of opioid pain medication was not formal exclusion criteria, no individual in the OIP or CON group recorded taking such medication (data not shown).

We defined hypopneas according to the 2007 *AASM recommended rules* as a 30% reduction in airflow accompanied by a 4% oxygen desaturation. Applying *AASM alternative scoring rules* (a 50% reduction in airflow accompanied by a 3% oxygen desaturation OR an arousal) may well have increased the difference in proportion of abnormal AHI and the mean AHI between individuals with occupational injuries and the controls. Thornton et al. have shown that using the *AASM recommended scoring rules* tends to yield lower mean and median AHI values compared to using the *AASM alternative scoring rules* (*Thornton* et al. 2012).

The analyzed study sample was rather small and decreased further due to data loss that occurred on our sleep laboratory computer. We lost data from six males and four females assigned to the CON group. Their mean BMI was similar, and their mean age was slightly higher than that of the analyzed individuals in the CON group (data not shown). In our sleep laboratory, we had limited capacity during weekends to investigate study participants. Therefore, we could only investigate patients who were able to undergo PSG during the weekend 2 weeks following injury. Therefore, while we cannot exclude a selection bias, we think that this would have affected OIP and CON groups in a similar fashion. Furthermore, the recruitment of study participants was limited to normal daytime working hours and our study sample mainly consisted of dayshift workers. Shift and night work are known to be associated with an increased OI risk (Wagstaff and Sigstad Lie 2011). We limited recruitment to patients with an emergency severity index of 3–4 and without trauma to the central nervous system or severe injury to the thoracic cage. Therefore, the observed associations need to be confirmed in future studies investigating patients with more severe OIs and other types of injury. Finally, we only included individuals with sufficient German language skills that allowed them to fill in the questionnaires used in this study.

Conclusion

In our study, individuals treated for OIs in the ER were shown to have more abnormal findings suggestive of OSAS or other sleep disorders compared with the control group of hospital outpatients. These results suggest that OSAS, as well as other sleep disorders, could be important risk factors for OI and therefore screening for these conditions should form part of the postaccident medical investigation. Furthermore, all individuals with known risk factors for OSAS such as male gender, higher age, and increased BMI should be counseled regarding OSAS, its adverse outcomes, and treatment options during regular health surveillance exams. Future studies are required to investigate the impact of OSAS screening and treatment on OI rate and how to approach high-risk workers with cost-effective diagnostic tests.

Abbreviations

AHI: Apnea-hypopnea-index; BMI: Body-mass-index; CI: Confidence intervall; CON: Controls; CPAP: Continous positive airway pressure; EDS: Excessive daytime sleepiness; ER: Emergency room; ESS: Epworth sleepiness scale; LMI: Limb movement index; ODI: Oxygen desaturation index; OI: Occupational injuries; OIP: Occupational injuries patients; OR: Odds ratio; OSAS: Obstructive sleep apnea syndrome; p: *p*-value; PSG: Polysomnography; SD: Standard deviation

Acknowledgments

The authors would like to thank all collaborating staff of the University Hospital of Basel, Switzerland, for their kind permission to recruit patients within their organization. We thank Dr. Werner Strobel for the analysis of the full-night attended PSG studies.

Funding

We gratefully acknowledge financial support from the Swiss National Accident Insurance Institution (Suva).

Authors' contributions

SS, KU, DM and JDL were responsible for the study conception and design; DM, WS, RB, SD, SM, SB and JDL carried out the data acquisition; SS conducted the data analysis; SS drafted the manuscript; KU, DM, RB, SD, SM, MH, SB and JDL critically revised the manuscript; and DM was responsible for primary supervision. All authors read and approved the final manuscript.

Competing interests

David Miedinger and Katrin Uehli were employed by Suva during the data collection and analysis phase of this study. Other authors declare that they have no competing interests.

Author details

[1]Cantonal Hospital Baselland, University Clinic of Medicine, CH-4410 Liestal, Switzerland. [2]Department of Pneumology, University Hospital of Basel, Basel, Switzerland. [3]Department of Emergency Medicine, University Hospital of Basel, Basel, Switzerland. [4]Medical Faculty, University of Basel, Basel, Switzerland.

References

Abrishami A, Khajehdehi A, Chung F. A systematic review of screening questionnaires for obstructive sleep apnea. Can J Anaesth. 2010;57(5):423–38.

Accattoli MP, Muzi G, dell'Omo M, et al. Occupational accidents, work performance and obstructive sleep apnea syndrome (OSAS). G Ital Med Lav Ergon. 2008;30(3):297–303.

Akkoyunlu ME, Altin R, Kart L, et al. Investigation of obstructive sleep apnoea syndrome prevalence among long-distance drivers from Zonguldak, Turkey. Multidiscip Respir Med. 2013;8(1):10.

Arita A, Sasanabe R, Hasegawa R, et al. Risk factors for automobile accidents caused by falling asleep while driving in obstructive sleep apnea syndrome. Sleep Breath. 2015;19(4):1229–34.

Barbe F, Sunyer J, de la Pena A, et al. Effect of continuous positive airway pressure on the risk of road accidents in sleep apnea patients. Respiration. 2007;74(1):44–9.

Barger LK, Rajaratnam SM, Wang W, et al. Common sleep disorders increase risk of motor vehicle crashes and adverse health outcomes in firefighters. J Clin Sleep Med. 2015;11(3):233–40.

Bundesamt für Statistik. International Standard Classification of Occupations - ISCO 88 (COM). 2017. https://www.bfs.admin.ch/bfs/de/home/statistiken/arbeit-erwerb/nomenclaturen/isco-88-com.html. Accessed 23 Mar 2018.

Castillo DN, Pizatella TJ, Stout NA. Injuries and Occupational Safety. In: Levy BS, Wegman DH, Baron SL, Sokas RK, editors. Occupational and envrionmental health - recognizing and preventing disease and injury. 6th ed. New York: Oxford University Press; 2011. p. 315–34.

Eijsvogel MM, Wiegersma S, Randerath W, Verbraecken J, Wegter-Hilbers E, van der Palen J. Obstructive sleep apnea syndrome in company workers: development of a two-step screening strategy with a new questionnaire. J Clin Sleep Med. 2016;12(4):555–64.

European Statistics on Accidents at Work (ESAW) - Summary methodology. 2013th. Luxembourg: Publications Office of the European Union; 2013. http://ec.europa.eu/eurostat/en/web/products-manuals-and-guidelines/-/KS-RA-12-102. Accessed 13 Mar 2018.

Fava C, Montagnana M, Favaloro EJ, Guidi GC, Lippi G. Obstructive sleep apnea syndrome and cardiovascular diseases. Semin Thromb Hemost. 2011;37(3):280–97.

Garbarino S, Traversa F, Spigno F, Bonsignore AD. Sleepiness, sleep disorders and risk of occupational accidents. G Ital Med Lav Ergon. 2011;33(3 Suppl):207–11.

Gharibeh T, Mehra R. Obstructive sleep apnea syndrome: natural history, diagnosis, and emerging treatment options. Nat Sci Sleep. 2010;2:233–55.

Grossmann FF, Nickel CH, Christ M, Schneider K, Spirig R, Bingisser R. Transporting clinical tools to new settings: cultural adaptation and validation of the emergency severity index in German. Ann Emerg Med. 2011;57(3):257–64.

Gurubhagavatula I, Fields BG, Morales CR, et al. Screening for severe obstructive sleep apnea syndrome in hypertensive outpatients. J Clin Hypertens (Greenwich). 2013;15(4):279–88.

Hamalainen P, Leena Saarela K, Takala J. Global trend according to estimated number of occupational accidents and fatal work-related diseases at region and country level. J Saf Res. 2009;40(2):125–39.

Hassani S, Rahnama N, Seyedmehdi SM, et al. Association between occupational accidents and sleep apnea in hospital staff. Tanaffos. 2015;14(3):201–7.

Heinzer R, Vat S, Marques-Vidal P, et al. Prevalence of sleep-disordered breathing in the general population: the HypnoLaus study. Lancet Respir Med. 2015; 3(4):310–8.

Hirsch Allen AJ, et al. Obstructive sleep apnoea and frequency of occupational injury. Thorax. 2016;71:664–6.

Johns MW. A new method for measuring daytime sleepiness: the Epworth sleepiness scale. Sleep. 1991;14(6):540–5.

Jokubauskas L, Baltrusaityte A. Relationship between obstructive sleep apnoea syndrome and sleep bruxism: a systematic review. J Oral Rehabil. 2017;44(2):144–53.

Kales SN, Straubel MG. Obstructive sleep apnea in north American commercial drivers. Ind Health. 2014;52(1):13–24.

Key figures on Europe. Luxembourg: eurostat; 2016. http://ec.europa.eu/eurostat/web/products-statistical-books/-/KS-EI-16-001. Accessed 13 Mar 2018.

Kling RN, McLeod CB, Koehoorn M. Sleep problems and workplace injuries in Canada. Sleep. 2010;33(5):611–8.

Li X, Sundquist K, Sundquist J. Socioeconomic status and occupation as risk factors for obstructive sleep apnea in Sweden: a population-based study. Sleep Med. 2008;9(2):129–36.

Lindberg E, Carter N, Gislason T, Janson C. Role of snoring and daytime sleepiness in occupational accidents. Am J Respir Crit Care Med. 2001; 164(11):2031–5.

Mazza S, Pepin JL, Naegele B, et al. Driving ability in sleep apnoea patients before and after CPAP treatment: evaluation on a road safety platform. Eur RespirJ. 2006;28(5):1020–8.

Melamed S, Oksenberg A. Excessive daytime sleepiness and risk of occupational injuries in non-shift daytime workers. Sleep. 2002;25(3):315–22.

Orth M, Duchna HW, Leidag M, et al. Driving simulator and neuropsychological [corrected] testing in OSAS before and under CPAP therapy. Eur Respir J. 2005;26(5):898–903.

Osman EZ, Osborne J, Hill PD, Lee BW. The Epworth sleepiness scale: can it be used for sleep apnoea screening among snorers? Clin Otolaryngol Allied Sci. 1999;24(3):239–41.

Parks P, Durand G, Tsismenakis AJ, Vela-Bueno A, Kales S. Screening for obstructive sleep apnea during commercial driver medical examinations. J Occup Environ Med. 2009;51(3):275–82.

Rabelo Guimaraes Mde L, Hermont AP. Sleep apnea and occupational accidents: Are oral appliances the solution? Indian J Occup Environ Med. 2014;18(2):39–47.

Ramachandran SK, Josephs LA. A meta-analysis of clinical screening tests for obstructive sleep apnea. Anesthesiology. 2009;110(4):928–39.

Reichmuth KJ, Austin D, Skatrud JB, Young T. Association of sleep apnea and type II diabetes: a population-based study. Am J Respir Crit Care Med. 2005; 172(12):1590–5.

Stevens MS. Restless legs syndrome/Willis-Ekbom disease morbidity: burden, quality of life, cardiovascular aspects, and sleep. Sleep Med Clin. 2015;10(3):369–73. xv-xvi

Suzuki K, Ohida T, Kaneita Y, Yokoyama E, Uchiyama M. Daytime sleepiness, sleep habits and occupational accidents among hospital nurses. J Adv Nurs. 2005; 52(4):445–53.

Swiss National Accident Insurance Fund (Suva). Accident Statistics (Federal Law on Accident Insurance (UVG)) 2003–2007. 2009.

Thornton AT, Singh P, Ruehland WR, Rochford PD. AASM Criteria for scoring respiratory events: interaction between apnea sensor and hypopnea definition. Sleep. 2012;35(3):425–32. https://doi.org/10.5665/sleep.1710.

Uehli K, Mehta AJ, Miedinger D, et al. Sleep problems and work injuries: a systematic review and meta-analysis. Sleep Med Rev. 2014;18(1):61–73.

Uehli K, Miedinger D, Bingisser R, et al. Sleep problems and work injury types: a study of 180 patients in a Swiss emergency department. Swiss Med Wkly. 2013;143:w13902.

Ulfberg J, Carter N, Edling C. Sleep-disordered breathing and occupational accidents. Scand J Work Environ Health. 2000;26(3):237–42.

Wagstaff AS, Sigstad Lie JA. Shift and night work and long working hours–a systematic review of safety implications. Scand J Work Environ Health. 2011; 37(3):173–85.

Yamamoto H, Akashiba T, Kosaka N, Ito D, Horie T. Long-term effects nasal continuous positive airway pressure on daytime sleepiness, mood and traffic accidents in patients with obstructive sleep apnoea. Respir Med. 2000;94(1):87–90.

25

Clarifying the link between sleep disordered breathing and tracheal collapse: a retrospective analysis

Christena A. Kolakowski[*] ⓘ, Donald R. Rollins, Theodore Jennermann, Allen D. Stevens, James T. Good Jr, Joshua L. Denson and Richard J. Martin

Abstract

Background: Symptoms of acquired tracheobronchomalacia (TBM) include wheezing, shortness of breath, and chronic cough, and can negatively affect quality of life. Successful treatment of TBM requires identification of the disorder and of contributing factors. Acquired TBM is generally associated with a number of conditions, including asthma, chronic obstructive pulmonary disease (COPD), and gastroesophageal reflux. Although a possible relationship with obstructive sleep apnea (OSA) has been observed, data illuminating such an interaction are sparse.

Methods: In the present study, we analyzed the percent tracheal collapse (as measured on dynamic chest CT) and detailed sleep reports of 200 patients that had been seen at National Jewish Health, half of which had been diagnosed with OSA and half which did not have OSA.

Results: Tracheal collapse ranged from 0 to 99% closure in the population examined, with most subjects experiencing at least 75% collapse. OSA did not relate significantly to the presence or severity of tracheobronchomalacia in this population. Sleep disordered breathing (SDB) did show a strong association with TBM ($p < 0.03$).

Conclusions: Tracheobronchomalacia may develop as a result of increased negative intrathoracic pressure created during attempts at inhalation against a closed or partially closed supraglottic area in patients experiencing apneic or hypopneic events, which contributes to excessive dilation of the trachea. Over time, increased airway compliance develops, manifesting as tracheal collapse during exhalation. Examining TBM in the context of SDB may provide a reasonable point at which to begin treatment, especially as treatment of sleep apnea and SDB (surgical or continuous positive airway pressure) has been shown to improve associated TBM.

Keywords: Sleep disordered breathing, Obstructive sleep apnea, Tracheobronchomalacia

Background

Tracheomalacia (TM) and tracheobronchomalacia (TBM) manifest clinically as wheezing, chronic cough, and shortness of breath, and can negatively affect quality of life (Choo et al. 2013). TBM and TM are characterized by the collapse of the trachea (and bronchi, in the case of TBM) during forced expiration. Untreated TM can progress to TBM over time (Nuutinen 1977), though little is known about the histopathological changes in TBM in adults (Majid 2017). The degree of severity of TBM can be described as the percentage of anterior-posterior narrowing of the tracheal or bronchial wall during forceful exhalation or as the percentage of reduction in tracheal or bronchial lumen cross-sectional surface area (Murgu and Colt 2013). There is not a consistent standard in the literature for the point at which tracheal collapse becomes clinically significant; 50 to 80% collapse has been reported as such (Murgu and Colt 2013; Carden et al. 2005). TBM is reported to occur in 4.5–23% of the population, but the true incidence is difficult to determine (Carden et al. 2005; Jokinen et al. 1977). Acquired TBM is often discussed in an overlapping fashion with TM, hyperdynamic airway collapse (HDAC) and excessive dynamic airway collapse (EDAC) (Majid 2017). TBM is diagnosed either by direct

* Correspondence: kolakowskic@njhealth.org
Department of Medicine, National Jewish Health, 1400 Jackson St, Room A642, Denver, CO 80206, USA

observation of the airway during bronchoscopy or by dynamic expiratory imaging with multidetector computed tomography (CT) (Carden et al. 2005). Observations in adults have commonly associated acquired TBM with asthma, chronic obstructive pulmonary disease (COPD) and upper gastrointestinal disorders (aspiration, laryngopharangeal reflux [LPR], gastroesophageal reflux disease [GERD], reflux), as well as chronic cough (Murgu and Colt 2013; Carden et al. 2005; Palombini et al. 1999). In addition, obstructive sleep apnea (OSA) and/or sleep disordered breathing (SDB) have been occasionally associated with TBM (Ehtisham et al. 2015; Peters et al. 2005).

Though a connection between OSA and TBM has been observed before (Ehtisham et al. 2015; Peters et al. 2005; Seaman and Musani 2012; Sundaram and Joshi 2004), there is a paucity of data elucidating a mechanism for such a relationship. We performed a medical record database search to review this relationship in more detail through analysis of sleep studies, dynamic expiratory imaging, respiratory function, and concomitant diagnoses. We hypothesized that OSA may be an important contributor to the development of TBM. Increased negative intrathoracic pressure that occurs as a result of attempting to maintain airflow during obstructive events may induce tracheal over-dilation, gradually leading to increased tracheal compliance and collapse during exhalation (Peters et al. 2005).

Methods

This study was approved by the National Jewish Health Institutional Review Board (IRB #HS2990). A target of 100 total subjects with OSA and 100 without OSA was selected. The medical records database at National Jewish Health was queried twice to find patients with orders for both a sleep study and a high resolution chest CT with dynamic expiratory imaging. The initial search for subjects with an ICD-10 code for OSA yielded 331 subjects. The second search, excluding the ICD-10 code for OSA, provided 185 subjects. From both groups, subjects were excluded from analysis for the following reasons: one or both necessary studies were ordered but not completed, chest CT and sleep studies were greater than 12 months apart, home sleep studies, and/or diagnosis of central sleep apnea in the absence of OSA. Records were reviewed until each cohort contained 100 subjects. During data analysis, one subject was moved from the non-OSA group to the OSA group due to an error in the medical record, making the final count 101 patients with OSA and 99 without OSA.

Data collected from scored sleep reports were: O_2 saturation (SaO_2) nadir and time below 88% saturation, Respiratory Disturbance Index (RDI), Apnea-Hypopnea Index (AHI), REM AHI, Supine AHI, Supine REM AHI,

total apneas, total hypopneas, and total sleep time. Whether or not a patient was given oxygen supplementation during the study was additionally noted. Severity of OSA was determined by the AHI; OSA was considered to be mild if the AHI was between 5 and 15, moderate if the AHI was 15 to < 30, and severe if AHI was ≥30 (Bibbins-Domingo et al. 2017). The AHI is calculated from both apneas and hypopneas, averaged per hour of sleep time. In a scored sleep report, the AHI is calculated during different phases of sleep and in different sleeping positions, including but not limited to: total supine sleep, supine REM sleep, and total REM sleep (including any supine REM sleep that occurs). The RDI measures the average number of apneas, hypopneas, and respiratory event-related arousals per hour of sleep. Sleep disordered breathing (SDB) has no standard definition, but is defined here as the RDI and/or any AHI score being ≥5 per hour of sleep.

All multi-detector computed tomographic (CT) scans were performed at National Jewish Health. Sequential acquisitions at end-inspiration and during forced expiration (dynamic expiration) were made available for analysis. All CT scans were evaluated for research by a single radiologist, using TeraRecon (Aquarius, iNtuition, Version 4.4.8; TeraRecon Inc., Foster City, CA) software. Because not all subjects' scans included B50 (lung algorithm) sequences, B35 (soft tissue algorithm) inspiratory and dynamic expiratory sequences were analyzed with lung windows (level, – 700 HU; width, 1500). On the dynamic expiratory sequences imaging, the minimum area of the trachea from the thoracic inlet through carina was identified, the tracheal perimeter was traced by hand at this level using an electronic tracing tool and its area was recorded. Next, the same anatomical cross-section of the trachea was identified on inspiratory imaging and its cross sectional area was recorded. All measurements were obtained orthogonal to the long axis of the trachea. The percentage of tracheal collapse was calculated as follows:

Percentage of Expiratory Tracheal Collapse

$$= (1 - (\text{Minimum Tracheal Area on}$$

Dynamic Expiration/Corresponding Tracheal Area on

$$\text{Inspiration})) \times 100.$$

Patients with congenital TBM were not present in either cohort. Acquired tracheobronchomalacia and tracheomalacia were grouped together under the label of TBM to include those subjects with greater than or equal to 75% airway collapse on dynamic CT, whether or not bronchial collapse was present. Severe TBM was defined as greater than or equal to 85% collapse. The cutoff of 75% was chosen after review of the literature, in which anywhere from 50 to 80% tracheal narrowing is referenced as the defining point for TBM (Murgu and Colt 2013; Carden et al. 2005), and a mean of 54.3% tracheal collapse is reported in healthy individuals (Boiselle et al. 2009).

Spirometry data from tests closest to the date of the CT were also collected on these subjects. Forced Expiratory Volume in 1 s (FEV1), Forced Vital Capacity (FVC), FEV1/FVC, Forced Expiratory Flow at 50% of the FVC (FEF50), Forced Inspiratory Flow at 50% of the FVC (FIF50), the FEF50/FIF50 ratio, and the percent predicted of the above were analyzed.

Differences in quantitative data (i.e. spirometry, percent collapse of the trachea, and AHI) were evaluated by calculation of correlation coefficients and Student's T-Test. Rates of various qualitative characteristics between cohorts were assessed using the Z-Test and the Z-statistic. A P value of less than 0.05 was considered to be statistically significant. Statistical analyses were performed in Microsoft Excel.

Results
Demographics
Two hundred patients were included in the study (Table 1). There were 70 males and 130 females (35% males, 65% females). Patients from 19 to 85 years of age were represented (mean 57.3 ± 13.83); 58% were between 51 and 70 years old. A full spectrum of BMI categories was present; 53.5% of the patients were in the obese

category with a BMI of ≥30. The average BMI was 31.0 ± 6.42.

The ages of males and females were not significantly different (males 56.5 ± 15.76, females 57.7 ± 12.65). Females, as compared to males, had a higher BMI (31.8 ± 6.85 vs 29.3 ± 5.15, $p = 0.009$; Fig. 1), higher FEV1/FVC ratio ($p < 0.001$), higher FEF50/FIF50% predicted ($p = 0.01$), and higher FEF 50% predicted ($p = 0.03$). Otherwise their respiratory functions did not differ significantly. Patients with OSA were older (59.9 ± 11.59 vs 54.7 ± 15.36, $p = 0.008$), had higher BMI (32.3 ± 6.59 vs 29.6 ± 5.97, $p = 0.003$), had higher FEV1% predicted (75.92 ± 20.85 vs 67.95 ± 26.24, $p = 0.019$) and FEV1/FVC (73.71 ± 10.81 vs 69.33 ± 12.97, $p = 0.01$) than those without OSA (Table 1). Smoking histories for male versus female, subjects with and without OSA, and subjects with and without TBM were not significantly different. There were no statistically significant differences in BMI between patients with and without TBM. There were no statistically significantly different pulmonary function test results between those subjects with and without TBM. Equal proportions of males and females had TBM (24.2% of males and 26.1% of females).

Concurrent diagnoses
Diagnoses other than OSA and TBM occurring within the population here are summarized in Table 2, and are as follows: Asthma, COPD, upper GI disorders (this includes aspiration, abnormal swallow, LPR, GERD, reflux, and dysmotility), chronic/recurrent infections (pneumonia, bronchitis and recurrent pulmonary infections),

Table 1 Patient characteristics

	All Subjects $n = 200$	With OSA $n = 101$	Without OSA $n = 99$
Age	57.3 ± 13.83	59.9 ± 11.59	54.7 ± 15.36
BMI[a]	31.0 ± 6.43	32.3 ± 6.59[‡]	29.6 ± 5.97[‡]
n < 25	38 (19.0)	13 (12.9)	25 (25.3)
n 25–29.9	55 (27.5)	23 (22.8)	32 (32.3)
n ≥ 30	107 (53.5)	65 (64.3)	42 (42.4)
Male, n (%)	70 (35.0)	45 (44.6)	25 (25.3)
Female, n (%)	130 (65.0)	56 (55.4)	74 (74.7)
Pulmonary Function Test			
FEV1% Predicted	71.98 ± 24.01	75.92 ± 20.85[‡]	67.95 ± 26.24[‡]
FEV1/FVC	71.55 ± 12.12	73.71 ± 10.81[‡]	69.33 ± 12.97[‡]
FEF50/FIF50% Predicted	42.75 ± 27.93	44.12 ± 25.36	41.34 ± 30.28
Smoker (current and former), n (%)	91 (45.5)	48 (47.5)	43 (43.4)
Smokers Pack Years	23.5 ± 21.96	23.6 ± 21.98	23.4 ± 21.95

Data are presented as mean ± SD or number (percentage)
Abbreviations: *BMI* body mass index, *FEV1* forced expiratory volume in 1 s, *FCV* forced vital capacity, *FEF* forced expiratory flow, *FIF* forced inspiratory flow, *OSA* obstructive sleep apnea
[a]Weight (kg)/height(m)^2
[‡]Significantly Different, $p ≤ 0.01$ (within the same row)

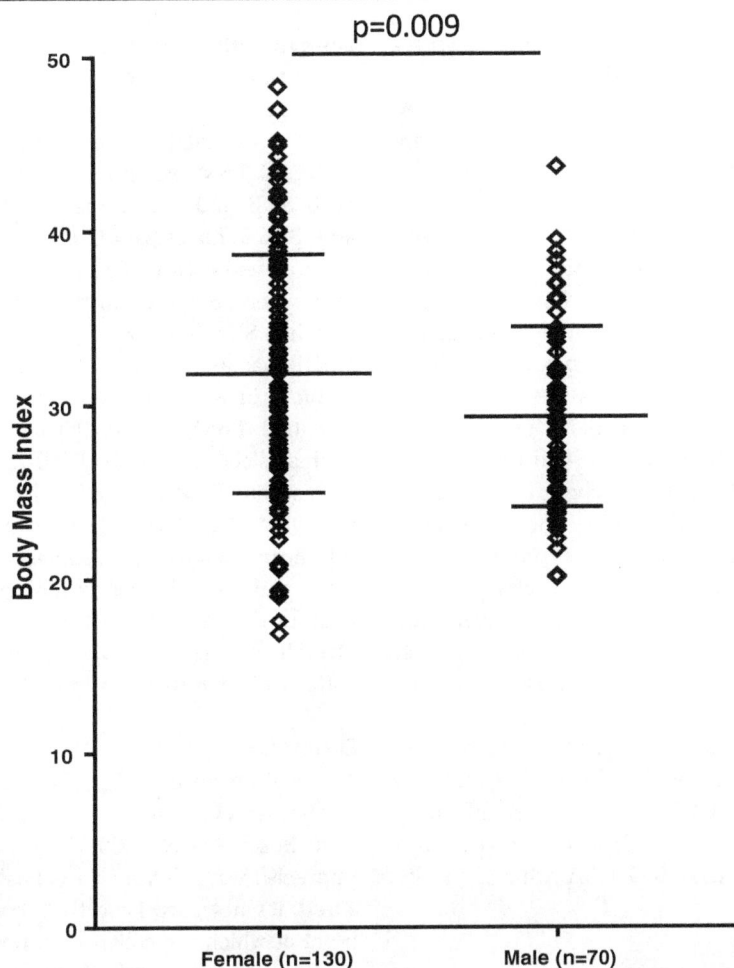

Fig. 1 Body mass index distribution by gender. Distribution of body mass index is shown for 130 females versus 70 males. Horizontal bars mark means and standard deviations for each group

VCD, and pulmonary hypertension. Pulmonary infections (OSA $N = 7$; non-OSA $N = 1$; $p = 0.03$), VCD (OSA $N = 12$; non-OSA $N = 2$; $p = 0.006$), and Pulmonary Hypertension (OSA $N = 5$; non-OSA $N = 0$; $p = 0.025$) occurred at significantly higher rates in patients with OSA than those without OSA. There were no statistically significant differences in the rates of comorbidities occurring between patients with and without TBM, in patients with both OSA and TBM, or in patients with Sleep Disordered Breathing (SDB) and TBM.

Table 2 Diagnoses observed in subject cohort

Diagnosis	Total Subjects $N = 200$ (%)	With OSA $N = 101$ (%)	Without OSA $N = 99$ (%)	With TBM $N = 51$ (%)	Without TBM $N = 149$ (%)
Asthma	110 (55.0)	54 (53.4)	56 (56.6)	27 (52.9)	83 (55.7)
COPD	33 (16.5)	13 (12.9)	20 (20.2)	9 (17.6)	24 (16.1)
Upper GI Disorders*	75 (37.5)	40 (39.6)	35 (35.4)	23 (45.0)	52 (35.0)
Chronic/Recurrent Infections**	15 (7.5)	7 (6.9) [‡]	1 (1.0) [‡]	3 (5.9)	12 (8.1)
VCD	14 (7.0)	12 (11.9) [‡]	2 (2.0) [‡]	4 (7.8)	10 (6.7)
Pulmonary Hypertension	5 (2.5)	5 (5.0) [‡]	0 (0.0) [‡]	1 (2.0)	4 (2.7)

Data are presented as number (percentage)
Abbreviations: *OSA* obstructive sleep apnea, *TBM* tracheobronchomalacia, *GI* gastrointestinal, *VCD* vocal cord dysfunction
*Upper GI Disorders: includes Reflux, Laryngopharangeal reflux, Gastroesophageal reflux disease, aspiration, dysmotility, and abnormal swallow
**Infections: Bronchitis, Pneumonia, Recurrent Pulmonary Infections
[‡]Significantly Different, $p \leq 0.05$ (within same row)

Sleep studies

All 200 patients had sleep studies with scored sleep reports, though not all subjects had sleep recorded in supine and/or REM sleep. Among patients with OSA, when comparing those with and without TBM, there were no significant differences in terms of oxygen saturation levels (SaO_2) or the number of patients requiring supplemental O_2 during sleep; however, patients with TBM spent a greater percentage of sleep time below 88% SaO_2 than those without TBM (46.4% vs 21.3%, $p = 0.009$). This pattern holds true within the group of patients with SDB as well (39.1% time below 88% SaO_2 with TBM vs 12.4% time below 88% SaO_2 without TBM $p = 0.003$). Forty-six (46.5%) of 99 patients in the cohort without OSA (overall AHI scores < 5) had at least one elevated AHI score on their sleep report (supine AHI, REM AHI, or supine REM AHI); 26 of those had multiple elevated AHI scores. Nine patients in this group had elevated RDI scores in the absence of elevated AHI scores. Overall, 156 patients had sleep disordered breathing (as defined by RDI and/or any individual AHI value of ≥5). Only 44 subjects had completely normal sleep studies.

Though the group of patients with OSA had roughly equal proportions of males and females, 64% of males in the entire cohort had OSA, which is significantly more than did not have OSA (36%; $p = 0.004$). Conversely, only 43% of females had OSA while 57% did not ($p = 0.004$).

Tracheal collapse

Tracheal collapse in this patient population ranged from 0 to 99.5%; 74.5% of subjects demonstrated less than 75% collapse. Thirty-one percent of obese (BMI ≥30) patients had TBM, and 18% of non-obese (BMI < 30) patients had TBM; these proportions are not statistically significantly different. Percent tracheal collapse did not correlate with BMI.

Severe TBM (≥85% collapse) was present at a significantly higher rate in subjects with OSA than without OSA (15 subjects vs 6, respectively, $p = 0.04$). Tracheal collapse correlated significantly with supine AHI ($r = 0.27$, $p < 0.001$) in all 200 subjects, as well as in the 101 subjects with OSA ($r = 0.311$, $p = 0.0015$). All 21 of the patients with severe TBM (> 85% collapse) had SDB. In subjects with SDB, supine AHI was significantly higher in subjects with TBM than those without TBM (33.9 ± 33.7 vs 20.0 ± 28.2; $p = 0.015$). Supine AHI was also significantly higher in those with TBM than those without TBM, as assessed by Student's T-Test (29.6 ± 33.3 vs 14.9 ± 25.9; $p = 0.015$; $p = 0.003$). Subjects with an elevated supine AHI had significantly higher collapse than those without an elevated supine AHI (60.0% ± 24.5 vs 52.0% ± 25.0; $p = 0.03$). Additionally, subjects with severely elevated supine AHI had far higher rates of collapse than those without an elevated supine AHI (51.8% ± 25.1 vs 69.2% ± 20.9; $p = 0.0004$).

Gender distribution in patients with both OSA and TBM was equal, but gender distribution in patients with SDB and TBM was not. This group of 44 subjects with both SDB and TBM was comprised of 61.4% females and 38.6% males ($p = 0.03$). One hundred percent of male patients with TBM had SDB; a significant proportion, when compared to the 79.4% of females with TBM who had SDB ($p = 0.04$).

SDB was associated with a higher rate of TBM; 28.2% of those in whom any AHI score, or RDI, was elevated (≥5) had TBM versus 20.0% of those with completely normal sleep studies had TBM. All 21 of the patients with severe TBM had SDB, while none of those with severe TBM had normal sleep studies; this is statistically significant ($p = 0.01$). In subjects with SDB, supine AHI was significantly higher in subjects with TBM than those without TBM (33.9 ± 33.7 vs 20.0 ± 28.2; $p = 0.015$). Overall, supine AHI was significantly higher in those with TBM than those without TBM ($p = 0.003$).

Discussion

Tracheal collapse is highly variable from one individual to another, even among healthy members of the population (Boiselle et al. 2009). When also accounting for the imprecise ways in which tracheal collapse is often measured, it's not surprising that it is difficult to define the point at which the collapse becomes significant. The lack of consistency in the literature regarding clinical significance lends credence to this theory; some sources report that 50% collapse is indicative of disease, while others suggest that it is well within the range of normal and that clinically significant TBM isn't present unless there is at least 70 or even 80% collapse (Murgu and Colt 2013; Carden et al. 2005; Boiselle et al. 2009). TBM does not exist in isolation; looking at tracheal collapse alone, and trying to decide an exact percent at which is becomes significant before trying to decide on treatment, may be irrelevant. It could, instead, be more helpful to look at patients with elevated supine AHI on their scored sleep reports. Should those individuals display moderate to severe (60% or higher) tracheal collapse alongside chronic cough and other symptoms of TBM, they should be considered for CPAP, even if their overall AHI score is normal (Seaman and Musani 2012; Sundaram and Joshi 2004; Ferguson and Benoist 1993).

Acquired TBM is most commonly seen in the middle aged and elderly (Nuutinen 1982), an observation which is borne out in the present cohort. Observations in adults have associated TBM with obesity, asthma, COPD and Upper GI Disorders (aspiration, LPR, GERD, reflux), as well as chronic cough (Murgu and Colt 2013; Carden et al. 2005; Palombini et al. 1999; Seaman and Musani 2012). It has been suggested that chronic/recurrent infections (pneumonia, bronchitis and recurrent pulmonary infections), and chronic inflammation are important contributors to the development of TBM (Feist et al. 1975); specific markers of such inflammation have not been examined (Carden et al. 2005). Acquired TBM clearly has multiple causes, but based on the observations in the group with SDB, it's possible that more than half of cases have SDB as a major contributing factor. There has not been a general appreciation of the high incidence of TBM in patients with OSA or SDB (Ehtisham et al. 2015), yet 30% of the patients in the present study with SDB also had TBM.

Throughout the analysis of the data gathered for this study, multiple theorized causes of TBM fell short. In this population, smoking, COPD, asthma, pulmonary infections and cough held no particular connection to TBM or tracheal collapse in general. BMI, pulmonary hypertension and infections did have a relationship with OSA, but not with TBM. Surprisingly, within the cohort examined here, severity of acquired TBM did not correlate with BMI, or with any particular BMI category. More than 50% of the patients in the present cohort were obese, and 52% of the obese subjects demonstrated moderate to severe tracheal collapse. Though the tracheal collapse observed in patients with BMI ≥30 was higher than that observed in patients with a BMI < 25, the average was still below 75% collapse (60.2% vs 49.5%, $p = 0.03$). This is supportive of the idea discussed by Seaman and Musani (Seaman and Musani 2012), who describe obesity as a contributor to TBM and suggest that weight loss would be an effective treatment in cases of TBM. Weight loss in obese patients improves OSA and SDB (Mitchell et al. 2014), which could then reduce the amount of tracheal collapse in those patients, thereby improving associated TBM.

In our exploration of the relationship between OSA and TBM, we found that TBM (≥75% tracheal collapse) corresponds more to abnormalities in other measures of sleep-disordered breathing than to the overall AHI score and diagnosis of OSA. Eighty-six percent of patients with TBM had sleep disordered breathing evident on the scored report – though not necessarily an abnormal overall AHI. However, the overall AHI does not always represent the extent of sleep disordered breathing present. The component AHI values (supine, REM, and Supine REM), as well as the RDI, should not be overlooked. These measures represent the most severely disordered aspects of sleep, but their significance may be diminished when averaged over an entire night of sleep (Punjabi 2016). In particular, supine AHI appears to be the best predictor of tracheal collapse within this dataset. Tracheal collapse correlated significantly with supine

AHI, and subjects with an elevated supine AHI had significantly greater tracheal collapse than those without an elevated supine AHI.

There are a number of limitations within this study. Because it was retrospective in nature, we were bound by the available records rather than a controlled patient selection. The relatively small cohort size of 200 patients total may preclude our finding significant differences among the subgroups. Data interpretation is limited to the impact of OSA/SDB on tracheal collapse, given that the study design was based around presence or absence of OSA rather than presence or absence of TBM.

Conclusion

In cases of moderate to severe tracheal collapse with no evident cause, it may be worthwhile to pursue a formal sleep study (Sundaram and Joshi 2004). The single subject in the present cohort with a history of tracheoplasty experienced total recurrence of TBM with a tracheal collapse of 80.9% within a year of surgery. Though this person was included in the non-OSA group due to an overall AHI of 4.1, all of the scores for AHI in supine and/or REM sleep were elevated (mean 18.8 ± 1.35). Because the patient had not had sleep testing done prior to the tracheoplasty, sleep disordered breathing was not identified. There was no sleep apnea treatment (i.e. CPAP) given, which may in part explain the relapse, as CPAP has been successfully used to treat TBM (Seaman and Musani 2012; Sundaram and Joshi 2004; Ferguson and Benoist 1993).

Though our original hypothesis was that OSA is an important contributor to the development of TBM, the data collected do not support a strong relationship between OSA and TBM. There are, however, evident connections between SDB and TBM, which support a modified hypothesis. Sleep disordered breathing, particularly in supine sleep, generates increased negative intrathoracic pressure during attempts at inhalation against a closed or partially closed supraglottic area, which contributes to excessive dilation of the trachea and proximal bronchi (Peters et al. 2005). Over time, increased airway compliance develops; this manifests as atrophy of and quantitative reduction in longitudinal elastic fibers, an increase in membranous tracheal diameter, and fragmentation of cartilaginous rings noted on histopathology and at autopsy in patients with TBM (Murgu and Colt 2013; Jokinen et al. 1977). In addition, because TBM can be successfully treated with CPAP (Sundaram and Joshi 2004; Ferguson and Benoist 1993), treating cases in which TBM occurs alongside borderline OSA, or instances where there is an elevated supine AHI, may be beneficial. Treatment of OSA either by surgical methods or CPAP has been shown to improve associated TBM (Peters et al. 2005; Sundaram and Joshi 2004).

Future studies should follow treatment of OSA with study of inflammatory markers and assessment of tracheal collapse as it coexists with OSA. Additional imaging studies, where the trachea can be visually monitored during apneic events, would shed light on this relationship more directly, though there are difficulties inherent in imaging a sleeping person. Many specific markers of inflammation have been found in OSA (Sundar and Daly 2011); however, though TBM is reported to occur with inflammation (Feist et al. 1975), specific markers have not been described. The link between upper airway inflammation and uncontrolled laryngopharyngeal reflux (LPR) (Lommatzsch et al. 2013) would be another possible avenue of research. There has not been discussion of LPR and a direct relationship with OSA (i.e. treating LPR and seeing an improvement in OSA), but it may be worth examining, given the recurring connection in the literature of OSA and upper gastrointestinal disorders.

Abbreviations
AHI: Apnea-hypopnea index; BMI: Body mass index; COPD: Chronic obstructive pulmonary disease; CPAP: Continuous positive airway pressure; CT: Computerized tomography; EDAC: Excessive dynamic airway collapse; FEF50: Forced expiratory flow at 50% of the FVC; FEV1: Forced expiratory volume in 1 s; FIF50: Forced inspiratory flow at 50% of the FVC; FVC: Forced vital capacity; GERD: Gastroesophageal reflux; HDAC: Hyperdynamic airway collapse; ICD-10: International Classification of Disease, Tenth Edition; IRB: Institutional Review Board; LPR: Laryngopharyngeal reflux; OSA: Obstructive sleep apnea; RDI: Respiratory disturbance index; REM: Rapid eye movement; SDB: Sleep disordered breathing; TBM: Tracheobronchomalacia; TM: Tracheomalacia

Authors' contributions
CK compiled and analyzed patient data, and wrote the manuscript and tables. DR initiated the project, and aided in project design, hypothesis development and manuscript preparation. TJ analyzed the patients' dynamic CT scan images and measured the percent collapse of the trachea. AS compiled data and provided insights during the data analysis process. JG contributed to study design and manuscript feedback. JD provided manuscript support and suggestions for analysis. RM guided the project from the start, including project design, hypothesis development, and manuscript preparation. All authors read and approved the final manuscript.

Competing interests
The authors declare that they have no competing interest.

References
Bibbins-Domingo K, Grossman DC, Curry SJ, Davidson KW, Epling JW, García FAR, et al. Screening for obstructive sleep apnea in adults. JAMA. 2017;317:407. https://doi.org/10.1001/jama.2016.20325.

Boiselle PM, O'Donnell CR, Bankier A, Ernst A, Millet ME, Potemkin A, et al. Tracheal collapsibility in healthy volunteers during forced expiration: assessment with multidetector CT. Radiology. 2009;252:255–62.

Carden KA, Boiselle PM, Waltz DA, Ernst A. Tracheomalacia and tracheobronchomalacia in children and adults: an in-depth review. Chest. 2005;127:984–1005.

Choo EM, Seaman JC, Musani AI. Tracheomalacia/tracheobronchomalacia and hyperdynamic airway collapse. Immunol Allergy Clin N Am. 2013;33:23–34.

Ehtisham M, Azhar Munir R, Klopper E, Hammond K, Musani AI. Correlation between tracheobronchomalacia/hyper dynamic airway collapse and obstructive sleep apnea. Am J Respir Crit Care Med. 2015;191:A5037–7.

Feist JH, Johnson TH, Wilson RJ. Acquired tracheomalacia: etiology and differential diagnosis. Chest. 1975;68:340–5. https://doi.org/10.1378/chest.68.3.340.

Ferguson GT, Benoist J. Nasal continuous positive airway pressure in the treatment of tracheobronchomalacia. Am Rev Respir Dis. 1993;147:457–61.

Jokinen K, Palva T, Sutinen S, Nuutinen J. Acquired tracheobronchomalacia. Ann Clin Res. 1977;9:52–7.

Lommatzsch SE, Martin RJ, Good JT Jr. Importance of fiberoptic bronchoscopy in identifying asthma phenotypes to direct personalized therapy. Curr Opin Pulm Med. 2013;19:42–8.

Majid A. Tracheomalacia and tracheobronchomalacia in adults. UpToDate. https://www.uptodate.com/contents/tracheomalacia-and-tracheobronchomalacia-in-adults. Accessed 1 Jan 2017.

Mitchell LJ, Davidson ZE, Bonham M, O'Driscoll DM, Hamilton GS, Truby H. Weight loss from lifestyle interventions and severity of sleep apnoea: a systematic review and meta-analysis. Sleep Med. 2014;15:1173–83.

Murgu S, Colt H. Tracheobronchomalacia and excessive dynamic airway collapse. Clin Chest Med. 2013;34:527–55.

Nuutinen J. Acquired tracheobronchomalacia: a bronchological follow-up study. Ann Clin Res. 1977;9:359–64.

Nuutinen J. Acquired tracheobronchomalacia. Eur J Respir Dis. 1982;63:380–7.

Palombini BC, Villanova CAC, Araújo E, Gastal OL, Alt DC, Stolz DP, et al. A pathogenic triad in chronic cough: asthma, postnasal drip syndrome, and gastroesophageal reflux disease. Chest. 1999;116:279–84.

Peters CA, Altose MD, Coticchia JM. Tracheomalacia secondary to obstructive sleep apnea. Am J Otolaryngol - Head Neck Med Surg. 2005;26:422–5.

Punjabi NM. COUNTERPOINT: is the apnea-hypopnea index the best way to quantify the severity of sleep-disordered breathing? No Chest. 2016;149:16–9. https://doi.org/10.1378/chest.14-2261.

Seaman JC, Musani AI. Tracheobronchomalacia and hyperdynamic airway collapse. Pakistan J Chest Med. 2012;18:65–70.

Sundar KM, Daly SE. Chronic cough and OSA: a new association? J Clin Sleep Med. 2011;7:669–77.

Sundaram P, Joshi JM. Tracheobronchomegaly associated tracheomalacia: analysis by sleep study. Indian J Chest Dis Allied Sci. 2004;46:47–9.

26

Quality of life, depression, and productivity of city government employees in Japan: a comparison study using the Athens insomnia scale and insomnia severity index

Masanori Takami[1], Hiroshi Kadotani[1*] (iD), Kohei Nishikawa[2], Yukiyoshi Sumi[3], Takao Nakabayashi[3], Yusuke Fujii[3], Masahiro Matsuo[3], Naoto Yamada[3] and the NinJaSleep Study Group

Abstract

Background: Insomnia has a high prevalence in modern society. Various tools have been developed to assess insomnia. We performed a direct comparison between the Insomnia Severity Index (ISI) and the Athens Insomnia Scale (AIS) in a Japanese population.

Methods: A cross-sectional questionnaire-based study was conducted in September 2017 as part of the Night in Japan Home Sleep Monitoring Study. In addition to insomnia, assessed using the AIS and ISI, depression, sleepiness, quality of life, and work performance were assessed using the Patient Health Questionnaire (PHQ)-9, a Japanese version of the Epworth Sleepiness Scale, the Short Form-8 Health Survey Questionnaire (SF-8), and the World Health Organization Health and Work Performance Questionnaire, respectively. Receiver operating characteristic (ROC) curves were constructed to compare the outcomes of the AIS and the ISI.

Results: A total of 1685 (81.9%) of all eligible employees were enrolled. The total scores of the AIS and ISI had a Pearson correlation coefficient (r) of 0.80 ($p < 0.01$). The area under the ROC curve for the AIS and ISI for the detection of depression (PHQ-9 $\geq$ 10) was 0.89 and 0.86, respectively. The prevalence of clinical insomnia (ISI $\geq$ 15) and definite insomnia (AIS $\geq$ 10) were 6.5 and 10.8%, respectively. Both the AIS and ISI showed a weak negative correlation with the physical component summary score of the SF-8 ($r = -0.37$, $p < 0.01$ and $r = -0.32$, $p < 0.01$, respectively) and absolute presenteeism ($r = -0.32$, $p < 0.01$ and $r = -0.28$, $p < 0.01$, respectively) and a moderate negative correlation with the mental component summary score of the SF-8 ($r = -0.53$, $p < 0.01$ and $r = -0.43$, $p < 0.01$, respectively).

Conclusions: A strong positive correlation was found between the total scores of the AIS and ISI. Both the AIS and ISI were found to be associated with low physical and mental quality of life, depression, and productivity loss at work. Moreover, they had a moderate accuracy for detecting depression. Both the AIS and ISI may serve as useful screening tools for both insomnia and depression in the Japanese working population.

Keywords: Insomnia, Receiver operating characteristic, Questionnaire, Depression, Quality of life, Presenteeism

* Correspondence: kadotanisleep@gmail.com
[1]Department of Sleep and Behavioral Sciences, Shiga University of Medical Science, Seta Tsukinowa-cho, Otsu City, Shiga 520-2192, Japan
Full list of author information is available at the end of the article

Background

Insomnia is highly prevalent in modern society. The Insomnia Severity Index (ISI) [Bastien et al. 2001] and Athens Insomnia Scale (AIS) [Soldatos et al. 2000; Okajima et al. 2013] were developed based on the standard diagnostic criteria for insomnia. These tools are widely used for assessing an individual's risk of insomnia [Lomeli et al. 2008].

To date, few studies have directly compared the ISI and AIS. One meta-analysis estimated and compared the diagnostic accuracy of the ISI and AIS and found that these tools yield comparable diagnostic properties for insomnia screening [Chiu et al. 2016]. However, this meta-analysis did not directly compare the ISI and AIS, but rather performed a comparison of sensitivity and specificity using references such as the International Classification of Sleep Disorders, Second Edition [American Academy of Sleep Medicine 2005] and the Diagnostic and Statistical Manual of Mental Disorders, Fourth Edition [American Psychiatric Association 2010]. A few studies have directly compared the ISI and AIS [Jeong et al. 2015; Sierra et al. 2008; Chung et al. 2011]. A strong positive correlation was found between the scores of the AIS and ISI in Korean firefighters ($r = 0.85$) [Jeong et al. 2015] and elderly Spanish individuals ($r = 0.93$) [Sierra et al. 2008]. Another study used the AIS and ISI simultaneously and assessed their internal consistency, reliability, and validity compared to individual clinical diagnoses [Chung et al. 2011].

Prior studies have confirmed that insomnia is associated with depression [Knekt et al. 2011], work productivity loss [Bolge et al. 2009], and reduced quality of life (QOL) [Ishak et al. 2012]. Patients with insomnia report experiencing a variety of symptoms, including daytime sleepiness, fatigue, cognitive impairment, symptoms of depression and anxiety, health decrement, and impairment in social and occupational function [Krystal 2007]. Insomnia is a frequent complaint of individuals with depression. Eighty five percent of patients with depression reportedly have insomnia [Sunderajan et al. 2010]. Insomnia remains the most common unresolved symptom of depression even after mood improvement by pharmacological treatment [Ishak et al. 2012]. Research has shown that patients with insomnia have 24.2% greater work impairment (work productivity loss) and 18.0% greater activity impairment than those without insomnia [Bolge et al. 2009]. It has also been reported that the individual-level decrements in work performance caused by insomnia have a human capital value of $2280, which is equivalent to an annualized population-level estimate of $63.2 billion in the USA [Kessler et al. 2011]. Clearly, impairments in health, function, and QOL are central features of insomnia, which can lead to significant economic burden. Therefore, diagnosing and treating insomnia appropriately by improving the perceived health, function, and QOL of patients with this condition is essential [Krystal 2007].

Significant economic and social burden is caused by depression [Global Burden of Disease Study 2013 Collaborators. 2015; Kadotani et al. 2014] and insomnia [Daley et al. 2009]. Questionnaire surveys are commonly used to assess depression and insomnia in large-scale community settings or in working environments. Increasing the response rate in surveys helps minimize bias and maximize the generalizability of the findings [Blair and Zinkhan. 2006]. To this end, minimizing the length of the questionnaire was reported to significantly increase the response rate [Sahlqvist et al. 2011]. Therefore, ff a questionnaire designed to measure insomnia can also detect depression with acceptable accuracy, it may help reduce the length of the questionnaires distributed in large-scale surveys and correspondingly increase the response rate.

Here, we performed a direct comparison between the ISI and AIS in a Japanese population. Both tools were expected to show a similar diagnostic performance with respect to the health outcomes associated with insomnia.

Methods

Participants

A cross-sectional questionnaire-based study was conducted as part of the Night in Japan Home Sleep Monitoring (NinJaSleep) sleep and mental health epidemiological study. Participants were government employees of Koka city, which is a rural city in the Shiga Prefecture of Japan. Employees for whom the consent of a legal representative was required for participation or who had taken extended leaves from employment were excluded. Among the 2119 employees, 62 were excluded because of extended leaves, including sick, maternity, and childcare leaves. Thus, a total of 2057 participants were included. Questionnaires were distributed on September 6, 2017.

Questionnaires

The AIS and ISI were used to assess insomnia. Depression, sleepiness, QOL, and work performance were assessed using the Patient Health Questionnaire (PHQ)-9 [Kroenke et al. 2001; Gilbody et al. 2007], a Japanese version of the Epworth Sleepiness Scale (ESS) [Johns 1991; Takegami et al. 2009], the Short Form-8 Health Survey Questionnaire (SF-8) [Ware et al. 2001; Fukuhara and Suzukamo 2004], and the World Health Organization Health and Work Performance Questionnaire (WHO-HPQ) [Kessler et al. 2003; Suzuki et al. 2014], respectively. Participants' bedtime, sleep latency, and waking time on weekdays were also recorded in the questionnaires.

The AIS evaluates the following eight items: AIS_1) sleep initiation; AIS_2) awakening during the night;

AIS_3) early morning awakening; AIS_4) total sleep duration; AIS_5) overall QOL; AIS_6) problems with sense of well-being; AIS_7) overall functioning; and AIS_8) daytime sleepiness [Soldatos et al. 2000; Okajima et al. 2013]. The ISI examines the following seven items: ISI_1) sleep-onset; ISI_2) sleep maintenance; ISI_3) early morning awakening; ISI_4) satisfaction with current sleep pattern; ISI_5) interference with daily functioning; ISI_6) noticeability of impairment attributed to sleep problems; and ISI_7) level of distress caused by sleep problems [Bastien et al. 2001]. For the ISI, total scores of 8–14 and ≥ 15 are classified as subthreshold insomnia and clinical insomnia, respectively [Bastien et al. 2001]. Subjects with AIS scores of < 6 can be reliably considered as not having insomnia [Soldatos et al. 2003]. An AIS score of 6 is the optimum cutoff based on the balance between sensitivity and specificity [Soldatos et al. 2003]. Subjects with AIS scores of ≥10 are expected to be diagnosed with insomnia [Soldatos et al. 2003]. Thus, we classified AIS total scores of 6–7 and ≥ 10 as suspected and definite insomnia, respectively.

The PHQ-9 is a reliable and valid instrument for screening individuals for major depressive disorder [Kroenke et al. 2001; Gilbody et al. 2007]. In previous studies, participants with a PHQ-9 ≥ 10 [Kroenke et al. 2001; Gilbody et al. 2007] were classified as having depression, and this same cutoff was used here. As for the ESS, in line with prior studies, a score of > 10 was considered to indicate sleepiness [Johns 1991; Takegami et al. 2009]. General health-related QOL was assessed using the SF-8, which consists of eight items and is divided into physical component summary (PCS) and mental component summary (MCS) scores [Ware et al. 2001; Fukuhara et al. 2004]. Higher PCS and MCS scores indicate better health. In the general Japanese population, scores > 50 and those < 50 are considered above and below the average, respectively [Fukuhara et al. 2004]. Here, poor physical and mental QOL were defined as the lowest tertiles of the PCS and MCS QOL scores from the SF-8, respectively. Productivity loss at work because of health problems is called presenteeism and this parameter can be measured using the WHO-HPQ [Kessler et al. 2003; Suzuki et al. 2014]. Absolute presenteeism in the WHO-HPQ represents actual performance. In the present study, we used absolute presenteeism to assess work productivity loss.

Participants in the lowest tertile of the absolute presenteeism score in the WHO-HPQ were classified as having poor work productivity [Suzuki et al. 2014]. Regarding participants' waking times and sleep latency, participants who woke up in the earliest tertile (before 06:00) and those in the shortest tertile for total sleep time (TST < 6 h) were classified as having early awakening and a short TST, respectively. Additionally, in adults, an onset

latency > 30 min typically has clinical significance [American Academy of Sleep Medicine 2014]; therefore, here, participants with a sleep latency > 30 min were classified as having a long sleep latency.

Statistical analyses

Pearson correlation coefficient analyses were performed to determine the strength of the association between two variables. One-way analyses of variance were used to identify differences among three or more groups, and post hoc testing was performed using Scheffé's method. Additionally, receiver operating characteristic (ROC) curve analysis was performed to compare the screening performance of the questionnaires. Pairwise comparisons of the ROC curves were performed by calculating the standard error of the area under the curve (AUC) and the difference between the two AUCs. Cohen's kappa coefficient was used for agreement evaluation. Statistical analyses were performed using MedCalc Version 17.9.7 (MedCalc Software, Mariakerke, Belgium). $P < 0.05$ was considered statistically significant.

Results

A total of 1685 (81.9%; 1685/2057) city government employees had returned the questionnaires by September 30, 2017. Fifty-two of the individuals who returned the survey worked the night shift. Data were missing for six participants. Data from the remaining 1627 (79.1%: 1627/2057) participants were analyzed in this study. Table 1 and Additional file 1: Figure S1 summarize the participant characteristics.

Both the AIS and ISI had moderate reproducibility (weighted kappa: 0.58). A strong positive correlation was found between the total scores of the AIS and ISI ($r = 0.80$, $p < 0.01$). The distribution of the AIS and ISI scores is

Table 1 Participant characteristics

	Mean		SD
Age, yrs.	45.30	±	12.22
Gender	Male: 39.30%		Female: 60.70%
BMI, kg/m^2	22.55	±	3.75
AIS	4.98	±	3.57
ISI	6.96	±	4.39
ESS	7.85	±	4.54
Sleep latency, h.	0.38	±	0.52
Wake-up time	06:00	±	00:46
Total sleep time, h.	6.51	±	1.13
Absolute presenteeism score	58.35	±	18.23
PHQ-9	4.65	±	4.54
PCS	47.77	±	7.20
MCS	47.35	±	7.51

presented in Fig. 1 and Additional file 2: Figure S2. When we compared the categories of the AIS (0–5: no pathological insomnia, 6–9: suspected insomnia, and 10–24: definite insomnia) and the ISI (0–7: no clinically significant insomnia, 8–14: subthreshold insomnia, and 15–28: clinical insomnia), the weighted kappa was 0.578 (Table 2). The prevalence of clinical insomnia (ISI ≥ 15) and definite insomnia (AIS ≥ 10) in this population was 6.5 and 10.8%, respectively.

Both the AIS and ISI were associated with low physical and mental QOL, depression, and productivity loss at work (Fig. 2 and Additional file 3: Table S1). Furthermore, both the AIS and ISI showed a weak negative correlation with the PCS ($r = -0.37$, $p < 0.01$ and $r = -0.32$, $p < 0.01$, respectively) and absolute presenteeism ($r = -0.32$, $p < 0.01$ and $r = -0.28$, $p < 0.01$, respectively) and a moderate negative correlation with the MCS ($r = -0.53$, $p < 0.01$ and $r = -0.43$, $p < 0.01$, respectively) (Additional file 3: Table S1).

We performed ROC analyses to compare the ability of the AIS and ISI to detect poor QOL (lowest tertiles of the PCS and MCS from the SF-8), depression (PHQ-9 ≥ 10), and poor work performance (lowest tertile of the absolute presenteeism score in the WHO-HPQ) (Fig. 2). All the ROC curves presented in Fig. 2 had significantly high AUCs ($p < 0.01$, compared with AUC = 0.5), which suggested that the AIS and ISI can identify low physical QOL, low mental QOL, depression, and productivity loss at

Table 2 AIS and ISI total scores

		AIS				
		0–5	6–9	10–24	Total	%
ISI	0–7	862	141	7	1010	60.10%
	8–14	174	295	92	561	33.40%
	15–28	2	25	82	109	6.50%
	Total	1038	461	181	1680	100%
	%	61.80%	27.40%	10.80%	100%	

The total scores of the AIS (0–5, 6–9, and 10–24) and ISI (0 7, 8–14, and 15–28) were compared. Weighted kappa: 0.58

work. The AIS had a significantly higher AUC than did the ISI for physical QOL, mental QOL, and depression. The AUCs to detect depression exceeded 0.85. The Pearson correlation coefficients were significantly different between the AIS and ISI compared with the PHQ-9 and MCS (Additional file 4: Table S2).

Each item of the AIS was compared with the corresponding item of the ISI. AIS_1 and ISI_1 assess problems with sleep initiation. AIS_3 and ISI_3 assess problems with early awakening (Additional file 5: figure S3). These items yielded similar AUCs ($p = 0.81$ comparing AIS_1 with ISI _1; $p = 0.50$ comparing AIS_3 with ISI_3) (Fig. 3). AIS_4, AIS_6, and AIS_8 assess sleep duration, problems with sense of well-being, and sleepiness, respectively (Additional file 5: Figure S3). The scores for these items were compared with the short TST (shortest tertile < 6 h), depression (PHQ-9 ≥ 10), and sleepiness (ESS > 10) data, respectively. The AUCs for AIS_4, AIS_6, and AIS_8 were 0.70, 0.84, and 0.67, respectively (Fig. 4).

A ROC analysis was performed using each item of the AIS and ISI as test variables with depression, poor physical QOL, poor mental QOL, and poor work performance as outcomes. Of these ROC analyses, only AIS_6 and AIS_7 had an AUC > 0.8 when compared with depression (Additional file 6: Table S3).

Discussion

In this study, the presence of insomnia and its outcomes were assessed simultaneously with the AIS and ISI in city government employees in Japan. A strong positive correlation was found between the AIS and ISI. Both tools were associated with QOL, depression, and productivity loss at work (Fig. 1), suggesting comparable properties.

Ten percent of the general population is expected to have chronic insomnia [American Academy of Sleep Medicine 2014]. Our prevalence of clinical insomnia (ISI ≥ 15: 6.5%) and definite insomnia (AIS ≥ 10.8%) may represent the prevalence of chronic insomnia in city government employees in Japan.

Major depressive disorder is commonly comorbid with insomnia [Riemann and Voderholzer, 2003; Tsuno et al. 2005; Kadotani et al. 2017]. Among the three outcomes

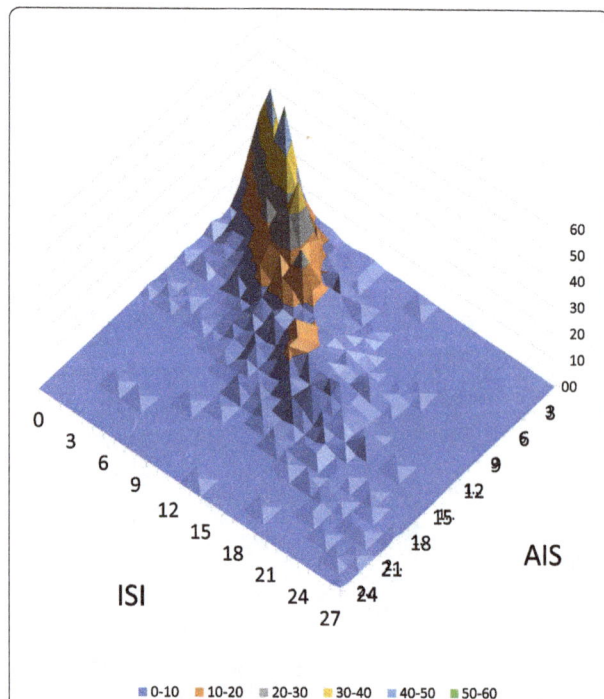

0-10   10-20   20-30   30-40   40-50   50-60

Fig. 1 Athens Insomnia Scale (AIS) and Insomnia Severity Index (ISI) three-dimensional histogramThe height (z-axis) represents the number of subjects, with the ISI and AIS scores shown in the x- and y-axis, respectively.

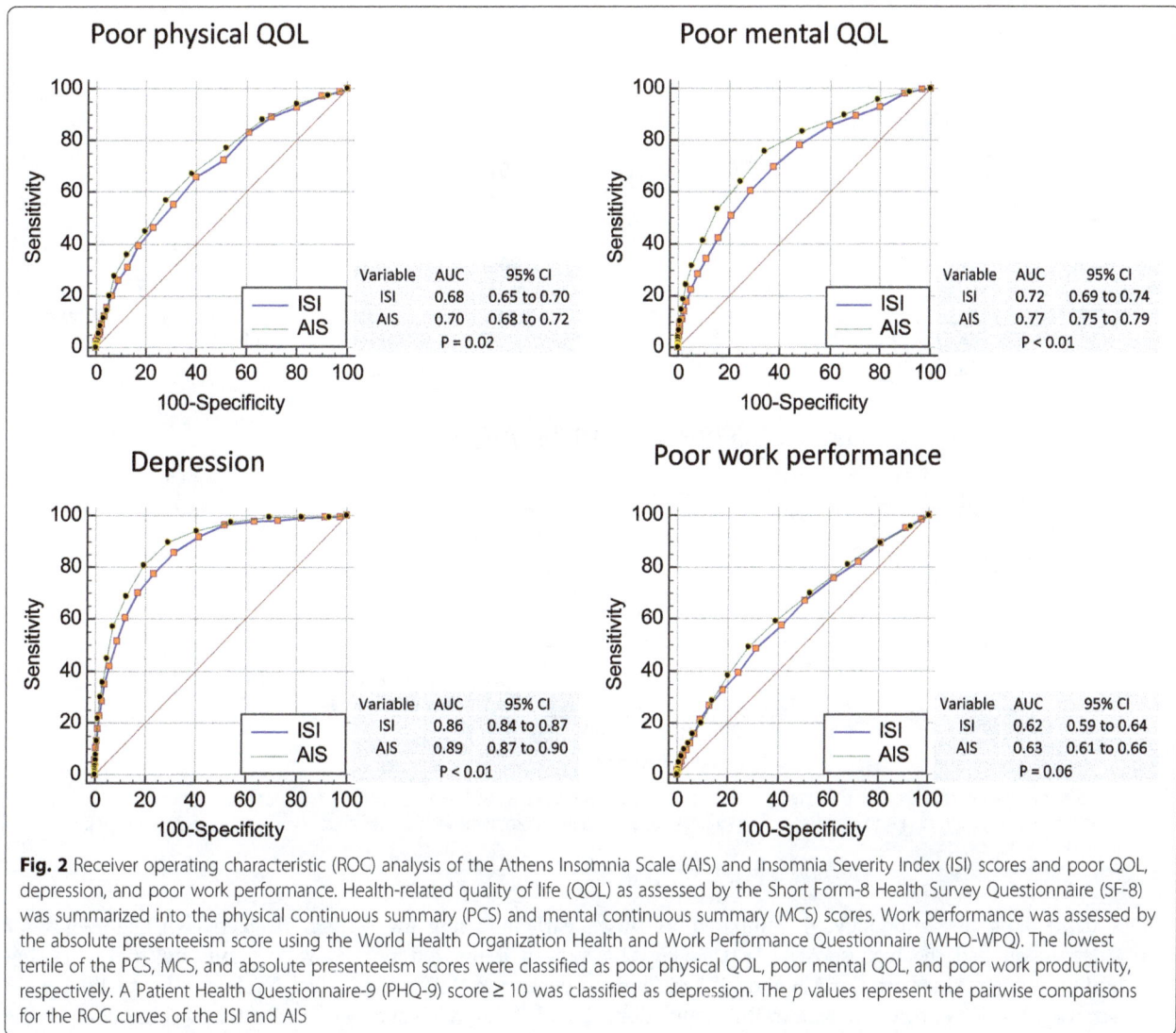

Fig. 2 Receiver operating characteristic (ROC) analysis of the Athens Insomnia Scale (AIS) and Insomnia Severity Index (ISI) scores and poor QOL, depression, and poor work performance. Health-related quality of life (QOL) as assessed by the Short Form-8 Health Survey Questionnaire (SF-8) was summarized into the physical continuous summary (PCS) and mental continuous summary (MCS) scores. Work performance was assessed by the absolute presenteeism score using the World Health Organization Health and Work Performance Questionnaire (WHO-WPQ). The lowest tertile of the PCS, MCS, and absolute presenteeism scores were classified as poor physical QOL, poor mental QOL, and poor work productivity, respectively. A Patient Health Questionnaire-9 (PHQ-9) score ≥ 10 was classified as depression. The p values represent the pairwise comparisons for the ROC curves of the ISI and AIS

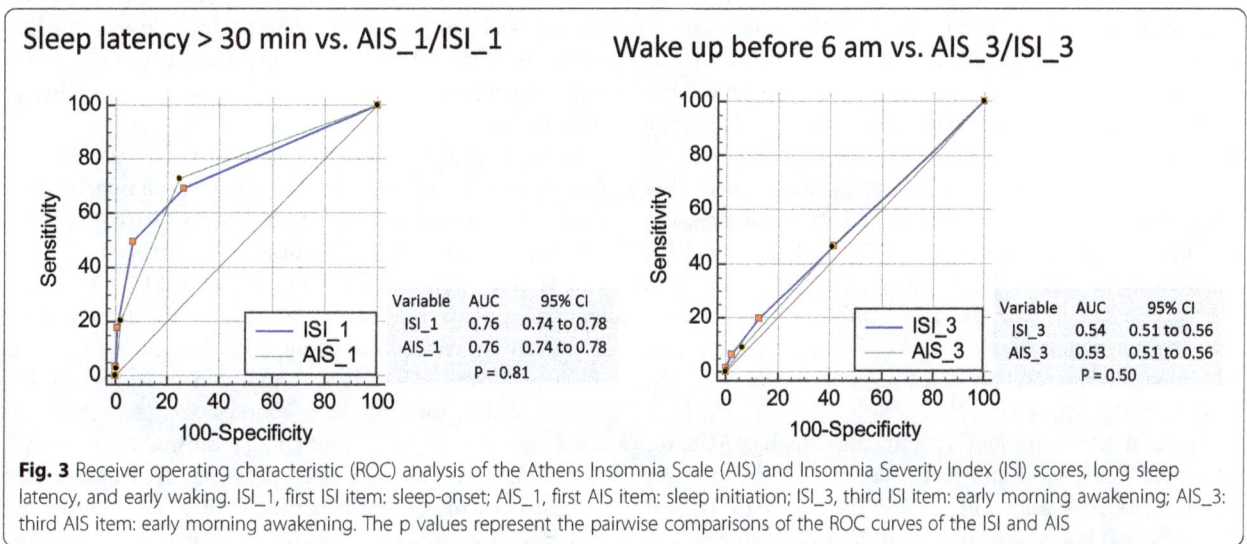

Fig. 3 Receiver operating characteristic (ROC) analysis of the Athens Insomnia Scale (AIS) and Insomnia Severity Index (ISI) scores, long sleep latency, and early waking. ISI_1, first ISI item: sleep-onset; AIS_1, first AIS item: sleep initiation; ISI_3, third ISI item: early morning awakening; AIS_3: third AIS item: early morning awakening. The p values represent the pairwise comparisons of the ROC curves of the ISI and AIS

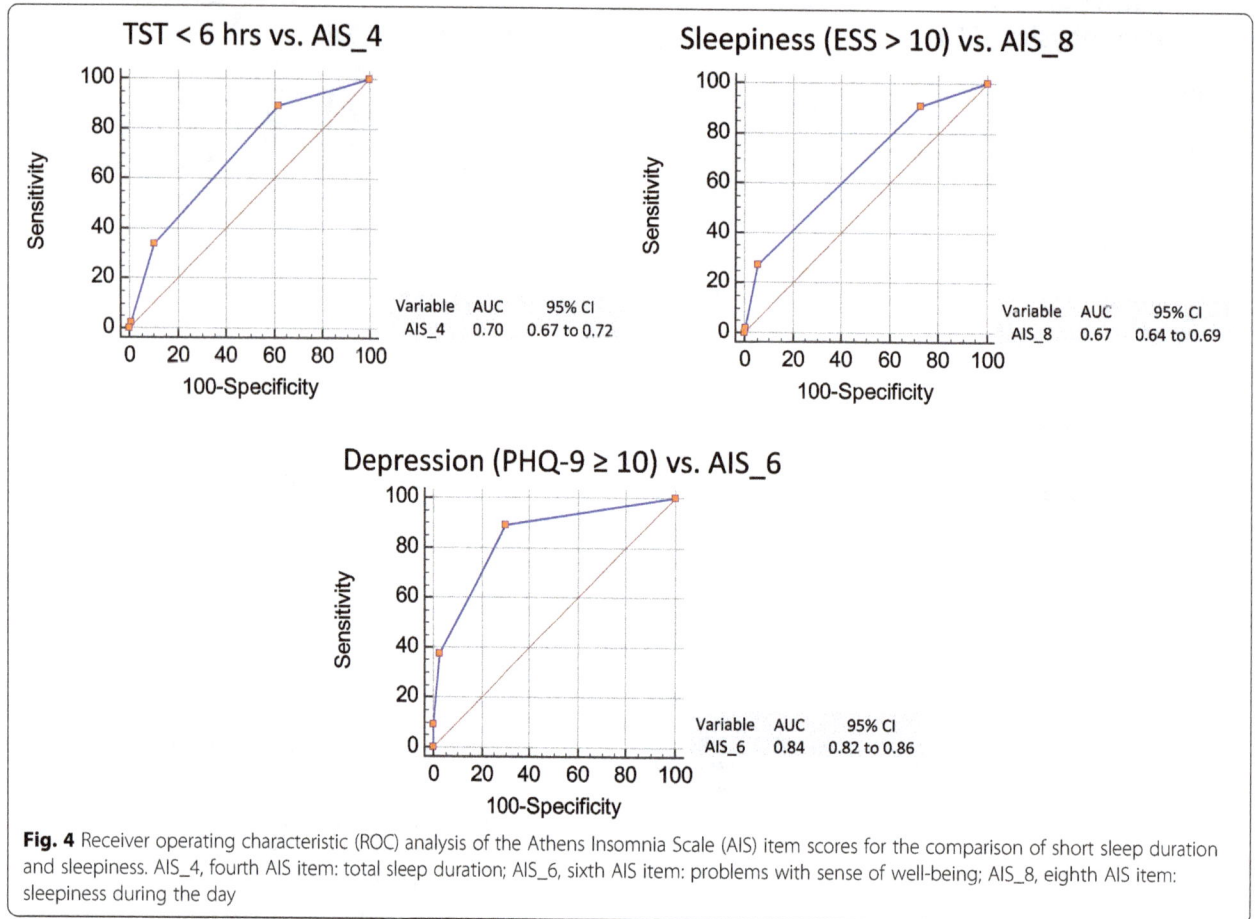

Fig. 4 Receiver operating characteristic (ROC) analysis of the Athens Insomnia Scale (AIS) item scores for the comparison of short sleep duration and sleepiness. AIS_4, fourth AIS item: total sleep duration; AIS_6, sixth AIS item: problems with sense of well-being; AIS_8, eighth AIS item: sleepiness during the day

(QOL, depression, and productivity) compared in this study, depression had the highest AUC (> 0.85; Fig. 2). This finding suggests that both the AIS and ISI had moderate accuracy for detecting depression in this population. AIS_6 and AIS_7 also had similar AUCs (0.84 and 0.82, respectively; $p = 0.05$; Additional file 6: Table S3 and Additional file 7: Figure S4). These items alone may be useful for screening for depression in the general population.

The present findings are in contrast to those of our previous study, which did not reveal an association between insomnia and depression when using the Pittsburgh Sleep Quality Index and clinical interview in a different population of working Japanese men (the Pittsburgh Sleep Quality Index values in the depression and control groups were 5.58 ± 2.28 and $4.76. \pm 1.97$, respectively; $p = 0.05$) [Kadotani et al. 2017]. However, the sample size of our previous study was 314. Therefore, the use of the AIS/ISI and/or the larger sample size may have been useful in detecting depression with the AIS/ISI in this study.

The total AIS score had a significantly higher AUC for QOL and depression and had a slightly higher AUC for productivity loss than did the ISI (Fig. 2). AIS_1/ISI_1 and AIS_3/ISI_3 assess problems in sleep latency and

early morning awakening, respectively. The AUCs for these items did not show a significant difference between the AIS and ISI (Fig. 3). The AIS and ISI have 8 and 7 items, respectively. Each item yielded comparable results and the total score had a higher AUC in the AIS than in the ISI. The AIS (AIS_6) assesses well-being, but the ISI does not. AIS_6 had the highest AUC among all the items of the AIS and ISI (Additional file 6: Table S3). Thus, the different AUCs for the AIS and ISI total scores might have been due to the differences in the number of their items.

In the current study, five items of the AIS (AIS_1, AIS_3, AIS_4, AIS_6, and AIS_8) were compared with the outcomes related to sleep latency, early morning awakening, short TST, sleepiness, and depression (Figs. 3 and 4). Two items in the ISI (ISI_1 and ISI_3) were also compared with the outcomes related to sleep latency and early morning awakening (Fig. 3). The other items in the AIS and ISI were not analyzed in this study because we did not have data sources for sleep maintenance problems (or awakening during the night), satisfaction with current sleep patterns (or sleep quality), or distress caused by sleep problems. Daily functioning (functional capacity during the day) may be associated with QOL; however, the SF-8 can only yield physical and mental summary scores, not a total summary score.

Our results showed that AIS_3 and ISI_3 were not associated with early awakening (earliest tertile of awakening time; Fig. 3). The earliest tertile of awakening time may not have been a suitable outcome for the comparison. The cutoff threshold using the tertile was earlier than 6:00 am, whereas the mean awakening time was 6:00 am (Table 1). We used this cutoff value because we used tertiles for most of the outcomes in this study. However, the awakening time or awakening time tertile may not have been suitable for detecting problems with early awakening.

This study had some limitations. First, our participants were city government employees in Japan. Therefore, while they may share similarities with the general population of their particular city, they may not have been representative of the general Japanese population. Second, this study used only questionnaire data; no objective data or clinical diagnoses were used. Although we plan to perform portable electroencephalography [Matsuo et al. 2016] and sleep respiratory monitoring to analyze sleep apnea in this population (NinJaSleep Study), such data were not collected in the present study. Finally, this was a cross-sectional study; thus, we could not show a causal relationship. We plan to conduct a longitudinal study in this population to further investigate this relationship.

Conclusions

The AIS and ISI were simultaneously administered to assess insomnia and its outcomes in Japanese city government employees. Both the AIS and ISI were associated with a low physical and mental QOL, depression, and productivity loss at work. A strong positive correlation was found between the total scores of the AIS and ISI. Moreover, the AIS, ISI, AIS_6, and AIS_7 showed a moderate accuracy for detecting depression in this population. Both the AIS and ISI may be useful for screening Japanese workers for not only insomnia, but also depression.

Additional files

Additional file 1: Figure S1. Histograms of participant characteristics.

Additional file 2: Figure S2. Distribution of the Athens Insomnia Scale (AIS) and Insomnia Severity Index (ISI). The numbers represent the count in each bin.

Additional file 3: Table S1. Pearson correlation coefficients (r) for the physical continuous summary (PCS), mental continuous summary (MCS), absolute presenteeism, Athens Insomnia Scale (AIS) and Insomnia Severity Index (ISI).

Additional file 4: Table S2. Comparison of correlation coefficients. The Pearson correlation coefficients were compared with the Athens Insomnia Scale (AIS) and Insomnia Severity Index (ISI) scores.

Additional file 5: Figure S3. Athens Insomnia Scale (AIS) and Insomnia Severity Index (ISI) items compared with sleep latency, wake-up time, total sleep time (TST), Patient Health Questionnaire-9 (PHQ-9), and Epworth Sleepiness Scale (ESS). A, b, c, d, and e represent p < 0.05 against scores in 0, 1, 2, 3, and 4, respectively, of the AIS and ISI items using one-way analysis of variance.

Additional file 6: Table S3. Receiver operating characteristic (ROC) analysis of the Athens Insomnia Scale (AIS) and Insomnia Severity Index (ISI) items compared with depression. The eight items from the AIS (from AIS_1 to AIS_8) and 7 items from the ISI (from ISI_1 to ISI_7) were compared with depression. A Patient Health Questionnaire-9 (PHQ-9) score ≥ 10 was classified as depression.

Additional file 7: Figure S4. Receiver operating characteristic analysis of the sixth and seventh items of the Athens Insomnia Scale (AIS) compared with depression.

Abbreviations

AIS: Athens Insomnia Scale; AUC: Area under the receiver operating characteristic curve; BMI: Body mass index; ESS: Epworth Sleepiness Scale; ISI: Insomnia Severity Index; MCS: Mental continuous summary; PCS: Physical continuous summary; PHQ-9: Patient Health Questionnaire-9; QOL: Quality of life; ROC: Receiver operating characteristic; SD: Standard deviation; SF-8: Short Form-8 Health Survey Questionnaire; TST: Total sleep time; WHO-HPQ: World Health Organization Health and Work Performance Questionnaire

Acknowledgments

We express gratitude to the participants of Koka City. We thank T Toyoda, R Matsumoto, A Toguchi, and H Nakayama for their assistance with data collection. We would like to thank Editage (www.editage.jp) for English language editing. The complete list of collaborators in the NinJaSleep Study is as follows: Hiroshi Kadotani, Masanori Takami, and Taeko Toyoda (Department of Sleep and Behavioral Sciences); Yukiyoshi Sumi and Masahiro Matsuo (Department of Psychiatry), and Hitoshi Nakayama (Koka City).

Funding

The present study was supported by MEXT/JSPS (KAKENHI Grant Number: 17H00872), MEXT Program for Building Regional Innovation Ecosystems, and a grant from the Investigator-Initiated Studies Program of Merck Sharp & Dohme Corp./MSD K.K.

Authors' contributions

HK conceived and designed the study and drafted the manuscript. HK was responsible for data collection. HK and MM performed the statistical analyses and interpreted the data. MT and YS assisted in manuscript drafting. MT, KN, YS, TN, YF, MM, and NY provided input on the manuscript drafts and assisted with data interpretation. All authors read and approved the final manuscript.

Competing interests

HK's laboratory is supported by a donation from Fukuda Lifetech Co., Ltd., Fukuda Life Tech Keiji Co., Ltd., Tanaka Sleep Clinic, Akita Sleep Clinic, and Ai Ai Care Co., Ltd. to the Shiga University of Medical Science. HK received grants from MEXT/JSPS (KAKENHI Grant Number: 17H00872), MEXT (Program for Building Regional Innovation Ecosystems), and Merck Sharp & Dohme Corp./MSD K.K. (the Investigator-Initiated Studies Program). The opinions expressed in this paper are those of the authors and do not necessarily represent those of Merck Sharp & Dohme Corp./MSD K.K. The other authors have no conflicts of interest directly relevant to the content of this article.

Author details
[1]Department of Sleep and Behavioral Sciences, Shiga University of Medical Science, Seta Tsukinowa-cho, Otsu City, Shiga 520-2192, Japan. [2]Shiga CBT center, 3-12 Chuou-cho, Hikone 522-0063, Japan. [3]Department of Psychiatry, Shiga University of Medical Science, Seta Tsukinowa-cho, Otsu City, Shiga 520-2192, Japan.

References

American Academy of Sleep Medicine. The international classification of sleep disorders: diagnostic and coding manual. 2nd ed. Westchester, IL: American Academy of Sleep Medicine; 2005.

American Academy of Sleep Medicine. The international classification of sleep disorders. 3rd ed. Darien, IL: American Academy of Sleep Medicine; 2014.

American Psychiatric Association. Diagnostic and statistical manual of mental disorders. 4th ed. Washington, DC: American Psychiatric Publishing; 2010.

Bastien CH, Vallières A, Morin CM. Validation of the insomnia severity index as an outcome measure for insomnia research. Sleep Med. 2001;2:297–307.

Blair E, Zinkhan GM. Nonresponse and generalizability in academic research. J Acad Marketing Sci. 2006;34:4–7. https://doi.org/10.1177/0092070305283778.

Bolge SC, Doan JF, Kannan H, Baran RW. Association of insomnia with quality of life, work productivity, and activity impairment. Qual Life Res. 2009; https://doi.org/10.1007/s11136-009-9462-6.

Chiu HY, Chang LY, Hsieh YJ, Tsai PS. A meta-analysis of diagnostic accuracy of three screening tools for insomnia. J Psychosom Res. 2016; https://doi.org/10.1016/j.jpsychores. 2016.06.010.

Chung KF, Kan KK, Yeung WF. Assessing insomnia in adolescents: comparison of insomnia severity index, Athens insomnia scale and sleep quality index. Sleep Med. 2011; https://doi.org/10.1016/j.sleep.2010.09.019.

Daley M, Morin CM, LeBlanc M, Gregoire JP, Savard J. The economic burden of insomnia: direct and indirect costs for individuals with insomnia syndrome, insomnia symptoms. and good sleepers Sleep. 2009;32:55–64.

Fukuhara S, Suzukamo Y. Manual of the SF-8 Japanese version (in Japanese). Kyoto: Institute for Health Outcomes and Process Evaluation Research; 2004.

Gilbody S, Richards D, Brealey S, Hewitt C. Screening for depression in medical settings with the patient health questionnaire (PHQ): a diagnostic meta-analysis. J Gen Intern Med. 2007;22:1596–602.

Global Burden of Disease Study 2013 Collaborators. Global, regional, and national incidence, prevalence, and years lived with disability for 301 acute and chronic diseases and injuries in 188 countries, 1990-2013: a systematic analysis for the global burden of disease study 2013. Lancet. 2015;386:743–800. https://doi.org/10.1016/S0140-6736(15)60692-4.

Ishak WW, Bagot K, Thomas S, Magakian N, Bedwani D, Larson D, et al. Quality of life in patients suffering from insomnia. Innov Clin Neurosci. 2012;9:13–26.

Jeong HS, Jeon Y, Ma J, Choi Y, Ban S, Lee S, et al. Validation of the Athens insomnia scale for screening insomnia in south Korean firefighters and rescue workers. Qual Life Res. 2015; https://doi.org/10.1007/s11136-015-0986-7.

Johns MW. A new method for measuring daytime sleepiness: the Epworth sleepiness scale. Sleep. 1991;14:540–5.

Kadotani H, Nagai Y, Sozu T. Railway suicide attempts are associated with amount of sunlight in recent days. J Affect Disord. 2014; https://doi.org/10.1016/j.jad.2013.08.040.

Kadotani T, Kadotani H, Arai H, Takami M, Ito H, Matsuo M, et al. Comparison of self-reported scales and structured interviews for the assessment of depression in an urban male working population in Japan: a cross-sectional survey. Sleep Sci Practice. 2017;1:9. https://doi.org/10.1186/s41606-017-0010-y.

Kessler RC, Barber C, Beck A, Berglund P, Cleary PD, McKenas D, et al. The World Health Organization health and work performance questionnaire (HPQ). J Occup Environ Med. 2003;45:156–74.

Kessler RC, Berglund PA, Coulouvrat C, Hajak G, Roth T, Shahly V, et al. Insomnia and the performance of US workers: results from the America insomnia survey. Sleep. 2011; https://doi.org/10.5665/SLEEP.1230.

Knekt P, Lindfors O, Renlund C, Sares-Jäske L, Laaksonen MA, Virtala E. Use of auxiliary psychiatric treatment during a 5-year follow-up among patients receiving short- or long-term psychotherapy. J Affect Disord. 2011; https://doi.org/10.1016/j.jad.2011.07.024.

Kroenke K, Spitzer RL, Williams JB. The PHQ-9: validity of a brief depression severity measure. J Gen Intern Med. 2001;16:606–13.

Krystal AD. Treating the health, quality of life, and functional impairments in insomnia. J Clin Sleep Med. 2007;3:63–72.

Lomeli HA, Pérez-Olmos I, Talero-Gutiérrez C, Moreno CB, González-Reyes R, Palacios L, et al. Sleep evaluation scales and questionnaires: a review. Actas Esp Psiquiatr. 2008;36:50–9.

Matsuo M, Masuda F, Sumi Y, Takahashi M, Yamada N, Ohira MH, et al. Comparisons of portable sleep monitors of different modalities: potential as naturalistic sleep recorders. Front Neurol. 2016; https://doi.org/10.3389/fneur.2016.00110.

Okajima I, Nakajima S, Kobayashi M, Inoue Y. Development and validation of the Japanese version of the Athens insomnia scale. Psychiatry Clin Neurosci. 2013; https://doi.org/10.1111/pcn.12073.

Riemann D, Voderholzer U. Primary insomnia: a risk factor to develop depression? J Affect Disord. 2003;76:255–9.

Sahlqvist S, Song Y, Bull F, Adams E, Preston J, Ogilvie D. iConnect consortium. Effect of questionnaire length, personalisation and reminder type on response rate to a complex postal survey: randomised controlled trial. BMC Med Res Methodol. 2011;11:62. https://doi.org/10.1186/1471-2288-11-62.

Sierra JC, Guillén-Serrano V, Santos-Iglesias P. Insomnia severity index: some indicators about its reliability and validity on an older adults sample (in Spanish). Rev Neurol. 2008;47:566–70.

Soldatos CR, Dikeos DG, Paparrigopoulos TJ. Athens insomnia scale: validation of an instrument based on ICD-10 criteria. J Psychosom Res. 2000;48:555–60.

Soldatos CR, Dikeos DG, Paparrigopoulos TJ. The diagnostic validity of the Athens insomnia scale. J Psychosom Res. 2003;55:263–7.

Sunderajan P, Gaynes BN, Wisniewski SR, Miyahara S, Fava M, Akingbala F, et al. Insomnia in patients with depression: a STAR*D report. CNS Spectr. 2010;15:394–404.

Suzuki T, Miyaki K, Sasaki Y, Song Y, Tsutsumi A, Kawakami N, et al. Optimal cutoff values of WHO-HPQ presenteeism scores by ROC analysis for preventing mental sickness absence in Japanese prospective cohort. PLoS One. 2014; https://doi.org/10.1371/journal.pone.0111191.

Takegami M, Suzukamo Y, Wakita T, Noguchi H, Chin K, Kadotani H, et al. Development of a Japanese version of the Epworth sleepiness scale (JESS) based on item response theory. Sleep Med. 2009; https://doi.org/10.1016/j.sleep.2008.04.015.

Tsuno N, Besset A, Ritchie K. Sleep and depression. J Clin Psychiatry. 2005;66:1254–69.

Ware JE, Kosinski M, Dewey JE, Gandek B. How to score and interpret single-item health status measures: a manual for users of the SF-8 health survey. Lincoln, RI: QualityMetric Incorporated; 2001.

Permissions

List of Contributors

Robson Capasso, Soroush Zaghi, Ryan Williams and Stanley Yung-Chuan Liu
Division of Sleep Surgery, Department of Otolaryngology-Head and Neck Surgery, Stanford Hospital and Clinics, Stanford, CA, USA

Carlos Torre
Division of Sleep Surgery, Department of Otolaryngology-Head and Neck Surgery, Stanford Hospital and Clinics, Stanford, CA, USA
Division of Sleep Medicine, Department of Psychiatry and Behavioral Sciences, Stanford Hospital and Clinics, Stanford, CA, USA
Department of Otolaryngology-Head and Neck Surgery, University of Miami, Miller School of Medicine, Miami, Florida, USA

Arlener D. Turner, Christine E. Smith and Jason C. Ong
Department of Neurology, Northwestern University Feinberg School of Medicine, 710 North Lake Shore Drive, Abbott Hall, Room 1005, Chicago 60611, IL, USA

Christopher J. Gouveia, Hannan A. Qureshi and Robert C. Kern
Department of Otolaryngology, Head and Neck Surgery, Northwestern University Feinberg School of Medicine, 676 N. St. Claire, Suite 1325, Chicago, IL 60611, USA

Stanley Yung-Chuan Liu and Robson Capasso
Department of Otolaryngology, Head and Neck Surgery, Stanford University Medical Center, Stanford, CA, USA

Kelly Glazer Baron
Department of Behavioral Sciences, Rush University Medical Center, 1653 W. Congress Parkway, Chicago, IL 60612-3833, USA

Heather E. Gunn
Department of Psychiatry, University of Pittsburgh, Pittsburgh, USA

Lisa F. Wolfe and Phyllis C. Zee
Center for Circadian and Sleep Medicine, Feinberg School of Medicine, Northwestern University, Chicago, USA

Shin-ichi Ando
Sleep Apnea Center, Kyushu University Hospital, Kyushu University, 3-1-1 Maidashi Higashiku, Fukuoka 812-8582, Japan

Hiroko Tsuda
Sleep Apnea Center, Kyushu University Hospital, Kyushu University, 3-1-1 Maidashi Higashiku, Fukuoka 812-8582, Japan
Department of General Dentistry, Kyushu University Hospital, Kyushu University, 3-1-1 Maidashi Higashiku, Fukuoka 812-8582, Japan

Naohisa Wada
Department of General Dentistry, Kyushu University Hospital, Kyushu University, 3-1-1 Maidashi Higashiku, Fukuoka 812-8582, Japan

Feihong Ding and Clete A. Kushida
Division of Sleep Medicine, Department of Psychiatry and Behavioral Sciences, Stanford Sleep Medicine Center, 450 Broadway Street, MC 5704, Pavilion C, 2nd Floor, Redwood City, CA 94063-5704, USA

Jimmy Kar-Hing Wong
Department of Anesthesia, Palo Alto Veterans Affairs, Stanford, CA, USA

Alice S. Whittemore
Division of Epidemiology, Department of Health Research and Policy, School of Medicine, Stanford University, Stanford, CA, USA

Erin L. Cassidy-Eagle
Department of Psychiatry and Behavioral Sciences, Stanford University School of Medicine, Stanford, CA, USA

Allison Siebern
Sleep Health Integrative Program Fayetteville NC Veterans Affairs Medical Center, Stanford University School of Medicine, Stanford, CA, USA

Robert Joseph Thomas
Division of Pulmonary, Critical Care, and Sleep Medicine, Beth Israel Deaconess Medical Center, Boston, MA, USA

Chol Shin
Institute of Human Genomic Study, Department of Respiratory Internal Medicine, Korea University Ansan Hospital, Ansan, South Korea

Matt Travis Bianchi
Division of Sleep Medicine, Department of Neurology, Massachusetts General Hospital, Boston, MA, USA

Clete Kushida
Psychiatry and Behavioral Sciences, Stanford Center for Sleep Sciences and Medicine, Stanford University Medical Center, Redwood City, CA, USA

Chang-Ho Yun
Department of Neurology, Seoul National University Bundang Hospital, Seongnam, South Korea

Parisa Adimi Naghan
Clinical Tuberculosis and Epidemiology Research Center, National Research Institute of Tuberculosis and Lung Diseases (NRITLD), Shahid Beheshti University of Medical Sciences, Tehran, Iran

Oldooz Aloosh
Chronic Respiratory Diseases Research Center, National Research Institute of Tuberculosis and Lung Diseases (NRITLD), Shahid Beheshti University of Medical Sciences, Masih Daneshvari Hospital, Darabad Avenue, Shahid Bahonar roundabout, Tehran, Iran

Hamze Ali Torang and Majid Malekmohammad
Tracheal Diseases Research Center, National Research Institute of Tuberculosis and Lung Diseases (NRITLD), Shahid Beheshti University of Medical Sciences, Tehran, Iran

Karuna Datta and Hruda Nanda Mallick
Department of Physiology, All India Institute of Medical Sciences, New Delhi, India

Manjari Tripathi
Department of Neurology, All India Institute of Medical Sciences, New Delhi, India

Andreas Ateke Njoh, Michel Karngong Mengnjo, Leonard Njamnshi Nfor, Leonard Ngarka, Samuel Eric Chokote, Julius Yundze Fonsah, Samuel Kingue, Felicien Enyime Ntone and Alfred Kongnyu Njamnshi
Faculty of Medicine and Biomedical Sciences, University of Yaoundé 1, Yaoundé, Cameroon

Eta Ngole Mbong
Faculty of Medicine and Biomedical Sciences, University of Yaoundé 1, Yaoundé, Cameroon
PC Great Soppo, Buea, Cameroon

Valeri Oben Mbi
ISEC Schools of Health Sciences, Yaoundé, Cameroon

Maria Comas
CIRUS, Centre for Sleep and Chronobiology, Woolcock Institute of Medical Research, University of Sydney, 431 Glebe Point Road, Glebe, Sydney, NSW 2037, Australia

Woolcock Emphysema Centre, Woolcock Institute of Medical Research, University of Sydney, Sydney, NSW, Australia
Central Clinical School, Faculty of Medicine, University of Sydney, Sydney, NSW, Australia

Ronald R. Grunstein
CIRUS, Centre for Sleep and Chronobiology, Woolcock Institute of Medical Research, University of Sydney, 431 Glebe Point Road, Glebe, Sydney, NSW 2037, Australia
Central Clinical School, Faculty of Medicine, University of Sydney, Sydney, NSW, Australia

Christopher J. Gordon
CIRUS, Centre for Sleep and Chronobiology, Woolcock Institute of Medical Research, University of Sydney, 431 Glebe Point Road, Glebe, Sydney, NSW 2037, Australia
Sydney Nursing School, University of Sydney, Sydney, NSW, Australia

Craig L. Phillips
CIRUS, Centre for Sleep and Chronobiology, Woolcock Institute of Medical Research, University of Sydney, 431 Glebe Point Road, Glebe, Sydney, NSW 2037, Australia
Woolcock Emphysema Centre, Woolcock Institute of Medical Research, University of Sydney, Sydney, NSW, Australia
Northern Clinical School, Faculty of Medicine, University of Sydney, Sydney, NSW, Australia
Department of Respiratory and Sleep Medicine, Royal North Shore Hospital, Sydney, NSW, Australia

Brian G. Oliver
Woolcock Emphysema Centre, Woolcock Institute of Medical Research, University of Sydney, Sydney, NSW, Australia
Respiratory Cellular and Molecular Biology, Woolcock Institute of Medical Research, University of Sydney, Sydney, NSW, Australia
School of Life Sciences, Faculty of Science, and Centre for Health Technology, University of Technology Sydney, Sydney, NSW, Australia

Nicholas W. Stow
Department of Otolaryngology, Mona Vale Hospital, Sydney, NSW, Australia

Gregory King
Woolcock Emphysema Centre, Woolcock Institute of Medical Research, University of Sydney, Sydney, NSW, Australia
Physiology and Imaging Group, Woolcock Institute of Medical Research, University of Sydney, Sydney, NSW, Australia

Northern Clinical School, Faculty of Medicine, University of Sydney, Sydney, NSW, Australia
Department of Respiratory and Sleep Medicine, Royal North Shore Hospital, Sydney, NSW, Australia

Pawan Sharma
Woolcock Emphysema Centre, Woolcock Institute of Medical Research, University of Sydney, Sydney, NSW, Australia
Respiratory Cellular and Molecular Biology, Woolcock Institute of Medical Research, University of Sydney, Sydney, NSW, Australia
School of Life Sciences, Faculty of Science, and Centre for Health Technology, University of Technology Sydney, Sydney, NSW, Australia

Alaina J. Ammit
Woolcock Emphysema Centre, Woolcock Institute of Medical Research, University of Sydney, Sydney, NSW, Australia
School of Life Sciences, Faculty of Science, and Centre for Health Technology, University of Technology Sydney, Sydney, NSW, Australia

Tomiko Kadotani
Horizontal Medical Research Organization, Graduate School of Medicine, Kyoto University, Yoshida-Konoe-cho, Sakyo-ku, Kyoto 606-8501, Japan
Department of Pediatrics, Takatsuki General Hospital, 1-3-13 Kosobe-cho, Takatsuki, Osaka 569-1192, Japan

Hiroshi Kadotani
Horizontal Medical Research Organization, Graduate School of Medicine, Kyoto University, Yoshida-Konoe-cho, Sakyo-ku, Kyoto 606-8501, Japan
Department of Sleep and Behavioral Sciences, Shiga University of Medical Science, Seta Tsukinowa-cho, Otsu City, Shiga 520-2192, Japan

Hiroyasu Ito
Department of Sleep and Behavioral Sciences, Shiga University of Medical Science, Seta Tsukinowa-cho, Otsu City, Shiga 520-2192, Japan

Honami Arai and Masanori Takami
Department of Sleep and Behavioral Sciences, Shiga University of Medical Science, Seta Tsukinowa-cho, Otsu City, Shiga 520-2192, Japan
Department of Psychiatry, Shiga University of Medical Science, Seta Tsukinowa-cho, Otsu City, Shiga 520-2192, Japan

Masahiro Matsuo and Naoto Yamada
Department of Psychiatry, Shiga University of Medical Science, Seta Tsukinowa-cho, Otsu City, Shiga 520-2192, Japan

Magdy Younes
Sleep Disorders Centre, Misericordia Health Centre, Winnipeg, Canada
YRT Ltd, Winnipeg, MB, Canada

Gaurav Nigam
Clay County Hospital, 911 Stacy Burk Drive, Flora, IL 62839, USA

Macario Camacho
Division of Otolaryngology, Sleep Surgery, and Sleep Medicine, Tripler Army Medical Center, 1 Jarrett White Road, Tripler AMC, Honolulu, HI 96859, USA

Muhammad Riaz
Sunnyside Community Hospital and Clinics, 208 N. Euclid, Grandview, WA 98930, USA

Huan Lu, Xiaodan Wu, Cuiping Fu, Jing Zhou and Shanqun Li
Department of Pulmonary Medicine, Clinical Center for Sleep Breathing Disorder and Snoring, Zhongshan Hospital, Fudan University, 180 Fenlin Road, Shanghai 200032, China

José Rafael P. Zuzuárregui
Division of Neurology, University of California, San Francisco, Fresno Center for Medical Education and Research, 155 N. Fresno St., Fresno 93701, CA, USA

Kevin Bickart
Department of Neurology, Stanford University School of Medicine, Stanford, USA

Scott J. Kutscher
Division of Sleep Medicine, Department of Psychiatry, Stanford University School of Medicine, Stanford, USA

Xi Mei, Qi Zhou, Xingxing Li and Zhenyu Hu
Ningbo Key Laboratory of Sleep Medicine, Zhuangyu South Road No.1, Zhenhai District, Ningbo City 315201, Zhejiang Province, China
Ningbo Kangning Hospital, Ningbo City 315201, Zhejiang Province, China

Pan Jing and Xiaojia Wang
Ningbo Kangning Hospital, Ningbo City 315201, Zhejiang Province, China

Q. Afifa Shamim-Uzzaman
VA Ann Arbor Heathcare Center and University of Michigan, 2215 Fuller Rd, Ann Arbor, MI 48105, USA

Sukhmani Singh
Oakland University, Rochester, MI, USA

Susmita Chowdhuri
John D. Dingell VA Medical Center and Wayne State University, Detroit, MI, USA

J. F. Pagel
University of Colorado School of Medicine, Couthern Colorado Residency Program, Pueblo, CO, USA. Rocky Mountain Sleep, 1306 Fortino Blvd, Pueblo, CO 81008, USA

Seithikurippu R. Pandi-Perumal
Somnogen Canada Inc, College Street, Toronto, ON, Canada

Jaime M. Monti
School of Medicine Clinics Hospital, University of the Republic, Montevideo, Uruguay

Abiodun O. Ayoka and Joseph G. Omole
Department of Physiological Sciences, Faculty of Basic Medical Sciences, College of Health Sciences, Obafemi Awolowo University, Ile-Ife, Nigeria

Benson A. Fadeyi and Adeniyi M. Oluwadaisi
Department of Physiological Sciences, Faculty of Basic Medical Sciences, College of Health Sciences, Obafemi Awolowo University, Ile-Ife, Nigeria
Department of Dental and Oral Surgery, Federal Teaching Hospital, Ido-Ekiti, Ekiti State, Nigeria

Quadri K. Alabi
Department of Physiological Sciences, Faculty of Basic Medical Sciences, College of Health Sciences, Obafemi Awolowo University, Ile-Ife, Nigeria
Department of Haematology and Blood Transfusion, Faculty of Basic Medical Sciences, College of Medicine, Afe-Babalola University, Ado-Ekiti, Ekiti State, Nigeria

Michael B. Fawale
Department of Medicine (Neurology Unit), Faculty of Clinical Sciences, College of Health Sciences, Obafemi Awolowo University, Ile-Ife, Nigeria

Cheng-Ann Wang
Department of Psychiatry and Behavioral Rhythms, Stanford University, Stanford, CA 94305, USA

Jamie M. Zeitzer
Department of Psychiatry and Behavioral Rhythms, Stanford University, Stanford, CA 94305, USA
Mental Illness Research Education and Clinical Center, VA Palo Alto Health Care System, Palo Alto, CA 94304, USA

Raymond P. Najjar
Department of Psychiatry and Behavioral Rhythms, Stanford University, Stanford, CA 94305, USA
Department of Visual Neurosciences, Singapore Eye Research Institute, Singapore 169856, Singapore

Mirelle Kass
Department of Psychiatry and Behavioral Rhythms, Stanford University, Stanford, CA 94305, USA
Connecticut College, New London, CT, USA

Joseph Cheung and Emmanuel Mignot
Stanford University Center for Sleep Sciences and Medicine, Palo Alto, CA, USA
Department of Psychiatry and Behavioral Sciences, Stanford University, Stanford, CA, USA

Jamie M. Zeitzer
Stanford University Center for Sleep Sciences and Medicine, Palo Alto, CA, USA
Department of Psychiatry and Behavioral Sciences, Stanford University, Stanford, CA, USA
Mental Illness Research Education and Clinical Center, VA Palo Alto Health Care System, Palo Alto, CA, USA

Haoyang Lu
Department of Psychiatry and Behavioral Sciences, Stanford University, Stanford, CA, USA

Stig Solbach, Katrin Uehli, Stefanie Brighenti-Zogg, Selina Dürr, Sabrina Maier and Michel Hug
Cantonal Hospital Baselland, University Clinic of Medicine, CH-4410 Liestal, Switzerland.

Jörg Daniel Leuppi and David Miedinger
Cantonal Hospital Baselland, University Clinic of Medicine, CH-4410 Liestal, Switzerland

Werner Strobel
Department of Pneumology, University Hospital of Basel, Basel, Switzerland

Roland Bingisser
Department of Emergency Medicine, University Hospital of Basel, Basel, Switzerland
Medical Faculty, University of Basel, Basel, Switzerland

Christena A. Kolakowski, Donald R. Rollins, Theodore Jennermann, Allen D. Stevens, James T. Good Jr, Joshua L. Denson and Richard J. Martin
Department of Medicine, National Jewish Health, 1400 Jackson St, Room A642, Denver, CO 80206, USA

Masanori Takami and Hiroshi Kadotani
Department of Sleep and Behavioral Sciences, Shiga University of Medical Science, Seta Tsukinowa-cho, Otsu City, Shiga 520-2192, Japan

Kohei Nishikawa
Shiga CBT center, 3-12 Chuou-cho, Hikone 522-0063, Japan

Yukiyoshi Sumi, Takao Nakabayashi, Yusuke Fujii, Masahiro Matsuo and Naoto Yamada
Department of Psychiatry, Shiga University of Medical Science, Seta Tsukinowa-cho, Otsu City, Shiga 520-2192, Japan

Index

www.ingramcontent.com/pod-product-compliance
Lightning Source LLC
Chambersburg PA
CBHW080509200326
41458CB00012B/4143